DIAGNOSIS AND TREATMENT OF THE SPINE

NONOPERATIVE ORTHOPAEDIC MEDICINE AND MANUAL THERAPY

DOS WINKEL, PT

Instructor, Scientific Society of Flemish General Practitioners
Antwerp, Belgium
Director, Dutch and German Academy of Orthopaedic Medicine
Delft, the Netherlands and Göttingen, Germany
President, International Academy of Orthopaedic Medicine

GEERT AUFDEMKAMPE, PT
Instructor, Physical Therapy School
Hogeschool Midden Nederland
Utrecht, the Netherlands

OMER MATTHIJS, PT
Instructor, International Academy of
  Orthopaedic Medicine
Instructor, American Academy of
  Orthopedic Medicine, Inc.
Tucson, Arizona

ONNO G. MEIJER, MD, PHD
Movement Scientist
Free University
Amsterdam, the Netherlands

VALERIE PHELPS, PT
Instructor, International Academy of
  Orthopaedic Medicine
Director and Instructor, American Academy of
  Orthopedic Medicine, Inc.
Tucson, Arizona

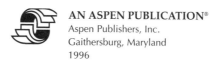

AN ASPEN PUBLICATION®
Aspen Publishers, Inc.
Gaithersburg, Maryland
1996

Library of Congress Cataloging-in-Publication Data

Diagnosis and treatment of the spine : nonoperative orthopaedic
medicine and manual therapy / Dos Winkel ... [et al.].
p.   cm.
Translation and adaptation of material previously published in
Dutch under the titles: Orthopedische geneeskunde en manuele
therapie (deel 4a-c) by Dos Winkel, Geert Aufdemkampe, and Onno G.Meijer
and Weke delen aandoeningen van het bewegingsapparaat (deel1)
by Andry Vleeming, Dos Winkel, and Onno G. Meijer.
Includes bibliographical references and index.
ISBN 0-8342-0731-1
1. Spine—Diseases—Treatment. 2. Spine—Diseases—Physical
therapy. 3. Spine—Diseases. I. Manipulation, Orthopedic.
II. Winkel, Dos. III. Winkel, Dos. Orthopedische geneeskunde en
manuele therapie. IV. Vleeming, Andry. Weke delen aandoeningen
van het bewegingsapparaat.
[DNLM: 1. Spinal Diseases—therapy. 2. Spinal Diseases—
diagnosis. 3. Orthopedics—methods. WE 725 D536 1996a]
RD768.D52 1996
617.3'75—dc20
DNLM/DLC
for Library of Congress
95-31860
CIP

The authors have made every effort to ensure the accuracy of the information herein. However, appropriate
information sources should be consulted, especially for new or unfamiliar procedures. It is the responsibility of
every practitioner to evaluate the appropriateness of a particular opinion in the context of actual clinical situations and with due consideration to new developments. Authors, editors, and the publisher cannot be held responsible for any typographical or other errors found in this book.

Editorial Resources: Ruth Bloom

Library of Congress Catalog Card Number: 95-31860
ISBN: 0-8342-0731-1

Printed in the United States of America

1 2 3 4 5

Table of Contents

Contributors

Geert Aufdemkampe, PT
Instructor, Physical Therapy School
Hogeschool Midden Nederland
Utrecht, The Netherlands

Fred G. van den Berg, MD
Radiologist
Department of Radiodiagnostics
Hospital of the Free University
Amsterdam, The Netherlands

Harry L.M.G. Bour, PhD
Neurobiologist
Faculty of Health Care
Department for Physical Therapy
Central Netherlands Polytechnic
Utrecht, The Netherlands

R. Deutman, MD
Orthopedic Surgeon
University Hospital
Groningen, The Netherlands

Albert de Jong, PhD
Psychologist/Psychotherapist
Voorburg and Delft, The Netherlands

Gert Jan Klein Rensink, PhD
Functional Morphologist
Department of Biomechanics and Anatomy
    of the Locomotor System
Erasmus University
Rotterdam, The Netherlands

Rutger der Kinderen, PT
Physical Therapist/Manipulative Therapist
Eindhoven, The Netherlands

Hans M. Lagas, MD
Anesthesiologist
Hospital of the Free University
Amsterdam, The Netherlands

Omer Matthijs, PT
Physical Therapist/Manipulative Therapist
Instructor, International Academy of
    Orthopaedic Medicine
Instructor, American Academy of
    Orthopedic Medicine, Inc.
Tucson, Arizona

Jan M.A. Mens, MD
Jan van Breemen Institute
Amsterdam, The Netherlands
Erasmus University
Rotterdam, The Netherlands

Onno G. Meijer, MD, PhD
Movement Scientist
Free University
Amsterdam, The Netherlands

Jacques de Moor, MD
Radiologist
Department of Radiology
University Hospital
Antwerp, Belgium

Didi G.H. van Paridon-Edauw, PT
Physical Therapist/Manipulative Therapist
Academy for Orthopedic Medicine
Stuttgart, Germany
Dutch Academy for Orthopedic Medicine
Delft, The Netherlands
American Academy of Orthopedic Medicine
Tucson, Arizona

Paul M. Parizel, MD
Radiologist
Department of Radiology
University Hospital
Antwerp, Belgium

Valerie Phelps, PT
Physical Therapist/Manipulative Therapist
Instructor, International Academy of
    Orthopaedic Medicine
Director and Instructor, American Academy
    of Orthopedic Medicine, Inc.
Tucson, Arizona

A.M. de Schepper, MD, PhD
Radiologist
Professor of Radiology
University Hospital
Antwerp, Belgium

Peter J.M. Scholten, PhD
Medical Technologist
Polytechnic of Utrecht
Utrecht, The Netherlands

Chris J. Snijders, PhD
Biomedical Technologist, Physicist
Erasmus University
Rotterdam, The Netherlands

Michel H. Steens, DDS
Department for Oral Diseases and Dental
    Surgery
University of Utrecht
Utrecht, The Netherlands

A.G. Veldhuizen, MD
Orthopedic Surgeon
University Hospital
Groningen, The Netherlands

Andry Vleeming, PT, PhD
Anatomist, Physical Therapist
Department of Biomechanics and the
    Anatomy of the Locomotor System
Erasmus University
Rotterdam, The Netherlands

Dos Winkel, PT
Instructor, Scientific Society of Flemish
    General Practitioners
Antwerp, Belgium
Director, Dutch and German Academy of
    Orthopaedic Medicine
Delft, The Netherlands and Göttingen,
    Germany
President, International Academy of
    Orthopaedic Medicine

Anton de Wijer, PT, PhD
Physical Therapist/Manipulative Therapist
Department for Oral Diseases and Dental
    Surgery
University of Utrecht, the Netherlands
Faculty of Health Care
Department for Physical Therapy, The
    Netherlands
Central Netherlands Polytechnic
Utrecht, The Netherlands

Preface

Orthopaedic medicine is a medical specialty that has gone through enormous changes during past decades. Research is being conducted worldwide in the various fields of movement science. This research includes arthrokinematics and dynamic electromyography, often with the aid of motion pictures. Because of such research, the causes of many disorders have become increasingly more apparent, thus facilitating a more causal approach to the treatment of patients. A direct consequence of this research is the decrease in the use of injection therapy, arthroscopy, and other surgical procedures. However, the opposite impression is gained when dealing with patients' histories.

This book concerns functional anatomy, clinical examination, pathology, and treatment of spinal disorders. The thorax and temporomandibular joint are also discussed. Although the temporomandibular joint does not belong strictly to the spine, from a functional point of view it falls within the realm of the topic, and in our opinion it warrants attention.

Actually there is a vast amount of literature available on the spine. On almost every one of the topics in this book, a book in itself could be written. The goal of this work is to offer a concise and practical overview of the most often seen pathology and the accompanying treatment possibilities for the physician and the physical therapist. Here the composite of patient symptoms and signs is the starting point for all therapeutic treatment. The results of the history, the inspection, and the clinical examination determine the treatment of choice.

Although many manual therapy examination and treatment techniques are described, this is not meant to be a handbook for manual therapy, and references are given for the appropriate resources. Rather, we have tried to present an overview of orthopaedic medicine for the spine and its associated structures. Because manual therapy plays an important role in nonoperative orthopaedic medicine, we chose to include this term in the title of the book.

Even though spinal research studies are not in agreement on every detail, it is generally accepted that approximately eight of every ten people experience back pain at least once in their lifetime. Complaints of neck pain are also common. Within orthopaedic medicine, complaints related to the spine and its associated structures hold a prominent place. With this in mind, thoracic outlet syndrome is discussed in detail as well.

General principles of orthopaedics in terms of examination and treatment are also discussed in this book. The general consensus is that one principally tries to treat the cause of a disorder, which also includes attempting to influence the disorder on a local level. Unfortunately, it is not always possible to determine the exact cause of a disorder. In such cases, patients are given a thorough explanation about the particular pathology and then, if possible, a local treatment. For instance, after a rotation manipulation of the spine, used to decrease pain and to increase range of motion, the patient is advised how to perform daily activities correctly, and a specific exercise program may be prescribed. The rotation manipulation should never be considered the "be all and end all" of treatments. It is really only part of a comprehensive treatment program in which a close working relationship between physicians and therapists must be sought. Even when the basic principle of the interdisciplinary teamwork is not directly described in each chapter, we view this as one of the standards of manual therapeutic conduct.

Intentionally, we divided this work into three parts. The first two parts give an insight into the daily application of pathology, diagnostics, and treatment. The third part offers the reader an introduction to the fundamental and applied knowledge regarding diagnostics and treatment of the spine and its associated structures.

Very often there are tensions or even conflicts between fundamental theories and practical views. We purposefully did not strive to remove these areas of discord. By leaving them intact, a vivid picture of the contemporary views of orthopaedic medicine and manual therapy of the spine is created. Although the sacroiliac joint, lumbar spine, thoracic spine, cervical spine, and temporomandibular joint are dealt with separately, the spine should be considered in its entirety. That is to say, for instance, the position of the lumbar spine will have an influence on the rest of the spine. In the treatment of posturally related problems, this can be of greater significance therapeutically.

Geert Aufdemkampe and Onno G. Meijer were co-editors of the 1991 Dutch edition. Their main focus was the scientific aspects that are in Chapters 8 through 17 of this text. The 1984 *Anatomy in Vivo* book, of which translated parts are included in the present volume, was written by Andry Vleeming, Dos Winkel, and Onno G. Meijer. Many people have contributed to earlier versions of the above two books. Without their contribution, the present volume would not have been possible.

The final text was created with intensive editorial reworking; therefore, the editors carry the end responsibility for this work. We particularly thank Didi van Paridon-Edauw and Omer Matthijs, whose critical contributions during the entire formation of this work were of considerable value. We also want to thank the publisher, who diligently followed the birth of this work. A personal word of thanks is due to Dr. Jacques de Moor, who provided many illustrations from his own unique collection of slides and X-rays, and who proved to be willing to give, in a relaxed but stimulating atmosphere, valuable information—especially about the relationship between clinical diagnostics and imaging diagnostics of the spine.

I am very grateful to Valerie Phelps, PT, who is the Director of the American Academy of Orthopaedic Medicine, for translation of this book. This was a monumental task, which she performed with excellence.

I am grateful, as well, to both Valerie Phelps and Omer Matthijs for having updated this book from both the Dutch and German versions. Omer Matthijs has for years been one of my closest co-workers and collaborators, as well as being a most excellent practitioner and teacher.

Recognizing that improvements in the field are constantly being made, it is necessary to provide updated information as well as hands-on practice via a series of instructional courses designed around the techniques described in this book. Therefore, in addition to individual use, this book supports and provides source material for instructional courses organized by the American Academy of Orthopaedic Medicine, Inc. For information about these courses, call 1-800-AAOM-305 (1-800-226-6305).

I hope that the use of this book will improve the effectiveness of making the diagnosis and providing the appropriate treatment techniques. To everyone who will use this book: I hope you enjoy great success in using this knowledge and these techniques to the benefit of your patients.

Dos Winkel

Part I

Surface Anatomy of the Spine and General Aspects of Back Pain

1

Surface Anatomy of the Spine

1.1 GENERAL INSPECTION OF THE HEAD, NECK, AND TRUNK

Superficial orientation is often difficult in the region of the head, neck, and trunk. Therefore, orientation lines and regions are used to describe features and locations during examinations of the surface anatomy. These orientation lines and regions are also used to locate and describe certain phenomena. However, while using these locational and descriptive aids, it is important to keep in mind that constructions of the head, neck, and trunk are subject to significant individual variance.

Position of the Patient: Sitting or prone

INSPECTION FROM THE DORSAL ASPECT

At the back of the head, the external occipital protuberance is easily palpable. The linea nuchae (nuchal line) extends from each side of the protuberance; the occipital region, with corresponding occipital bone, bulges cranially (Figures 1–1, 1–2, and 1–8). The examiner is usually not able to discern the border between the occipital bone and parietal bone (with its corresponding parietal region).

On each side of the occiput, just below the ears, the mastoid process can be palpated. The mastoid process is a bony prominence of the temporal bone. The lateral part of the occiput is bordered bilaterally by the temporal region.

The neck starts just below the occipital bone. The nuchal region is filled, to a great extent, by the trapezius muscle. The posterior median line is well visible at the neck and indicates the course of the nuchal septum. At each side, the nuchal region is bordered by the similarly named sternocleidomastoid region and muscles.

In the back, orientation begins with the help of the usually evident posterior median line. The vertebral column and erector spinae muscles together form the vertebral region.

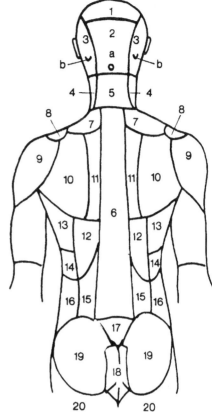

Figure 1–1 Regions at the back of the head, neck, and back. The terms in parentheses are seldom used. *a*, External occipital protuberance; *b*, mastoid process; *1*, parietal region; *2*, occipital region; *3*, temporal region; *4*, sternocleidomastoid region; *5*, nuchal region; *6*, vertebral region; *7*, suprascapular region; *8*, (acromial region); *9*, deltoid region; *10*, scapular region; *11*, (interscapular region); *12*, infrascapular region; *13*, (lateral pectoral region); *14*, hypochondriac region; *15*, lumbar region; *16*, (lateral region); *17*, sacral region; *18*, anal region; *19*, gluteal region; *20*, posterior region of the thigh.

The scapula is easy to see and palpate on the thorax. The contour of the scapula corresponds to the scapular region. The scapular line runs along the medial border of the scap-

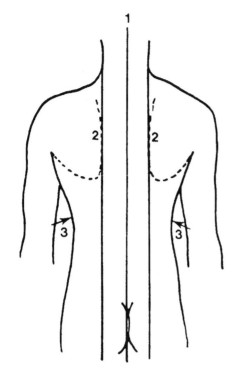

Figure 1–2 Orientation lines at the back of the head, neck, and back. *1*, Posterior median line; *2*, scapular line; *3*, axillary line.

ula. If the medial border does not stand vertically, the line runs through the inferior angle of the scapula. The suprascapular region is above the scapula, and the infrascapular region is below the scapula.

The back is bordered at the sides by the axillary line, which is a vertical line passing through the middle of the axilla. The axillary line divides the body into anterior and posterior surfaces. The hypochondriac region begins at the laterodistal aspect of the thorax and ends bilaterally at the ventral aspect of the trunk.

The lumbar region comprises the lower back area, to the left and right of the vertebral region.

The contours of the gluteal region generally are determined by subcutaneous fat tissue, not by the gluteus maximus muscles. The lower edge of the muscle runs diagonally from

its origin, in a lateral and distal direction, whereas the lower border of the gluteal region runs horizontally. The sacral region corresponds to the sacrum. Distally it runs to the gluteal fold.

Petit's Triangle

Petit's* triangle (lumbar trigone) is located between the dorsal part of the iliac crest, the lateral edge of the latissimus dorsi, and the dorsal edge of the external oblique muscle of the abdomen. It is the only site where the internal oblique muscle of the abdomen is palpable, because it is not covered by other muscles. Hernias can occur in Petit's triangle, but they are rare.

Michaelis' Diamond

Michaelis'[†] diamond lies between the lowest point of the lumbar lordosis, both posterior superior iliac spines, and the upper end of the gluteal fold. In instances of leg length differences or pelvic "torsion," this region will be asymmetrical.

INSPECTION OF THE PERINEUM

The perineum begins in the gluteal fold. When inspecting the back, the anal region can be made visible by positioning the patient on all fours. Keep in mind that inspection of this region can be uncomfortable for the patient.

The nomenclature regarding the perineum itself (perineal region) can be confusing. Previously, in surface anatomy, the area between the anal region and the urogenital region typically was called the perineum. Presently, the perineum is considered to consist of *both* the anal and urogenital regions (Figure 1–3).

The anal region surrounds the anal opening. It is bordered by the sacral, gluteal, and

*Petit, Jean Louis. Anatomist and surgeon, Paris, 1664–1750.
[†]Michaelis, Gustav Adolf. Gynecologist, Kiel, Germany, 1778–1848.

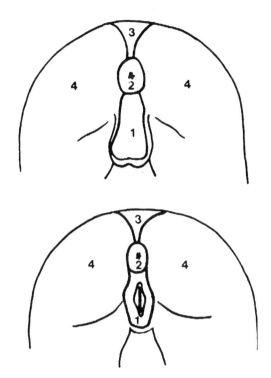

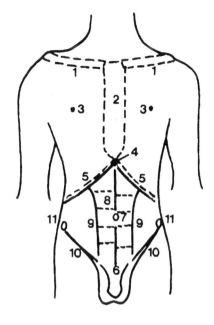

Figure 1–3 Perineum of male and female. **1**, Urogenital region; **2**, anal region; **3**, sacral region; **4**, gluteal region.

Figure 1–4 Orientation on the ventral trunk wall. **1**, Clavicle; **2**, sternum; **3**, nipple; **4**, xiphoid process; **5**, costal arch; **6**, linea alba; **7**, umbilicus; **8**, tendinous intersection; **9**, semilunar line; **10**, inguinal ligament; **11**, anterior superior iliac spine.

urogenital regions. The latter includes the area of the external sex organs. The urogenital region is bordered by the anal, gluteal, and pubic (abdominal wall) regions, as well as the lower extremities.

Inspection of the perineal area generally does not fall within the scope of examination of the musculoskeletal system.

INSPECTION FROM THE VENTRAL ASPECT

The abdominal wall is bordered cranially by the costal arches and the xiphoid process. Distally, it is bordered by the inguinal ligament and urogenital region. Usually, orientation is made with the help of the clearly visible linea alba (the tendinous sheath between the two rectus muscles), which forms the lower part of the median line (Figures 1–4 to 1–6).

The semilunar lines are the slightly laterally convex outer borders of the rectus abdominius. The lateral border of the abdominal wall is formed by the axillary line.

The axillary line is sometimes called the middle axillary line. In this instance, it is differentiated from anterior and posterior axillary lines, which run vertically through the anterior and posterior axillary walls.

The epigastrium (epigastric region) is found below the xiphoid process. It is an important area in the palpation of the stomach and abdominal aorta. To the right and left of the epigastrium lies the hypochondrium, which is considered to lie on the wall of the thorax rather than the abdomen. The subcostal plane, a transverse plane through the lower edge of the 10th costal cartilage, forms the lower border of this region. Caudal to the subcostal plane, the umbilical and lateral re-

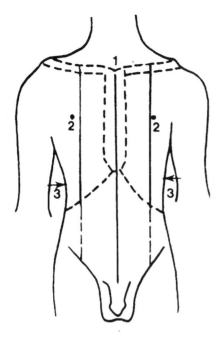

Figure 1–5 Orientation lines on the ventral trunk wall. *1*, Anterior median line; *2*, medioclavicular line; *3*, axillary line; *4*, semilunar line.

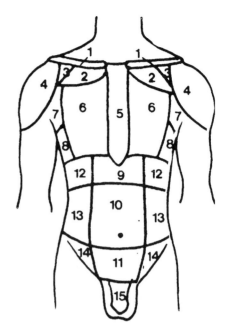

Figure 1–6 Regions on the ventral trunk wall. The terms in parentheses are rarely used. *1*, (Clavicular region); *2*, infraclavicular region; *3*, (trigonum deltoideopectorale); *4*, deltoid region; *5*, sternal region; *6*, mammary region; *7*, (axillary region); *8*, (lateral pectoral region); *9*, epigastric region; *10*, umbilical region; *11*, pubic region; *12*, hypochondriac region; *13*, (lateral region); *14*, inguinal region; *15*, genital region.

gions are found. These regions are bordered distally by the supracrestal plane, a transverse plane at the level of the proximal edge of the iliac crest, which also runs through the fourth lumbar vertebra. Underneath this plane lie the pubic and inguinal regions.

The clavicle and upper edge of the sternum are clearly visible at the upper part of the thorax. They form the upper border of the ventral trunk wall, which is bordered at the sides by the deltoideopectoral sulcus and axillary line. The costal arch and xiphoid process form the lower border of the thorax. At the ventral aspect of the thorax, commonly used orientation lines are: anterior median, medioclavicular (through the midpoint of the clavicle), and axillary. Structures lying at the edge of the sternum are called parasternal.

In men, the nipples (mamillae) generally lie just lateral to the midclavicular line. Each breast covers an area that lies between the second and sixth ribs and extends between the parasternal line and anterior axillary line. This is the mammary region, which is bordered above by the infraclavicular region and below by the hypochondriac region.

Superficial anatomy in the throat area is complex (Figure 1–7). Precise orientation is necessary. It is best to start by locating the sternocleidomastoid muscle, which is usually easy to see and palpate. The corresponding skin area is termed the sternocleidomastoid region, which is bordered by the nuchal region and temporal region from above.

The lateral neck region lies dorsal to the sternocleidomastoid region, which has a distal border with the clavicle and dorsal border with the trapezius muscle (nuchal region). The lateral neck region is in the shape of a tri-

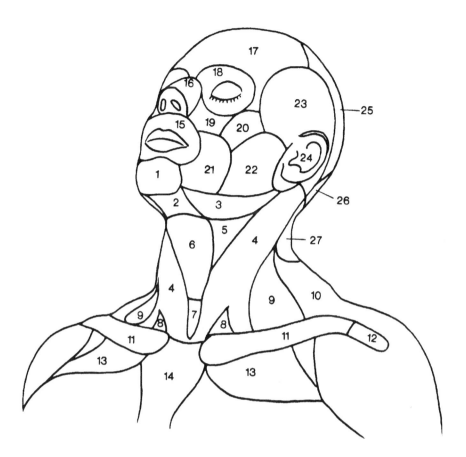

Figure 1–7 Regions of the head and throat/neck. The terms in parentheses are rarely used. *1*, Mental region; *2*, (submental region); *3*, submandibular trigone; *4*, sternocleidomastoid region; *5*, carotid triangle; *6*, anterior neck region; *7*, jugular fossa; *8*, lesser supraclavicular fossa; *9*, lateral neck region; *10*, (suprascapular region); *11*, (clavicular region); *12*, (acromial region); *13*, (infraclavicular region); *14*, (sternal region); *15*, oral region; *16*, nasal region; *17*, frontal region; *18*, orbital region; *19*, infraorbital region; *20*, zygomatic region; *21*, buccal region; *22*, parotideomasseteric region; *23*, temporal region; *24*, auricular region; *25*, parietal region; *26*, occipital region; *27*, nuchal region.

angle standing on its base and contains a number of palpable structures. Some authors divide this region again, into a ventral greater supraclavicular fossa and a dorsal occipital fossa. The edge of the levator scapulae muscle forms the border between these two fossae.

The space between both insertions of the sternocleidomastoid on the clavicle and sternum is called the lesser supraclavicular fossa. It fits like a small wedge in the sternocleidomastoid region.

In observing the neck ventrally, an intricately formed triangular space is found between both sternocleidomastoid muscles and the floor of the mouth. This area is divided into four regions. Just proximal to the sternal manubrium lies the jugular fossa; farther proximal lies the anterior neck region, in which the larynx is found. On each side of the larynx, at its dorsolateral aspect, the neurovascular bundles of the neck run cranially. The region in which the neurovascular bundles are found is called the carotid triangle, a triangular space between the sterno-cleidomastoid, submandibular triangle, and anterior neck region.

Regions of the head are generally much easier to identify. The chin is known as the mental region. The area lying under the chin is the submental triangle. Behind this region, and below the maxilla, lie both submandibular trigones, in which the submandibular glands are palpable.

The area around the lips is the oral region. The nose area is called the nasal region. The forehead is termed the frontal region, which corresponds to the borders of the frontal bone. It is impossible to locate exactly the borders of these regions in adults. The area around the hollows of the eyes is called the orbital region; the area underneath, the infra-orbital region. To the right and left of the in-fraorbital regions, the zygomatic arches in the zygomatic regions are found. The cheeks are called the buccal regions, behind which are found the parotideomasseteric regions with the parotid glands and masseter muscles. The ear is surrounded by the temporal region, the borders of which cannot be identified clearly. In this region the temporal muscle and artery can be palpated.

1.2   PALPATION OF THE HEAD, NECK, AND TRUNK

PALPATION OF THE STRUCTURES AT THE BACK OF THE HEAD

Position of the Patient: Sitting
Position of the Examiner: Sitting behind the patient

External Occipital Protuberance

The external occipital protuberance (Figure 1–8) is a bony prominence at the middle of the back of the head (occiput). It is easily palpable, and its size varies greatly.

From here, the linea nuchae, the lateral bony ridge of the occiput, can be felt. Caudal to the linea nuchae, there are two indentations, which can be extremely tender to the touch.

Mastoid Process

The mastoid process of the temporal bone lies behind the ear at each side of the occiput. This prominence is the insertion of the ster-nocleidomastoid muscle.

Inflammations of this region make the mastoid process very tender. Inflammations in the scalp area can lead to irritation of the lymph nodes lying over the mastoid process, which will also cause tenderness in this area. Such inflammations require careful treatment by a specialist and can be treated with medication.

The transverse process of the atlas can be palpated approximately 1 cm distal, and slightly ventral, to the mastoid process.

Occipital Artery and Vein, and Greater Occipital Nerve

Approximately one third of the distance between the external occipital protuberance and the mastoid process, the occipital artery and vein, along with the greater occipital nerve, become superficial (Figure 1–8). However, palpation of these structures is difficult. Patients with occipital migraines have severe pain in this region. The physical therapist can apply local massage (transverse friction) along with other therapeutic measures in order to achieve relaxation in this region.

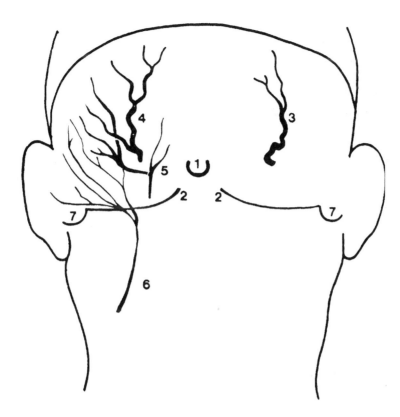

Figure 1–8 *1*, External occipital protuberance; *2*, linea nuchae; *3*, occipital artery; *4*, occipital vein; *5*, greater occipital nerve; *6*, lesser occipital nerve; *7*, mastoid process.

PALPATION OF THE NECK STRUCTURES

Position of the Patient: Sitting
Position of the Examiner: Sitting behind the patient

Spinous Processes

During palpation of the spinous processes in the neck region, the patient should try to relax the neck musculature. The examiner can promote relaxation in this area by resting the hand on the back of the patient's neck for a short time before beginning the palpation.

The first cervical vertebra (atlas) does not have a spinous process. In palpating from the external occipital protuberance in a distal di-

rection, the first spinous process encountered is the second cervical vertebra (axis). The spinous processes from C2 to C6 are split in two at their ends, those from C3 to C5 are palpable only with relaxed musculature, while C6 and C7 are almost always easy to locate. The latter two can be identified during neck extension; the spinous process of C6 "disappears."

It is often said that C7 has the most prominent spinous process in the neck region. However, it is just as possible that the spinous process of T1 is the most prominent. Thus, "the most prominent spinous process" should not be used as the only reference point in counting the vertebrae without first determining whether it belongs to C7 or T1. When placing the palpating fingers on either side of the C7 spinous process, significantly more motion (in a rotation direction) can be felt during cervical sidebending than when the T1 spinous process is palpated. In addition, by exerting alternating pressure dorsally against the sternal manubrium, the T1 spinous process is pushed dorsally via the first ribs; this can be felt easily during palpation of the T1 spinous process.

The small zygapophyseal joints of the cervical spine can be palpated by placing the finger lateral to the spinous process and performing a sidebending motion to the opposite side. This palpation can be difficult if the cervical musculature is not relaxed.

Transverse Process

The transverse processes of C2 to C7 are palpable in the lateral neck region. They are found further ventrally than the inexperienced examiner would expect, and can be palpated in front of the trapezius muscle rather than through the muscle from behind. Both sides can be palpated at the same time. The palpating fingers are placed in the lateral neck region, just in front of the trapezius, and exert pressure in a medial direction.

Palpation of the dorsal aspect of the C1 transverse process is more difficult. It is indirectly palpable underneath the splenius capitis (cranial) or levator scapulae (caudal). This site is sometimes painful and uncomfortable; thus any palpation should be gentle.

Splenius Capitis

The splenius capitis muscle (Figure 1–9) forms the cranial continuation of the splenius cervicis muscle. It runs from the first three thoracic spinous processes (and nuchal ligament of the C4(5) to C7 spinous processes) to the lateral aspect of the linea nuchae (superior) and external occipital protuberance. It contracts in ipsilateral rotation, which differentiates it from the semispinalis capitis muscle. During right rotation, if a muscle in the right side of the neck can be palpated, it is

the splenius capitis and not the semispinalis.

The splenius capitis is found just beneath the trapezius muscle at the lateral aspect of the neck. During ipsilateral rotation, the cranial and lateral sides of the contracting muscle can be recognized. In the upper part of the lateral neck region (occipital fossa), the insertion of the splenius capitis on the mastoid process can be palpated at the point where it has shortly before exited from underneath the trapezius.

Semispinalis Capitis

The semispinalis capitis muscle (Figure 1–9) forms the cranial continuation of the semispinalis cervicis muscle. The semispinalis capitis originates from the transverse processes of the third cervical to fifth (or sixth) thoracic vertebrae and inserts between the superior and inferior linea nuchae at the occiput. It contracts in contralateral rotation, and thus can be differentiated from the already mentioned splenius capitis.

Hidden underneath the trapezius muscle and partly covered by the splenius capitis, the semispinalis capitis lies very deeply in the nuchal region. Thus, it is palpable only during one specific motion, in which the other mentioned muscles remain relaxed. In contralateral rotation, the craniomedial edge of the contracting muscle often can be palpated in the upper corner of the lateral neck region (Figure 1–9).

Levator Scapulae

The levator scapulae (Figure 1–9) runs from the transverse processes of the first four cervical vertebrae to the superior angle of the scapula. It can be palpated in the lateral neck region further ventrally than usually expected. The muscle covers the distal part of the cervical vertebral transverse processes, which are simultaneously palpated in this area. The levator scapulae contracts specifically through internal rotation of the scapula; the patient is asked to move the arm (which is lying against the back) backward. During this

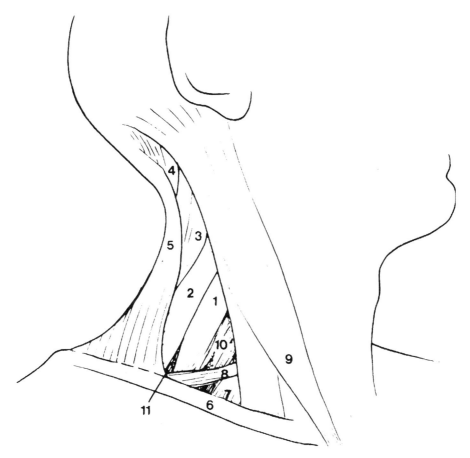

Figure 1–9 Palpable structures of the lateral cervical region. *1*, Middle scalene muscle; *2*, levator scapulae; *3*, splenius capitis; *4*, semispinalis capitis; *5*, trapezius muscle; *6*, clavicle; *7*, anterior scalene muscle; *8*, omohyoid muscle; *9*, sternocleidomastoid muscle; *10*, brachial plexus; *11*, posterior scalene muscle.

maneuver the neighboring muscles relax. Palpating the distal part of the levator scapulae is much more difficult. It can be palpated next to the C7 spinous process as a rolling cord under the fingers. From there, the muscle can be followed (through the trapezius) distally to the inferior angle of the scapula. The insertion on the scapula is a frequent site of referred pain.

PALPATION OF THE BACK STRUCTURES

Position of the Patient: Standing or on the side, lying with maximally flexed hips and chin to chest

Spinous Processes

Palpation of the thoracic and lumbar spinous processes must take into account great individual variance. Sometimes the spinous processes are easy to palpate; sometimes only tough resistance is met whereby the individual processes can hardly be identified.

In general, the iliac crest is at the level of the fourth lumbar vertebra. This generalization is often used in further orientation of the spinous processes. However, as with the generalization that C7 is the most prominent spinous process, there are significant individual differences in the height of the iliac crest. Thus, the spinous processes should be counted both from above and again from below. Only when the results are in agreement can one be certain that the spinous processes have been identified correctly.

In counting the vertebrae, use two fingers. With one finger resting on the spinous process of one vertebra, the other finger searches for the next spinous process. Then the first finger follows, while the second finger palpates further for the next spinous process, and so on. Often it is helpful to outline the individual spinous processes with a skin marker. Keep in mind, however, that the patient's movements will shift the position of the markings.

If the results are still doubtful, the examiner should either palpate every spinous process of the cervical spine (excepting the first, of course) or begin with the spinous process of S2. The S2 spinous process is always found on the horizontal line connecting both posterior superior iliac spines.

Remember that the thoracic spinous processes point diagonally downward. The corresponding vertebral body always lies slightly higher.

Transverse Processes

Palpation of the transverse processes is made significantly more difficult by the covering musculature. However, identifying these processes can be very important, for instance, in order to reposition a rib in its costovertebral joint. Keep in mind, like the vertebral body, the thoracic transverse processes lie cranial to their corresponding spinous processes.

In general, the "finger rule" can be applied in locating the thoracic transverse processes:

- Transverse processes of T1 and T2 lie approximately one fingerwidth cranial to the caudal tip of the corresponding spinous process.

- Transverse processes of T3 and T4 lie approximately two fingerwidths cranial to the caudal tip of the corresponding spinous process.

- Transverse processes of T5 to T8 lie three fingerwidths cranial to the caudal tip of the corresponding spinous process.

- Transverse processes of T9 and T10 lie two fingerwidths cranial to the caudal tip of the corresponding spinous process.

- Transverse processes of T11 and T12 lie one fingerwidth cranial to the caudal tip of the corresponding spinous process.

Palpate approximately 5 cm lateral to the midline. If the patient complains of clearly localized tenderness next to a thoracic transverse process, with simultaneous radiating pain between the ribs during breathing, there may be a (sub)luxation of a rib. By careful palpation, the affected rib can be identified and the appropriate technique applied to bring about pain relief.

The other parts of the vertebrae are not palpable.

The lumbosacral junction occasionally can be palpated from ventral, but only in very thin people with completely relaxed abdominal musculature. This junction can be felt approximately one handwidth below the navel.

Thoracolumbar Fascia

Both layers of the thoracolumbar fascia (Figure 1–10) surround the erector spinae muscle. The superficial layer is the area of origin for the latissimus dorsi, while both layers together serve as the origin for the abdominal wall muscles (except for the rectus abdominis). The deep fascial layer with the underlying quadratus lumborum and psoas major muscles are not palpable (Figure 1–10). In contrast, the erector spinae, covered by the superficial fascial layer, is easily palpable. At the widest part of the lower lumbar fascia, the

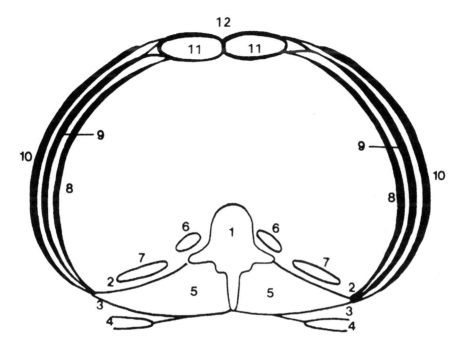

Figure 1–10 The trunk musculature with thoracolumbar fascia and rectus sheath. *1*, Vertebra; *2*, thoracolumbar fascia, deep layer; *3*, thoracolumbar fascia, superficial layer; *4*, latissimus dorsi; *5*, erector spinae; *6*, psoas major; *7*, quadratus lumborum; *8*, transverse abdominal muscle; *9*, internal oblique abdominal muscle; *10*, external oblique abdominal muscle; *11*, rectus abdominis with rectus sheath; *12*, linea alba.

origins of the latissimus dorsi and gluteus maximus can be palpated.

Erector Spinae

The erector spinae muscle consists of a complex system of muscle fibers. It lies between the two layers of the thoracolumbar fascia and runs cranially into the neck musculature. Identification of the separate parts is rarely necessary.

The medial tract consists of short muscles that connect the spinous processes (interspinales muscles), somewhat longer muscles running over the spinous processes (spinalis muscles), and short muscles between the transverse processes (intertransversarii muscles). The medial tract is active, particularly during back extension. Specific palpation is difficult.

The diagonal system (transversospinal system) also belongs to the medial tract. It consists of small muscles that run from the transverse processes to the adjacent cranial spinous process (rotatory muscles). Longer muscles extend over one to three vertebrae (multifidi muscles), the longest muscles extend over three to six vertebrae. The diagonal system rotates the vertebral column to the opposite side and thus is specifically palpable during this motion. In the lumbar region particularly the strongly developed multifidi can be palpated, and in the neck particularly the semispinalis capitis can be palpated.

The lateral tract of the erector spinae consists of the longissimus and iliocostalis muscles. The first runs from the sacrum upward to the transverse processes of the vertebral column; the latter runs from the iliac crest to the posterior angle of the ribs. Palpation of the lateral tract is easier than palpation of the medial tract.

Of the numerous ligaments connecting the vertebrae, only the interspinal and supraspinal ligaments are palpable. They are felt as band-shaped structures along the posterior midline.

PALPATION OF THE PERINEAL STRUCTURES

Position of the Patient: Kneeling, or in a sidelying or prone position with knees pulled up

Anal Region

The examination of the anal region (Figures 1–3 and 1–11) is not part of a routine examination of the musculoskeletal system. Here, besides the possible presence of hem-

orrhoids, the tonus of the external anal sphincter muscle can be assessed. Furthermore, the anus is the port for internal body examinations. This examination is uncomfortable for both the patient and the examiner. Therefore, it should be performed only by the appropriate specialist when specifically indicated. The general illustrations in Figures 1–11 and 1–12 are provided for orientation.

Urogenital Region

The female urogenital region (Figures 1–3 and 1–11) is surrounded by the labia majora, which continue ventrally into the mons pubis and dorsally into the posterior commissure. This examination can be significant in the diagnosis of an inguinal hernia. The labia majora enclose the labia minora, between which the ventrally located clitoris is found. Behind the

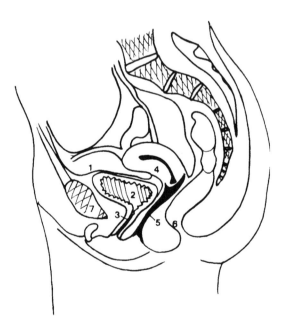

Figure 1–11 Sagittal section through the female lesser pelvis. *1*, Peritoneum; *2*, bladder; *3*, urethra; *4*, uterus; *5*, vagina; *6*, rectum; *7*, pubic symphysis.

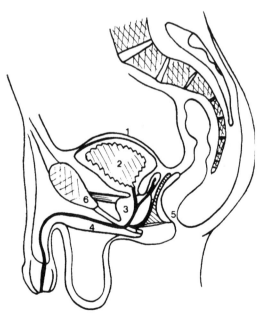

Figure 1–12 Sagittal section through the male lesser pelvis. *1*, Peritoneum; *2*, bladder; *3*, prostate; *4*, urethra; *5*, rectum; *6*, pubic symphysis.

clitoris lies the external urethral orifice. Even further dorsally, but in front of the posterior commissure of the labia, lies the vaginal orifice.

Through the male urogenital region runs a median ridge, the raphe penis and the raphe scroti. This ridge runs from the underside of the penis to the ventral edge of the anus. The bulb of the penis is covered by the bulbocavernous muscle and on both sides by the ischiocavernous muscle. The bulb of the penis can be palpated as a round, balloonlike elastic structure, which merges into the penis. On both sides the inferior pubic ramus is palpable. The scrotum is located ventral in the urogenital region. Both testicles are easy to palpate. The scrotal examination can be important in the diagnosis of an inguinal hernia.

PALPATION OF THE ABDOMINAL WALL AND ABDOMINAL ORGANS

Position of the Patient: Supine

In the abdominal examination, the patient should be as relaxed as possible. The palpation should not be threatening to the patient. Generally, the patient lies in a supine position. The examiner's hands should not be too cold. Before beginning the palpation, the examiner can place both hands on the patient's stomach and ask the patient to concentrate on the hands. At the same time, the examiner concentrates on the patient's stomach. Usually, the musculature relaxes, and the respiration rhythms of both individuals become synchronous.

Occasionally both hands are needed in the abdominal examination. If only one hand is used in a certain palpation, the other hand should rest on the patient's abdomen.

Rectus Abdominis

The rectus abdominis muscle and the ventral layer of the rectus sheath (Figures 1–10 and 1–13) are often clearly visible and always easily palpable. Begin in the midline just un-

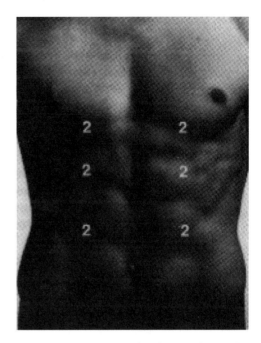

Figure 1–13 Rectus abdominis. *1*, Linea alba; *2*, intersectiones tendineae.

derneath the sternum, and palpate the tendinous part, linea alba, to the pubic bone. In so doing, palpate in the navel region for an umbilical hernia; this occurs rather frequently. The thickness of the linea alba varies; sometimes weak areas and tears can be palpated. The muscle itself has several tendinous intersections. They are transversely running, palpable tendons. They are best palpated during contraction of the abdominal muscles. Between left and right sides, these tendinous intersections are not always found at the same level (Figure 1–13).

The outlying border of the rectus abdominis (linea semilunaris) serves as an important orientation line in the abdominal region.

External Oblique Muscle of the Abdomen

The patient lies supine with both knees slightly flexed; the head rests on a small pillow. Place the flat hand on the trunk, sideways under the caudal border of the pectoralis major, whereby the fingers point medially. By now palpating between the heads of the serratus anterior, the upper edge of the external oblique abdominal muscle is reached (Figures 1–10 and 1–13). By shifting the hand caudally, the entire muscle can be palpated.

Generally seen, the muscle fibers run from craniolateral to caudomedial (the same direction as the hand points in a pants pocket). The function of the external oblique muscle is rotation of the trunk to the opposite side. The rotation motion serves to differentiate the external from the internal oblique muscle (trunk rotation to the same side). Palpation of the external oblique abdominal muscle is simplest in the sidebent trunk; however, this motion does not allow for differentiation of the internal oblique muscle.

Internal Oblique Muscle of the Abdomen

The internal oblique abdominal muscle (Figure 1–10) is hidden underneath the external oblique, making it very difficult to palpate. Its fibers run from caudolateral to craniomedial (except the horizontally running lower fibers), and contraction functions to rotate the trunk to the same side. During active right rotation, if contraction of a deeper-lying muscle is felt at the right abdominal wall, this is likely the internal oblique abdominal muscle. A second method of palpating the muscle is by placing the hand on the abdomen, perpendicular to the running of the muscle fibers, and moving the fingers gently back and forth.

In the lower back region, a small part of the internal oblique abdominal muscle is palpable near its origin just above the iliac crest, where it is not covered by the external oblique abdominal muscle. This area is called Petit's triangle. Here the muscle is directly palpable, but this is of little practical value.

The transverse abdominal muscle lies too deep to palpate and is not discussed further in this book.

Inguinal Canal

In its course, the inguinal canal penetrates the abdominal wall just proximal to the inguinal ligament (Figures 1–14 and 1–15). It originates from a position laterally in the deep inguinal annulus, an opening in the fascia of the transverse abdominal muscle, approximately 1 cm above the midinguinal point (in other words, halfway between the anterior superior iliac spine and the pubic tubercle). From here, the canal runs medial and becomes superficial after penetrating the transverse and internal oblique abdominal muscles. Some fibers of the internal oblique muscle join the structures already located in the canal. Finally, the canal runs through the superficial inguinal annulus, which is formed by the aponeurosis of the external oblique muscle and is found approximately 1 cm proximal to the pubic tubercle.

Thus, the inguinal canal runs above the medial half of the inguinal ligament. In contrast to this, the lacuna vasorum, which contains the femoral artery and nerve, runs under the ligament. Furthermore, the lacuna vasorum runs in a straight line from dorsal to ventral, while the inguinal canal runs diagonally from laterodorsal to medioventral. The inguinal ligament forms the floor of the canal. The aponeurosis of the external oblique abdominal muscle forms the ventral wall. The dorsal wall is formed by the aponeurosis of the transverse abdominal muscle and the "ceiling" from fibers of the internal oblique abdominal muscle.

In men, the canal empties with the spermatic cord and deferent duct into the scrotum. In women, the canal contains the teres ligament of the uterus and ends at the labia majora. In both men and women, the ilioinguinal nerve is found in the inguinal canal.

When an inguinal hernia is present, the abdominal contents protrude into the canal.

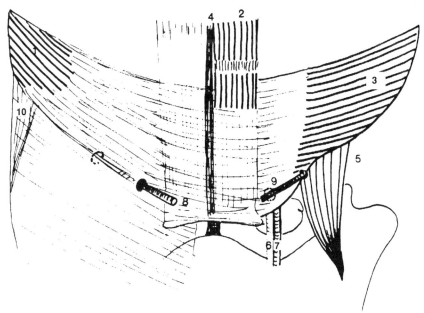

Figure 1–14 Course of the abdominal muscle fibers (fascia removed). *1*, External oblique muscle; *2*, rectus abdominis muscle; *3*, internal oblique and transverse abdominal muscles; *4*, linea alba; *5*, iliopsoas muscle; *6*, femoral vein; *7*, femoral artery; *8*, spermatic cord in superficial inguinal annulus; *9*, spermatic cord in deep inguinal annulus; *10*, tensor fascia latae. **Source:** Reprinted with permission from Rozendal RH. *Inleiding in de Kinesiologie van de Mens*. Culemborg, Netherlands: Stam-Kemperman; © 1974.

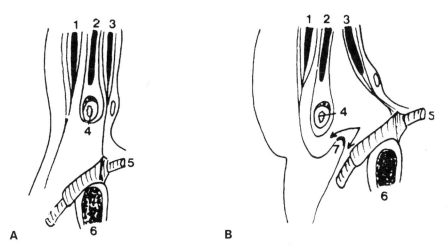

Figure 1–15 Sagittal views through the inguinal canal. *1*, External oblique abdominal muscle; *2*, internal oblique abdominal muscle; *3*, transverse abdominal muscle; *4*, spermatic cord; *5*, femoral artery with vessel sheath; *6*, pubic bone; *7*, inguinal ligament. **A**, In the presence of a normal abdominal wall. **B**, In the presence of a weak abdominal wall. The inguinal ligament is not clearly visible. Arrows indicate an inguinal hernia (above) and a femoral hernia (below). **Source:** Reprinted with permission from Rozendal RH. *Inleiding in de Kinesiologie van de Mens*. Culemborg, Netherlands: Stam-Kemperman; © 1974.

When an indirect inguinal hernia is present, the abdominal contents protrude through the deep inguinal annulus into the inguinal canal and can follow the canal down into the scrotum or labia majora. When a direct hernia is present, the abdominal contents protrude ventrally, directly through the superficial inguinal annulus, avoiding the inguinal canal. Such a protrusion is surrounded by the transverse and internal oblique abdominal muscles. The diagnosis of an inguinal hernia is the responsibility of a specialized physician; however, the possibility of a hernia should not be overlooked in the routine examination of the musculoskeletal system. Thus, the inguinal canal and its contents (spermatic cord or teres ligament of the uterus) should be palpated. If an inguinal hernia is suspected, the scrotum and labia majora should be palpated as well.

PROJECTION OF THE ORGANS IN THE ABDOMINAL CAVITY

Although examination of the abdominal organs is not part of the routine examination of the musculoskeletal system, indirect contact with the abdominal contents is unavoidable during palpation of the abdominal wall. Thus, the examiner should have an idea of the orientation of the abdominal organs and be able to interpret palpation findings in this region (Figures 1–16 and 1–17). For this reason, it is appropriate to discuss the projection of the abdominal cavity organs in relation to the abdominal wall.

The intestinal organs are found, for the most part, "within" the peritoneum (Figure 1–16). In other words, they are surrounded by membraneous duplications of their own structures. In peritonitis, the abdominal wall is extremely taut and very tender to palpation.

The palpable part of the stomach is found in the epigastric region (region underneath the xiphoid process). The lower edge of the liver is usually at the level of the right costal arch

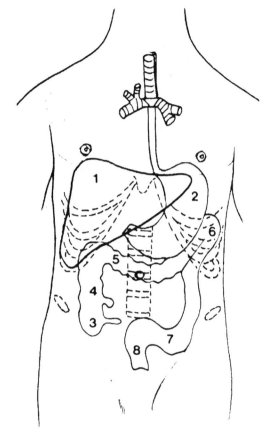

Figure 1–16 Digestive tract (ventral view). *1*, Liver; *2*, stomach; *3*, cecum and appendix; *4*, ascending colon; *5*, transverse colon; *6*, descending colon; *7*, sigmoid colon; *8*, rectum.

and extends left into the epigastric region. The gallbladder can be palpated at the lower edge of the liver. The pancreas and duodenum lie too far dorsally to be able to palpate. Generally, the appendix is oriented between the outer and middle thirds of a line connecting the right anterior superior iliac spine to the navel. Often, however, this point is not tender in appendicitis. Sometimes, the ascending colon and the sigmoid colon are palpable in the left inguinal region or in the lower lateral trunk region.

Besides parts of the digestive tract, parts of the urogenital tract are also palpable in the

left hand grasps the patient's flank and remains there without moving for the remainder of the palpation. The fingers of the right hand lie horizontally on the abdominal wall (perpendicular to the ascending colon); the fingertips are at the level of the right linea semilunaris. The palpating hand now presses gently into the abdominal cavity and slides, with the fingers moving slightly back and forth, slowly in a lateral direction. In a relaxed abdominal wall, the ascending colon can be felt deeply in the abdominal cavity as a vertically running structure. In certain intestinal disorders, this structure can be very tender.

Sigmoid Colon

In palpation of the sigmoid colon (Figures 1–16 and 1–17), the examiner again rests one hand against the patient's flank, while the other hand is placed on the abdomen in the umbilical region, perpendicular to the expected course of the sigmoid colon (45° angle to the long axis of the trunk). The palpating hand moves slowly laterally and caudally, feeling the sigmoid colon as a deeply lying and diagonally running soft cord.

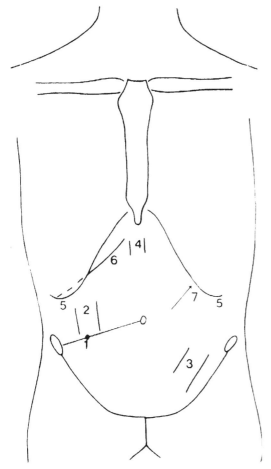

Figure 1–17 Palpation of the organs in the abdominal cavity (ventral view). **1**, McBurney's point; **2**, ascending colon; **3**, sigmoid colon; **4**, abdominal aorta; **5**, kidneys; **6**, lower edge of the liver; **7**, palpation area for an enlarged spleen.

Abdominal Aorta

The examiner places both hands, one on top of the other, on the patient's epigastric region. The top-lying hand gently pushes the other hand into the abdominal cavity. Generally, the pulsation of the abdominal aorta is felt deeply in the cavity with only slight pressure (Figures 1–17 and 1–18). Without an urgent indication to palpate more deeply, the palpation remains superficial in order not to injure the deeper-lying structures. Often the abdominal pulse is visible at the abdominal wall, making palpation unnecessary.

Painful conditions of the stomach or other epigastric organs can make palpation in this region very painful, and it is performed only when necessary.

abdominal cavity. The kidneys lie deep in the lateral trunk region. A full bladder is palpable above the pubic symphysis. The uterus can be palpated in the pubic region.

Ascending Colon

The ascending colon is palpable in the right lateral trunk region (Figures 1–16 and 1–17). The patient lies in a supine position, and the examiner stands to the right. The examiner's

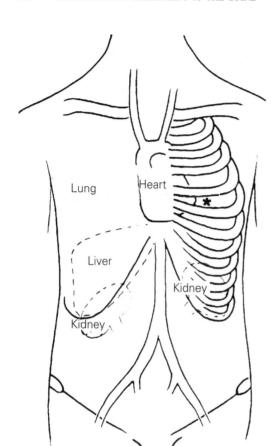

Figure 1–18 Projection of several organs on the ventral trunk wall.

Kidneys

In very thin people, the kidneys can be palpated (Figures 1–17 and 1–18). The examiner grasps the patient's flank with one hand, whereby the fingers lie dorsally in the lateral trunk region. The other hand gently presses into the lateral trunk region from ventrally. Sometimes it is possible to "dance" the kidneys between the two hands (ballottement). Pain in the flank during palpation may indicate pathological changes in the kidney and requires examination by a specialist. However, most of the time, the kidneys are not palpable. Palpation of the kidneys is not within the scope of routine musculoskeletal examinations.

Liver

The patient lies in a supine position. The examiner stands at the right side. With the left hand, the examiner grasps the patient's flank and the hand remains there for the rest of the palpation. The fingertips of the right hand are placed approximately 3 cm below the right costal arch. The fingers are pointed craniolaterally in a 45° angle. The subject is now asked to breathe deeply in and out several times. During the exhalation, the palpating hand pushes carefully craniolaterally into the abdominal cavity; at the level of the costal arch, the fingers come against a firm resistance. This is the lower edge of the liver (Figures 1–16 and 1–17). Due to various pathological processes, this organ can become enlarged; in this case, the lower edge is found farther caudally.

Spleen

The spleen lies in the upper left half of the abdomen, where it is hidden deeply dorsally under the costal arch (Figure 1–17). Thus, under normal conditions, it is not palpable. However, in certain disorders, the spleen can be significantly enlarged, at which time it is accessible to palpation underneath the left costal arch. The same technique is used to palpate the spleen as was used in palpation of the liver.

The patient lies in the supine position. The examiner stands at the patient's right side. The examiner grasps the patient's flank with the right hand, where the hand remains for the rest of the palpation. The fingertips of the left hand are placed approximately 3 cm below the left costal arch. The fingers are pointed craniolaterally in a 45° angle. The subject is now asked to breathe in and exhale deeply several times. During the exhalation, the palpating hand pushes carefully, craniolaterally into the abdominal cavity. If firm resistance is encountered at the level of the costal arch, an enlarged spleen should be suspected.

PALPATION OF THORACIC STRUCTURES

Position of the Patient: Supine

Sternum

Palpation of the sternum is a simple procedure. The cranial border (jugular notch), sternal manubrium, junction between the manubrium and the body of the sternum (sternal angle), body of the sternum, and the xiphoid process are clearly palpable.

The sternal angle can be palpated approximately 4 cm caudal to the sternal notch as a horizontally running plateau. Generally the second rib is found at the same level as the sternal angle; however, occasionally the third rib is at this level. In such instances, mistakes can be avoided by noticing that the sternal angle in these individuals is farther than 4 cm caudal to the sternal notch. Because the pectoralis major muscle originates on the sternum, palpation of the entire sternum takes place indirectly (through the pectoralis major muscle).

Ribs

The ribs and costocartilage are easily palpable for the most part. Nevertheless, locating the individual ribs without making mistakes requires a great amount of practice.

Before beginning the palpation, ensure that the sternal angle is indeed at the level of the second rib. The first rib is completely covered by the clavicle, which makes palpation of this rib more difficult. By passively bringing the shoulder girdle into elevation, part of the first rib can sometimes be palpated.

Begin counting ribs from the second rib. In so doing, place two fingers horizontally against the sternal angle and slide the fingers laterally. The cranial-lying finger now lies in the first intercostal space and the caudal finger lies in the second intercostal space. Between both fingers is the second rib. The cranial finger then shifts into the second intercostal space, while the other finger locates the third intercostal space, and so on. Actually, the fingers "walk" over the thorax. In the course of the "walk," the fingers wander further laterally. In female patients the palpation is made more difficult due to breast tissue. In males, the nipple generally lies directly over the fifth rib.

Generally, palpation to the 12th rib is possible. If the 12th rib is "missing" or there is a "13th" rib, there has likely been a mistake in the palpation and counting. The inexperienced examiner may have an easier time of orienting the intercostal spaces by using a skin marker.

Breasts

We have included the orientation of the breasts in the section discussing the ventral trunk wall. Needless to say, the breasts are usually clearly visible and their identification should not be a problem.

Examination of the female breast is not part of a routine examination of the musculoskeletal system. However, in the scope of the general physical examination, the early discovery of pathological changes can be of great importance. During this palpation, the woman lies in a supine position. Her hands are placed behind her head. Attention is given to the appearance of the nipples (pulled in), the presence of secretions, changes in the skin (orange-peel appearance), and the presence of nodules. Nodules can be benign or malignant, but in every case should be further evaluated by a physician. Serious and infectious processes in the breast can lead to swelling of the lymph nodes in the infraclavicular region, lateral neck region, and axillae.

Ictus Cordis

As an exception to the other thoracic structures, the ictus cordis (heartbeat) is not palpated, but rather percussed and auscultated. Often the pulsation of the heartbeat can be seen in the left half of the thorax, just to the right of the medioclavicular line in the fifth in-tercostal space, 7 to 8 cm away from the median line (Figure 1–18).

The ictus cordis can also be found at other sites. In children it usually lies more cranial. The visible ictus cordis is generally found approximately 2 cm medial to the actual apex cordis (apex of the heart). Visible pulsation in the epigastric area does not necessarily come

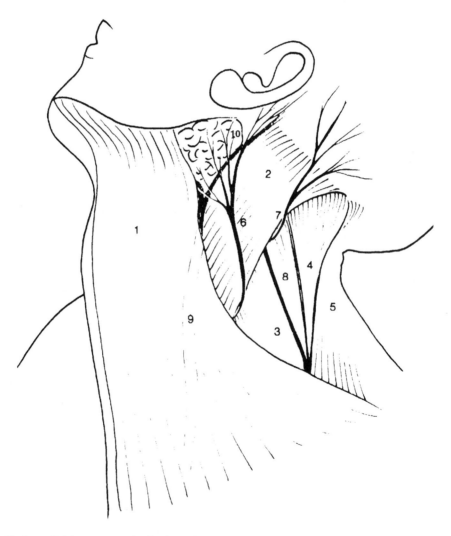

Figure 1–19 Superficial structures in the lateral throat and neck region. **1**, Platysma; **2**, sternocleido-mastoid; **3**, levator scapulae; **4**, splenius capitis; **5**, trapezius muscle; **6**, greater auricular nerve; **7**, lesser occipital nerve; **8**, accessory nerve; **9**, external jugular vein (under the platysma); **10**, submandibular gland.

from the abdominal aorta; it can also be caused by the ictus cordis.

PALPATION OF THE STRUCTURES LYING IN THE THROAT REGION

Position of the Patient: Sitting or supine

Platysma

The platysma, a cutaneous muscle, lies over the sternocleidomastoid muscle, directly under the skin of the throat (Figure 1–19). The patient is asked to open the mouth as wide as possible. In so doing, contraction of the platysma is observed.

Hyoid Bone

In order to locate the hyoid bone (Figure 1–20), the mandible is grasped from each side with thumb and index finger of the same hand. By sliding the fingers caudally along the contour of the throat, a horseshoe-shaped

bone is felt—the hyoid. When swallowing, the hyoid bone moves downward. Because the hyoid bone lies at the level of the third cervical vertebra, it can be used as an orientation point in locating the latter structure.

Trachea

The jugular fossa lies just above the sternal notch. Palpation of this fossa can be very uncomfortable for the subject. Deep in the fossa, the trachea can be felt (Figure 1–20). It is covered by several muscles, which are not further discussed.

Larynx

The larynx is found between the hyoid bone and trachea (Figure 1–20). It is composed of nine cartilages: the single thyroid, cricoid, and epiglottic cartilages and the paired arytenoid, cuneiform, and corniculate cartilages. Ridged collagenous connective tis-

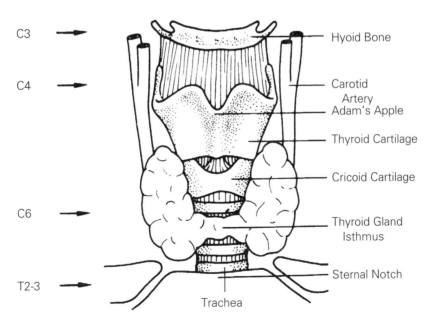

Figure 1–20 Structures in the anterior neck region. *Source:* Reprinted with permission from Ellis H. *Clinical Anatomy.* London: Blackwell Scientific Publications Ltd, © 1992.

sue is found between the hyoid bone and thyroid cartilage.

When the index finger slides approximately one fingerwidth caudally from the midpoint of the hyoid bone, it comes against the median indentation of the thyroid cartilage, at the level of the fourth cervical vertebra. The edge just below the indentation is the so-called Adam's apple, the meeting point of both clearly palpable cartilage plates.

By following the sharp edge of the thyroid cartilage caudally, the finger runs into a cartilage ring just below the thyroid cartilage—the cricoid cartilage. Its wider part is found more dorsally. The trachea begins caudally to the cricoid cartilage. The cricoid cartilage is an important reference point in the neck region, because it lies at the level of the sixth cervical vertebra. Found at the same level are the junctions between the larynx and trachea, and between the pharynx and esophagus. This is also where the vertebral artery enters the foramen transversum of the sixth cervical vertebra (carotid tubercle). The middle cervical ganglion is also found at this level as well.

Thyroid Gland

The thyroid gland is palpated at the anterior neck region (Figure 1–20). Hold the cricoid cartilage between thumb and index finger, and ask the patient to swallow. Larynx and thyroid gland move up and down. In this way, the consistency and mobility of the thyroid gland can be assessed. A pathological palpatory finding should be evaluated by a specialist.

Carotid Tubercle

In the lower tip of the carotid triangle, behind the cricoid ring, the carotid tubercle can be palpated. The palpating finger is placed against the anterior aspect of the sternocleidomastoid muscle and exerts slight pressure dorsally at the level of the cricoid ring. In order to prevent the so-called carotid reflex (sudden bradycardia due to bilateral clamping of the carotid arteries), this palpation should never be performed bilaterally.

Neurovascular Bundle

Slightly farther cranially, the pulsation of the carotid artery can be palpated in the carotid triangle (never palpate bilaterally). At this site the common carotid artery divides into the internal and external carotid arteries (Figure 1–21). The latter is palpable.

The external carotid artery forms a common neurovascular bundle with the nonpalpable internal jugular vein and the vagus nerve.

Scalenic Triangles

The scalenic triangles are found in the ventrocaudal part of the lateral neck region. The nonpalpable subclavian vein runs through the anterior scalenic triangle, formed by the anterior scalene and sternocleidomastoid.

The easily palpable brachial plexus runs through the posterior scalenic triangle, between the anterior and middle scalenes. The subclavian artery, which runs along the floor of this triangle, is also palpable at this site. The omohyoid muscle runs diagonally over the posterior scalenic triangle.

With the patient in a state of maximal inhalation, the posterior scalene is recognizable behind the middle scalene.

Punctum Nervosum

The punctum nervosum (Erb's* point) can be palpated by following the middle scalene cranially, directly below the sternocleidomastoid (Figure 1–21). This site is usually tender to palpation. The following nerves arising from the cervical plexus can be palpated here:

- greater auricular nerve, which runs over the sternocleidomastoid cranially to the cheek and ear area

---

*Erb, Wilhelm Heinrich. Neurologist, Heidelberg, Germany, 1840–1921.

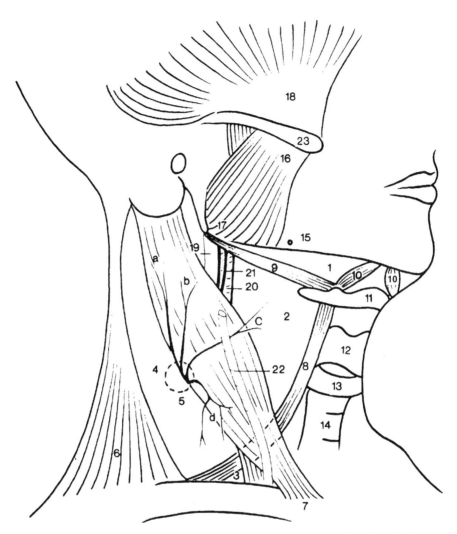

Figure 1–21 Structures in the lateral head and neck region. *1*, Submandibular triangle; *2*, carotid triangle; *3*, supraclavicular fossa; *4*, lateral neck region; *5*, punctum nervosum; *a*, lesser occipital nerve; *b*, greater auricular nerve; *c*, transverse colli nerve; *d*, supraclavicular nerve; *6*, trapezius muscle; *7*, sternocleidomastoid muscle; *8*, omohyoid muscle; *9*, stylohyoid muscle; *10*, digastric muscle; *11*, hyoid bone; *12*, thyroid cartilage; *13*, cricoid cartilage; *14*, trachea; *15*, palpation site for the facial artery; *16*, masseter muscle; *17*, mandibular arch; *18*, temporal muscle; *19*, internal jugular vein; *20*, external carotid artery; *21*, vagus nerve; *22*, external jugular vein (after excision of the cranial part); *23*, zygomatic arch.

- lesser occipital nerve, which runs behind the ear to the back of the head
- transverse colli nerve, which runs over the sternocleidomastoid ventrally and innervates the skin (sensory) in the platysma area

- suprascapular nerve, which is superficial and runs caudally to innervate the skin (sensory) in the clavicle area

At the punctum nervosum, pain and tenderness from the cervical plexus can be assessed. Also, brachial plexus problems can be treated here.

External Jugular Vein

The external jugular vein arises at the level of the mandibular angle and runs distally between the platysma and sternocleidomastoid muscles (Figures 1–19 and 1–21). It empties into the subclavian vein behind the clavicular insertion of the sternocleidomastoid.

The external jugular vein is often visible in the throat region. Its caudal part can often be seen to be filled. Farther up, it is flat and not palpable. The amount of fullness depends on the level of pressure in the right atrium.

Omohyoid Muscle

The omohyoid muscle originates from the superior scapular border, between the superior angle and the scapular notch (Figure 1–21). The inferior belly then runs in the direction of the cervical neuromuscular bundle. There the muscle consists of a tendinous

junction that is covered by the sternocleidomastoid. The superior belly of the muscle runs toward the head and inserts on the lower outer edge of the hyoid bone.

A small part of the pars inferior is palpable, superficial to the cervical plexus, at the level of the anterior scalenic triangle. The patient is asked to close the mouth forcefully. The muscle is now palpable as a diagonally running cord. By following the muscle farther ventrally, a small part of the tendinous junction is palpable underneath the sternocleidomastoid.

PALPATION OF THE STRUCTURES AROUND THE HEAD

Position of the Patient: Supine

Mandible

Palpation of the outer mandibular edge is easy (Figures 1–21 and 1–22). The mandibular angle serves as an important orientation point. The mandibular ramus is covered by

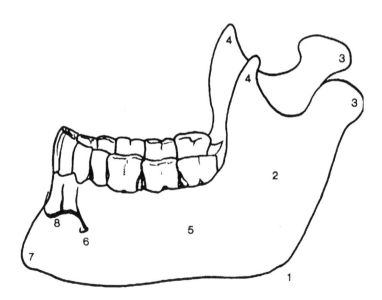

Figure 1–22 Mandible. *1*, Mandibular angle; *2*, mandibular ramus; *3*, condylar process; *4*, coronoid process; *5*, body of the mandible; *6*, mental foramen; *7*, mental protuberance; *8*, mental nerve.

the masseter muscle. The condylar process of the mandible is palpable just in front of the ear.

By palpating along the cheek dorsally, the mandibular coronoid process is the first bony structure the palpating finger meets.

At the ventrolateral aspect of the mandible, the mental foramen is found, where the mental nerve, a sensory branch of the trigeminal nerve, is palpable.

Atlantal Transverse Process

The transverse process of the atlas can be palpated in the tip of the carotid triangle, where it lies between the mandibular angle and the mastoid process, and is covered by the sternocleidomastoid muscle.

The transverse process of the atlas is also indirectly palpable. It is felt as a hard structure through the overlying musculature. This palpation is seldom necessary, and because it can be painful and uncomfortable, it is performed with great care and only when necessary.

Temporomandibular Joint

Movement of the mandibular condylar process can be felt by placing the finger in the patient's external auditory meatus and asking for jaw movement. The same palpation (and for the patient a more comfortable palpation) is possible approximately 0.5 cm farther ventrally, just in front of the ear.

As the mouth is opened, one can feel how the condylar process shifts in a ventral-caudal direction and then rests on the articular tubercle.

Submandibular Gland

The submandibular gland is palpable in front of the mandibular angle and underneath the mandibular body in the submandibular triangle (Figures 1–19 and 1–23). If there is inflammation of the salivary gland, a painful swelling can be found.

Facial Artery

The pulse of the facial artery can be palpated at the border between the first and second thirds of the mandible, in front of the mandibular angle (Figures 1–21 and 1–23).

Parotid Gland

The parotid gland lies superficially in front of the ear and reaches as far as the mandibular ramus (Figure 1–23). In inflammations of the parotid gland, the ear lobe moves outward.

Zygomatic Arch

When palpating ventrally from the condylar process of the mandible, the finger comes against the zygomatic arch, which is formed by the temporal and zygomatic bones (Figure 1–21).

The temporal muscle lies above and the masseter muscle lies below the zygomatic arch.

Masseter Muscle

The masseter muscle closes the mouth. Both superficial and deep parts run from the zygomatic arch to the mandibular ramus (Figures 1–21 and 1–23). It is easily palpable at the level of the ramus. After placing the palpating finger against the ramus, the patient is asked to close the mouth forcefully.

Pterygoid Muscles

The medial pterygoid muscle also closes the mouth. The lateral pterygoid muscle opens the mouth. Both muscles lie deeply and are difficult to palpate; they are not discussed further.

Temporal Muscle

The temporal muscle runs from the temporal fossa, underneath the zygomatic arch, to the coronoid process (Figure 1–21). It also functions in closing the mouth.

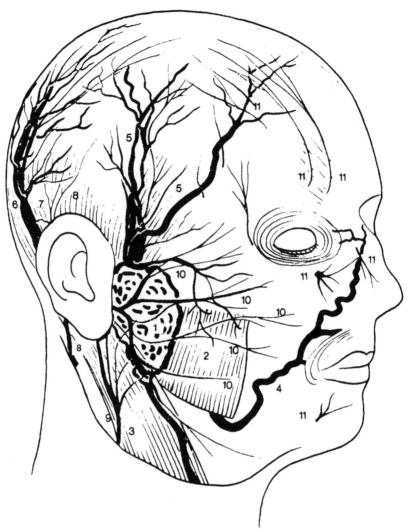

Figure 1–23 Blood vessels and nerves of the head. *1*, Parotid gland; *2*, masseter muscle; *3*, sterno-cleidomastoid muscle; *4*, facial artery; *5*, superficial temporal artery; *6*, occipital artery; *7*, greater occipital nerve; *8*, lesser occipital nerve; *9*, greater auricular nerve; *10*, branches of the facial nerve; *11*, branches of the trigeminal nerve.

In front of the ear the muscle is very easy to palpate, and above the ear it is still relatively easy to palpate. Place the palpating finger against the temporal region and ask the patient to close the mouth forcefully.

Superficial Temporal Artery

The pulsation of the superficial temporal artery is palpable above the temporal muscle in the temporal region (Figure 1–23). Particu-larly in elderly individuals, the vein is often tortuous and visible to the naked eye. Certain blood vessel disorders can make palpating this structure extremely painful. In these cases, examination by a specialist is indicated.

Trigeminal Nerve

The trigeminal nerve innervates the masticatory muscles and is responsible for the sensory innervation of the face (Figure 1–23).

Trigeminal neuralgia can be extremely painful.

Branches of the trigeminal nerve are rarely palpable individually. The mental nerve is easily palpable after it leaves the mental foramen (Figure 1–22). The auriculotemporal and zygomaticotemporal branches of the trigeminal nerve can sometimes be palpated in the region of the superficial temporal artery.

Branches of the frontal nerve that run over the forehead are sometimes palpable at the upper edge of the orbita. At this site they become superficial.

The external nasal rami (which innervate the nose), the infraorbital nerve (which lies under the orbita), and the zygomaticofacial ramus (which runs lateral to the orbita) are rarely palpable.

Facial Nerve

Branches of the facial nerve enter the subcutaneous layer in front of the ear and then run over the parotid gland (Figure 1–23). Occasionally they can be palpated individually at this site.

Oral Cavity

Inspecting the oral cavity is generally not a part of the examination of the musculoskeletal system.

The color of the tongue is sometimes an indication of the general health of the individual being examined.

Tongue movements give information about the function of the hypoglossal nerve; an intact glossopharyngeal nerve ensures the symmetrical curvature of both halves of the hard palate.

Orbital Region

The oculomotor, trochlear, and abducens nerves are responsible for the movement of the eyeballs.

Pupil reactions to light are an indication of the function of the oculomotor nerve.

The color of the connecting skin of the lower eyelids gives an indication of the hemoglobin content of the blood. In anemia, the connective skin can be very pale.

Sometimes branches of the frontal nerve can be palpated at the upper edge of the orbitae.

1.3 SCHEMATIC TOPOGRAPHY OF THE BLOOD VESSELS AND NERVES OF THE HEAD, NECK, AND TRUNK

CRANIAL NERVES

The topography and function of the cranial nerves are described in this section, although most cannot be palpated. The function of a cranial nerve generally can be assessed through clinical examination. Disturbances in function always require further examination by a specialist. Such functional disturbances can indicate pathological processes in the brain and should always be taken seriously.

Olfactory Nerve

The olfactory nerve connects the olfactory mucosa in the nasal cavity to the olfactory bulb in the frontal lobe. If damaged, the sense of smell is affected.

Optic Nerve

The optic nerve connects the eye with the midbrain. If damaged, vision decreases. The site of the lesion generally can be located through precise diagnostics.

Oculomotor Nerve

This nerve runs from the brain stem to the orbita. It innervates most of the eye muscles and the pupils. A deficit of this nerve causes ptosis (hanging down of the eyelid), fixed pupil, dilated pupil, and a caudolaterally deviated position of the eyes.

Trochlear Nerve

The trochlear nerve runs from the brain stem to the superior oblique muscle of the orbita. A deficit of this nerve makes looking in a caudolateral direction impossible. In order to compensate, the nonaffected side may develop torticollis.

Trigeminal Nerve

The trigeminal nerve originates in the brain stem. One branch, the mandibular nerve, leaves the skull through the oval foramen of the sphenoid bone and innervates the mastication muscles. In addition, it sends sensory branches to the cheek, temporal region, and the mandibular and tongue areas (from rami such as the mental nerve).

A second branch (mostly sensory) is the maxillary nerve, which innervates the maxilla, zygomatic arch, and the infraorbital region.

Finally, the ophthalmic nerve, the third branch of the trigeminal nerve, leaves the skull through the orbita. Its most important twig is the frontal nerve, which supplies sensory innervation to the forehead. Other rami run to the nasal region (to the superficial branches of the trigeminal nerve).

Trigeminal neuralgia, which is seen rather frequently, can be extremely painful.

Abducens Nerve

The abducens nerve runs from the brain stem to the rectus lateralis muscle in the orbita. Deficits of this nerve cause the eye to be directed medially (cross-eyed). The nerve is often the first to be affected in space-occu-

pying processes within the skull, as well as in instances of increased intracranial pressure.

Facial Nerve

The facial nerve runs from the brain stem, past the inner ear, and through the temporal bone, where it becomes superficial. The facial nerve innervates the muscles of expression. This nerve is also partly responsible for the sense of taste and several salivary glands.

Deficit of the facial nerve (peripheral paresis) can be caused not only by inner ear infections, but also by trauma (operations) in the parotid gland area. This nerve is also often affected (central paresis) by vascular disturbances of the brain. These deficits can vary. In a peripheral paresis, the patient cannot completely close the eye or wrinkle the forehead. A unilateral deficit leads to a deviation of the mouth (the corner of the mouth hangs down). (See Figure 1–23 for superficial branches of the facial nerve.)

Vestibulocochlear Nerve (Acoustic Nerve)

The vestibulocochlear nerve runs from the brain stem to the inner ear and innervates the auditory and equilibrium systems.

Glossopharyngeal Nerve

The glossopharyngeal nerve originates in the brain stem and leaves the cranium through the jugular foramen, together with the vagus and accessory nerves. It partially innervates the pharynx, tongue, and gustatory epithelium. In addition, it innervates the parotid gland.

Vagus Nerve

The vagus nerve runs from the brain stem through the jugular foramen to the neurovascular bundle of the neck. It belongs to the parasympathetic system and innervates the smooth muscles in several parts of the pharynx, esophagus, larynx, and digestive tract. It also assists in regulating heartbeat.

Accessory Nerve

The accessory nerve runs from the brain stem caudally through the jugular foramen and can be palpated dorsally in the lateral neck region, superficial to the levator scapula. It innervates the trapezius and sternocleidomastoid muscles.

Hypoglossal Nerve

The hypoglossal nerve runs from the brain stem caudally through its own opening in the base of the skull and provides motor innervation to the tongue.

CERVICAL PLEXUS

The cervical plexus is formed from the ventral spinal nerves above C4, together with the hypoglossal and accessory nerves. The cervical plexus, which is covered by the sternocleidomastoid muscle, exits between the origins of the anterior scalene, middle scalene, and levator scapulae muscles. The following branches go through the punctum nervosum:

- The greater auricular nerve gives sensory innervation to the ear region and is occasionally palpable superficial to the sternocleidomastoid muscle.
- The lesser occipital nerve can be palpated dorsally. It gives sensory innervation to the lateral part of the occipital region.
- The transverse nerve of the neck is sometimes palpable in front of the greater auricular nerve. It is a sensory nerve and partially innervates the skin of the neck.
- The suprascapular nerve, covered by the platysma, runs caudally with several branches and partially innervates the skin in the clavicular region.

Various branches of the cervical plexus innervate the scalene muscles. The phrenic nerve (mainly C4) arises in the cervical plexus. This nerve runs along the medial pleural layer from the anterior scalene muscle to the diaphragm.

DORSAL RAMI OF THE SPINAL NERVES

Of the dorsal spinal nerves, the two most cranial are the suboccipital and greater occipital nerves. The first innervates the semispinalis capitis muscle. The latter is palpable lateral to the external occipital protuberance (Figure 1–8).

The other dorsal spinal nerves innervate the entire erector spinae muscles. They are not palpable.

VENTRAL RAMI OF THE SPINAL NERVES

From T1 caudally, the trunk wall is innervated by the ventral rami of the spinal nerves. In the thoracic area, the intercostal nerves (ventral rami) innervate the intercostal spaces. They innervate both the intercostal muscles and the skin. The lower intercostal nerves innervate the musculature and skin of the upper abdominal wall. They are not palpable.

The lumbar ventral rami (excluding L5) form the lumbar plexus. Several nerves emerging from this plexus innervate the lower abdominal wall. The uppermost lumbar branch is the iliohypogastric nerve, which runs over the iliac crest through the abdominal wall. The branch caudal to the iliohypogastric nerve is the ilioinguinal nerve. Both nerves innervate the outer abdominal wall, as well as parts of the legs and the external genitalia. The genitofemoral nerve has almost no role in the innervation of the abdominal wall.

Sympathetic innervation of the head, neck, and trunk occurs with the help of countless networks, which, to a large extent, travel alongside the blood vessels. In the neck, there are several sympathetic ganglia. In the trunk, the ganglion chain lies in front of the vertebral column. In the area of the large abdominal vessels there are several plexuses. However, none of these structures are palpable.

ARTERIAL VASCULARIZATION

Thoracic Aorta

The ascending aorta arises from the left ventricle (Figure 1–24). Its first branches are the coronary arteries. To the left of the sternum, at approximately the level of the second intercostal space, the aortic arch curves first dorsally and then caudally. The descending aorta begins dorsally in the thorax at the level of the fourth thoracic vertebra and pierces through the diaphragm in its distal course.

The brachiocephalic trunk arises at the right side of the aortic arch and bifurcates into the right subclavian and common carotid arteries. The left common carotid and subclavian arteries spring from the aortic arch, just to the left of the brachiocephalic trunk. Numerous intercostal arteries spring from the descending thoracic aorta and supply blood to the intercostal spaces, the greater part of the thoracic wall, and the upper abdominal wall.

The subclavian artery exits the thorax through the posterior scalenic triangle and then divides into a number of branches supplying the neck region with blood. The internal thoracic artery is a branch from the subclavian artery. It runs distally along the inner side of the thoracic wall, which it partially vascularizes. The vertebral artery is a dorsal branch of the subclavian artery. It originates in front of the posterior scalenic triangle and runs directly dorsal to the carotid tubercle of the sixth cervical vertebra. From there, it traverses through the transverse processes of the cervical spine to the skull. It is responsible for vascularization of the posterior part of the brain.

In cases of cervical arthrosis, the vertebral artery can become compressed because of its position in the cervical spine. This could lead to a decrease in the blood supplied to the posterior part of the brain.

Carotid Arteries

The common carotid arteries run cranially on each side of the trachea. At the level of the carotid tubercle, the arteries divide into an internal carotid artery and an external carotid artery. The internal carotid artery runs behind the external carotid artery and enters the skull through the carotid canal. Its branches vascularize the anterior and middle parts of the brain. The orbita also receives its blood supply from this artery.

The external carotid artery runs cranially with the neurovascular bundle of the neck. Deep in the neck, it crosses the mandibular angle. From below the mandible, branches go to the larynx and thyroid gland; the upper part provides branches to the tongue and part of the pharynx. Another branch from the external carotid artery is the facial artery, which perforates the submandibular gland on its way anterior and then spirals upward around the body of the mandible. It is palpable at this site (Figure 1–23). This artery supplies blood to part of the face.

Still farther cranially, the external carotid artery gives off a dorsal branch, the occipital artery, which runs from the origin of the sternocleidomastoid muscle to the back of the head (occiput). The occipital artery is palpable at this site (Figure 1–8). Finally, the external carotid artery provides the posterior auricular artery for vascularization of the ear region.

The uppermost section of the carotid artery cannot be palpated; it lies deeply behind the mandibular ramus. Somewhat above the zygomatic arch, it divides into two final branches, the maxillary artery and superficial temporal artery. The first artery runs anteriorly in the infratemporal region, an area of intricate topography lying deeply underneath the zygomatic arch. This artery is not palpable. It supplies blood to part of the tem-

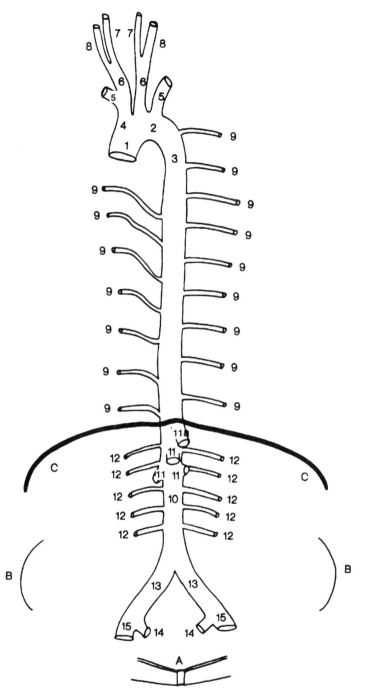

Figure 1-24 Schematic illustration of the arterial blood supply. **A**, Pubic symphysis; **B**, Iliac crest; **C**, diaphragm; **1**, ascending aorta; **2**, aortic arch; **3**, descending aorta; **4**, brachiocephalic trunk; **5**, subclavian artery; **6**, common carotid artery; **7**, external carotid artery; **8**, internal carotid artery; **9**, abdominal aorta; **10**, arteries of the intestinal tract; **11**, celiac trunk; **12**, lumbar arteries; **13**, common iliac artery; **14**, internal iliac artery; **15**, external iliac artery.

poromandibular joint, jaw, masticatory muscles, and part of the meninges. The second artery curves around the mandibular ramus on its course anteriorly and runs superficially above the parotid gland. It then runs over the zygomatic arch and supplies the frontal and parietal regions of the skull. In the temporal fossa it is easily palpable (Figure 1–23).

Abdominal Aorta

The abdominal aorta runs caudally below the diaphragm, to the left and in front of the vertebral column. It divides into the common iliac arteries at the level of the iliac crest. These arteries run over the edge of the lesser pelvis in their caudolateral course. They divide again, into an internal iliac and external iliac artery, at the level of the sacroiliac joint. The internal iliac artery supplies blood to the lesser pelvis, part of the legs, and the external genitalia. The external iliac artery runs along the edge of the lesser pelvis to the lacuna vasorum, where it is called the femoral artery. The femoral artery becomes the inferior epigastric artery shortly before the lacuna vasorum. The epigastric artery runs cranially along the inner side of the abdominal wall. Finally, it anastomoses with the end branches of the internal thoracic artery. Posterior in the abdominal cavity, the abdominal aorta produces several lumbar arteries. At its anterior aspect, the large arteries of the digestive tract originate. Somewhat farther below, to the left and right, a renal artery branches off to the kidneys. Still farther, to the right the testicular (ovarian) artery runs to the testicles (or ovaries) along the posterior wall of the abdominal cavity.

VENOUS SUPPLY

The venous blood of the cranium drains into a cranial venous sinus, from which the jugular vein originates in the jugular foramen. The jugular vein exits the skull together with the glossopharyngeal, vagus, and accessory nerves. These four structures enter the neurovascular bundle of the neck, where they run distally next to and behind the arteries. Most of the branches of the common carotid artery are accompanied by a similarly named vein; all these veins flow into the internal jugular vein. The venous tributaries of the nasal region run though the skull. Inflammation in this region must be carefully treated to prevent the spreading of infectious germs into the skull.

The external jugular vein drains the occipital region, outer ear, and submandibular triangle. The vein originates underneath the mandibular angle, where it runs distally, covered only by the platysma (Figure 1–19). An anterior jugular vein runs in front of the larynx, on each side. The topographical location of this vein varies greatly. The anterior jugular vein drains either into the end of the external jugular vein or directly into the subclavian vein.

The internal, external, and anterior jugular veins unite with the brachiocephalic vein behind the clavicular insertion of the sternocleidomastoid muscle, where they lie in front of the arteries. Somewhat above and to the right, in front of the aortic arch, both brachiocephalic veins drain into the superior vena cava, which runs farther to the right atrium of the heart. Most of the intercostal veins empty into the azygos vein, which runs cranially to the right of the thoracic vertebral column and finally drains into the superior vena cava.

The large pelvic arteries are accompanied by veins of similar names. To the right of the aortic bifurcation these veins unite with the inferior vena cava, which runs cranially on the right side of the abdominal aorta. The inferior vena cava gathers blood from the lumbar, renal, and testicular (or ovarian) veins. The left testicular (or ovarian) vein drains into the left renal vein. Almost all of the blood in the digestive tract runs through the portal vein to the liver, where it is "cleaned" in a massive network of capillaries. Finally it collects in the hepatic veins, which drain into the inferior vena cava, cranially in the abdominal cavity. The inferior vena cava pierces the diaphragm and ends in the right atrium of the heart.

In a venous obstruction of the abdomen (for instance, due to a pathological process in the liver), the venous tributaries of the abdominal cavity can run through portocaval anastomoses. In these instances, the cutaneous veins of the abdominal wall are swollen and clearly visible (caput medusae).

SUGGESTED READING

Clain A, ed. *Hamilton Bailey's Demonstrations of Physical Signs in Clinical Surgery.* Bristol, England: John Wright & Sons; 1965.

Crawford Adams J. *Outline of Orthopaedics.* 6th ed. London: Churchill Livingstone; 1967.

Cyriax J. *Textbook of Orthopaedic Medicine.* 7th ed. London: Baillière Tindall; 1978;1.

Elias N. *Über den Prozeß der Zivilisation.* 5th ed. Baden-Baden, Germany: Suhrkamp; 1978;1, 2.

Gardner E, Gray DJ, O'Rahilly R. *Anatomy.* Philadelphia: WB Saunders; 1975.

Gray H, Williams PL, Warwick R. *Gray's Anatomy.* 36th ed. London: Churchill Livingstone; 1980.

Haak A, Steendijk R, de Wijn IF. *De Samenstelling van het menselijk Lichaam.* Assen, Netherlands: Van Gorcum; 1968.

Hafferl A. *Lehrbuch der topographischen Anatomie des Menschen.* Berlin: Springer Verlag; 1957.

Hamilton WJ, Simon G, Hamilton SGI. *Surface and Radiological Anatomy.* 5th ed. London: Macmillan Press Ltd; 1976.

Healy EJ, Seybold WD. *A Synopsis of Clinical Anatomy.* Philadelphia: WB Saunders; 1969.

Heerkens YF, Meijer OG. *Tractus-Anatomie.* Interfaculty Physical Education. Amsterdam; 1980.

Hoppenfeld S. *Physical Examination of the Spine and Extremities.* New York: Appleton-Century-Crofts; 1976.

Janis JL, Mahl GF, Kagan J, Holt RR. *Personality, Dynamics, Development, and Assessment.* New York: Harcourt, Brace and World, Inc; 1969.

Lohman AGM. *Vorm en beweging: Leerboek van het bewegingsapparaat van de mens.* 4th ed. Utrecht, Netherlands: Bohn, Scheltema & Holkema; 1977;1, 2.

McMinn RMH, Hutching RT. *A Color Atlas of Human Anatomy.* London: Wolfe Medical Publications Ltd; 1977.

Russe O, Gerhardt JJ, King PS. *An Atlas of Examination, Standard Measurements and Diagnosis in Orthopaedics and Traumatology.* Bern, Switzerland: Hans Huber Verlag; 1972.

Sobotta J, Becher PH. *Atlas of Human Anatomy.* 9th English ed. Berlin: Urban & Schwarzenberg; 1975;1, 2, 3.

Winkel D, Fisher S. *Schematisch handboek voor onderzoek en behandeling van weke delen aandoeningen van het bewegingsapparaat.* 6th ed. Delft, Netherlands: Nederlandse Akademie voor Orthopedische Geneeskunde; 1982.

2

General Aspects of Examination and Treatment

EDITOR'S PREFACE

In 1989, a supplement written by Allan and Waddell[1] with regard to the history of low back pain and the resulting limitations in the activities of daily living was published in the journal Acta Orthopaedica Scandinavica. *Even though low back pain is not the sole subject of this book, the ideas from Allan and Waddell are mentioned in this introduction because of their general implications.*

The history of low back pain dates back to the Bible. Allan and Waddell cite a text from 1500 BC: "When you examine a man with a dislocation of a vertebra of the spinal column, say to him: 'Extend your legs and contract both legs.' Immediately he contracts both legs because of the pain which is caused in the vertebra of the spinal column, which is the cause of his suffering."[1]

Throughout the course of history, explanations for low back pain have changed. For conservative treatment, however, little has changed. Compared with 2500 years ago, today's thermal baths, heat applications, and bed rest still belong to the arsenal of treatment.

*Since the 18th century, people from the Western hemisphere have related low back symptoms to anatomical causes. However, the interpretation of the cause has changed several times over the years. Low back pain has been ascribed as coming from diseases of the sciatic nerve, arthritic changes in the spinal column (at the end of the 19th century called fibrositis), and changes in the form of the spinal column (mainly scoliosis). In the 20th century these diseases were initially replaced by the sacroiliac disorders and, after the important publication by Mixter and Barr in 1934,[2] by lesions of the disc. However, there are still authors who emphasize the significance of the sacroiliac joint,[3] or those who find the zygapophyseal joints respon-*sible for low back pain, although this has not yet been proven.[4]*

*Through modern imaging techniques, it has been recognized that correlation between anatomical disturbances and complaints is often very poor. Therefore, low back pain should be observed not only as an anatomical disturbance but also, because of restrictions in daily movement behavior, as a disabling experience. This especially counts for chronic low back pain. From the analysis of Allan and Waddell,[1] it is clear that **disability** based on low back pain first appeared at the end of the 19th century, more or less simultaneously with the first appearance of labor laws and insured medicine. Back problems into the 19th century were mainly interpreted as having a rheumatic origin; they are now perceived as diseases that are treatable with prolonged bed rest and that alone can lead to disability. The latter perception coincides with the fact that low back pain is often ascribed to a (severe) trauma, with or without degenerative changes. In this sense, much of the disability due to low back pain can be interpreted as iatrogenic because this "disability" is the result of a medical interpretation.*

These contemplations could lead to future consideration of low back pain as being independent of morphological-physiological changes. However, this book has been written with the conviction that with the help of professional functional and anatomical thinking, at least some of the complaints can be treated successfully.

Controlled studies on treatment effectiveness have indicated that substantial parts of the complaint patterns can be treated conservatively. Some treatment methods have shown greater effectiveness than others. It is the therapist's task to use the treatment methods offering the greatest possibility for success. Of course, this does not rule out the probability that effective treatment methods are based partially on placebo effects. However, it is not important to the patient whether the success of the treatment is based on a placebo effect or on specific parts of the therapy. What counts is the treatment success.

Only the use of technical conservative treatment of back pain, such as described in this book, is incomplete. Information concerning movement and posture is at least as important as therapy. This also counts for the maintenance of intensive contact between therapist and patient in order to facilitate long-term changes in behavior of the patient. Often the significance of the complaints can be interpreted correctly only when taking into consideration the personal situation of the patient. Keeping these aspects in mind when applying the various treatment measures, with or without the cooperation of other disciplines, will greatly improve the effectiveness of therapeutic management.

Nonoperative treatment and prevention are emphasized in this book. However, this is not a statement against operative treat-ment, which is discussed briefly in the following chapters. Unfortunately, some surgeons still apply their scalpels too early, often resulting in an increase rather than a decrease in the complaints.[4] Conservative therapy and preventive measures are preferred as long as the patient is able to manage the symptoms. The decision for surgery, if necessary, should be made based on a discussion between therapist/physician and patient.

Our preface ends with a warning: no single theoretical or empirical framework is sufficient to alleviate all complaints present in our society. Excessive belief in one treatment form is harmful. The caregiver should be aware of the many available treatment methods. This also means that the existing techniques should be mastered in order to give the patient the best possible treatment. Applying this concept will yield great success. However, it is far from our goal to suggest that this is the only concept that should be used to understand and treat every symptom.

2.1 FUNCTIONAL ANATOMY

INTRODUCTION

The spine is artificially divided into three sections for easy reference throughout this book. The sections are the lumbar spine, the thoracic spine, and the cervical spine. Transitional areas such as the sacroiliac joints (SI joints) and the atlanto-occipital joints are also described. Although it does not really belong to the vertebral column or its transitional areas, the temporomandibular joint is also discussed.

Many anatomical structures overlap the sections that we use; these structures connect the various parts of the spine with each other. The specific functional anatomy of each spinal region is discussed at the beginning of the corresponding sections. Some general aspects of spinal anatomy are highlighted in the following section.

SPINAL COLUMN

A large part of the body is constructed segmentally, and the stratification of the spinal column is one expression of that segmental construction. Keeping this in mind, one realizes that the term *segment* changes its meaning according to the topic of discussion. From the osteological point of view, the various vertebrae can be seen as segments. In studying spinal movement , one speaks of the "motion-segment," which is the connection between two adjacent vertebrae.

The sacrum consists of 5 sacral vertebrae. The lumbar spine has 5 vertebrae, the tho-

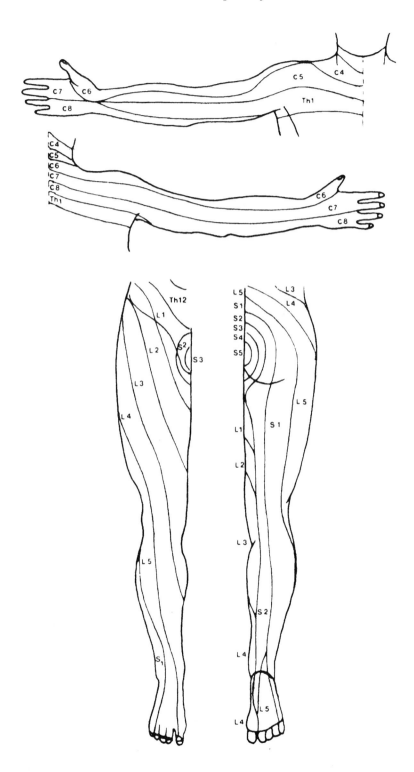

Figure 2–1 Segmental distribution of the dermatomes of the extremities. A considerable overlap exists between the different dermatomes. In addition, there are considerable interindividual differences.

racic spine has 12 vertebrae, and the cervical spine has 7 vertebrae, of which the upper 2 (axis and atlas) have a different morphology.

The spine consists of 31 nerve pairs: 8 cervical, 12 thoracic, 5 lumbar, 5 sacral, and 1 in the coccygeal area. Every spinal nerve is formed by a dorsal nerve root and a ventral nerve root. The spinal nerves from C1 to C7 leave the spinal canal above the vertebra with the same number. The spinal nerve C8 lies

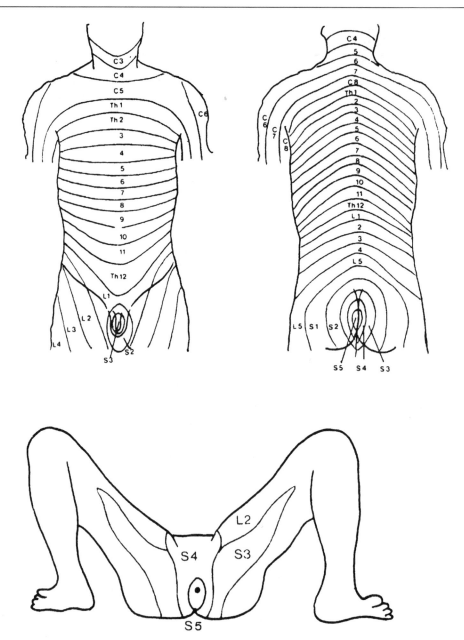

Figure 2–2 Segmental distribution of the dermatomes of the trunk. This classification reflects the average description by various authors. Here also, considerable interindividual differences are possible.

above the first thoracic vertebra. The other spinal nerves lie caudal from the vertebra with the same number.

With increased pressure in the spinal canal, symptoms can manifest themselves in specific neurologically defined segments: local pain and disturbances in the related dermatome and/or myotome (Figures 2–1 and 2–2). These segments are defined by the nerve roots they belong to. In the cervical region, the neurological segment is situated at the level of the cranial aspect of the spinous process of the vertebra with the same number. In the upper and midthoracic regions, the tip of the spinous process indicates a neurological segment of two levels more caudal (in other words, the tip of the Nth spinous process is at the level of the neurological segment $N + 2$). In the lower thoracic region there is a difference of three levels; the neurological segment L3 is found at T11, and the neurological level S1 is located at T12. At the caudal end of the spinal column the neurological segments are situated relatively high in relation to the vertebra of the same number. (See Figure 8–2.)

A typical vertebra has a ventral body and a dorsal vertebral (or neural) arch, which together enclose the spinal canal (Figure 2–3). Within this framework the spinal cord is situ-

ated with its surrounding membranes, arteries, etc. The pedicles comprise both sides of the ventral part of each vertebral arch and have a small vertical diameter. Between the pedicles of adjacent vertebrae, the intervertebral foramen is found, through which the spinal nerves and blood vessels run. Also, part of the vertebral arch, situated dorsal of the pedicles, are the laminae and seven major prominences: two superior and two inferior articular processes, two transverse processes, and one spinous process.

FUNCTIONAL OVERVIEW

In women, the sacrum is the part of the pelvis on which specific demands are placed during childbirth. During childbirth, the pelvic joints become more mobile, while at the same time stability remains important.

Considered vertically, the pelvis is the connection between the lumbar spine and the legs. Describing the motions of the pelvis is often difficult. Motions of the pelvis in relation to the lower extremities do not have to conform with its movements in relation to the lumbar spine.

The SI joints, the L5–S1 disc, and numerous ligaments, connect the sacrum to the lumbar spine. These structures are the most heavily loaded and strongest part of the spine. Despite its strong morphology, the lumbar spine is the site of frequent pathology, particularly the intervertebral discs. The normal lumbar spine curves ventrally, forming a lordosis (Figure 2–4).

The thoracic spine is part of the thorax. Protection of the respiratory organs is of importance here. Mobility in the thoracic spine is minimal, although not insignificant. During breathing the rib-vertebra connections play an important role in their relation to the spinal column. The normal thoracic spinal column curves dorsally, forming a kyphosis (Figure 2–4).

The cervical spine has a considerable amount of mobility designed to serve the head. In a normal standing or sitting posi-

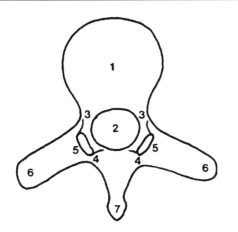

Figure 2–3 Typical features of a vertebra (cranial view). **1**, Vertebral body; **2**, spinal canal; **3**, pedicle; **4**, lamina; **5**, superior articular process; **6**, transverse process; **7**, spinous process.

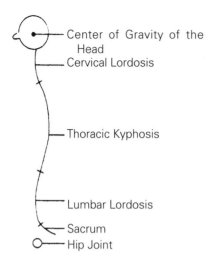

Figure 2–4 The normal curves of the spinal column.

tion, the head's center of gravity is situated ventral of the spinal column. Therefore, relatively large forces play a significant role in cervical spine pathology. The normal cervical spine curves ventrally, forming a lordosis (Figure 2–4).

COUPLED AND COMBINED MOVEMENTS

The motions in the spinal column consist of the following:

- flexion and extension around a fronto-transverse axis (the x axis),
- sidebending around a sagittotransverse axis (the z axis), and
- axial rotation around a frontosagittal axis (the y axis).

Because of the specific morphology of the zygapophyseal joints and ligaments, it is normally impossible to perform a sidebending motion without a simultaneous axial rotation. These are called *coupled movements*. (See Chapter 9.) A coupling is termed ipsilateral if the sidebending induces an axial rotation in the same direction, and contralateral if the sidebending induces an axial rotation in the

opposite direction. Axial rotations are appointed according to the direction of the motion of the vertebral body, thus opposite to the direction of motion of the spinous process.

Within the practical framework that is offered in later chapters, the following coupled movements are accepted:

- lumbar spine: ipsilateral in flexion; contralateral in extension
- lower thoracic spine: same as lumbar spine
- midthoracic spine: sometimes as lower, sometimes as upper thoracic spine
- upper thoracic spine: same as cervical spine
- cervical spine: ipsilateral in both flexion and extension
- upper cervical spine (C0 to C2): contralateral in flexion and extension

Movements contrary to the coupled movements are called *combined movements*. In principle

- Coupled movements are mainly restricted by ligamentous structures.
- Combined movements are mainly restricted by zygapophyseal joint compression.

CONNECTIONS

The vertebrae are connected to each other by means of zygapophyseal joints (between the articular processes), the intervertebral discs, and the ligaments. Of course, the muscles also play a significant role in the mobility and stability of the spinal column.

Zygapophyseal Joints

In relation to the parasagittal plane, the zygapophyseal joints have a vertical orientation in the lumbar spine, an oblique inclination (approximately 60°) in the thoracic spine, and along an oblique imaginary line connecting the motion segment and the orbitae in the cervical spine. Likewise, the zygapophyseal joints have different orientations in the transverse plane: in the lumbar spine they are primarily oriented in the sagittal plane, in the thoracic spine their orientation approaches the frontal plane, and in the cervical spine they lie in the frontal plane. Left-right asymmetry is almost always present in the zygapophyseal joints. (See Chapter 4.) Interindividual differences are also considerable.

According to some manual therapy "schools," the zygapophyseal joints are thought to be primarily responsible for most of the problems in the lumbar spine; others strongly refute this view. Recent literature[5] concludes that zygapophyseal facet degeneration actually does not occur without disc degeneration occurring first. Therefore, we have classified the lumbar spine pathology in relation to the intervertebral disc. Furthermore, the form and position of the zygapophyseal joints are not related to disc pathology.[6]

The existence of "coupling patterns" is due chiefly to the form and position of the zygapophyseal joints. (See Chapter 9.) The joints "guide" the movement on a precise track. Because of the intraindividual asymmetry and the interindividual differences, one cannot expect exactly the same coupling pattern in each person. Theoretically, it is even possible for a coupling to the right to behave differently from a coupling to the left in the same person. The variability is significant, especially in the midthoracic region.

Motions contrary to the coupling patterns (combined movements) do not, per definition, follow the specific track guided by the zygapophyseal joints. These combined movements are primarily restricted by compression in the zygapophyseal joints. Thus, zygapophyseal joint pathology manifests itself in a painful limitation of motion in the combined movement patterns. In such pathology pain is felt "deep," with little chance of referred symptoms, and it has no clear segmental pattern because of the considerable overlap of the innervation pattern.[7]

Intervertebral Discs

From C2 down to and including S1, an intervertebral disc is apparent between the vertebral bodies. This disc functions as a shock absorber and plays an important role in the mobility of the spinal column as well. In dealing with pathology of the spine we presume that this pathology is either directly (primarily) or indirectly (secondarily) related to the intervertebral disc.[8–10]

Based on histological characteristics, a division can be made between the nucleus pulposus (the center of the disc) and the annulus fibrosus (the peripheral part of the disc). However, this division is not so extreme as to say that there exist two separate, independently functioning structures between the two vertebral bodies. Macroscopically, the transition between annulus and nucleus is very smooth. Functionally, the division is present in the sense that the nucleus pulposus primarily deals with compressive forces, while the annulus predominantly deals with tensile forces. The nucleus pulposus of a healthy disc occupies between 30% and 60% of the horizontal cross-section of the center of the disc. It acts as a noncompressible fluid; the amount of fluid varies from 70% to 90%.[10]

The annulus fibrosus is formed by layers of fibers surrounding the nucleus. Each layer consists of strong collagen fibers embedded in a cartilaginous matrix. The fibers are oriented in a specific angulation in relation to the transverse plane. Various investigators have found different degrees of angulation varying from 24° up to 45°.[11] Gracovetsky and Farfan[12] indicate that in the inner layers the fibers have an inclination of 37°, whereas in the outer layers they have an inclination of 24°. They attribute a special mechanical function to this feature.

— Meniscoid folds present in cerv. + lumbar ZAJ capsule, not in Th. area (Ty-8),

Galante[13] states that the amount of collagen in a disc is about 16% of the total volume of the disc. Eyre[14] found that the fibers in the inner layers are of the type I collagen, a type that is abundant in tendons and has to resist strong tensile forces. Fewer fibers are present in the dorsal aspect of the disc, compared with the ventral aspect, leading to the conclusion that the dorsal part of the disc is less stiff than the ventral part.[15]

The collagen fibers of the outer layers of the disc are connected to the bone of the adjacent vertebral bodies. The fibers of the inner layers insert into the hyaline end-plates, the original growth centers of the vertebral bodies, which normally form an impenetrable barrier.

Nutrition

The avascular disc depends on two systems for nutrition. The blood vessels near the ligaments at the level of the outer fibrous layers are responsible for a part of the nutrition. Nutrition also takes place from within the end plates. Seventy percent of the glucose enters the disc through the end plates, while 30% enters via the outer layers of the annulus. In contrast, 70% of the sulfates enter through the annulus, while 30% enter via the end plates.[4] The mechanism of diffusion is stimulated through an alternating compression and decompression of the disc, a so-called pump mechanism.[16]

After a disc rupture, vascularization of the dorsal aspect of the disc often takes place. These blood vessels alone can be a possible source for nocisensoric afferent pain.[17]

Innervation

It has become evident that in the cervical disc there are a certain number of free nerve endings present, although in the past it was assumed that the intervertebral disc was not innervated.[7] Innervation at the lumbar level had been noticed much earlier, at first in the outer layers,[18,19] and later in the more central layers of the annulus fibrosus[20] as well. The innervation consists of free nerve endings and Vater-Pacini corpuscula. In fetuses and young children they are more abundant than in adults.

Ligaments

The long ligaments of the spine are structures that span the entire vertebral column. They play an important role in the stability of the spinal column.

The ligamentum flavum runs along each side of the spine between the vertebral arches. It is very elastic (the ratio of elastic to collagen fibers is about 2:1). At rest there is also a certain tension on these ligaments; during flexion they are stretched. The ligamentum flavum is part of the capsule of the zygapophyseal joints.[17]

The anterior longitudinal ligament runs from the atlas to the sacrum at the ventral aspect of the vertebral bodies, with which the ligament has a close connection. It widens from cranial to caudal. The posterior longitudinal ligament runs from the occiput to the sacrum. In contrast to the anterior longitudinal ligament, this ligament has a stronger connection to the intervertebral discs and a looser connection with the vertebral bodies. The ligament narrows from cranial to caudal and consists of only a thin collagenous filament at the lumbosacral junction.

The supraspinous ligament runs from the spinous process of C7 caudally. However, it never reaches the sacrum.[21] At the lower lumbar levels, the homologue of the supraspinous ligament consists of fibers derived from the thoracolumbar fascia.

Upon close examination, the interspinous ligaments consist of three parts. The ventral (or deep) part can be seen as a continuation of the flaval ligament. The middle part is more developed than the other parts and runs between the spinous processes. Finally, the dorsal (or superficial) part is connected with the supraspinous ligament (Figure 2–5).

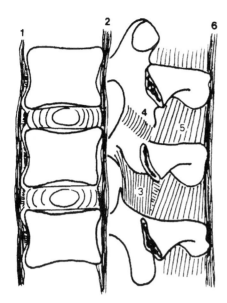

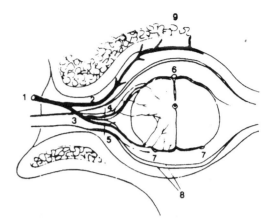

Figure 2–5 The ligaments of the spinal column. *1*, Anterior longitudinal ligament; *2*, posterior longitudinal ligament; *3*, ligamentum flavum; *4*, capsule of the zygapophyseal joint; *5*, interspinous ligament; *6*, supraspinous ligament.

Figure 2–6 Arterial vascularization of the spinal canal. *1*, Arteria radicularis; *2*, arterial branch to the vertebral body; *3*, arterial branch to the spinal nerve and the roots; *4*, arterial branch to the ventral root; *5*, arterial branch to the dorsal root; *6*, ventral spinal artery; *7*, dorsal spinal artery; *8*, arachnoid and dura mater; *9*, vertebral body.

Innervation

With the exception of the ligamentum flavum, all ligaments are nociceptively innervated. Nociceptive free nerve endings are the most abundant in the posterior longitudinal ligament. The innervation is multisegmental, with recurrent branches of the recurrent nerve (meningeal nerve) running within the spinal canal several segments cranially or caudally. (See Chapter 8.) This situation can account for the fact that pain is very often perceived in a diffuse manner.

Lesions of the ligaments occur mostly as a result of trauma. In systemic diseases such as rheumatoid arthritis or ankylosing spondylitis, softening of the ligamentous complex can develop. This is of major significance in the upper cervical region. In such cases mobilization, particularly manipulation, can have disastrous consequences.

In general, the dorsal structures, including the posterior longitudinal ligament, are considered restrictive to the flexion motion. The

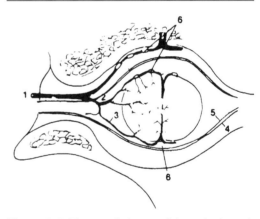

Figure 2–7 Venous drainage of the spinal canal. *1*, Intervertebral vein; *2*, ventral radicular vein; *3*, dorsal radicular vein; *4*, dura mater; *5*, arachnoid; *6*, internal and external vertebral venous system.

anterior longitudinal ligament restricts extension. Sidebending is limited by the contralateral ligamentous structures. As mentioned previously, the coupled movements are guided in particular patterns due to the form and position of the zygapophyseal joints. At the end of their trajectory these movements are mainly limited by the ligaments from the motion segment concerned. Thus, ligamentous lesions can manifest themselves by pain at the end of the range of motion of the coupled movements. Limitation of motion occurs only in patients with severe pain.

VASCULARIZATION

The spinal canal is vascularized from the spinal branches of the vertebral, deep cervical, intercostal, and lumbar arteries. Ventral and dorsal spinal branches anastomose in long longitudinal vessels. From the spinal branches of the anastomosing structures, radicular arteries arise that are responsible for the vascularization of the segment's most important structures (Figure 2–6). The anastomosing pattern varies considerably; however, the arteria radicularis magna is consistently present and is responsible for the vascularization of the contents in the caudal two thirds of the spinal canal. Compression of these large radicular arteries can give rise to pathology of the spinal cord.

The radicular veins drain into anastomosing networks with several large longitudinal vessels (Figure 2–7). Through intervertebral veins, the blood leaves the spinal canal.

2.2 EXAMINATION

INTRODUCTION

In 1978 Macnab and McCulloch[22] stated that many concepts concerning the pathogenesis of low back pain were still largely based on hypotheses. Now, many years later, the situation has hardly changed. For instance, a patient with an acute rupture of a lumbar intervertebral disc shows an obvious spasm of the sacrospinal musculature along with a decreased lumbar lordosis. However, the sacrospinal muscles are extensors of the lumbar spine. How can a decreased lumbar lordosis exist when there is a spasm of the sacrospinal muscles? Obviously the discussion concerning this matter is not yet closed.

Another point of discussion concerns specific changes observed on radiological examination, such as disc narrowing, osteophytes, spondylarthrosis, and so on. Unfortunately, too often these radiological changes alone are used in making the "diagnosis."

By far, most symptoms that develop from the lumbar spine occur in persons between 35 and 55 years of age. In this age span, the above-mentioned radiological "aberrations" almost always exist. On one hand, the incidence of complaints related to the lumbar spine decreases significantly with aging (from approximately the 45th year on); on the other hand, the radiological changes increase at that time. What is the significance of these radiological changes? For the time being, this specific question will not be answered.

A diagnosis should always be made by means of a thorough history and functional examination. Radiological examination and other imaging techniques (such as magnetic resonance imaging [MRI]), as well as other forms of technical examination (laboratory testing, electromyography [EMG], arthroscopy, and others) change or supplement the diagnosis in only about 10% of all cases. Thus, the functional clinical examination, at least for now, is the most important diagnostic measure.

The fact that many health caregivers are inadequately educated in the diagnostics of the musculoskeletal system is a significant problem. Presently, caregiver initiative is required in order to become acquainted with the necessary evaluation techniques.

OVERVIEW

In assessing the spine, the examination should be directed to the affected region. Of course, a general orientation takes place first.

The examination consists of the following:

- general inspection
- history
- specific inspection
- palpation prior to the functional examination
- functional examination
- if possible, palpation after the functional examination
- if necessary, additional tests

In the general inspection the entire spine is observed. Note how the patient enters the room, sits down, shakes hands, etc.

The significance of a thorough history of complaints of the spine is of utmost importance—in many cases, even more important than in complaints of the peripheral joints. From the history, one can already form an idea about a likely diagnosis.

During the specific inspection, the static posture is always observed.

The first palpation is directed mainly at any apparent swelling. The temperature of the skin can also be judged by palpation.

The most substantial support for the suspected diagnosis (as a result of the history) takes place within the framework of the functional examination. After the functional examination, if the working diagnosis has been confirmed, palpation follows, that is, if the affected structure is accessible to palpation. At this point a treatment plan is instituted.

In cases of doubt, or when the results of the treatment are disappointing, an additional examination is performed. This may consist of a segmental functional examination or an additional neurological examination. The help of other specialists is sought in every case where severe pathology is suspected. Other additional examinations consist mostly of imaging diagnostics: particularly computed tomography (CT) scanning or MRI and, in some cases, EMG or laboratory tests.

With the diagnosis an idea about the cause of the complaints emerges, so that a causal therapy can be instituted. Of course, it is of-

ten necessary first to treat the acute symptoms. If possible, the long-term treatment is directed at eliminating the cause as well as to preventing recurrence.

Exclusively treating the site of local pain almost never leads to a positive result in disorders of the spine (Figure 2–8) and often has disastrous consequences for the patient.

ASPECTS OF THE CLINICAL EXAMINATION

General Inspection

The clinical examination begins with a general inspection. The examiner observes the patient, especially the manner in which the patient enters the examination room, sits down and—after the history—stands up again. In some cases one can also obtain information from the way the patient gets undressed. Unfortunately, often the patient is first seen by the examiner when he or she is already sitting undressed in an examination room. Thus, a great deal of important information is lost.

History

Why the patient seeks your consultation is determined during the introduction phase. This introduction phase precedes the systematized history. The examiner tries to gain insight into the patient's main complaint. In this phase, the examiner also tries to get an impression about motives and goals of the patient in seeking medical assistance.[23]

Goal

During the history, the examiner gathers facts that could lead to the diagnosis. The examiner also looks for the nature and possible causes of the complaints.

In complaints of the spine, the history is one of the most important parts of the diagnostic process. At the same time, it is the most difficult part of the clinical examination because one has to know not only which ques-

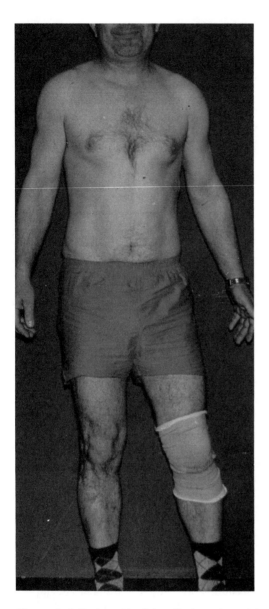

Figure 2–8 Patient who felt radicular pain mainly in the left knee. He was "treated" with a knee bandage. **Source:** Courtesy of Dr. Peter Hirschfeld and Liz Longton, Bremen, Germany.

a skill that one can learn, too, but something else also plays an important role—experience. Experience is not learned from a textbook; it is obtained after years of seeing patients.

Content

In the history, attention is given to the following:

- personal data
- history, nature, and location of the complaints
- factors that influence the complaints
- family history

Information regarding the following topics should be noted in the patient history:

- age
- occupation, hobby (sport)
- chief complaints
- onset
- duration
- location of complaints
- factors that influence the symptoms
- medication
- patient's reaction to symptoms

Depending on experience, one's system of questions can vary slightly from those listed above. If the entire clinical examination does not lead to a clear diagnosis, one can delve into specific aspects of the history in order to obtain a specific working diagnosis.

Age

Many disorders of the musculoskeletal system are, more or less, age related. This factor should play a relatively important, but not absolute, role in the history: the typical ages mentioned in this book for the various disorders are general indications. The individual patient is all too often an exception to these carefully set rules.

Occupation, Hobby (Sport)

Based on ergonomic research, some professions can place an enormous load on the

tions to ask but, more importantly, how to interpret the patient's answers correctly.

Performing the functional examination is a technical skill that generally can be acquired in a very short period of time. Of course, taking the history and interpreting the answers is

low back. The nature of the load often depends on the working posture and on the working environment: squatting versus stooping over, use of chairs with wheels versus those without wheels, use of an adjustable reading surface versus a flat desk, adjustable table height, etc. (See Chapter 12.)

An important peculiarity of hobbies and sports is that many people exert themselves in an unusually intense manner after a long period of rest. In these instances, with inadequate preparation, disorders of the musculoskeletal system can occur easily.

Chief Complaints

Does the patient complain primarily of pain, paresthesia, numbness, loss of strength, the inability to perform activities, or vertigo with or without tinnitus?

In complaints of pain, it is important to obtain information about the nature of the pain: possible radiation, day and night cycle, and so forth. To a large degree, the answer to the question "What are the complaints?" should determine the remainder of the history as well as the choice of treatment plan.

Unfortunately, all too often a certain "aberration" is found (such as a limitation of motion) and the entire treatment is then directed to that problem. In itself, this can be an effective way to treat the patient's symptoms; however, the goal still has to focus on the complaint itself. For instance, if the patient complains of pain and a limitation of motion is found, then the treatment of the limitation of motion should never be the definitive goal of the therapy; instead, the relief of pain is the goal.

Onset

In disorders of the musculoskeletal system, the complaints are often related to certain postures or positions and movements.

It is important to distinguish whether the onset was sudden or gradual. Sustained traumas and fractures are significant in terms of subsequent changes in the "loadability" of the affected structures.

Besides the local aspect, the examiner also should consider possible influences from other regions. Endogenous factors that can lead to an irritation of the local structure and/or maintain this irritation include stress, systemic diseases, or internal pathology such as metabolic disturbances. Exogenous factors, such as (micro)traumas and specific working conditions, should be taken into account as well. From the psychological literature, it is known that the personal life history plays an important role in the development of complaints in certain regions. (See Chapter 17.)

Duration

In general, the chance for immediate therapeutic success is great if the symptoms are of short duration. If this entails symptoms that normally lead to a spontaneous recovery, then the duration of the complaints can be used in making the prognosis.

In the case of chronic complaints that are related to posture and movement, it is often difficult to change the patient's movement patterns in such a way that the symptoms will not recur. Unfortunately, these patterns often involve very strong habits in the patient's behavior. Seeing the patient on a regular basis over a long period seems to be the best way to achieve the desired behavioral change. (See Chapter 16.)

Localization of Symptoms

Paresthesia always indicates pathology of a neurological structure. The localization of the paresthesia gives information about the approximate localization of the lesion. Pressure on the nerve root can cause paresthesia, which is generally experienced far distally. In this instance, there is usually a very clear segmental distribution but without a sharp border. (See Chapter 8.) The further distal in the body these neurological structures are irritated, the more distinct is the localization of the paresthesia (Figure 2–9).

Following are some basic rules that are used in relation to the localization of pain.

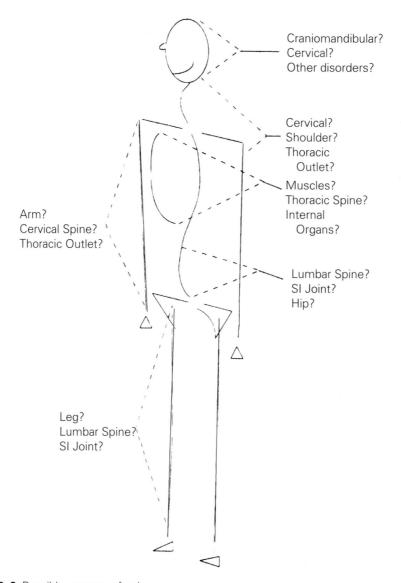

Figure 2–9 Possible sources of pain.

Keep in mind that these rules are general and not absolute.

Pain in the Extremities.

- The more distal the pain is localized in an extremity, the greater the chance that the location of the lesion corresponds to the localization of the pain.
- The more proximal the pain is localized in the extremity, the greater the chance

that the location of the lesion does not correspond to the localization of the pain.

Pain in the Lower Extremity.

- If the pain is localized solely in the lower extremity, pathology of the lower extremity is generally considered; the appropriate functional examination is thus performed.

- If pain in the lower extremity is associated with pain in the low back, a problem in the lumbar spine is suspected. However, the diagnosis can be established only after performing the functional examination of the lumbar spine. In more rare cases it may involve pathology of the SI joint.

Pain in the Low Back.

- Pain in the low back is generally caused by problems in the sacroiliac joint(s), the hip(s), and/or the lumbar spine. The history and the functional examinations are decisive for the diagnosis.
- If the sacroiliac provocation tests are positive, the diagnosis can be established (with a high probability) as a sacroiliac joint problem.
- If the passive functional examination of the hip is positive, one should first consider hip pathology and perform the entire hip functional examination. One then suspects a lesion of the lumbar spine if the hip examination is negative.

Differentiating Lumbar Spine Problems.

- If there is radicular pain (pain that radiates in a segmental distribution), one first suspects primary or secondary discogenic lesions. (See section 2.3.)
- If there is referred pain (pain that does not have an obvious segmental radiation into the leg, the paravertebral region of the thorax, or the upper arm), and if the pain is felt deep in the spine and cannot be clearly localized by the patient, one should consider a zygapophyseal joint problem.
- If the pain is not dependent on posture or movement, and there is also percussion pain and/or pain when falling back on the heels from a tiptoe position, one should suspect severe pathology, such as inflammations or tumors.

Pain in the Thorax.

- In instances of local pain in the thorax, which is mainly related to positions and/or movement of the arm, one should consider problems of the pectoralis major, pectoralis minor, or latissimus dorsi.
- If intercostal pain increases with movement and there is tenderness to palpation, one first thinks of a lesion of the ribs, the connections between the rib and the vertebra(e), or the intercostal musculature.
- If thoracic pain exists that is not clearly postural or movement related, and there is no percussion pain and/or pain when falling onto the heels from a tiptoe position, one should suspect pathology of the internal organs.

Pain in the Neck-Shoulder Region.

- If the pain is particularly influenced by neck movements, one should consider problems of the cervical spine.
- If the pain is mainly dependent on arm movements, one should consider shoulder problems.
- The Roos test is pathognomonic for thoracic outlet syndrome.

Pain in the Region of the Head.

- If pain in the head region is particularly influenced by neck movements, one should consider problems of the cervical spine.
- If pain in the head region is mainly dependent on movements of the temporomandibular joint, one first thinks of a craniomandibular dysfunction.
- In all other cases, examinations other than orthopaedic examinations are indicated.

Factors That Influence Symptoms

Very important diagnostic information can be gained from the fact that the symptoms are dependent on particular positions and movements. In instances of constant pain, infections or tumors should be suspected—the latter especially if the pain is experienced only at night.

If thoracic pain is related to exertion, but not to certain positions or movements, a cardiac consultation is indicated.

Medication

Continuous use of anticoagulants is a contraindication for manipulation.

The use of medications gives an indication as to the general progression in the treatment of the complaint. Earlier medications and their results are noted. If the medications did not offer satisfactory results, then one should question the reason.

Attention is also given to previous advice that the patient has received as well as to the types of assistive devices that the patient uses. Empiricism shows that patients generally do not use their assistive devices reliably. Above all, if there is not regular contact between patient and therapist or physician, the patient's faith in therapy is very low. (See Chapter 16.)

Patient's Reaction to Symptoms

The patient's reaction to symptoms gives a clear indication of how the patient copes with the complaints in daily living. Symptoms that severely affect the patient's daily activities demand fast and adequate treatment.

The way in which the patient deals with the complaints—continues versus stops working, goes on bed rest versus remains active, etc.—can also indicate whether or not to involve a psychotherapist in the treatment. This applies not only to situations in which the patient's specific life history explains the occurrence of the complaints, but also to situations whereby the symptoms severely disrupt the patient's daily life. It cannot be emphasized enough that the whole existence of the one who "was always healthy" can be completely disrupted by a sudden physical problem.

The medical history is concluded with the family history.

Conclusions Related to History

After concluding the history, the examiner now knows why the patient sought help. In-sight has been given into some etiological factors, and into the character, the localization, and the course of the complaints. This information leads to a decision as to the nature and the progression of additional examinations as well as to the choice of a treatment plan.

Specific Inspection

The specific inspection is directed at the posture, whereby the following points are noted:

- the position of the feet and both legs
- the position of the pelvis
- the position of the lumbar and thoracic spines
- the position of the cervical spine and the head
- the position of the shoulder girdle
- obvious changes in the skin, muscles, and joints

Trophic disturbances are significant in relation to influences of the sympathetic nervous system.[24]

Inspection during Motion

Special attention is given to the symptom provoking and/or inhibiting activities.

Palpation before Functional Examination

Palpation before the functional examination of the spine is performed only if swelling and/or local warmth is noted. However, this is observed much less frequently in lesions of the spine than in lesions of the peripheral joints.

Swelling can be expected after a trauma (with a resultant local hematoma), or in the rare instance of a tumor or inflammation. With the exception of superficial tumors such as skin and subcutaneous tumors (e.g., lipoma), tumors are seldom visible.

Local warmth may be present in the case of a superficial inflammatory process or in a more deeply located severe inflammation.

Palpating to localize the patient's pain, before performing the functional examination, is useless because almost all patients experience "misleading" (referred or radicular) pain. Thus, patients with lumbar pain almost always indicate pain in the region of the posterior superior iliac spine and, in instances of radiating pain, deep in the gluteus maximus region. In lesions of the cervical spine the pain is usually localized in the trapezius region and at the level of the scapula. These are also examples of referred pain. Because of the phenomenon of referred pain, if treatment subsequently is directed to these trigger points, not much success can be expected.

Functional Examination

After the general inspection, the history, the specific inspection, and possible palpation, the structures of the affected spinal region are examined. This takes place by means of an active and a passive examination of motion, resistance tests, and, if necessary, joint-specific translatory tests. Additional imaging examinations can also be performed.

General Examination of Motion

The general examination of motion consists mainly of the following:

- active movements
- passive movements
- tests against resistance

Local Examination of Motion

The local examination of motion consists mainly of the following:

- translatory tests in a traction direction
- translatory tests in a gliding direction
- examination of local coupled passive movements
- compression (especially when fractures or osteolytic processes are suspected)

Palpation

Palpation of the affected structure takes place after the functional examination and only if the structure is accessible to palpation.

Korr[25] gives an extensive description of the specific tissue changes that are based on increased orthosympathetic activity. Under certain circumstances (a selectivity or nonselectivity of the nervous system[26]), continuous nocisensoric activity can cause specific tissue changes in trophic-sensitive structures such as connective tissue. Oostendorp[24] describes the importance of palpation in order to determine these specific tissue changes.

Additional Examinations

An additional examination may consist of the following:

- additional specific functional examination (such as neurological)
- special technical procedures such as EMG, imaging techniques, and/or laboratory tests

Conclusions Regarding Examination

After performing the clinical examination, the examiner reaches a summarized conclusion in which a direct relationship can be determined between the complaints of the patient and the findings of the examination. If this is the case, a clear (although temporary) diagnosis can be made. This diagnosis is considered "confirmed" if the chosen treatment plan offers the expected results.

If no clear conclusion can be drawn after the examination, or if the results of the treatment are disappointing, one can still decide to perform further testing. If this additional examination does not offer any obvious results, treatment should not be initiated.

With the initiation of therapy, as well as in cases in which it is not possible to formulate a treatment plan, frequent consultation between the various caregivers is necessary. The family physician is often better acquainted than the therapist with the life story, the social circumstances, and the medical data of the patient. Depending on the nature of the pathology, cooperation with other specialists may be indicated. Because of the fact that the disorders described in this book almost always have multiple causes, such cooperation quite often contributes to the effectiveness of the therapeutic management. In this way, the role of the psychotherapist can also be of great importance. (See Chapter 17.)

Once the treatment has been determined, it is discussed with the patient. The patient should receive a thorough explanation of the findings and the treatment possibilities. The numbers of treatments and the appointments for follow-up (and reassessment) are decided. In this stage, the patient's further wishes are incorporated into the final treatment plan. If appropriate, advice regarding proper posture and body mechanics is also given.

2.3 PATHOLOGY

INTRODUCTION

In this book, the most common disorders of the sacroiliac joint, the spine, and the craniomandibular joint are discussed. Pathologies of both the sacroiliac and the craniomandibular joints present, as a matter of speaking, a case apart. Thus, the specific disorders related to these joints are described in the corresponding chapters. Some general thoughts concerning the pathology of the lumbar, thoracic, and cervical spines are appropriate in this introductory chapter, however.

As a result of recent improvements in imaging diagnostics (CT scan and MRI), it has been confirmed that a large number of spinal disorders are related to disc pathology. In the authors' opinion, this has brought about a number of consequences that have been given insufficient attention.

First, a reclassification of the established classifications of spine pathology has to occur—of course, bearing in mind the earlier warning. For instance, a disorder such as acute low back pain (lumbago), earlier considered to be a muscle spasm or a nerve inflammation, is now more likely involvement of the disc. Thus, "acute low back pain" as a *symptom* remains; however, thoughts concerning the *etiology* have changed.

Second, a reorientation is currently taking place in the literature concerning the ques-

tion of whether or not changes in the disc are pathological. In the process of aging, it is certainly normal (and therefore physiological) that ultimately the nucleus pulposus (almost) completely disappears. This is called a physiological "discosis." This physiological discosis occurs at a slow rate. The rate is so slow that within the motion segment, a physiological process of adaptation is able to take place that prevents the occurrence of symptoms. Thus, the "radiological" presence of disc narrowing, osteophytosis, and spondylarthrosis does not have to be an indication for pathology at all.

However, it is a different matter when these processes occur too quickly. Every process that occurs too quickly in one aspect of the motion segment results in too little time for the other aspects of the involved segment to adapt; thus symptoms may arise. Root compression is a classic example of this phenomenon (see Appendix A, Algorithms for Diagnosis and Treatment)..

After the age of approximately 45 years, the physiological discosis has progressed to such a degree, accompanied by sufficient (physiological) adaptation, that the further occurrence of pathology becomes less likely. Therefore, beyond this age, although disorders occur much less often, the radiological appearances make a larger pathological impression.

A large number of spinal disorders have a (micro)traumatic origin: a moment in which a sudden high load leads to a "marching out of step" of one aspect of the motion segment. Because of the sudden moment, there is no time for physiological adaptations; thus, symptoms occur.

Therefore, it becomes understandable that *acute* complaints very often "heal" by themselves, although this recovery can be enhanced by therapy. (See Chapters 14 to 16.) However, this does not mean that traces of this acute lesion do not remain in the affected part of the spine. On the contrary, there is a high probability that a "weak area" develops; now a smaller amount of overload than before will lead to a recurrence of the lesion.

One can also have *chronic* symptoms consisting of recurrent episodes, in which each episode has an acute onset. Differentiating between *acute* and *chronic* symptoms can be ascertained by a thorough history. In chronic pain, the problem lies more in the "loadability" of the segment. Perhaps this explains the finding that acute symptoms, especially those of the low back, are best treated with compression-decreasing measures, while the treatment of chronic complaints must include measures aimed at increasing the loadability. (See Chapter 16.)

Nevertheless, even in the above discussion of the literature, there are still (particularly in relation to the lumbar spine) a lot of uncertainties. For instance, the precise parts of the intervertebral discs, the capsules of the zygapophyseal joints, and the ligaments responsible for the development of pain are still unclear.

This continued uncertainty explains the fact that there are still "schools" for manual therapy. The chiropractor has treatment principles based on foundations different from those of the osteopath, who often has other foundations different from those of the physical therapist. One claims to be treating the facet joints, the other the disc. However, one must ask the question: Is it possible to treat the disc solely, without moving the facet joints as well, and vice versa?

Based on convincing theoretical grounds, a treatment that moves a part of the motion segment results in movement in the whole segment. (See Chapter 13.) Butler et al[5] published a study that clearly demonstrated that discs degenerate before the zygapophyseal joints. When the disc is primarily affected, all other structures belonging to the same motion segment consequently will be affected. In the same way, when one directs the treatment primarily to the zygapophyseal joints, the treatment will also have an effect on all the other structures of the motion segment.

CLASSIFICATIONS OF DISORDERS

The above-mentioned discussion leads to a classification of disorders of the lumbar, thoracic, and cervical spine. Of course, attempts to make such a classification will result in some discrepancies, but it is a practical classification that remains very close to the recent developments in medical literature.

The fact that this book deals primarily with orthopaedic medicine influences this classification system. The incidence of each disorder is not a main criterion for classification. Thus, some of the often-occurring disorders (such as rheumatoid arthritis), in which orthopaedic medicine cannot be of significant help, play a subordinate role in this book. On the other hand, disorders with a low incidence (such as Tietze's syndrome), in which orthopaedic medicine can play a pre-eminent role, are discussed extensively.

Primary Discogenic Disorders

In primary discogenic disorders, the disc protrusion and the disc prolapse are of particular importance. Since they involve the consequences of overload, the primary discogenic disorders are closely related to several postural syndromes.

The symptomatology occurs mainly through root compression.*Treatment consists primarily of decompression ("taking the load off"). Concise information must be given to the patient regarding the nature of the disorder, and advice must be given regarding

*In cerv. & lumbar.

See Addendum p. 20-22 { In thoracic, large post. hern. may compress cord, others - irritate dura, oft c vague non-radicular sx. Also Discitic or disc fissure → pains.

correct posture and body mechanics. After healing, the subsequent weak area carries an implication that the next episode could occur with a relatively low load.

Secondary Discogenic Disorders

Secondary discogenic disorders occur as a result of degenerative changes due to a prior disc lesion. As already noted by Verbiest[27] in 1955, the relation between the structures in the spinal canal and the lateral recess, along with the available space, is of utmost importance in the development of symptoms.

For instance, patients with a small spinal canal can experience more symptoms from a small (primary) disc protrusion than other patients with a large disc prolapse in a large spinal canal. The same applies to the secondary discogenic disorders. Large "arthrotic" changes that will narrow the spinal canal give rise to symptoms only when the spinal canal is already small by nature (congenital).

Traumatic Disorders

Strictly speaking, *traumatic disorder* is too broad a term for its category, because the primary as well as the secondary discogenic disorders can be interpreted as being traumatic. In this book, "traumatic disorders" are discussed after the discogenic disorders and include only the non–discogenic traumatic disorders.

Fractures occur fairly frequently as a result of sports injuries and accidents, especially in the cervical and lower thoracic spines. However, keep in mind that the fracture and/or subluxation within the spinal column will almost always occur in conjunction with a disc lesion. This classification includes not only disorders in which the patient recalls a traumatic onset, but also includes the so-called "spontaneous" fractures. Such fractures (especially in osteoporosis) are similar to the secondary discogenic disorders in regard to their etiology: they are disorders that develop as a result of an overload in an already degenerated part of the musculoskeletal system.

Finally, a number of disorders are known to occur traumatically, even without the patient's being able to recall a trauma. These disorders are also classified under the category "traumatic."

Form Aberrations

During a certain period in the 19th century, a significant amount of spinal column pathology was thought to be based on "posture." One assumed to know the ideal posture, which was particularly based on esthetics. Scolioses and kyphoses were halted through "mechanical violence," and the ideal "posture" formed an important aspect of one's upbringing.

Today we think more in dynamic terms: form aberrations of the spine have an "evolutionary" process-like character rather than a static character. Therefore, the "classic" forms of aberrations—kyphosis, lordosis, scoliosis—are discussed together with chronic disorders that concern the morphology of the entire spine, such as ankylosing spondylitis.

Other Disorders

The discrepancies in this classification system—or in any other system of classification—are shown by the presence of a category termed other disorders. This classification does not mean that these disorders are of less importance or have a lesser incidence. Again, the criteria are based on the fact that this is a manual of orthopaedic medicine, and in this context less attention is given to the various tumors of the spinal column. However, it must be emphasized that complaints caused by tumors almost always appear at first to be an apparently benign syndrome of the spinal column. In these cases, the history is of utmost importance. Often the complaints are not specifically position or movement dependent. Therefore, additional imaging examinations (CT scan, MRI) and laboratory examinations are necessary.

2.4 TREATMENT

INTRODUCTION

There are trends within manual therapy in which the entire spinal column is always examined and treated (segmentally) regardless of localization of the complaints. Frequently, there are disadvantages to this approach. For example, patients treated elsewhere seek help for cervical spine complaints that occurred after a mobilization "treatment" of the cervical spine, even though the patient initially sought medical help concerning complaints of the lumbar spine.

Manual therapy (mobilization or manipulation of the spinal column) should never be the sole therapeutic measure. The patient for whom manual therapy is indicated should be informed extensively about the disorder before the first treatment is even applied. Afterward, exercises are given with the goal of maintaining the mobility achieved through the mobilization. This applies not only to the spinal column, but to the peripheral joints as well. When treatment consists of only mobilization or manipulation, there is a significant chance that the problem will recur.

Although this is not a book for manual therapy, a number of mobilization techniques are described and depicted. Of these techniques, the so-called general mobilization techniques have been the most extensively researched. They are mobilization techniques with an axial separation component.

Historically, local (segmental) manual therapy techniques have not been thoroughly researched. These techniques are applied only when

- manual therapy is indicated and the general techniques do not provide any improvement, or
- when the complaints are constantly recurring *and the complaints are not primary disc-related*. (Discogenic lesions should be treated only with axial separation techniques.)

Primarily, treatment should be aimed at alleviating the pain, not the hypomobility. In other words, small limitations of motions that are not painful do not usually have clinical relevance. Humans are not symmetrical. In examining mobility of the spine, almost everyone will have one side in which the movement is greater and more elastic than the other side. Furthermore, everyone has a slight degree of torsion in the spinal column (scoliosis). If a vertebra has a (physiological) rotated position, rotation in that direction will be greater than that in the opposite direction.

THE MULTIDIMENSIONAL APPROACH

Medical literature indicates that in chronic disorders, it is necessary to apply a multidimensional approach from the onset of the treatment.[28-31] Trott[32] states: "The cause of the symptoms is multifactorial and therefore requires treatment directed at each facet of the problem." (See Chapter 17 for more detailed information.) However, acute problems often can be considered in terms of monofactorial etiology.

In recent years it has become clear that there are differences between acute and chronic pain in relation to etiology, mechanism, function, diagnostics, and treatment.[33] Chronic persistent pain does not have any biological function; instead it is a debilitating process that often exerts severe emotional, physical, economical, and social stress on the patient, family, and society. Adequate pain management is essential. The examiner must possess knowledge about the most current pain theories and must be willing to invest his or her time and knowledge in discovering the causes of pain through the patient's history and functional examination.[33,34]

In 1980, Post stated: "The modern human being sees pain exclusively as something that has to be fought against. This person is so involved with the fight against the pain, that he barely thinks about the meaning of the pain."[35]

Adequate pain treatment does not necessarily require the mastering, and application, of highly sophisticated techniques (Figure 2–10). Primarily, one must be able to deal with the patient in pain in an appropriate way.[36] The history is chiefly focused on the musculoskeletal system. However, considering the points just mentioned, the visceral[28] and the social aspects of the patient's life should be examined as well.[30,37]

In regard to the multifactorial etiology, the (family) physician, dentist (in craniomandibular dysfunctions), and physical therapist are part of the treatment team. In some cases, a psychologist also belongs to the team. The physician pays particular attention to the visceral and psychological dimensions, and the physical therapist focuses particularly on the somatogenic trail. Each discipline has to take into account the etiological factors. If the pain is influenced by movement, even in the form of a vicious cycle, the prescription of physical therapy is worthwhile.

Within this framework, physical therapy consists of two kinds of measures, which complement each other. First, direct pain-relieving measures are performed. Next, the therapeutic exercise treatment program begins. At the same time, the tissue-specific changes must also be treated.[24]

The amount of selectivity within the nervous system determines the choice of trigger. Bernards[26] indicates that doubt, fear, and uncertainty of the patient are factors that influence the healing process in a negative way. The therapist can address these factors through explanation, reassurance, and encouragement.

Treatment by the physical therapist is mostly directed at relaxation, mobilization, pain relief, and influencing pain tolerance and the patient's physical condition. By relieving the pain and dealing with specific tissue changes, better conditions are created for ex-

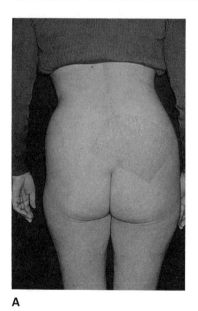 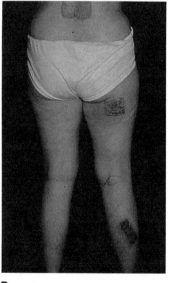

A   **B**

Figure 2–10 **A** and **B**, Two patients with diagnosed lumbar disc protrusions and radiating pain into the leg. They were "treated" with electrotherapy. The consequences of this therapy are clearly visible. Causal therapy in combination with mobilization and/or traction would have been indicated. *Source:* Courtesy of Dr. Peter Hirschffeld and Liz Longton, Bremen, Germany.

ercise therapy. Trying to influence pain behavior by improving the patient's physical condition is a very important goal. The therapy has to carry a clear preventive character as well.

Fricton et al.[34] support the interdisciplinary approach and indicate that: "A well-defined evaluation and management system that is outpatient, while focusing on a self-care approach, is a typically more efficient, less costly, and highly viable and recommended approach to patient management."

Bonica[33] states that over the years no obvious improvement in the treatment of the patient has occurred, due to the following:

- a shortage of knowledge, or inadequate use of the available knowledge, due to a lack of organization
- a progressive trend for specialization
- the impossibility or unwillingness of the therapist to make the necessary time available for the patient

In order to describe the contribution of the physical therapist in more detail, the various goals of the physical therapy treatment plan are briefly described in the following section.

Relaxation

Relaxation techniques generally fall into one of two basic categories: Jacobson's "progressive relaxation"[38] and the "autogenic training" of Schultz.[39] One significant difference between the two techniques is that the former achieves relaxation through exercising the separate muscle groups, while the latter achieves a more general relaxation by means of suggestion. The relaxation exercises of Mitchell[40] and Jacobson may actually be preferable.

Mitchell[40] developed the "simple relaxation" technique, which is based on the principle of reciprocal innervation. Although it is the result, the exercises do not emphasize relaxation. The techniques are directed at the muscles, teaching the patient the difference between tension and relaxation.

Because of a lack of comparative research, the best approach has not yet been proven. However, in sports in which relaxation techniques are often used, it appears that it makes little or no difference what techniques are applied.[41]

Instruction in home relaxation exercises is important, and the following suggestions should be taken into account:

- Exercise areas that do not cause any problems during the treatment sessions.
- In order to prevent "demotivation" it is important to emphasize to the patient that in the beginning the effect of the exercise (relaxation) is often not very well achieved.
- Be specific about duration and frequency of the exercises.
- If the patient has difficulty performing the exercises at home, an instructional tape can be very helpful.

Other frequently used forms of therapy in which relaxation can be achieved include biofeedback, breathing exercises, and massage.

Massage

Massage therapy has many indications. Its influence is especially noted in the following areas:

- general tension (relaxation)
- local muscle tension (increasing tone or inhibiting tone)
- local metabolism and circulation (arterial, venous, and lymphatic)[42]

Pain is usually accompanied by muscle spasms and protective muscle hypertonicity. This increased tone leads to progressive joint dysfunction, which then leads to more pain. Muscle spasms and hypertonicity have the tendency to decrease the flow of circulation to the muscles and to inhibit the removal of metabolites, resulting in increased pain.

Stress pushes the body into an alarm situation, with a nonspecific increase in the activity of several mechanisms of the nervous system. As a result, the ergotropic mechanisms, which are stimulated during such an alarm phase, remain constantly active. The entire body no longer goes back into a state of rest. Instead, it remains ergotropically tuned. Because of this, the trophic situation of several tissue structures worsens.[26]

Warmth and massage can be an effective treatment for the circulatory status and accumulation of metabolites, as well as for muscle hypertonicity. Application of heat causes a local hyperemia, vasodilatation, and increased metabolism.

Indications for heat and massage in the head and neck region include general and local problems such as the following:

- manifestations of stress in the form of stiffness
- local muscle symptoms, such as fatigue
- pain as a result of prolonged or too forceful muscle tension
- local "knots" in the muscle tissue, fasciae, septa, etc.
- cramps
- adhesions in muscle or muscle fibers
- traumatic swelling

Special forms of massage therapy include connective tissue massage and lymph drainage. Connective tissue massage can be chosen as a form of treatment in disorders with a clear vegetative component, in which reflex zones are found within the subcutaneous connective tissue. The goal of this form of therapy is to restore the vegetative balance, especially the balance between trophotropic and ergotropic situations.[43] Focus is initially placed on the tissue-specific changes within the subcutaneous connective tissue.[44]

At first this massage is applied daily for 3 to 4 days; after 2 days of rest, it is then continued two or three times weekly until the specific changes in the subcutaneous tissue have disappeared. According to the symptoms and findings from the examination, the intensity of the treatment as well as the frequency can be adjusted.

Lymph drainage is a form of treatment directed at activating the lymph vessels and enhancing the transport capacity within the lymph vessels and lymph nodules. Indications for therapeutic lymph drainage include the following:

- post-traumatic swelling
- edema due to an obstruction of lymph vessels and/or nodules after cancer surgery
- acute aseptic inflammatory processes (for instance, rheumatoid arthritis)

The massage is always performed in the direction of the flow: this means the outlet of the right lymphatic duct into the right angulus venosus and the outlet of the thoracic duct into the left angulus venosus. Because of the mild, large surface covering and the repetitive maneuver by the hands, this treatment is both relaxing and pain inhibiting.[44]

Mobilization

Mobilization is never the sole treatment strategy. In order to prevent recurrence, it must be supported by exercise therapy directed at muscular balance, posture (and movement), coordination, improvement of proprioception, and the static and dynamic muscle stability.[45]

Mobilization may take place via neuromuscular techniques through use of the following:

- direct muscle force
- post-isometric relaxation
- reciprocal innervation

The technique whereby the therapist uses direct muscle force is often given in the form of self-mobilization as a home exercise for the patient. The post-isometric relaxation technique is also indicated as a home program for the patient. An extensive practical manual is described by Evjenth and Hamberg.[46] The reciprocal innervation techniques consist of a passive mobilization after isometric contraction in the direction of the limited motion.

In order to restore function other techniques are also available, such as the following:

- passive translatory movements (traction, gliding)
- passive angular movements
- combination of both mobilization forms
- soft tissue techniques
- regional mobilization, performed actively and/or passively

Mobilization techniques with an impulse (manipulations) consist of a fast, precise movement that passes the pathological, but not the anatomical, movement range. In this way, one tries to resolve the limitation of motion in one movement impulse. Controlled research,[47] mostly in regard to the spinal column, indicates that there is a tendency for faster improvement in the manipulation group in comparison to other forms of physical therapy.

In treatment, including mobilization, the choice of technique and how it is performed depends entirely on the goal that has to be reached. For instance, in the case of a joint dysfunction, restoring the normal function is the primary goal. It is achieved through a normalization of the translatory motions (in other words, of the play in the joint). In this way, the normal roll-gliding is restored. After that, the reflexively related changes can be influenced through soft tissue mobilization, electrotherapy, or vibration. These skin and muscle changes can also be treated before the joint mobilization and before initiating a further exercise treatment plan. Normal muscle function is restored not only by restoring the muscle balance (muscle length, force, and coordination), but also by improving posture and movement patterns.

Immobilization

Unfortunately, plaster immobilization is still frequently applied. Because of the severe atrophy and loss of tension of the back and abdominal muscles, the decalcification of bone, and the cartilaginous damage to the zygapophyseal joints, immobilization by plaster should be obsolete.

Concerning the application of corsets, the opinions are strongly divided. This is a form of partial immobilization which does not have the disadvantages of plaster immobilization. Because this form of treatment is not applied by the authors it is not discussed further.

Another form of partial immobilization is taping. For various disorders of the back in which flexion has to be avoided for a short duration, one can apply strips of "reminder" tapes on the back. This is a very useful method for patients who have difficulty maintaining the appropriate posture. In several disorders of the cervical spine, a firm collar can be useful. This gives stability because the movements are kept limited. At the same time, a good collar gives continuous slight traction and the cervical spine is kept warm. In instances of instability, a hard collar should be applied for stabilization (frequently in rheumatoid arthritis).

Posture

Authors Brügger[48] and Rocabado[49] indicate that many syndromes of the musculoskeletal system, such as back, shoulder, and cervical pain, are caused by diminished force of the postural muscles and continuing postural faults. Brügger[48] describes the so-called sternal overload syndrome, characterized by a strong thoracic kyphosis, increased cervical flexion, and an anterior position of the head. Brügger states that nociceptive activity exists because of prolonged overload of the tissue structures of the musculoskeletal system. This prolonged nociceptive activity can lead to the development of orthosympathetic manifestations in the head-neck region. Ultimately this will cause tissue-specific changes.

Thus, instruction concerning posture is an important part of the therapeutic program. The necessary additional requirements in order to achieve this postural correction are dealt with by the physical therapist. For example, it may be necessary to correct muscle length and/or mobilize the joints in the involved arthrogenic and myogenic chains. Muscle strengthening and improvement of the proprioceptive capabilities are also part of these additional requirements.

Pain Relief

Pain relief can be attained with the postisometric relaxation technique previously discussed. According to Sansiesteban,[50] pain relief can also be achieved with the following:

- fast and moderate rhythmically performed traction and gliding techniques
- oscillation and vibration techniques[51]
- soft tissue techniques[52]
- the aforementioned relaxation and mobilization techniques
- physiotechnical applications[37,53–56]
- massage therapy, to include transverse friction[42]

Neuromodulation techniques, such as pressure, massage, vibration, cold, warmth, gel, transcutaneous electrical nerve stimulation (TENS), exercise therapy, and manual therapy, can be applied in accordance to the principles of the "gate control theory of pain." Wall[56] writes: "That a gate control exists is no longer open to doubt, but its functional role and its detailed mechanisms remain open for speculation and experiment." Until today this statement has remained unchanged. For instance, electrical triggering of the myelinated afference of type II fibers from the skin and type III fibers from the muscle can be used to normalize orthosympathetic activity. Melzack et al.[57] indicate a high correlation (71%) between trigger points and acupuncture points,

especially regarding their localization and the associated pain patterns. These authors indicate that the same mechanisms play a role. Trigger points are also associated with visceral structures. However, the occurrence of trigger points is still unexplained.

Trigger points can be treated with vibrating modalities,[51] ultrasound,[37] TENS,[58] spray and stretch techniques, and injection therapy.[59] In applying electrotherapy, nonpolarized currents, such as interferential current and TENS, are preferred. Stimulation of the trigger points with TENS results in significantly more pain relief than a placebo treatment.[58] Based on sound foundations, the pain-relieving effect of conventional TENS is due to inhibition of the nociceptive transmission in accordance with the gate control theory.[24] Selective stimulation of thick myelinated nerve fibers, especially the type II and the low-threshold type III nerve fibers, is responsible for this.[24,60] The pain-relieving effect of the "acupuncture-like TENS" is based on activation of the descending endogenic nociceptive modulation system, in accordance with the "endogenous pain control theory."[11] Stimulation of thin, nonmyelinated nerve fibers (especially the high-threshold type III and type IV nerve fibers) is responsible for the effect achieved. This kind of stimulation is best applied if conventional, high-frequency TENS has no effect.[61]

The electrodes are placed on the tender points or areas. These points, or areas, generally include the paraspinal skin areas (innervated by the dorsal rami of the spinal nerves), superficial peripheral nerves, cutaneous branches of peripheral nerves, acupuncture points, motor points, "trigger points," and "trigger areas."[24] In addition, the stimulation can also be applied to areas that correspond segmentally with the spinal level of entry and processing of the nociceptive impulses from the head, neck, shoulder, arm, and upper trunk regions.

Transcutaneous nerve stimulation is a safe treatment. Contraindications are minimal, and there are generally no side effects.[61] In patients who have an "on-demand" pacemaker, TENS is contraindicated. "Fixed-rate" pacemakers do not constitute a contraindication for the application of TENS.[62] In addition, stimulation should never be applied in the area of the carotid sinus because this could lead to bradycardia and hypertension. Study results of the effectiveness of TENS in the treatment of patients with chronic pain give rise to moderate optimism.[24,63]

In the application of shortwave diathermy for pain relief, metal objects must be kept out of the electric field. Metal concentrates the electric field, resulting in energetic density with overheating. Side effects are described for shortwave diathermy in its application to the orofacial area.[64,65] Beneficial effects of diathermy and TENS are reported in muscular problems.[54]

Cryotherapy can be indicated for a pain-relieving and tone-decreasing effect.

Oscillating techniques in manual therapy also provide pain relief. Oscillations are alternating motions with a small amplitude, performed in a fast rhythm, for a duration of 15 to 30 seconds. Depending on the actuality of the pain, and the reaction and the tolerance of the patient, the technique can be repeated several times. As the pain decreases during the oscillation, the intensity of the oscillation is increased until either no further adaptation takes place or until the pain disappears completely. Of course, if the pain increases, the intensity is correspondingly decreased. Oscillations follow the principles of the "gate control theory."[56]

Gentle traction and gliding manual therapy techniques often result in pain relief for the patient. By changing the techniques, the direction of translation, and the frequency of the oscillations the best pain-relieving effect can be achieved.

Relaxation, pain relief, and functional improvement are attained through gentle resisted exercises, for instance, in the form of "hold-relax" techniques. Furthermore, the "rhythmic stabilization" techniques from proprioceptive neuromuscular facilitation can be used to improve proprioceptive control, resulting in increased postural and movement awareness.

In approaching pain through manual techniques, the physical therapist emphasizes movement. Improvement remains permanent only when the manual therapy is supplemented with an appropriate exercise program.[66]

INFLUENCE OF PHYSICAL CONDITION ON PAIN TOLERANCE

Pain tolerance and physical condition appear to be closely related.[30] A patient with a "weak" neck or back should be encouraged to perform specific exercises in order to optimize the condition of the musculoskeletal system. When activity decreases, there is a subsequent decrease in the physical condition, with a resulting decrease in pain tolerance. Therefore, advice such as "give the back or neck some rest" is not always very sensible. In practice, the physical therapist is confronted daily with pain and functional disturbances of the musculoskeletal system that are, for a large part, due to a disturbed relationship between load and loadability.[15]

Decreased effectiveness of restoring mechanisms diminishes the average level of loadability. The vegetative environment also influences the effectiveness of this local restoration mechanism. For instance, if a patient with manifestations of bruxism is put under continuous stress, the nervous system puts itself in an alarm phase, with a resulting ergotropic reaction. This means that the periods of rest, during which tissues can recover, can no longer be optimally used. All restoration mechanisms work more slowly and less effectively, leading to a situation of increased vulnerability (relative overload).[26]

Knowledge regarding the nature of functional disturbance and the factors that influence it, together with a gradual increase of the load, decreases the vulnerability for lesions. Besides the local loading of the affected structure, attention should also be given to the general physical condition. The use of elements from sports is a positive experience for many patients. In addition, prolonged physical therapy is often not reasonable. The "physical attention" often leads to an increase of the pain behavior.[30] Therefore, mutual consultation with the patient, in order to determine precise goals and the termination of treatment, is highly recommended.

REFERENCES

1. Allan DB, Waddell G. A historical perspective on low back pain and disability. *Acta Orthop Scand Suppl.* 1900;234.

2. Mixter WJ, Barr JS. Rupture of the intervertebral disc with involvement of the spinal canal. *N Engl J Med.* 1934;211:210–215.

3. Vleeming A. *The Sacro-Iliac Joint: A Clinical-Anatomical, Biomechanical and Radiological Study.* Rotterdam: Erasmus University; 1990. Dissertation.

4. Nachemson A. Rational work-up for Differential Diagnosis. Presented at the Lumbar Spine Instructional Course, organized by the International Society for the Study of the Lumbar Spine; May 11, 1991; Zürich, Switzerland.

5. Butler D, Trafimov JH, Andersson GB, McNeill TW, Huckman MS. Discs degenerate before facets. *Spine.* 1990;15:111–113.

6. Hägg O, Wallner A. Facet joint asymmetry and protrusion of the intervertebral disc. *Spine.* 1990;15:356–359.

7. Bogduk N, Windsor M, Inglis A. The innervation of the cervical discs. *Spine.* 1988;13:2.

8. Krämer J. *Bandscheibenbedingte Erkrankungen.* Stuttgart: Georg Thieme Verlag; 1978.

9. Porter RW. *Management of Back Pain.* Edinburgh: Churchill Livingstone; 1986.

10. White AA, Panjabi MM. *Clinical Biomechanics of the Spine.* Philadelphia: JB Lippincott; 1978.

11. Fields HL, Basbaum AJ. Brainstem control of spinal pain transmission neurons. *Annu Rev Physiol.* 1978;40:217–248.

12. Gracovetsky S, Farfan H. The optimum spine. *Spine.* 1986;15:543.

13. Galante JO. Tensile properties of the human annulus fibrosus. *Acta Orthop Scand Suppl.* 1967;100:1–91.

14. Eyre DR. Biochemistry of the intervertebral disc. *Int Rev Connect Tissue Res.* 1979;8:227.

15. Blumenkrantz N, Sylvest J, Asboe-Hansen G. Local low-collagen content may allow herniation of intervertebral disc: biochemical studies. *Biochem Med.* 1977;18:282.

16. Junghanns H. *Die Wirbelsäule unter den Einflüssen des täglichen Lebens, der Freizeit, des Sportes.* Stuttgart: Hippocrates Verlag; 1986.

17. Rauschning W. Three dimensional anatomy. Presented at the Lumbar Spine Instructional Course, organized by the International Society for the Study of the Lumbar Spine; May 11, 1991; Zürich, Switzerland.

18. Jackson HC, Winkelman RK, Bickel WM. Nerve endings in the human lumbar spinal column and related structures. *J Bone Joint Surg [Am].* 1966;48:1272.

19. Pederson HE, Blunck CFJ, Gardner E. The anatomy of the lumbosacral posterior rami and meningeal branches of spinal nerves (sinuvertebral nerves). *J Bone Joint Surg [Am].* 1956;38:377.

20. Bogduk N, Tynan W, Wilson AS. The nerve supply to the human lumbar intervertebral discs. *J Anat.* 1981;132:39.

21. Heylings DJA. Supraspinous and interspinous ligaments of the human lumbar spine. *J Anat.* 1978;125:127.

22. Macnab I, McCulloch J. *Backache.* 2nd ed. Baltimore: Williams & Wilkins; 1990.

23. Schouten JAM. *Anamnese en Advies.* De Nederlandse bibliotheek der Geneeskunde, Alphen a/d Rijn, Netherlands: Stafleu; 1982.

24. Oostendorp RAB. *Functionele Vertebrobasilaire Insufficiëntie.* Nijmegen, Netherlands: Catholic University; 1988. Dissertation.

25. Korr JM. *The Neurobiological Mechanisms in Manipulative Therapy.* New York: Plenum Press; 1978.

26. Bernards ATM. Relaties tussen belasting en belastbaarheid. *Issue 5.* 1988;4:1–5.

27. Verbiest H. Further experiences on the pathological influence of a developmental narrowness of the bony vertebral canal. *J Bone Joint Surg [Br].* 1955;37:576–583.

28. Cranenburgh B van. *Inleiding in de toegepaste neurowetenschappen.* Part 3: *Pijn.* Lochem, Netherlands: De Tijdstroom; 1987.

29. Flor H, Turk DC. Etiological theories and treatments for chronic back pain, I: somatic models and interventions. *Pain.* 1984;19:105–121.

30. Meyler WJ. *Preventie van het Chronisch Pijnsyndroom.* Werkgroep preventie chroniciteit; Nederlandse Vereniging ter Bestudering van Pijn. Groningen, Netherlands: Academisch Ziekenhuis; 1984.

31. Noordenbos W, Wall PD, Melzack R, eds. *Textbook of Pain.* Edinburgh: Churchill Livingstone; 1984.

32. Trott PH. Tension headache. In: Grieve GP, ed. *Modern Manual Therapy of the Vertebral Column.* Edinburgh: Churchill Livingstone; 1986:336–342.

33. Bonica JJ. In: Pauser G, Gerstenbrand F, Gross D., eds. *Gesichtsschmerz.* Stuttgart: Gustav Fischer Verlag; 1979.

34. Fricton JR, Hathaway KM, Bromaghim C. Interdisciplinary management of patients with TMJ and craniofacial pain: characteristics and outcome. *J Craniomandibular Disord.* 1987;1,2:115–123.

35. Post D. *De Huisarts en zijn Hoofdpijnpatiënten.* Alphen a/d Rijn, Netherlands: Stafleu's Wetenschappelijke Uitgeversmaatschappij B.V.; 1980.

36. Schulkes-van de Pol J. Pijn en pijnbehandeling. In: Cranenburgh B van, Dekker JB den, Meerwijk GM van, Wessel HFM, Wijer A de, eds. *Jaarboek Fysiotherapie.* Utrecht, Netherlands: Bohn, Scheltema & Holkema; 1987.

37. Wijma K Duinkerke ASH, Reitsma B. Behandeling van patiënten met somatische fixatie in de tandheelkundige pradtijk. *Nederlands Tijdschrift Tandheelkunde.* 1987;94:101–104.

38. Bernstein DA, Douglas A, Borkovec D, Thomas D. *Progressive Relaxation Training: A Manual for the Helping Professions.* Champaign, Ill: Research Press X; 1973.

39. Kruithof WM. Psychologisch geschrift. Subfaculteit Psychologie. Utrecht, Netherlands: Rijks University.

40. Mitchell L. *Simple Relaxation: The Physiological Method for Easing Tension.* London: Murray; 1985.

41. Bakker FC. Relaxatietechnieken in de sport: een overzicht. *Geneeskde Sport.* IV;1987:145–151.

42. Patist JA. *Massagetherapie.* Lochem, Netherlands: De Tijdstroom; 1982.

43. Teirich-Leube H. *Grundriss der Bindegewebsmassage.* Stuttgart: Gustav Fischer Verlag; 1968.

44. Boomsma A. *Dictaat Massage.* Postbus 14211. Utrecht, Netherlands: Stichting Nederlandse Hogeschool Centraal; 1988.

45. Gutmann G, Vele F. *Das Aufrechte Stehen.* Opladen, Norway: Westdeutscher Verlag; 1978.

46. Evjenth O, Hamberg J. *Muscle Stretching in Manual Therapy: A Clinical Manual.* Alfta, Sweden: Alfta Rehab I/II; 1984.

47. Ottenbacher K, Difabio RP. Efficacy of spinal manipulation/mobilization therapy. *Spine.* 1985;10:833–837.

48. Brügger A. *Die Erkrankungen des Bewegungsapparates und seines Nervensystems.* Stuttgart: Gustav Fischer Verlag; 1980.

49. Rocabado M. Biomechanical relationship of the cranial, cervical and hyoid regions. *J Craniomandibular Pract.* 1983;3:62–66.

50. Sansiesteban A. The role of physical agents in the treatment of spine pain. *Clin Orthop.* 1983;179:24–30.

51. Lundeberg T, et al. Pain alleviation by vibratory stimulation. *Pain.* 1984;20:25–44.

52. Tilscher H, Eder M. *Die Rehabilitation von Wirbelsäulen Gestörten.* Berlin: Springer Verlag; 1983.

53. Chung JM, et al. Prolonged inhibition of primate spinothalamic tract cells by peripheral nerve stimulation. *Pain.* 1984;19:259–275.

54. Esposito CJ, et al. Alleviation of myofascial pain with ultrasonic therapy. *J Prosthet Dent.* 1984;51,1:106–108.

55. Hoogland R. Elektrotherapie als reflextherapie bij pijn en functiestoornissen van de spier. *Geneeskde Sport.* 1987;2:74–78.

56. Wall PD. The gate control therapy of pain mechanisms: a re-examination and restatement. *Brain.* 1978;101:1–18.

57. Melzack R, Stillwell DM, Fox EJ. Triggerpoints and acupuncture points for pain: correlation and implications. *Pain.* 1977;3:3–23.

58. Melzack R, Vetere P, Finch L. Transcutaneous electrical nerve stimulation for low back pain. *Phys Ther.* 1983;63:489–493.

59. Rubin D. Myofascial triggerpoint syndromes: An approach to management. *Arch Phys Med Rehabil.* 1981;62:107–111.

60. Howson DC. Peripheral neural excitability: implications for transcutaneous electrical nerve stimulation. *Phys Ther.* 1978;58:12.

61. Besse TC. Pijnbehandeling door middel van elektrostimulatie. In: *Reeks Informatiegidsen voor de Gezondheidszorg.* Utrecht, Netherlands: Medifo, Bohn, Scheltema & Holkema; 1987:37–45.

62. Eriksson MBE, Schuller H, Sjolund BH. Hazard from transcutaneous nerve stimulators in patients with pacemakers. *Lancet.* 1978;1:1319.

63. Aufdemkampe G, Meijer OG. Effect-onderzoek in verband met TENS. In: Mattie H, ed. *Pijn Informatorium.* Alphen a/d Rijn, Netherlands: Stafleu Samson; 1986.

64. Hargreaves AS, Wardle JJM. The use of physiotherapy in the treatment of temporomandibular disorders. *Br Dent J.* 1983;155:121–124.

65. Taube S, Ylipaavalniemi P, Perkki K, Oikarinen VJ. Side-effects of electrical physiotherapy treatment in the orofacial region. *Proc Finn Dent Soc.* 1983;79:168–171.

66. Aufdemkampe G, Meijer OG, Winkel D, Witmaar GC. Manuele pijnbenaderingen. In: Mattie H, ed. *Pijn Informatorium.* Alphen a/d Rijn, Netherlands: Stafleu Samson; 1985.

SUGGESTED READING

Bogduk N. Cervical causes of headache and dizziness. In: Grieve GP, ed. *Modern Manual Therapy of the Vertebral Column.* Edinburgh: Churchill Livingstone; 1986.

Bremer GJ, Janssen JJ, Veenstra A, de Planque BA, Sedee GA. Hoofdpijn. Leiden, Netherlands: Stafleu's Wetenschappelijke Uitgeversmaatschappij N.V.; 1970.

Cranenburgh B van. *Segmentale Verschijnselen.* Utrecht, Netherlands: Bohn, Scheltema & Holkema; 1985.

Duinkerke ASH. Biofeedback training en "habit reversal" techniek (gewoonte omdraaiing). *Bulletin N.V.G.* 1985:3.

Flor H, Turk DC. Etiological theories and treatments for chronic back pain, II: somatic models and interventions. *Pain.* 1984;19:209–233.

Frisch H. *Programmierte Untersuchung des Bewegungsapparates.* Berlin: Springer Verlag; 1983.

Hagenaars LHA, Dekker LJ, Plaats J van der, Bernards ATM, Oostendorp RAB. Effecten van het orthosympathische zenuwletsel op de dwarsgestreepte spier. *Nederlands Tijdschr Fysiother.* 1985;95:77–88.

Hijzen TH, Slangen JL. Myofascial pain dysfunction: subjective signs and symptoms. *J Prosthet Dent.* 1985;54,5:705–711.

Ihalainen U, Perkki K. The effect of transcutaneous nerve stimulation on chronic facial pain. *Proc Finn Dent Soc.* 1978;74:86–90.

Levit K. *Manuelle Medizin im Rahmen der Medizinischen Rehabilitation.* Leipzig, Germany: Joh. Ambrosius Barth; 1987.

Mink RJF, Veer HJ ter, Vorselaars JACT. *Extremiteiten, functie-onderzoek en manuele therapie.* Eindhoven, Netherlands: Educational Foundation for Manual Therapy; 1983.

Paris SV. Clinical decision making: orthopaedic physical therapy. In: Wolf SL, ed. *Clinical Decision Making in Physical Therapy.* Philadelphia: F.A. Davis Co; 1985;215–255.

Rugh JD, Solberg WK. Psychological implications in temporomandibular pain and dysfunction. In: Zarb GA, Carlsson GE, eds. *Temporomandibular Joint Function and Dysfunction.* Copenhagen, Denmark: Munksgaard; 1979.

Steenks MH, Touw WD. In: Cranenburgh B van, Dekker JB den, Meerwijk GM van, Wessel HFM, Wijer A de, eds. *Jaarboek Fysiotherapie.* Utrecht, Netherlands: Bohn, Scheltema & Holkema; 1987.

Travell J, Simons G. *Myofascial Pain and Dysfunction: The Trigger Point Manual.* Baltimore: Williams & Wilkins; 1983.

Zutphen HCF. *Nederlands Leerboek der Fysische Therapie in Engere Zin.* Utrecht, Netherlands: Bunge; 1982.

Part II

The Spine and Transitional Joints

Chapter 3

Sacroiliac Joint

3.1 FUNCTIONAL ANATOMY

INTRODUCTION

The sacroiliac (SI) joints build the connection between the sacrum and the right and the left ilium (innominate). The joint surface consists of the auricular surfaces on the sacrum and on the ilium (Figure 3–1). In contradiction to what many expect, the SI joints cannot be palpated at their dorsal aspect because they are covered by muscles and multiple fibrous layers. At the dorsal aspect of the SI joint, the distance between the skin and the SI joint itself averages about 5 cm at the cranial part and about 2 cm at the caudal part.

OVERVIEW

The lumbar spine, the sacrum, both innominates, and the hip joints form a functional unit. Almost every movement of the lumbar spine has an influence on the pelvic joints, which consist of both SI joints and the pubic symphysis. Through the sacrum and the SI joints, forces are transmitted to the hip joints and then to the other parts of the lower extremities (and vice versa).

The weakest link in this kinetic chain is the lumbosacral junction. The caudal intervertebral discs are exposed to rather considerable forces. The angle between L5 and the sacrum

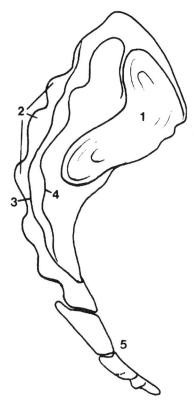

Figure 3–1 Auricular surface of the sacrum. **1**, Auricular surface of the sacrum; **2**, medial sacral crest; **3**, intermediate sacral crest; **4**, lateral sacral crest; **5**, coccyx.

has a ventral opening, and it widens under loads that cause the sacrum to tip ventrally.[1,2] Much of a ventral directed force is absorbed by the strong anterior longitudinal ligament, which is connected to the sacrum.

There is an extensive number of strong collagenous connections between the sacrum and the surrounding bony structures: the interosseous sacroiliac ligaments, the ventral and dorsal sacroiliac ligaments, and the sacrotuberous and the sacrospinous ligaments. In addition, the iliolumbar ligaments connect the ilium with L4 and L5 without being directly connected to the sacrum. This well-developed connective tissue complex around the SI joints, together with the construction of the joint, is responsible for the fact that the sacroiliac motion is very limited.

Because many of the ligamentous and muscular connections bridge a certain number of vertebrae, motion between adjacent vertebrae can result in simultaneous movement of vertebrae located farther away. In the same way, movements between L5 and S1 (and also in some levels located more cranial) will also be influenced by motions of the sacrum between the innominate bones. Every motion of the sacrum induces movement in the L5-S1 segment.

In most books dealing with anatomy, the connective tissue complex of the lumbar spine is described separately from the connective tissue complex of the sacroiliac connections. Unfortunately, important information is lost in making this separation. In the following section, the anatomy of these regions is discussed as a whole. The anatomical description is based on the author's observations[3] and on research by Bakland and Hansen.[4]

ANATOMICAL STUDY OF THE DORSAL ASPECT OF THE SI JOINT

After removing the skin and the subcutaneous connective tissue one sees the fascia of the gluteus maximus, the gluteus medius, and the erector spinae (Figure 3–2). The fascia of the gluteus maximus inserts partly into the thoracolumbar fascia, making it possible for the muscle to tighten this fascia. Some fibers of the gluteus medius fascia and of the iliotibial tract are also connected to the thoracolumbar fascia. Upon removal of the superficial connective tissue, tendinous structures of the erector spinae become visible (Figure 3–3).

At the spinous processes it is impossible to distinguish the superficial fascia from the underlying tendinous tissue: there are superficial fibers that have a deep insertion and deep fibers inserting superficially. The most caudal part of the erector spinae is located in the depression between the medial sacral crest and the posterior superior and posterior inferior iliac spines. The muscular and tendinous tissue in this region consists of two layers, a superficial layer mainly from the iliocostalis and a deep layer mainly from the multifidus. Based on the structure of the fascia in this region, one can conclude that the gluteus maximus and the erector spinae have a mutually dependent influence on the forces exerted by the sacrum and ilium upon each other.

When the gluteus maximus muscle is removed, the sacrotuberous and the sacrospinous ligaments become visible. In every cadaver examined by the authors the dorsal fascia of the piriformis appeared to be continuous with the sacrotuberous ligament. Therefore, to some extent, the piriformis can deform the sacrotuberous ligament. However, in our opinion (reinforced by valid scientific studies) the clinical relevance of the piriformis muscle and the sacrotuberous ligament, as well as the sacrospinous ligament, as possible sources of pain remains hypothetical.

In 5 female cadavers and 1 male cadaver from a total of 23, the biceps femoris inserted bilaterally into the sacrotuberous ligament without having a direct connection with the ischial tuberosity. In five other cadavers, the biceps femoris on one side inserted partly into the sacrotuberous ligament and partly into the ischial tuberosity. In such cases, the

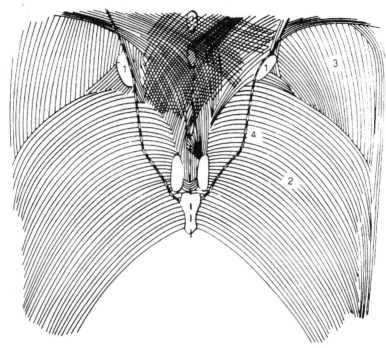

Figure 3–2 The superficial connective tissue dorsal to the sacrum. **1**, Posterior superior iliac spine; **2**, fascia of the gluteus maximus; **3**, fascia of the gluteus medius and the iliotibial tract; **4**, lateral sacral crest.

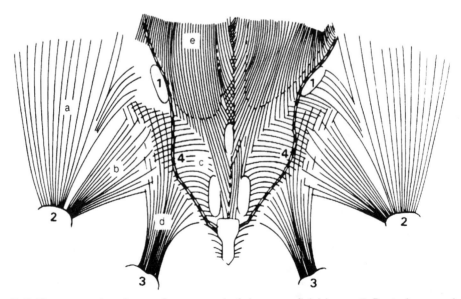

Figure 3–3 The connective tissue after removal of the superficial layer. **1**, Posterior superior iliac spine; **2**, greater trochanter; **3**, ischial tuberosity; **4**, lateral sacral crest; **a**, gluteus medius; **b**, piriformis with dorsal continuation into the sacrotuberous ligament; **c**, insertion of the gluteus maximus into the sacrum and the back muscles; **d**, sacrotuberous ligament; **e**, aponeurosis of the erector spinae.

biceps femoris is capable of tightening the sacrotuberous ligament.[5] It is important to keep the possible existence of these connections in mind when performing the straight leg raise (SLR) test, because in this test the biceps femoris (among other structures) is being stretched. This offers a possible explanation for the fact that the SLR test is positive in a number of sacroiliac disorders (especially in the various forms of sacroiliitis).

Because of the interwoven character of most of the collagenous connections of the ilium, sacrum, L5, and L4, a prolonged kyphotic (sitting) posture can result in nonradiating low back pain. (See Chapter 4, section 4.3.) The deepest ligaments at the dorsal aspect, the dorsal and interosseous sacroiliac ligaments, have several strong connections with the gluteus maximus. This is clinically significant because this muscle represents the only contractile structure bridging the sacroiliac joint. The gluteus maximus plays a very important role in the treatment of the instability of this joint.

The dorsal SI capsuloligamentous structures are innervated by the medial branches of the dorsal rami, particularly from S1 and S2. (See Chapter 8.) Here there also exists a considerable variability (L3 to S3). Therefore, during the functional examination, if pain is provoked as a result of stretch or compression of the sacroiliac joint complex, the patient can experience pain in a number of different dermatomes.

VENTRAL ASPECT OF THE SI JOINT

At the ventral aspect of the SI joint, the less developed ventral sacroiliac ligament can be found. This ligament is clinically important; in cases of arthritis, if this ligament is stretched, the patient will experience pain. The pain localization varies because of differences in innervation patterns. Usually the ligament is innervated by the neurological segments L3 to S1, but the innervation can also occur from L1 to S2. (See Chapter 8.)

The psoas major is located ventral to the SI joint. Other structures in the immediate surroundings include the cranial insertions of the internal obturator muscle, the lumbosacral trunk (part of the fourth and all of the fifth lumbar ventral rami), the obturator nerve, and the iliac artery and vein.

CONSTRUCTION OF THE SI JOINT

The sacroiliac joint surfaces are generally described as having the shape of an ear; hence they are called the auricular surfaces. However, there is significant variability in form. The differences are considerable both interindividually and intraindividually[4] (Figure 3–4). In addition, the range of motion in the SI joint is very small and barely measurable without sophisticated equipment. These fundamental concepts are of great importance when interpreting the findings in the physical examination. With some exceptions, clinically relevant interpretation of possible findings in the manual mobility examination is almost impossible.

According to Bakland and Hansen,[4] an axial joint is found dorsal to the auricular surfaces (Figure 3–5). The function of this joint is unclear for the time being. The term *axial*—indicating that it is located at the level of the nutation/counternutation of the SI joint—is not an indication for the large variability in the location of the sacroiliac axes.

The structural development of the cartilage in the SI joint is not the same as in other joints of the body.[3] First, the normal smooth hyaline cartilage is absent. From the end of puberty on, the cartilaginous covering of the sacrum is relatively soft and thick. Microscopically, the SI cartilage, especially of the ilium, develops a rougher tissue than the cartilage in other synovial joints. Second, macroscopic ridges develop on the auricular surfaces with complementary grooves on the opposite joint surface. Thus with this combination of microscopic roughness as well as macroscopic ridges and grooves, one can as-

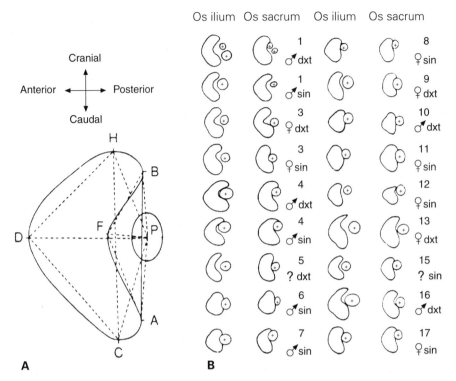

Figure 3–4 Intra- and interindividual differences in sacroiliac morphology. Indicated are the numbers, the sex, and the difference left to right. From cadavers 1, 3, and 4 the left and the right joint surfaces are displayed; these cadavers provide intraindividual comparison. The small circles containing a + refer to the so-called axial SI joint: an extra joint connection which, according to Bakland and Hansen,[4] is located dorsal to the auricular surfaces. **A**, Coordinate system; **B**, geometric differences of the auricular and axial regions.

sume that the function of the SI joint consists much more of providing "springing" stability than in providing for motion.

During pregnancy the mobility of the joint increases due to hormonal changes. This increase in mobility occurs at the cost of some stability, which in turn can lead to complaints of pain both during and after the pregnancy. (See section 3.3.)

NUTATION AND COUNTERNUTATION

In the SI joint, there is one main motion possible, along with a number of accessory movements.[6] This main motion can be performed in two directions, starting from the zero position, nutation and counternutation.

In the nutation movement the cranial aspect of the ilium moves dorsal in relation to the sacrum, or the cranial aspect of the sacrum moves ventral in relation to the ilium. This happens, for instance, in standing on one leg: the SI joint on the side of the weight-bearing leg moves into an almost maximally nutated position. During the nutation motion, the pelvic entrance (the distance between the promontory and the pubic symphysis) becomes smaller and the pelvic exit (the distance between the sacral apex and the pubic symphysis) increases. With counternutation the opposite occurs: the pelvic entrance becomes larger and the pelvic exit becomes smaller (Figure 3–6).

Sturesson et al.[6] performed a radiological

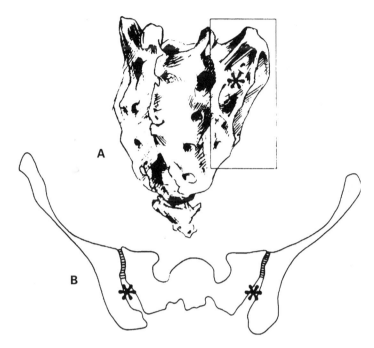

Figure 3–5 The axial sacroiliac joint (indicated by *). **A**, Lateral dorsal view; **B**, cross-section; the hatched areas indicate the articular surface.

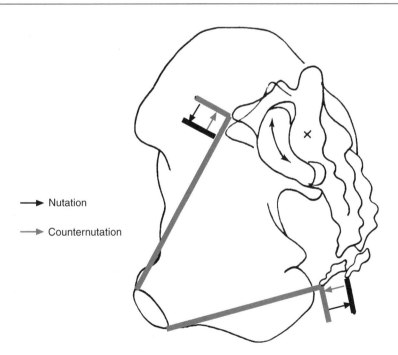

Figure 3–6 Nutation and counternutation of the SI joint.

stereophotogrammetric study of the SI joint movements in 25 patients. The largest motion occurred around the transverse axis (nutation–counternutation). The average range of motion was 2.5° (ranging from 0.8° to 3.9°). This is equal to a translation of 0.7 mm (ranging from 0.1 to 1.6 mm). The motions around the other axes were so small that they could not be measured.

BIOMECHANICAL CONSIDERATIONS

The SI joint is a relatively strong joint with limited mobility. Often it is considered a physiologically unimportant joint. Unfortunately, the functions of this joint are insufficiently researched and described. Lavignolle et al.[2] state, "The sacroiliac joints remain quite a mystery, and knowledge of their precise model of function is still incomplete."

This chapter is not meant to be a clinical lesson but rather an overview of the most important biomechanical aspects of the pelvis, and more specifically of the SI joint. In biomechanics, a number of methods from general mechanics are applied: the structure under examination is excised from its environment, forces induced by the environment are calculated, and then the conditions of equilibrium are postulated.

EQUILIBRIUM AROUND THE SI JOINT

The pelvic region can be divided into three bony parts, the left ilium, the right ilium, and the sacrum. The sacrum articulates with both ilia by means of both left and right sacroiliac joints. Both ilia are connected to each other through the pubic symphysis.

The weight of the mass above the pelvis (the upper body) averages approximately 65% of the total body weight and is mostly transferred via the sacrum to both SI joints. The SI joints are responsible for a further transfer of the forces to both lower extremities (Figure 3–7). Because of the location of

the upper body's center of gravity, not only the equilibrium of force but also the equilibrium of moments is important for the maintenance of static posture. This becomes particularly important in a nonupright position, as depicted in Figure 3–8.

The following question should now be asked: Is the SI joint sturdy enough to be able to handle the equilibrium of forces as well as an equilibrium of moments?

Equilibrium of Forces

Because of the earth's gravity, the mass of a body acquires weight. This weight is a force that always works vertically, in other words in the same direction as the force of gravity. For each part of the body this force (the body weight) can be considered as a concentrated force acting upon the center of gravity within that part itself. If we call this force the action force, then according to the law of equilibrium an equal but opposite reactive force acts on the specific body part as well.

Analysis of the orientation of the SI joint surfaces shows that their orientation has a beneficial influence on the transfer of forces. Forces acting on the SI joint consist of the reactive forces caused by the weight, G, of the mass located above the SI joint and the resulting force generated by the muscles bridging this joint (Figure 3–9). Depending on the amount and magnitude of the muscle forces between the lumbar spine and the pelvis, the direction of this resulting reactive force in the SI joint can vary from vertical to an angle of approximately 30° directed dorsally in relation to the vertical.

Resolution of the reactive forces in the SI joint results in a vertical vector and a dorsally directed horizontal vector, depending on the contracting lumbar muscles (Figure 3–10). Because the resulting muscle force, S_l, of the lumbar muscles in an upright posture forms an angle of approximately 30° to the vertical, the horizontal component of this muscle force is equal to $S_l \times \sin 30 = \frac{1}{2} \times S_l$. This means that

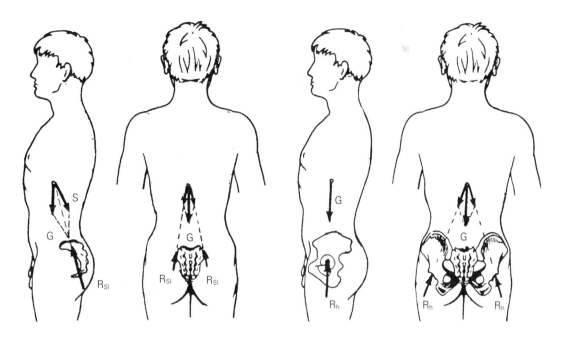

Figure 3–7 The force $\boldsymbol{R_{SI}}$ on the SI joint and $\boldsymbol{R_h}$ on the hip joint caused by the weight of the upper body. $\boldsymbol{G}$ = weight, $\boldsymbol{S}$ = muscle force, $\boldsymbol{R}$ = reactive force.

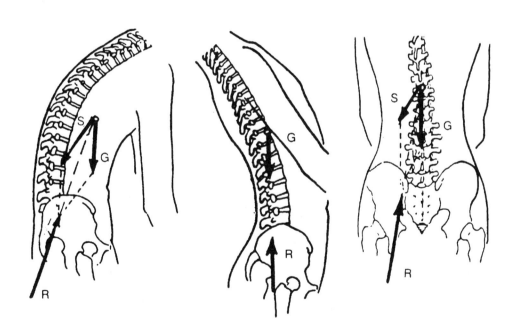

Figure 3–8 The force $\boldsymbol{R}$ on the SI joint in flexion and extension and in standing on one leg. $\boldsymbol{G}$ = weight, $\boldsymbol{S}$ = muscle force, $\boldsymbol{R}$ = reactive force.

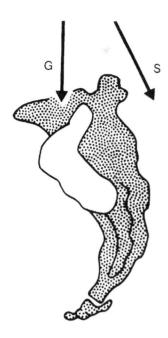

Figure 3–9 Load components in the SI joint. **G** = weight, **S** = muscle force.

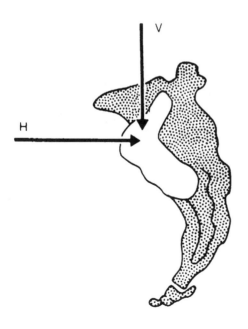

Figure 3–10 The joint load in the SI joint resolved into horizontal **(H)** and vertical **(V)** components.

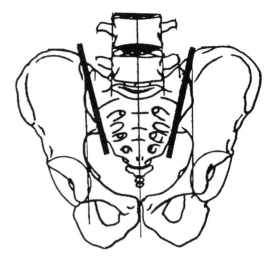

Figure 3–11 Frontal view of the pelvic bones indicating the average orientation of the SI joint surfaces in the frontal plane.

the horizontal component in an upright posture will never be more than about half of the force generated by the lumbar muscles. For the horizontal, H, and the vertical, V, components of the load in the SI joint, the following applies: $H = \frac{1}{2} \times S_l$ and $V = \frac{1}{2} \times \sqrt{3} \times S_l + G$.

In the frontal plane the SI joint surfaces converge caudally, as pictured in Figure 3–11. This converging position of both joint surfaces is beneficial in supporting the body weight. Suppose that the weight of the mass above the SI joints equals 500 N. In symmetrical body posture (equal weight on both feet), this weight is equally divided over both SI joints. If the lumbar muscles are not contracting, the load, F, on each SI joint surface equals $500/2 = 250$ N and has a vertical direction. This force, F, can be resolved into a vector, K, perpendicular to the joint surface and a vector, S, parallel to the joint surface (Figure 3–12). If the angle α that the joint surface forms to the vertical is equal to 25°, then the following can be applied:

$$K = F \sin \alpha = 250 \sin 25 = 105 \text{ N}$$

$$S = F \cos \alpha = 250 \cos 25 = 226 \text{ N}$$

Because the joint surface makes only a small angle to the vertical, the force, S, paral-

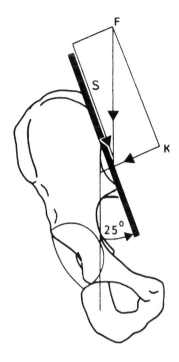

Figure 3–12 The force components, **K** and **S**, of the weight, **F**, acting in the frontal plane on the joint surface.

lel to the joint surface is of the same magnitude as the weight it has to bear. This force, S, has to be absorbed by the resistance of the joint, partly by the strength of the joint capsule and ligaments and partly by the friction between both joint surfaces.

The form of the joint surfaces helps to provide friction. In reality, the joint surfaces are not flat but instead have different curves in a variety of different directions. In other words, the joint consists of a number of facets with different orientations.

The force, K, is a compression force acting perpendicular to the joint surface. Due to bony structures this force can be absorbed easily. If the joint were to have a cranially converging form in the frontal plane, then the force acting perpendicular to the joint surface would not be of a compressive nature, but instead of a tensile nature. This tensile force could be absorbed only by the joint capsule

and the ligaments. Because of the much larger resistance of the bony structures against compression than the resistance of the joint capsule against tensile force, it is obvious that a compression force is much more favorable for the joint. It pushes both innominates away from each other, as illustrated in Figure 3–13. Both ilia are held in place by the capsules and ligaments connecting them either directly or indirectly to each other.

However, the construction is much stronger than the elements alone that bridge the SI joint. In a transverse plane the SI joint has a dorsally converging form, as illustrated in Figure 3–14. Because of this the dorsally acting component D of the reactive force in the SI joint can be absorbed. For the sake of simplicity, assume that the force, S_l, generated by the lumbar muscles equals the weight of the upper body with $S_l = 500$ N. As already demonstrated in Figure 3–9, the resulting force S_l generated by the lumbar muscles forms an angle of 30° with the vertical. Therefore, in a symmetrical loading of both SI joints, the dorsally acting horizontal component, D, in every SI joint is $D = (500/2 \times \sin 30) = 125$ N. This dorsally acting component, D, can be resolved into a compression force, K, perpendicular to the joint surface and the force, S, which is parallel to the joint surface (Figure 3–15). The angle that the joint surface forms with the sagittal plane at the level of S1 is about 20°. The following applies:

$$K = 125 \sin 20 = 43 \text{ N}$$
$$S = 125 \cos 20 = 117 \text{ N}$$

In addition, the load applied by the sacrum drives both ilia away from each other. As already mentioned, these forces are much smaller than the forces in the vertical plane in an upright position. With a ventral converging joint form in the transverse plane, the compression force in the SI joint would change into a tensile force which, as in the frontal plane, would create a less favorable situation for the joint.

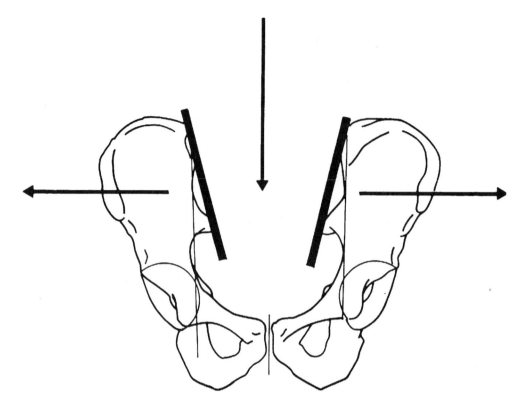

Figure 3–13 The caudally converging form pushes both ilia away from each other.

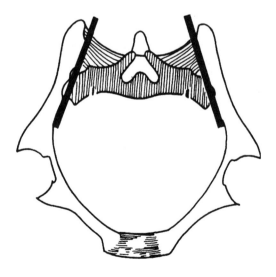

Figure 3–14 Orientation of the surfaces of the SI joints in the transverse plane.

Equilibrium of Moments

The upper body's center of gravity is ventrally located in relation to the SI joint. Therefore, the weight of the upper body induces a ventrally directed moment, M, in which $M = G \times a$ in relation to the sacroiliac joint (Figure 3–16). In order to meet the requirements necessary for an equilibrium of moments there has to be a dorsally directed moment evident in the same magnitude. This moment is supplied by the resistance in the SI joint, the ligaments, and the muscles (erector spinae) bridging this joint at its dorsal aspect.

It is generally accepted that the muscles around a joint are primarily meant to maintain an equilibrium in relation to the joint, and that the capsuloligamentous complex has a guiding function or a motion-restricting function (especially under extreme load situations).

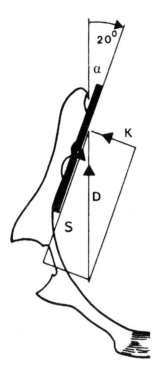

Figure 3–15 The force components **K** and **S** act on the joint surface in the transverse plane.

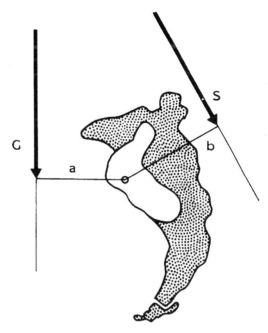

Figure 3–16 The equilibrium of moments in relation to the SI joint.

The question remains whether this assumption holds true for the SI joint, given the small amount of mobility in this joint. In the following section, the physical properties of the SI joint are discussed, as well as how the joint is able to provide enough resistance in order to establish a countermoment.

If only the active elements, in other words the dorsally located lumbar muscles, are providing the equilibrium of moments the following applies: $G \times a = S \times b$, in which $G \times a$ is the ventrally directed moment and $S \times b$ the dorsally directed moment. S is the magnitude of the force furnished by the lumbar muscles, with b being the moment arm of this force in relation to the SI joint (Figure 3–16).

From the equation above the following applies: $S = G \times a/b$. If a and b are equal in magnitude, then the force, S, supplied by the lumbar muscles is of the same magnitude as the weight, G, of the upper body. This assumption has already been mentioned. With a change in the position of the pelvis there will also be a change in the moment arms a and b. The relation between a and b directly determines the magnitude of the muscle force that must be supplied. Therefore, it is possible that through a change of posture the lumbar muscles can be more or less brought into relaxation. Taking into consideration the location and dimension of the lumbar back muscles, it is obvious that these muscles can supply enough force to meet the necessary requirements in maintaining the equilibrium of moments.

PHYSICAL BEHAVIOR OF THE SI JOINT

In order to be able to assess a change in the mobility of the SI joint, it is important to have an idea of the normal mobility in the joint. Every SI joint consists of two bony parts connected by means of a joint capsule and ligaments. Because this capsuloligamentous complex possesses some elastic properties, a relative movement in the joint can take place

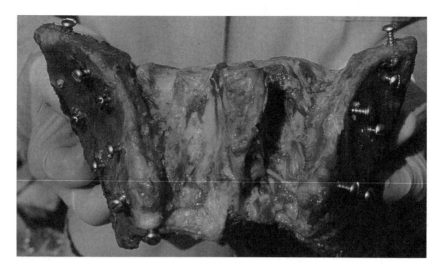

Figure 3–17 A cadaver section of the SI joint.

through an elastic deformation of the composing parts. If the properties of both SI joints are different, a difference in relative motion of both innominates in relation to the sacrum may occur. In the end, this could result in an asymmetrical pelvis.

In order to determine the mobility in the SI joint quantitatively, the elastic properties of the SI joint were determined in 10 fresh cadavers (Figure 3–17). Because the average age of the human material was 55 years, the resulting values for the elastic properties were relatively low. In the biological material of young people the elasticity is greater, and therefore the stiffness is less.

The relations between forces and moments on one side and displacement and rotation on the other side determine the physical properties of the SI joint, as we consider it here. Six kinds of stiffness can be distinguished. Three of these types of stiffness are created by the force-translation relationship and the other three describe the relation between moment and rotation in each of the three directions.

During the experimental determination of the different kinds of stiffness an innominate was placed in a clamp whereby only a connection between ilium and sacrum was apparent.

All other ligaments were removed, along with the connection at the pubic symphysis. A load of 300 N was applied along the x, y, and z axes, respectively, and then a moment of 40 Nm, was applied around these axes, as illustrated in Figure 3–18.

The x axis is a horizontal axis located in the frontal plane. The y axis is a vertical axis located in the frontal plane, and the z axis is perpendicular to both the x and y axes and points in an anterior-posterior direction. The origin of this coordinate system is located at the level of S1. The forces were applied at the origin of this coordinate system, and then the corresponding displacements along, and the rotations around, the three axes were measured.

The relation between the load on the sacrum and the displacement of this load is defined as the stiffness of the joint. Expressed in a formula, load = stiffness × displacement. In illustrating the relation between load and displacement in a graph, the stiffness is equal to the angle of the slope of the line showing this relation (Figure 3–19).

The six kinds of stiffness of the SI joint, three translations and three rotations, are illustrated in Figure 3–20 by six graphs. The loads and the moments are depicted along

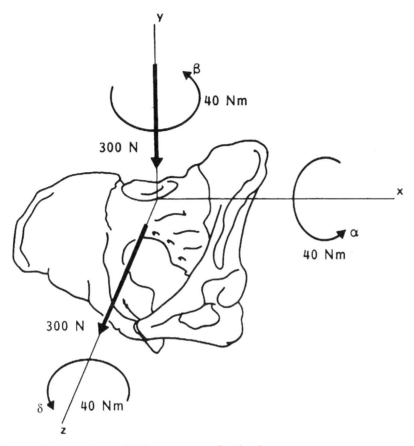

Figure 3–18 The coordinate system with the corresponding loads.

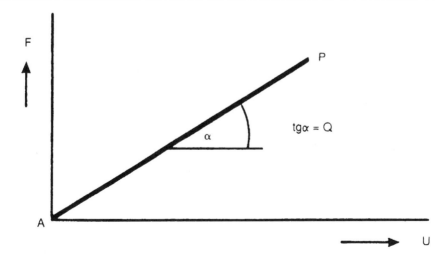

Figure 3–19 The relation between the load, **F**, and the displacement, **U**. For stiffness, **Q** applies (**Q** = **F/U**) and is equal to the slope of the line.

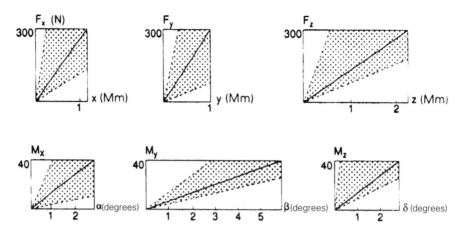

Figure 3–20 The six stiffness quotients of the sacroiliac joint.

the vertical axes. The translations and rotations are indicated along the horizontal axes. These correspond to the direction of the load. In each graph the dotted lines represent the area of the dispersion of the forces. Within the area of dispersion, 90% of all observations are localized. The solid straight line in each graph can be regarded as a representative amount of the average stiffness. These average amounts of stiffness are used in a following section for a biomechanical model of the pelvis. According to the data from Figure 3–20, the following average amounts are given:

Translation stiffnesses in N/mm:
Medial-lateral direction Qx: 260
Vertical direction Qy: 300
Anterior-posterior direction Qz: 133

Rotation stiffnesses in Nm/degree:
Flexion/extension $Q\alpha$: 14.7
Axial rotation $Q\beta$:   6.8
Lateral bending $Q\delta$: 14.7

In comparing the six graphs one notes that the stiffness quotients, Qx and Qy, in the frontal plane (the X-Y plane) are about equal. In the anterior-posterior direction (the Z direction) the stiffness is approximately half the

stiffness in the frontal plane. Thus in an equal load the displacement will be twice the displacement in the frontal plane. However, in an upright posture, the load in the anterior-posterior direction is much smaller than in the vertical direction. Therefore, the translations in all three directions are of the same magnitude. From this one sees that the structures have adapted to the demands placed on them. Throughout the musculoskeletal system this pattern is often encountered. Structures adapt to the demands placed on them—adaptation is a phenomenon that repeats itself.

Of the rotation stiffness quotients of the sacrum in relation to the ilium, the side-bending and the flexion have the same magnitude. The torsion stiffness in flexion and sidebending is half the rotation stiffness. This means that with the same moment, the axial rotation is twice the amount of flexion and sidebending. Here too, under normal circumstances, the torsion load is much smaller than the load in the frontal or sagittal planes.

The most important stiffness quotients are now known for the SI joint: these are the stiffness quotients according to the direction of the applied load. With the help of the available stiffness quotients, it is now possible to determine movement in the SI joint as a result of an arbitrary load on the sacrum. For a weight of the upper body of 500 N and a symmetrical posture (weight distributed equally on both legs), there is a vertical load on each SI joint of 250 N. The vertical displacement, Y, of the sacrum in relation to the ilium is as follows: $Y = Fy/Qy = 250/300 = 0.83$ mm.

Because of the location of the upper body's center of gravity in relation to the SI joint, a ventrally directed moment will be present. Suppose the working arm of this weight in relation to the SI joint in an upright position equals 0.1 m, then the moment will be 500 N × 0.1 m = 50 Nm. With a passive countermoment of both SI joints—without muscle activity—there will be a flexion moment of 25 Nm induced on each joint. Based on the given rotation stiffnesses this will be a ventral rotation of the sacrum of 25/14.7 = 1.7°. With a simultaneous active countermoment supplied by the back muscles, this rotation will be much smaller.

With less rotation due to the countermoment of the back muscles, the SI joint is loaded with a larger force, resulting in an increase in the translation.

The amount of rotation is greater in forward bending. A maximally flexed position can be attained without activity of the back muscles. The working arm of 0.1 m is tripled or quadrupled in this position, which can increase the rotation of the sacrum up to 5°.

Two points should be mentioned here. First of all, the various stiffness quotients of the SI joint were determined by means of relatively old material (cadavers). In younger individuals the average value for the different stiffness quotients will be smaller. Furthermore, the amounts given for the range of motions apply when only the capsuloligamentous complex of the SI joint is taken into consideration. Taking into account the structures connecting both innominates, and the structures connecting the lumbar spine to both innominates, the given range of motions are the maximal range of motions according to the clinical studies.

An often-used clinical method of determining pelvic stability was described by Chamberlain in 1930.[7] While the patient stands with the entire body weight on one leg, whereby the other leg hangs freely, an anterior-posterior (AP) radiological image is obtained. Movement noted at the symphysis is used as a tool in determining motion in the SI joint. An upper margin of this relative movement is 2 mm. Increased movement at the pubic symphysis is usually accompanied by pain from the SI joints.

INFLUENCE OF THE GEOMETRICAL AND PHYSICAL FACTORS ON THE MECHANICAL BEHAVIOR OF THE SI JOINT

In studying different stiffness quotients of the SI joints, the large range in the observations is striking. From a practical point of view, it is important to know whether a deviating behavior in relation to the average is caused by a deviated behavior of the elastic in the joint or by a deviated geometry. Insight can be gained, only by experimental means, first by carrying out a large number of observations and then by analyzing these observations statistically.

Through a mathematical description of the pelvic system one can gain, in a simple and quick manner, insight into the influence of the various parameters on the total behavior of the SI joint. Scholten et al.[8,9] developed a biomechanical model of the pelvis. An overview of the most important findings is given without going too deeply into the mathematical aspects, the suppositions, and the limitations of this model. The following influencing factors are discussed:

- the orientation of the surface of the SI joint represented by an angle, B, in the transverse plane, and an angle, C, in the frontal plane (Figure 3–21)
- the width of the sacrum
- the horizontal distance between both hip joints
- the influence of the physical properties of the SI joint

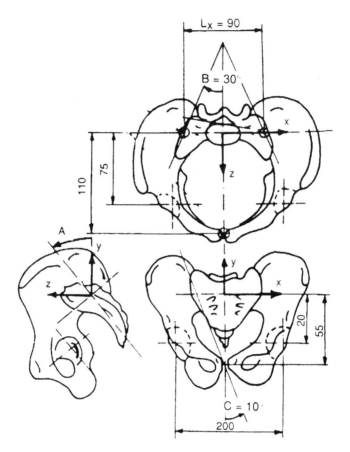

Figure 3–21 The geometrical parameters of the pelvis.

- the influence of the position of the pelvis and the inclination of the sacrum

Through experimental research it has been found that the SI joint shows a strong linear behavior. This means that with an increase in the load, the displacement will decrease proportionally. Furthermore, the displacements in a combined load can be seen as the sum of the displacements of the separate loads.

The presence of a leg length difference can serve as an example. If there is no leg length difference, the pelvis is symmetrically loaded by a force that acts upon the sacrum. This force is from the portion of body weight above the pelvis. With a leg length difference, a lateral tilt of the pelvis occurs. If the spine compensates for this tilt in such a way that the head is positioned vertically above the pelvis, the center of gravity of the mass above the pelvis will not be located perpendicular above the pelvis, but instead at a small distance from the vertical through the sacrum and the head. The weight of the mass above the pelvis results not only in a vertical force but also in a lateral moment acting upon the sacrum. This moment is equal to the product of the weight and the distance of the center of gravity to the vertical through the sacrum and pelvis. The effect of both loads can now be interpreted as the sum of the separate loads.

Orientation of the Pelvis

The orientation of the surface of the SI joint has a large influence on the translations in the joint. By increasing the orientation angle, B, of the joint surface in the transverse plane by 10°, from 30° to 40°, the displacement of the sacrum in a lateral direction in relation to the ilium will become five times smaller. This behavior can be explained by the fact that the resistance against compression in the SI joint is much smaller than the resistance against the translation of both joint surfaces in relation to each other. An increase of the transverse wedge angle, B, of the sacrum means that with lateral loading of the SI joint, part of the translation of both joint surfaces in relation to each other increases despite the large resistance to translation, whereas the amount in compression of both joint surfaces, with a lesser stiffness, decreases. This results in less mobility in the lateral direction.

Another consequence of enlarging this angle, B, is an increased mobility in an AP direction. Part of the relative movement in the SI joint decreases by increasing the transverse wedge angle, B. Thus the joint becomes more loaded either in a tensile or in a compressive way. Also, the flexion-extension movement of the sacrum in relation to the ilium increases when angle B increases. However, this influence is much smaller than the influence on the lateral displacement.

The decrease in the orientation angle, C, of the joint surface in the frontal plane from 10° to 0° causes a decrease in lateral mobility by 25%. This parameter does not bear any influence on the other movements.

Width of the Sacrum

The width of the sacrum has a significant influence on the relative motions of the sacrum in the sagittal plane, in other words, in a vertical and in an AP direction. The average width of the sacrum is 90 mm. A narrowing to 70 mm or a widening to 110 mm results in a decrease or an increase of the vertical mobility by approximately 30%, respectively. In an AP direction the effect is well over 40%. This influence can be explained through a load in the SI joint: when a vertical or horizontal force

acts upon the sacrum, the force results not only in a force in the SI joint but also in a moment that is dependent on the width of the sacrum. With a wide sacrum, a larger moment acts in the SI joint. This moment leads to extra motion of the sacrum in relation to both innominates.

Horizontal Distance between Both Hip Joints

The horizontal distance between both hip joints has an influence on the translation of the sacrum in the sagittal plane, in the vertical plane, and also in an AP direction. An increase of the distance by 20% results in an increase of the displacements by 40%. This increased mobility of the sacrum is caused by the fact that the moment arm of the force acting upon the sacrum becomes larger when the distance between both hip joints increases. As a result, both innominates tilt, causing a lateral displacement of both hip joints. Because of the tilting of both innominates, the sacrum translates more.

A change in the distance between both hip joints has almost no influence on the displacement of the sacrum in the lateral direction, on the flexion-extension movement, on the lateral bending, or on the torsion.

Physical Properties of the SI Joint

Of all the physical properties of the SI joint, the resistance against a relative motion of both joint surfaces in relation to each other has a great effect. This resistance is partly determined by the strength of the joint capsule and the ligaments located around the joint and partly by the resistance between both joint surfaces. The latter is determined by the roughness of the joint surface and can be interpreted as a friction resistance. A 25% decrease in the resistance against the relative motion of both joint surfaces in relation to each other in an arbitrary direction results in an increase of the sacral translation in the sagittal plane by 100%. The sidebending and axial rotation of the sacrum in lateral bending and in torsion increases by 150% to 200%.

In vivo, a significant increase in this resistance occurs in an osteoarthritic joint. This increase, which can be seen mainly as a friction resistance, has a strong influence on the displacement in the sagittal plane, the lateral bending, and the torsion. However, it has much less influence on the flexion-extension motion.

A change in the physical properties of the pubic symphysis has almost no influence on the mobility of the SI joints. This is due to the relatively large distance between the SI joints and the symphysis. Therefore, a relative translation of both innominates in the pubic symphysis will result in only a small rotation in the SI joint.

Position of the Pelvis and Inclination of the Sacrum

Further findings in this study indicate that in an upright position, if the sacrum has an average angle of inclination of 40° to 50°, the SI joints possess the greatest stiffness against translations and lateral bending. This corresponds to the pelvic position assumed by most human beings. A more dorsally or ventrally tilted pelvis results in greater mobility in the SI joint. Increased mobility of the SI joint places a larger load on the symphysis. This may explain why people with a hyperlordosis, and thereby a ventrally tilted sacrum, have more frequent complaints of pain in the pubic symphysis.

KINEMATICS OF THE SI JOINT

The relative movements in the previously described SI joint mobility measurements are of the same magnitude as the ones that are palpable in vivo in younger individuals (see section 3.2, Examination). It is of particular clinical and therapeutic importance to know how the different motion possibilities are mu-

tually coupled. Movement of the sacrum in space in relation to both ilia can be interpreted as a rotatory motion around an axis and a translation along that axis. In kinematical terms this axis is called a helical axis.

In a uniplanar or two-dimensional motion one speaks of a rotational pole. The motion, then, is a rotation around this pole. It is obvious that an arbitrary two-dimensional motion of a body will not always rotate around the same point. Translation of this body occurs due to the fact that the motion pole changes its place. This means that in a three-dimensional movement the helical axis is not a fixed axis. This conclusion is supported by the previously described mobility measurements. Besides rotatory motions there are also translatory motions in the SI joint.

One helical axis in the motion of two bony structures moving in relation to each other can be determined—the relative helical axis. This means that there are three relative helical axes present: (1) one axis describes the motion of the right ilium in relation to the sacrum or the motion of the sacrum in relation to the right ilium (this is one and the same axis); (2) a second axis is found for the movement between the sacrum and the left ilium; and (3) a third axis is found by observing the movement of both ilia in relation to each other.

The localization and position of a helical axis is determined by three factors: the load, the geometry of the joint surfaces, and the physical properties of the connecting elements between both joint parts. Because of the variation in these three influencing factors and the relatively small mobility in the SI joint, it is not easy to give a clear description of the position of the helical axis of the sacrum in relation to the ilium.

Presence of arthrosis in the SI joint makes the description of the motions particularly difficult. First, the relative motion is significantly diminished. Second, an arthrosis in the SI joint can be very localized, and this will influence the position of the helical axis. The position of the helical axis will move, usually in the direction of the joint affected.

The above-mentioned influencing factors have led to different theories concerning the location and the direction of the axes of rotation when the sacrum moves in relation to one or both ilia. Most of these theories are supported more by presumptions than by scientific research. Faraboeuf[10] and Bonnaire and Bue[11] describe the movement of the sacrum in relation to both ilia after measuring the different pelvic diameters in various positions of the human body. According to Faraboeuf, the rotation axis is a transversal axis located dorsal to the sacrum at the level of the axillary ligament. In a ventral tilting of the sacrum in relation to both ilia, the promontory moves in a ventrocaudal direction and the apex of the sacrum moves in a dorsocranial direction (Figure 3–22).

The sagittal diameter of the pelvic outlet, measured from the pubic symphysis to the coccyx, increases. According to Faraboeuf,[10] this motion is possible in the other direction as well. Therefore, in a dorsal tilting of the sacrum in relation to both ilia, an opposite motion will occur in relation to both ilia around the same transverse axis.

This contradicts the findings of Weisl.[12] Based on X-ray findings, Weisl determined the location of the rotational axis in a motion of the sacrum in relation to both ilia. In this way, the axis of rotation was located about 10 cm below the promontory and changed its position more than 5 cm in different positions of the body. However, a uniform localization as a function of body position could not be determined, as illustrated in Figure 3–23. One disadvantage in Weisl's research is that the X-ray plate was affixed to the pelvis by means of a sturdy band. If one bears in mind the successful results (in terms of decreased SI joint motion and diminished pain) obtained by wearing a so-called "pelvic girdle" in patients with an SI joint instability, then the results of the measurements by Weisl could be seriously compromised.

According to Kapandji[13] both innominates make an abduction during a ventral tilting of the sacrum in relation to both ilia. This abduction movement is chiefly determined by the caudally and dorsally converging surfaces of both SI joints. In a dorsal tilting of the sacrum, both ilia make the opposite motion, an adduction. However, according to Kapandji, the ventral tilting of the sacrum is limited early in the movement by the sacrotuberal, sacrospinous, and ventral sacroiliac ligaments.

Until now only symmetrical motions of the pelvis have been discussed. The kinematics of the SI joints become even more complex when there is an asymmetrical motion due to, for instance, an asymmetrical support of both innominates. According to Lewit[14] each ilium performs an opposite motion during sacral tilting. During walking or standing on one leg, the sacrum is asymmetrically loaded and there is an asymmetrical support of both ilia. This results in different motions in each of the SI joints. The axes of rotations of both SI joints, which merge together in a symmetrical motion, now have their own position and direction. Their location is now determined by the relative motions of both ilia and thus by the mobility of the pubic symphysis.

Because the support of both innominates has an effect on the SI joint kinematics, one

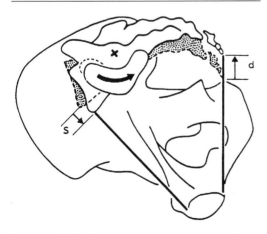

Figure 3–22 Direction of movement of the sacrum during ventral tilting.

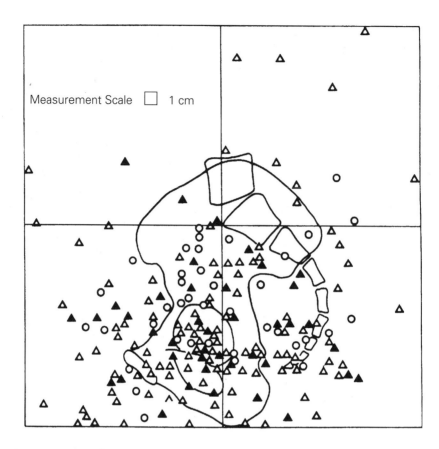

Figure 3–23 Position of the poles of motion in movements from different positions of the body, according to Weisl.[12]

can easily imagine that the mobility in the SI joints is influenced by the hip joints. In time, hip joint pathology may cause a change in the mechanical behavior of the SI joint.

CONCLUSION

In summary, the direction and the location of the axis of rotation in the SI joint depends on three factors: the load and support of the pelvis, the geometry of the joint surfaces, and the physical properties of the connecting elements between both joint parts. The large variety of loads on the SI joint, the possible variations occurring in the joint morphology, and the great variability in the physical properties make kinematics of the SI joint a complex unit. In the clinic, knowledge about the movement of a joint is important. More important, however, is the knowledge of which factors influence the mobility and how these factors are mutually related.

3.2 EXAMINATION

INTRODUCTION

It has been emphasized that the SI joints should not be looked at and examined as an isolated entity. The sacrum is connected to L5 through an intervertebral disc and two zygapophyseal joints, and it is connected with the ilium via the SI joints. Also, the ilium is directly connected to the lumbar spine by the iliolumbar ligaments. Therefore, movement of the ilium in relation to the sacrum will have a direct effect on the lumbar spine, as well as on the segments located more cranially. If one includes the hip flexors, hip adductors, hamstrings, and back and abdominal muscles, in reality the kinematic chain of the legs, pelvis, and back is much more complex than presented here. Directly and indirectly these muscles can influence the movement of the pelvis. In general we are discussing an area that has not received enough attention in orthopaedic medicine. *Examination of the SI joints must be part of the functional examination of the lumbar spine and hips.*

SI JOINT TESTS

Taking into consideration the above philosophy, tests with the sole purpose of testing the SI joints have to be looked at with great suspicion. This is not a new vision. Most schools for manual therapy—where tests of this joint are taught—are more or less aware of and acknowledge this fact. Many of these so-called specific SI tests are not specific at all. In some cases the SI joints are not even tested.

In a roundtable discussion published in the *Newsletter of the North American Academy of Manipulative Medicine* (Volume 3, No. 2, March 1972), Maigne is quoted as saying:

> We once had a meeting and there were very few thinking my way. The diagnostic session dealt with sacroiliac problems and motion testing. One of our fellows was a very good technician in manipulation. I brought two patients. One was a woman, about 30 years of age. I knew she had a problem as she had been a patient with me for some time. I presented her, she was examined by the others, and when I asked for their impressions, I got 10 quite different answers. Anterior sacrum on the left side, anterior sacrum on the right side, posterior sacrum on both sides, etc. In fact, this young lady had no sacroiliac at all. She had congenital fusion of the sacroiliac. But the "tests" were very positive!

Because of Maigne's statement, we examined some of the SI tests more closely. It appears that the most often described tests for SI mobility in the literature, for example, the "leg-length rotation test," can be positive (indicating movement of the joint) in people with a bony junction between the sacrum and the ilium (proven by radiological or computed tomography [CT] scan examination). This is frequently seen in men older than 55 years of age. However, our youngest patient with this finding was 30 years old. Thus, our experiences are comparable with those of Maigne. In addition, it appears that of the 54 various tests described in the literature, only 20 of these are really different from each other.

Tests of the SI joint can be categorized into provocation tests and mobility tests. Amplitudes of movement are examined either in the immediate area of the joint or from a distance. With the provocation tests one tries to ascertain whether the specific pain of the patient can be reproduced by means of either stretching or compressing the SI joint capsuloligamentous structures. With the mobility tests one looks specifically for the amount of movement in the joint.

SI joint tests are rarely the subject of research. Regarding some of the tests, the impression appears to be justified that an expert probably developed a nice idea concerning the SI joint on a Sunday afternoon, and after publication this concept was very often accepted as a new test without any critique. As an example, consider the test whereby the examiner stands at the end of the examination table and asks the patient to come to a sitting position from a supine position. The examiner then determines whether a leg length difference has occurred during this movement into a sitting position. One can easily refute this SI test by having patients perform oblique abdominal exercises. If these patients are tested before and after this exercise, there is sometimes an obvious difference between the two tests. In other words, a right positive result can change over into a left positive result. In view of the fact that the result can be affected by asymmetrical muscle tone at another level, this test is not specific for the SI joints. This means that this test also can be positive in patients in whom one or both SI joints are totally or partially ossified whereby movement is no longer possible (Figure 3–24). It seems to be senseless to learn the many SI tests until there has been adequate research on what these tests are, in fact, based on. Through anatomy and biomechanics, we will try to discuss these tests in general and without pretension. We realize that this is not the critical discussion that everyone has been waiting for.

Provocation Tests

Both the lower lumbar spine and the SI joint are innervated by sensory nerves de-

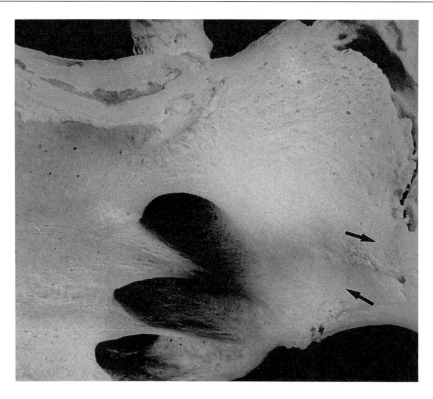

Figure 3–24 Bony bridge between the sacrum and the ilium in a 48-year-old man. Similar bridges can occur even at the age of 30 years.

rived from the L3 to S2 segments. Thus pain provoked through mobilization of the SI joint is not always caused by SI joint structures. This is of particular significance when the lumbar spine is not fixed or is insufficiently "locked." Nevertheless, it is not known at which exact moment the movement in the SI joint ends, thereby initiating movement in the lumbar spine. From the moment the sacrum starts to move, movement in the lower lumbar spine can occur. Even if the sacrum could be optimally fixed, there could still be a transfer of load to the lumbar spine via the iliolumbar ligaments and back muscles. Because of the similar innervation pattern, the pain elicited cannot be specifically accredited to the SI joint. Therefore, even in the absence of movement in the lumbar spine, pain could still be elicited in structures derived from the L5-S1 segment.

The biomechanical background of most of the tests for the SI joint ligaments is often seen too simply. The idea that when putting load on the leg in different directions only certain parts of the ligaments are being stressed is erroneous; other parts of these ligaments and other tissues are also being stressed.

In our view the most reliable tests for the SI joints are the provocation tests described under Provocation Tests in the section Functional Examination. During these tests parts of the capsuloligamentous complex are tested as selectively as possible by bringing these structures either under stretch or under compression. Through one test, stretch can occur at one part of the capsuloligamentous complex while compression results at another part (Figure 3–25). In these tests, both innominates are moved either away from or toward each other. If this test is positive for pain, then one can assume that there is pathology in the capsuloligamentous complex. Furthermore, it should be kept in mind that the symphysis is also being loaded during this test. In addition, this test can provoke pain due to distortion or stress of bone and/or muscles. Nonetheless, although one must

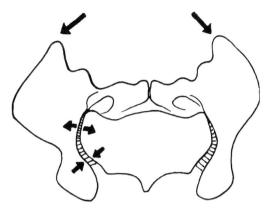

Figure 3–25 By pushing both anterior-superior iliac spines in a dorsolateral direction, stretch occurs on part of the capsuloligamentous complex while other structures are compressed.

also critically judge the findings of this test, empirically this test is the most sensitive test of all.

Mobility Tests

It is accepted that there are chiefly two movements in the SI joints, and there are also accessory movements that are almost not measurable.[6] The main movements are nutation and counternutation. During nutation the ilium moves dorsal in relation to the sacrum, or the sacrum moves ventral in relation to the ilium. This happens, for example, when one moves from a bipodal into a unipodal position. At that moment, the range of motion in nutation of the weight-bearing side's SI joint is partially or totally taken up. In the nutation movement, the distance between the promontorium and the pubic symphysis diminishes at the level of the pelvic entrance, whereas the distance between the sacral apex and the pubic symphysis increases at the level of the pelvic exit. With the counternutation movement the exact opposite will occur (Figure 3–26). The amount of movement in the SI joint is very small. Interindividual differences are the rule due to significant variations in form. In addition, there is always a left-right asymmetry. There-

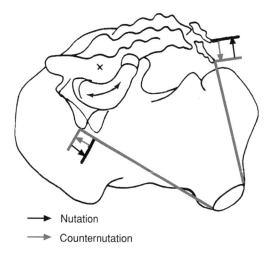

→ Nutation

→ Counternutation

Figure 3–26 The main movements of the SI joint: nutation and counternutation.

fore, assessment of SI joint movement without complicated equipment is almost impossible. After an accident, mobility of one or both joints can pathologically increase, thus making measurement possible at that moment (see the Vorlauf tests). Mobility of the SI joints also increases during pregnancy.

SI joint mobility tests that are performed with a fixed sacrum while moving the ilium are less misleading. Even if one tries to lock the vertebral column, when basing the assessment on a moving sacrum, one will almost inevitably test the spinal segments lying cranial to the SI joints. We performed research on two cadavers without rigor mortis, with intact SI joints (as confirmed during autopsy). Under radiological control 6-in steel pins were inserted into the sacrum at different locations: into both posterior superior iliac spines and into the L4 and L5 spinous processes. We then performed a nutation test as well as a counternutation test. The discussion here is limited to the pins that were inserted at the lumbar level. The movement of these pins clearly demonstrated that there was, without a doubt, no selective SI joint movement. With "purely" performed nutation and counternutation tests, the largest movement occurred in the lumbar spine. An obvious axial rotation occurred at the L4-L5 level as well as at L5-S1 (Figures 3–27 to 3–32).

The simultaneous movement of the lumbar spine can be explained by the fact that the zygapophyseal joints of the L5-S1 segment do not lie entirely in the parasagittal plane. The data of this limited research have to be interpreted with some care; however, the simultaneous movement of the spinal segments lying cranial of the SI joints during mobilization of the sacrum was obvious. By "locking" the lumbar spine (positioning against the coupling movement pattern), one can selectively influence the SI joint. (See section 3.4, Treatment: Manual Mobilization.)

As already mentioned, mobility tests based on a fixed sacrum are more specific. However, there is also a problem here due to the fact that the lumbar spine can be influenced through the iliolumbar ligaments. In addition, the back and the abdominal muscles can transfer forces to the spinal column via the ilium.

Whether one takes the sacrum or the ilium as the moving part, in both situations the examiner tries to determine amplitudes of movement. Therefore the fingers are placed as close as possible to the joint, for instance, one finger on the spinous process of S2 and another finger on the posterior superior iliac spine. *Palpation of the joint itself is impossible; the distance between the skin and the joint line amounts to approximately 2 in in the cranial part and approximately 1 in in the caudal part.* Although this may seem a good method to evaluate movement amplitude, it also has some apparent problems. First of all, the spinous process of S2 is not always easily palpable. Very often the examiner believes to be interpreting firm tissue as "bone" without realizing that the fingers are placed on a moving fascia covered by skin.

This misinterpretation can be illustrated very well by the following small experiment. With the forearm supinated, palpate both the anterior and the posterior aspects of the ulnar

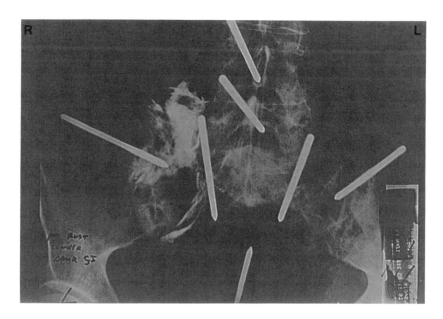

Figure 3–27 X-Ray of a cadaver without rigor mortis with pins in the sacrum, innominate, and the spinous processes of L5 and L4.

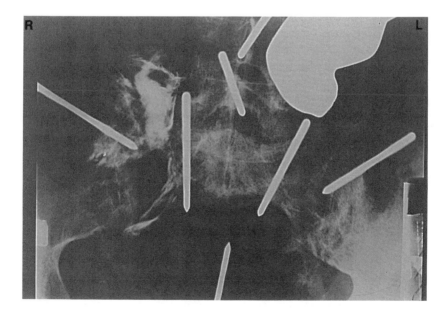

Figure 3–28 The same cadaver as in Figure 3–27 but now a nutation movement (sacrum ventral) is induced at the left side (thumb in lead glove).

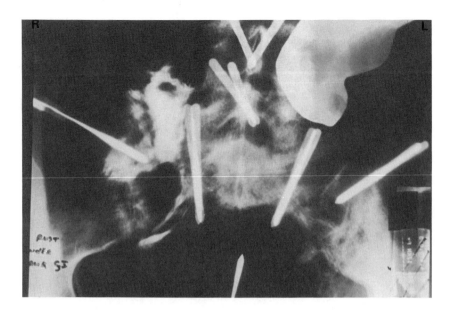

Figure 3–29 Here the X-rays of Figures 3–27 and 3–28 are projected over each other. The greatest amount of motion occurred in the lumbar spine, particularly at L4.

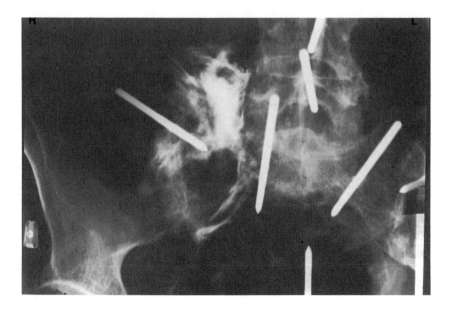

Figure 3–30 X-Ray of a cadaver, without rigor mortis, with pins in the sacrum, innominate, and the spinous processes of L5 and L4.

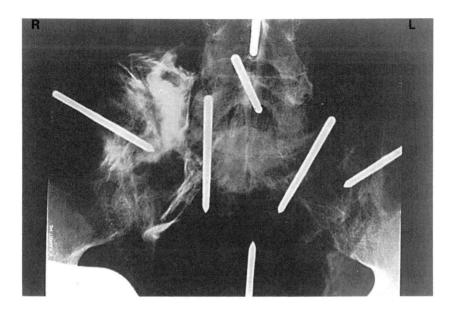

Figure 3–31 The same cadaver as in Figure 3–30, but now a counternutation movement is induced at the left side (innominate rotated ventrally).

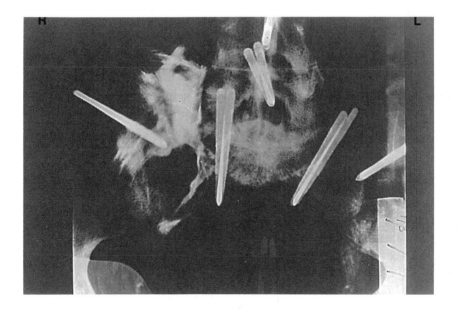

Figure 3–32 Here the X-rays of Figures 3–30 and 3–31 are projected over each other. The greatest amount of motion occurred in the lumbar spine, especially at L5.

head with thumb and index finger. Position the fingers so that no tendons are palpated. The ulnar head is an ideal bony palpation point whereby the bone can be "directly" palpated underneath the fingers. When one pronates the arm one feels that the palpating fingers are moving. It should be very clear that this cannot be caused by a real bony movement because the ulna does not rotate during pronation. The induced torsion of the fascia is interpreted here as the movement of bone.

Recent research has shown that not only the interindividual but also the intraindividual reliability in testing of minimal movements is very small.[15] In SI joint tests, there is also the factor of skin and fascial movements. Differences in the mobility of fascia between the left and right sides may also be of interest but should not be interpreted as a hypo- or hypermobility of an SI joint. If there is a real difference in movement between the left and right SI joints, one still does not know whether this is a pathological condition. SI joints are almost never symmetrical.

In lumbar spine pathology (whatever the cause), hyper-and/or hypotonus and possibly muscle shortening can occur. These muscle changes can alter the movement pattern of the lumbar spine and the SI joints. Tension differences in the fascia should also be included in this consideration. Because of this, one might have the impression that changes in the SI joint itself have taken place. The examiner should be aware of the possibility of a false interpretation due to movements of the fascia and skin.

The SI joint tests experience even another kind of "interference." One tends to "sentence" the living human body to a construction similar to the skeletons studied in school. Too often, one fails to realize that a skeleton, at its best, is only a calcium artifact in which most of the collagen has disappeared. Because the living human skeleton contains a large amount of collagen, it has plastic properties and can be deformed. Also,

until approximately 25 years of age there is palpable movement in the sacrum because the sacral vertebrae are not yet completely fused. If one pushes on the cranial or caudal aspect of the sacrum in fresh cadavers, this results (according to our research) in a significant deformation of the sacrum. Thus, in the interpretation of SI joint tests, one must always realize that bone deformation can play a role. During testing, when one pushes on the sacrum, the palpating fingers are feeling not only the movement but also the deformation of the sacrum.

Furthermore, as we observed during our research, the ilium can also deform slightly during the SI joint mobility tests.

Sacroiliac Instability and Joint Locking

In a sacroiliac instability and/or locking of the SI joint a triad must be evident:

1. a history that is typical for either an instability or a locking of the joint (or a combination)
2. one or more positive provocation tests
3. a Vorlauf phenomenon

Generally these cases are easy to diagnose. This also counts for most inflammatory SI joint pathology. Making a diagnosis becomes more difficult when a dysfunction arises in one or both SI joints based on pathology of the lumbar spine and/or one or both hip joints. In this instance, one can best work by eliminating other problems. In orthopaedic medicine it is customary that the most obvious findings are treated first, for instance, a lumbar disc protrusion. If the symptoms (too) quickly recur or if some of the symptoms remain, the SI joint may be contributing to the problem and a trial treatment of the SI joint(s) can be given.

Summary

In general, findings from the SI joint tests can be used, at best, in careful combination with the information from the patient history. The step from observation to judgment is much easier to make in other joints. In other joints, the various parts of the kinetic chain can be more easily isolated during the examination. For instance, when a positive Lachman test is found during examination of the knee, one can be almost certain of an anterior cruciate ligament lesion.

As previously mentioned, movement of the fascia and deformation of bone can influence the SI joint mobility tests. Above all, the asymmetrical form of the lumbar spine and the SI joints should be kept in mind when interpreting these mobility tests. If a specific disorder of the SI joint(s) can be observed, this pathology may be caused by pathology at another level of the kinematic chain. In this instance, the clinician has to decide at which level to start treating the disturbance.

Experienced therapists take a specific history and then by means of thorough observation and a series of tests, establish the appropriate and logical treatment plan. In so doing, the patient is not being sentenced to a specific pathology but instead to a disturbance in the movement chain that can be treated on different levels.

FUNCTIONAL EXAMINATION

SI tests are an inseparable part of the examination of a patient with low back pain. For the history, general inspection, palpation, and specific inspection refer to Chapter 4, section 4.2, Examination of the Lumbar Spine. Always compare the affected side with the nonaffected side. The examination is performed in the lying position (the provocation tests) as well as in the standing and sitting positions (the mobility tests).

Provocation Tests

Supine

1. Dorsolateral provocation test (Figure 3–33)

Sidelying

2/3. Ventromedial provocation test (Figure 3–34)

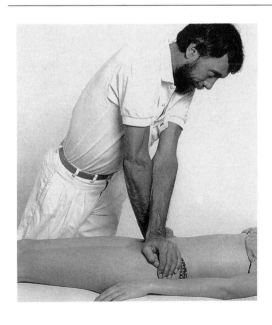

Figure 3–33

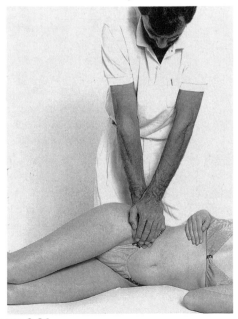

Figure 3-34

4. Counternutation mobilization as provocation test

5. Nutation mobilization as provocation test

Mobility Tests

Standing

6. Vorlauf test in normal standing position (Figure 3–35: 3–35A is initial position and 3–35B is the end position)

7/8. Vorlauf test in standing position on one leg (left/right) (Figure 3–36)

Sitting

9. Vorlauf test in sitting position (Figure 3–37)

In some cases, an additional examination is indicated, as follows:

- laboratory tests when an inflammatory disease is suspected
- plain X-rays and oblique tomography
- Chamberlain view when an instability is suspected (See section 3.3, Pathology.)
- CT scan (This gives more information than the plain X-rays.)

DESCRIPTION OF THE PROVOCATION TESTS

1. Dorsolateral Provocation Test
(Figure 3–33)

Position of the Patient

The patient lies supine with the hips in approximately 15° flexion. The arms are relaxed along the side of the body.

Position of the Examiner

The examiner stands beside the patient at the level of the patient's pelvis.

Performance

The examiner places one hand on each of the patient's anterior superior iliac spines.

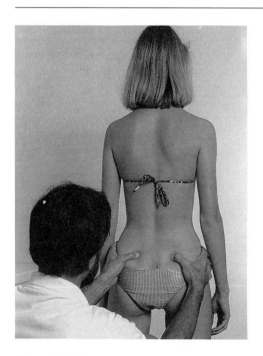

Figure 3–35A

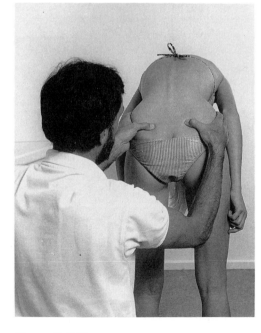

Figure 3–35B

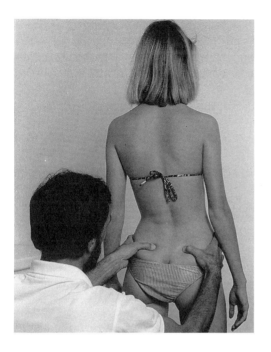

Figure 3–36

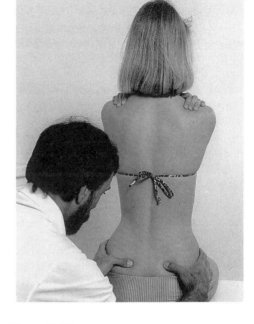

Figure 3–37

The examiner's arms are extended and crossed. The crossing point of the arms is located above the midline of the patient's body. The examiner now exerts pressure downward on both iliac spines with a resultant dorsolateral direction. The patient should be completely relaxed and the pressure maintained until the symptoms are reproduced or for at least 40 seconds in order to be certain that all collagenous structures have undergone a stretch. Then, if the symptoms still have not been provoked, an abrupt overpressure is performed.

Assessment

If the patient's pain is elicited in the midline, the test of the SI joint is negative. If the patient indicates his or her specific unilateral pain, however, the test is repeated with a stabilized lordosis. This can be done very simply by positioning the patient's hand or forearm (depending on the amount of the patient's normal lordosis) under the lumbar spine, tak-

ing care to avoid any increase in the normal lordosis. If the same pain is again provoked, then this test is determined to be positive for the SI joint.

2/3. Ventromedial Provocation Test
(Figure 3–34)

Position of the Patient

The patient lies on either side with the pelvis in a vertical position. The hips are flexed approximately 15° and the knees are in a comfortable amount of flexion to stabilize the sidelying position. The patient lies with the back as close as possible to the edge of the treatment table.

Position of the Examiner

The examiner stands behind the patient at the level of the patient's pelvis. The treatment table is positioned to a height of the therapist's patellas.

Performance

The examiner places the palm of the hand as flat as possible on the ventrolateral aspect of top innominate, reinforced by the other hand. Now the patient's pelvis is rolled slightly forward (out of a pure vertical position) in order to have the most effective compression from both sides of the pelvis. The examiner extends both arms with the shoulders positioned perpendicular above the hands. The test is performed twice, once on each side.

Assessment of the Provocation Tests

The test is positive when the patient's specific pain is provoked. Pain at the midline cannot be caused by the SI joints.

Because of the complex innervation of the SI capsuloligamentous structures, pain can be experienced in various regions. This can vary from pain in the back (paravertebral) and the gluteal region to pain in the groin and/or lower abdomen. In principle the pain can be felt in one or more dermatomes ranging from L3 to S2. The provocation tests can be positive in different disorders of the SI joints: in the active stage of an arthritis (for example, ankylosing spondylitis, Reiter's disease, rheumatoid arthritis, and gout), in a sacroiliac instability, and in a locking of the SI joint.

The two remaining provocation tests (test 4, counternutation mobilization as provocation test, and test 5, nutation mobilization as provocation test) are discussed under section 3.4, Treatment: Manual Mobilization. If the nutation motion is forced upon the joint and the SI joint is locked in a nutation position, the patient will experience (more) pain. In this case treatment consists of mobilization in the counternutation direction. On the other hand, if the counternutation is forced upon the joint when the SI joint is locked in a counternutation position, more pain will be elicited. Here the treatment consists of mobilization in the opposite direction.

The SLR test can also be positive in various SI joint pathologies. This is especially true when the tendon of the biceps femoris either partly or totally inserts on the sacrotuberal ligament.

From the tests described above, the first test will *always* be positive in an *active* stage of an arthritis in the SI joint. The same holds true for a (radiologically proven) SI instability. For now, in order to diagnose a locked SI joint we will take the view that the provocation tests must also be positive in combination with the specific history and the sometimes less obvious Vorlauf phenomenon at the locked side in both standing and sitting positions.

DESCRIPTION OF THE MOBILITY TESTS

Sometimes the so-called Vorlauf phenomenon can be of diagnostic significance. The Vorlauf phenomenon is examined in four different positions of the patient:

6. Normal standing position (Figure 3–35) (Figure 3–35A is initial position and Figure 3–35B is end position)
7/8. Standing position on one leg (left/right) (Figure 3–36)
9. Sitting position (Figure 3–37)

The results of these four tests are combined with the history and the results of the provocation tests.

6. Vorlauf Test in Normal Standing Position

Position of the Patient

The patient stands in normal standing position (feet about shoulder width apart) with weight equally distributed on each leg and with the posterior aspect of the heels in the same frontal plane.

Position of the Examiner

The examiner sits or squats behind the patient. The examiner palpates the caudal aspect of each of the patient's posterior superior iliac spines (PSISs) (Figure 3–35A).

Performance

The patient is asked to bend forward slowly in the sagittal plane. He or she is instructed to flex the head first, followed by the thoracic spine, then the lumbar spine, and finally the hips. In this way emphasis is placed on flexion with the SI joints in relation to their location in the kinetic chain, the spine cranial and the hip joints caudal. By means of palpation, the examiner tries to determine the movement of both PSISs during the flexion motion (Figure 3–35B).

Because the skin becomes stretched over the iliac spines during lumbar flexion, before the patient starts to bend forward, the examiner's thumbs push some of the more caudal lying skin in a cranial direction. This way there will be enough play in the skin to avoid misinterpretation through movement of the skin.

Assessment

One speaks of a Vorlauf phenomenon during forward flexion when one PSIS moves cranially earlier than the other. The interpretation is not easy. A Vorlauf phenomenon occurs in many people without any clinical significance. This can be the result of the following:

- asymmetry of the SI joints
- asymmetry of both innominates
- rotational position and/or torsion of the lumbar vertebrae
- leg length differences

If the provocation tests are negative, then the Vorlauf phenomenon cannot be interpreted as a positive SI joint test. In combination with the positive provocation test(s) the Vorlauf phenomenon can be relevant. The amount of translation in the SI joint is very small; even in the case of an instability it still consists of only a few millimeters. However, the trajectory of the PSIS is much greater

than what takes place in the joint itself. If the Vorlauf phenomenon is observed at the nonpainful side, one can assume that there is probably an SI instability. If the Vorlauf phenomenon is seen on the painful side, there is probably a locked SI joint.

7/8. Vorlauf Test in Standing Position on One Leg (Left/Right)

Position of the Patient

The patient stands on one leg. The foot of the other leg has contact with the floor, but it has no weight on it. The transfer of weight occurs through a horizontal shift of the pelvis and trunk in the direction of the weight-bearing leg.

Position of the Examiner

Same as for test 6.

Performance

Same as for test 6, except the patient is now weight bearing on one leg.

Assessment

When the body weight is transferred onto one leg, a nutation movement occurs in the SI joint on that side, which takes up the slack in that joint. This means that a Vorlauf phenomenon at the weight-bearing side is physiological. In cases of an instability (regardless of which side is affected) the physiological Vorlauf phenomenon will occur during flexion. In cases of a locked SI joint, there will be no Vorlauf phenomenon during the forward bending with unipodal weight bearing on the nonaffected side.

9. Vorlauf Test in Sitting Position

Position of the Patient

The patient sits on the treatment table with the upper legs slightly abducted and with both popliteal fossas in contact with the edge of the table. The feet rest flat on the floor.

Position of the Examiner

Same as for test 6.

Performance

Same as for test 6.

Assessment

Same as for test 6. The advantage of testing in this position is that a leg length difference, which is present in almost everyone, is eliminated. Also a possible hamstring shortening cannot influence the test in an adverse way. Thus, in the instance of either an unstable or a locked SI joint, a positive Vorlauf test in standing must be reconfirmed in sitting. (See Appendix A, Interpretation of the Vorlauf Phenomenon in Sacroiliac Joint Locking and Instability.)

3.3 PATHOLOGY

INTRODUCTION

Sacroiliac joint pathology can be classified into four different groups:

1. inflammatory disorders
2. instability
3. intra-articular derangement (locking)
4. other mechanical disturbances

Inflammations of the SI joint generally are not difficult to diagnose. The same is true for instability and intra-articular locking. Other mechanical disturbances involve problems that arise as a result of disorders in the other joints of the pelvic girdle. In most cases, this concerns the hip joint or lumbar spine disease.

Several rheumatoid-related illnesses can involve symptoms of the SI joint. The variety of clinical disorders, however, has been proven to be very small. In this section, the most frequently seen pathological conditions are described. When possible the differential diagnosis is discussed.

Despite the fact that an infectious sacroiliitis is extremely rare, it is thoroughly discussed in this section. In these disorders it is possible to prove that the SI joint alone is affected. Therefore, the symptomatology is helpful in the description of other SI joint disorders.

ACUTE SACROILIITIS

In attempting to classify the symptoms in an acute sacroiliitis a problem arises because some therapists make their diagnosis based exclusively on clinical appearances. The most useful classifications come from studies in which the diagnosis is also based on aspiration, biopsy, or imaging techniques. However, in purulent sacroiliitis one should always take into account that aspirated joint fluid is usually mixed with blood. If the blood cultures in these patients are positive, this means an aspiration that also tests positive cannot be used to confirm the existence of a purulent sacroiliitis.

Etiology

Infection is the most common cause for an acute sacroiliitis, in which there is almost always a unilateral involvement. Although it rarely happens, gout as well as pyrophosphate arthropathies can also cause an acute arthritis in the SI joint.

Only with great exception is a severe acute sacroiliitis encountered in ankylosing spondylitis and its related diseases. The chronic sacroiliitis seen in patients with ankylosing spondylitis is usually clinically and radiologically symmetrical. However, especially in the initial stage of the disease, the sacroiliitis can be acute (severe) and unilateral.

Clinical Findings

- Generally, in an acute severe sacroiliitis the patient complains mostly of pain at the site of the affected joint. This is usually accompanied by ipsilateral radiating pain into the buttock and posterior aspect of the thigh to the popliteal fossa. Some patients experience pain in the calf and even into the heel. Pain in the lower abdomen and groin are the main symptoms in 1% to 2% of patients.

- Every motion causing movement in the SI joint is avoided by the patient. The patient limps during walking, but prefers to lie flat in bed with the hip and knee joints of the affected side in a relaxed position (usually slightly flexed). Children often lie more on the nonaffected than on the affected side. Children who are too young to express themselves refuse to stand or walk.

- Because there are no monoarticular muscles that can selectively "lock" the SI joint, every shock causes pain. Therefore, coughing, sneezing, walking, and even (if the patient is a child) being carried are painful. Running into an object (such as the bed) is also painful.

- In the functional examination, every motion in the SI joint exacerbates the pain. Not only are the specific SI joint provocation tests positive, but also the passive hip motions (from both the ipsilateral and the contralateral hips) are painful at end-range as well. The same is found with the lumbar spine motions. Except for hip flexion, the mobility of the hip joints is normal.

- The total motion of bringing the thigh to the trunk in hip flexion is limited; however, this motion does not take place exclusively in the hip joint. In more than about 70° flexion (depending on the flexibility of the hip joint), increasing pain is provoked. Depending on the length of the hamstrings, the SLR test causes increased pain from approximately 50° on. This combination of a limited and painful SLR test with limited and painful hip flexion is known as the "sign of the buttock."[16]

- Sometimes local warmth and/or swelling is palpable in the upper inner quadrant of the buttock. There is almost always pain on percussion of the soft tissue covering the bony prominences of the innominate and the greater trochanter of the affected side. The gluteals, the piriformis, and the iliopsoas (as far as this muscle is accessible to palpation), as well as the sciatic nerve along its course in the buttock and thigh, are also tender to palpation.

- On rectal examination the ligaments connecting the sacrum and the innominate are often tender to palpation (sacrotuberous and sacrospinous ligaments).

Acute Severe Infectious Sacroiliitis

In an infectious sacroiliitis the patient not only shows the signs and symptoms described above, but also shows signs of an infection. Usually the patient has a fever (varying from subfebrile to 104°) and complains of a general feeling of malaise. In addition, the blood tests indicate an infection: a high erythrocyte sedimentation rate (ESR) (50 to 130 mm/h is not exceptional) and leukocytosis (12 to 15×10^9/L, sometimes up to 30).

Strangely enough, a large number of patients with severe sacroiliitis do not demonstrate leukocytosis. In some studies, besides severe pain, high temperature, and high ESR, approximately half of the patients have a leukocyte number under 10×10^9/L. Through blood culture and joint aspiration it is possible to isolate the cause of the disease in about 50% of all patients.

Radiological examinations do not show any pathological findings within the first few weeks of the onset. However, it is very wise to take X-ray films of the SI joints in order to have the ability to compare later X-ray films with the initial ones.

After 2 weeks, the radiological findings are rather nonspecific (Table 3–1). Particularly in the initial stage of a suspected sacroiliitis, a bone scan with technetium or gallium might provide additional information. However, its usefulness should not be overestimated. Possibly a leukocyte scan or a CT scan can be helpful if local complications are suspected.

Etiology

Bacteria can reach the SI joint through hematogenic or lymphatic pathways or directly from the surrounding tissues.

In about 30% of all patients it is impossible to determine a clear cause. A hematogenic pathway is obvious in patients with infections elsewhere in the body: throat, nose, or ear infections; abscesses in the roots of the teeth; and endocarditis. A pathway can also be found in intravenous drug users. Lymphatic dissemination through the Batson's venous plexus seems to be the cause for an incidental sacroiliitis caused by infections in the lesser pelvis. Possibly increased pressure within the pelvis, such as during pregnancy, is an extra risk (Table 3–2).

In the literature, it was once reported that a patient had a bacterial sacroiliitis and an infection of the great toe on the same side. The same bacterium was cultured from the SI joint and the great toe. Of course, bacterial sacroiliitis can be caused by an osteomyelitis of the surrounding bony structures (usually the ilium). Another case report described an infection that arose after the patient received an injection in and around the SI joint.[16]

Treatment

Treatment for infectious sacroiliitis consists of administration of antibiotics, preferably guided by the culture. The nature of the cause depends on the port of entry. The most common causes of infection are bacteria from the *staphylococcus* group (Table 3–3). If treatment is started early enough, the illness can usually be cured without any residual complications.

If the diagnosis is made too late, the infection can easily cause further complications of osteomyelitis (mainly of the ilium) and formation of abscesses that can spread underneath the gluteal muscles as well as the iliopsoas (with peritoneal irritation). In rare cases, the infection can spread to the hip joints or to the lumbar spine. Sometimes fistulas to the skin, intestines, or vagina develop. In the days when antibiotics were not available, one of every three patients died of this disorder.

Surgical intervention is necessary if formation of abscesses, fistulas, or a sequestration occurs. An arthrodesis is generally performed at the same time.

Table 3–1 Radiological Abnormalities in Acute Sacroiliitis

Time after Infection	Findings
0–2 wk	None
2–4 wk	Fading of the joint contours, especially caudal; decalcification of subchondral bone with pseudowidening of the joint line
4–6 wk	Erosions (mainly at the iliac side), sometimes visible only on tomograms (sometimes only on oblique views) or CT scan
After 6 wk	Increased density of the subchondral bone (mainly at a certain distance away from the joint); this phenomenon is often accompanied by decalcification and erosions, just underneath the joint cartilage
6–12 mo after healing	Stabilized situation with ankylosis (totally or partially); permanent erosion with or without subchondral increased density

Table 3–2 Risk Factors for Infectious Sacroiliitis

- Infections somewhere in the body, especially within the intestinal region
- Medical procedures that can cause bacteremia
- Intravenous use of drugs
- Pregnancy and childbirth
- Increased mobility of the joint
- Trauma
- Immunodeficiency

Predilection age: 20–30 y

In the instance of poor reaction to the treatment, or when there is uncertainty about the correct diagnosis (for instance, if tuberculosis cannot be ruled out), a biopsy is indicated. Bacteriological and histological examinations should be performed on the biopsied tissue. High doses of antibiotics should be administered for 3 to 10 weeks (depending on the severity and the duration of the disorder).

If the treatment period is too short, there is a chance either for recurrence or that the disease may become a less severe chronic condition. These risks are also present when the dosage is too low and/or the wrong antibiotic is administered.

In the preantibiotic era, the incidence of acute infectious sacroiliitis was much higher than it is nowadays. Recently, however, an increased incidence has been observed because heroin users have a relatively high risk of contracting this disease. In this high-risk group, any of the joints in the body can be affected, but the SI joints are a particular predilection site.[17] Other risk factors are mentioned in Table 3–2.

Table 3–3 The Most Common Bacterial Causes of Acute Infectious Sacroiliitis

- *Staphylococcus* (approximately 65%)
- *Streptococcus* (approximately 20%)
- Enterococcus (approximately 10%)
- *Pseudomonas aeruginosa*
- Pneumococcus

Differential Diagnosis

Confusion between infectious sacroiliitis and many other diseases is possible. Usually it is very difficult to differentiate this condition from osteomyelitis (Table 3–4). In osteomyelitis of the ilium, the functional examination can be less clearly positive. However, it is only possible to differentiate through CT scan and radioisotope scan. Magnetic resonance imaging may also be helpful in this matter.

Distinguishing between ankylosing spondylitis and related diseases can be difficult if the infection is not manifested by fever or blood toxicity. However, an ankylosing spondylitis seldom presents with a severe sacroiliitis and above all is almost always bilateral. In most instances, a thorough history, clinical examination of the other joints, and further radiological findings will be helpful in making the diagnosis. In cases of doubt, it is best to treat the condition as if there were an infection.

Differentiating a disorder of the SI joint from pain with a lumbar origin is always difficult. Patients with pain of lumbar origin often indicate the same localization and the same tender points. Because of the mechanical coupling of the movements of the lower lumbar vertebrae with the SI joints, differentiation through functional tests can sometimes be very difficult. Naturally, in instances of paresthesia, paresis, sensory disturbances, or changes in reflexes of the affected side there is a strong indication of neurological complications from the lumbar spine. However, a sacroiliitis can also cause neurological complications when the formations of abscesses compress the sciatic or femoral nerves.

Because of the fact that such neurological complications very seldom occur in sacroiliitis (and only do occur when the illness has spread to such an extent that there is no longer any doubt about the diagnosis), it can be assumed that in cases of doubt, neurological symptoms indicate a lesion of the lumbar spine. Because the SLR test is often very painful and therefore severely limited in a sacroiliitis, one cannot use this sign for differentiation. In that case, it is better to stretch the tibial nerve at the popliteal fossa by manually hooking it with the knee in a slightly bent position and the hip in 90° flexion (bowstring sign). Also, the absence of pain during the segmental mobility examination of the lumbar spine makes a lumbar disorder less probable.

Sometimes disorders of the retroperitoneal organs or of the organs in the lesser pelvis are also suspected in patients with sacroiliitis. Usually peritoneal irritation, fever, and general malaise are the chief signs of these disorders. When a sacroiliitis is suspected, it is usually not difficult to make an exact diagnosis with the help of a clinical examination and additional laboratory testing.

Be aware, however, that diseases of the pelvic organs can cause a sacroiliitis. On the other hand, as already mentioned, complications from a sacroiliitis include abscesses of the psoas and/or gluteal muscles or a septic arthritis of the hip or lumbar spine. Sometimes a urinary obstruction arises as a result of an abscess formation (with pyelitis).

Acute Noninfectious Sacroiliitis

In analogy to inflammations in other joints, an acute sacroiliitis can also have a variety of causes, including trauma, gout, pyrophosphate arthropathy, and rheumatoid arthritis. Some of the patients described in the literature with suspected infectious sacroiliitis probably actually fall into this category, particularly those patients without fever and/or without significant aberrations in their blood counts. Ankylosing spondylitis and related disorders must be mentioned again here; in this instance, the radiological examination does not provide any additional information.

The local findings in noninfectious sacroiliitis are basically the same as those in infectious arthritis. In a pyrophosphate arthropathy a chondrocalcinosis is sometimes visible within the SI joint on radiological imaging. Further differentiation for the cause of the sacroiliitis is based on laboratory findings and

Table 3–4 Differential Diagnosis in Acute Infectious Sacroiliitis.

- Osteomyelitis of the ilium
- Gluteal abscess
- Appendicitis, diverticulitis, adnexitis, pyelitis
- Coxitis
- Herniated disc, discitis, meningitis
- Ankylosing spondylitis, rheumatoid arthritis, Reiter's disease, psoriatic arthritis, gout, pyrophosphate arthropathy

clinical examination, including examination of the other joints.

CHRONIC SACROILIITIS

In analogy to the classification of inflammations in peripheral joints, the term *chronic sacroiliitis* is indicated when the disorder exists longer than 6 weeks. Although the adjectives *chronic* and *acute* do not indicate the severity of the inflammation, in the clinic (and often in word usage) a chronic arthritis is considered less severe than an acute arthritis. Thus, the symptoms of a chronic arthritis are essentially no different from those of an acute arthritis.

The pain is experienced at the same sites as in the acute form; however, the pain generally radiates less distally. Often the pain remains minimal for long periods, with an occasional exacerbation of the pain lasting a few days or months.

Because the symptoms are less intense, most patients are able to walk without problems. A classic feature in this disorder is the "misstep pain": severe pain in the buttock with radiating pain in the leg the instant that the patient either missteps or, for instance, stubs a toe.

Increased pain after prolonged lying is also a characteristic phenomenon. Often the patient wakes up because of pain after having been asleep for 2 to 4 hours. The patient tries to resume sleeping in a different position, but this is usually unsuccessful. Only after getting up and walking for a short period does the pain decrease and allow another short period of sleep.

Whether or not the symptoms are constant and/or are always located on the same side is clinically significant. A general feeling of malaise is almost always present, partly due to the underlying cause of the disease and partly because the patient does not sleep well and experiences pain in many daily activities.

In a long-existing sacroiliitis, signs of instability can occur. Thus the patient's history can change. Initially the patient experiences an exacerbation of the symptoms without any clear cause. Once an instability has arisen, mechanical factors seem to be of greater influence on the pain.

Radiological Findings

The same changes observed in the acute infectious sacroiliitis will eventually also occur in a chronic sacroiliitis. Years can pass before an ankylosing of the joints occurs. Some patients remain in stage 2 or stage 3 for decades (Table 3–1).

It must be emphasized that X-ray films do not reveal the inflammation, but rather the consequences of the inflammation.

Chronic Unilateral Sacroiliitis

A chronic unilateral sacroiliitis should be considered a tuberculosis until the opposite is proven. Tuberculosis is suspected particularly if there are indications of tuberculosis somewhere else in the body (chest X-ray, Mantoux reaction, tuberculosis spondylodiscitis).

Chronic infectious sacroiliitis can also be caused by brucellosis and by an ineffectively treated acute sacroiliitis. Brucellosis is suspected if the history and further examination do not give any indication for tuberculosis. Brucellosis occurs mainly in patients who handle cattle, sheep, or goats or who work with meat, milk, or dairy products of infected animals.

Serological examination is usually necessary in order to make the differentiation between chronic infectious sacroiliitis and brucellosis. An aspiration or a biopsy will settle the matter. Richter and Nübling[18] saw a bilateral involvement of the SI joints in 43 patients with severe tuberculosis of the SI joint. Probably in earlier days tuberculosis was too often thought to be the cause for a bilateral chronic sacroiliitis.

Chronic Bilateral Sacroiliitis

Analogous to the first statement made under chronic unilateral sacroiliitis, the following applies: a chronic bilateral sacroiliitis should be considered as coming from ankylosing spondylitis until the opposite is proven.

In the initial stage of ankylosing spondylitis, however, the sacroiliitis is sometimes unilateral. Sometimes exacerbations cause symptoms that alternate sides. If the disorder has already been present for a long period of time, ossification of the ligaments surrounding the joints and an ankylosis of the joints can develop. In that instance, the signs and symptoms occurring due to the inflammation rapidly decrease and the patient no longer has symptoms. Of course the disorder can become active at other sites in the spinal column and peripheral joints, but a sacroiliitis will never occur again.

Bilateral (sometimes also unilateral) sacroiliitis has a high incidence in rheumatoid-related disorders: psoriasis (Figure 3–38), Reiter's disease, Crohn's disease, ulcerating colitis, juvenile chronic arthritis, reactive arthritis (after intestinal infections), and Behçet's disease. It is seldom seen in rheumatoid arthritis, Whipple's disease, sarcoidosis, Gaucher's disease, ochronosis, and pustulosis palmaris plantaris. In these rare disorders it is sometimes difficult to decide whether there is a causal relation with the additional disease or whether a coincidental finding is the case.

The course of the sacroiliitis in these systemic diseases is slightly different from a sacroiliitis caused by tuberculosis or ankylosing spondylitis, not only clinically but

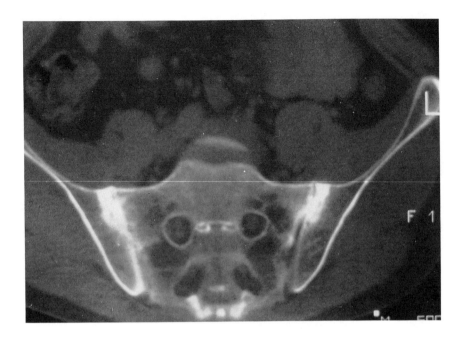

Figure 3–38 CT scan of a patient with back and groin symptoms as a result of a bilateral psoriatic sacroiliitis.

also radiologically. However, this is of minimal importance for the diagnosis. The question of whether the cause for the sacroiliitis is ankylosing spondylitis or another rheumatological disease is better determined by abnormalities elsewhere in the body or in the blood than by the local clinical and radiological differences.

In principle, disorders that affect the SI joint can also affect the pubic symphysis. In many cases this can be misleading because the patient presents with the same complaints often seen in a primary disorder of the SI joint, particularly concerning the symptom of groin pain (see Figure 3–39).

DISORDERS RELATED TO INCREASED MOBILITY

Assessing motion in the SI joint is not easy. Determining a limitation of motion is even more difficult. The most reliable information

concerning the mobility is obtained if one can ascertain movements of the ilium in relation to the sacrum itself. Sometimes this is possible in palpation of very slender people with a lot of mobility. However, if one finds decreased mobility, the question will always remain whether the test was adequate for such a patient, in other words, whether or not the test was reliable. (See section 3.2 Examination.) Furthermore, when a disturbance or a dysfunction is found, it is not completely clear which of the two SI joints is the cause of the ascertained dysfunction. Thus, localization of pain is of utmost importance.

Sometimes the mobility can be objectified by the X-ray views proposed by Chamberlain.[19] Three pelvic X-rays are made in this procedure:

1. one in left unipodal position
2. one in right unipodal position
3. one with equal weight on both legs

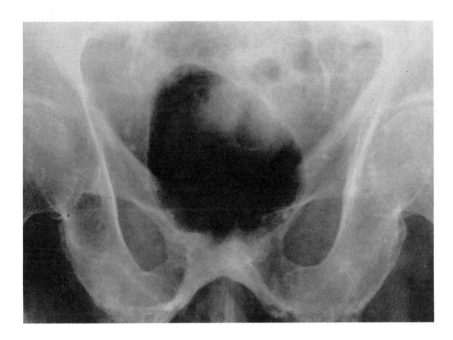

Figure 3–39 Conventional X-ray of the symphysis of a 35-year-old male with a history of groin pain. There is an ankylosis of the symphysis as the result of a psoriatic arthritis.

The mobility of the innominates in relation to each other is well visualized at the symphysis.

The terminology surrounding *instability* and *hypermobility* is often confusing. Within the scope of orthopaedic medicine, *hypermobility* is defined as an increased amount of mobility in a joint whereby the patient does not necessarily have complaints related to this large amount of mobility. Thus, *hypermobility* is a relative term. Criteria used in order to define hypermobility are the patient's other joints, and the same joints in other individuals. For some joints, parameters have been determined that must be met before one can speak of hypermobility. For instance, only when there is more than 15° of hyperextension in the knee or elbow is the finding interpreted as a sign of hypermobility.

Instability is defined as a pathological form of hypermobility causing symptoms from the joint or periarticular structures. Joint structures farther away can also become involved. Instability mostly concerns motions in a nonphysiological direction, for example, a large varus or valgus mobility in hinge joints. Because of the instability the joint has the tendency to subluxate/dislocate or repeatedly track incorrectly, resulting in traumatic arthritis and irritated ligaments after activity.

Of course the amount of activity also plays a role, whereby *instability* becomes a relative term as well. For example, a varus hypermobility in the knee will cause symptoms of instability earlier in a heavy person who jogs than in a well-trained biker.

Hypermobile joints have a greater tendency toward instability than joints with normal mobility.

Important Terminology in Dealing with the SI Joint

Capsular pattern limitation: a pathological form of decreased mobility in a disorder in which the whole capsule is equally involved.

One thinks of an arthritis, an osteoarthrosis, or increased pressure within the joint due to effusion or hemarthrosis.

Internal derangement (locking): a pathological form of decreased mobility that differs from a capsular pattern limitation. Internal derangements can have an intra-articular or an extra-articular cause, or both. Intra-articular causes include loose bodies, meniscal lesions, subluxations, intra-articular adhesions. Extra-articular locking can occur as a result of hypertonic or shortened muscles or space-occupying processes near the joint (such as an inflammation, an infection, or a tumor).

Nutation position: position of the SI joint in which the sacrum is tilted forward in relation to the ilium (or the ilium backward in relation to the sacrum). *Nutate:* movement in the direction of the nutation position.

Counternutation position: position of the SI joint in which the sacrum is tilted backward in relation to the ilium (or the ilium forward in relation to the sacrum). *Counternutate:* movement in the direction of the counternutation position.

The terms *nutation* and *counternutation* are based on the concept that the axis of rotation is located near the SI joint. It is obvious that, for instance, the right innominate cannot tilt forward and backward around a frontotransversal axis (right-left horizontal axis); the symphysis would never allow this. Also, the position and the form of the joint surfaces prevent such a movement. Therefore these tilting motions have to be accompanied by minimal rotations around the frontosagittal axis (vertical) and a sagittotransversal axis (dorsal-ventral horizontal). In addition, a slight translation along each of the mentioned axes occurs.

Internal and external rotation of the innominate: a rotation of the innominate around the vertical axis in which the innominate moves with its ventral aspect either toward the center or away from the center of the body.

As with nutation and counternutation, these movements cannot take place without accessory motions in other directions. Because of the rotation of the innominate, the position of the acetabulum also changes and with it the mobility of the thigh in relation to the trunk. Again these movements are extremely small.

Instability

Theoretically (and in analogy to instability of other joints), a patient with a sacroiliac instability will develop an irritation of one or more ligaments, or even an arthritis of the SI joint, after a relatively stressful activity. Pain is usually experienced lateral to the sacrum with radiation to the innominate of the same side (lower abdomen, greater trochanter, iliac crest and spines, groin) and, if the intensity is great enough, to the posterior aspect of the thigh.

Literature dealing with the SI joint often mentions the occurrence of hypermobility during pregnancy and within the first months after childbirth. This is related to an increase in the width of the pubic symphysis. A large study by Abramson et al. from 1933[20] indicated an increase in width from an average of 4 mm to 7.8 mm during this period.

The amount of fluid in a normal SI joint is almost nil. In pregnancy and the postpartum period a small amount of fluid is found within the joint, causing an increase in mobility. In a "traumatic" arthritis, an increase in fluid also occurs, therefore resulting in increased mobility for a certain period of time.

Severe post-traumatic instability usually occurs after significant trauma in which fractures and/or symphysiolysis is often involved. Nevertheless, the authors have also seen patients with an unstable SI joint after insignificant traumas. Yet within the framework of orthopaedic medicine, it is the general opinion that instability or recurrent mechanical arthritis of the SI joint is rare.

Patients with condensing iliitis almost never have an unstable SI joint. Symptoms experienced from the SI joint are probably due to an "overload" of the joint with or without a disturbance in the tracking. On X-ray, sclerosis is visible in the subchondral bone of the ilium. Condensing iliitis almost always involves patients who have a disturbance of mobility around the pelvis (limitation of hip motion, leg length difference, etc) or women who have given birth. Interestingly, these patients normally do not complain about the affected SI joint.

In an unstable SI joint, an obvious phenomenon at the nonaffected side is seen in the functional examination. In most cases, the provocation tests are also positive. When diagnosing an SI joint instability, one looks for a triad:

1. a typical history (the patient complains of pain with prolonged sitting, prolonged standing, strolling, carrying heavy objects, etc)
2. positive provocation tests
3. Vorlauf phenomenon at the non-affected side

By means of the radiological examination described by Chamberlain, the instability can be demonstrated on an AP view at the level of the symphysis. When standing on the affected leg, the pubic bone at the symphysis of the affected side is positioned higher than the nonaffected side (Figure 3–40). This phenomenon occurs because the ilium makes an abnormally large dorsal rotation at the affected side whereby the sacrum and the other ilium remain relatively behind.[7]

An unstable SI joint can easily develop an internal derangement due to an insignificant trauma. The rough cartilage of the ilium "catches" in the soft thick cartilage of the sacrum. The history changes from one of instability to one of internal derangement (locking). In the latter, the patient complains of pain during movement (in contrast to the former, in which movement generally decreases the symptoms). The faster the movements are performed and the more the movement is repeated (jumping, sprinting) the more pain the patient experiences. In this case the Vorlauf phenomenon is now observed at the affected side.

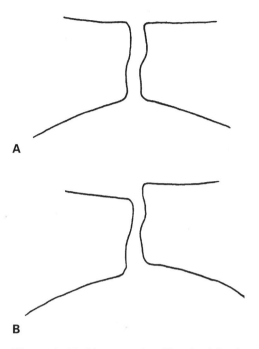

A

B

Figure 3–40 Diagram of a Chamberlain view. **A**, The patient stands with equal weight bearing on each leg; **B**, the patient stands on the left leg, causing nutation in the left SI joint. In turn, the sacrum takes the right innominate, resulting in a lower position of the right pubic bone.

Treatment

In general, conservative treatment of an SI joint instability takes a lot of time; the patient's motivation to exercise daily is very important. The gluteus maximus is the only muscle that (indirectly) attaches to the sacrum as well as to the ilium. Thus, strengthening this muscle is an essential component of the treatment. Strengthening of the abdominal muscles is also indicated. Walking on a daily basis is good training for the gluteus maximus.

Besides an appropriate exercise program, wearing a so-called "pelvic belt" in order to stabilize the SI joints and the symphysis is generally very beneficial (Figures 3–41 and 3–42). Because these belts are more often prescribed for pregnant women, it is necessary for the belt to run over the ventral aspect

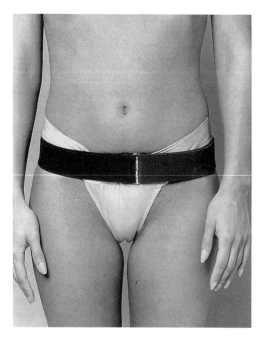

Figure 3–41 Narrow pelvic belt.

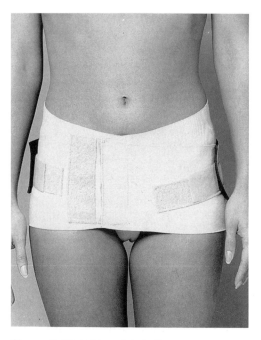

Figure 3–42 Wide pelvic belt.

of the pubic bone. When a sacroiliac belt is worn in direct contact with the skin, irritation often occurs due to small shifts of the belt. Therefore the belt is best worn over the underwear. Various types of belts are available; in practice it is mostly a matter of trying them out. Some patients prefer a narrow one; others prefer a wide one. Usually the patient is able to decide within a week whether the belt is a success or not. The principle of a belt or a tight cloth around the pelvis has been applied for centuries in many Third-World countries. The force necessary in order to obtain stability varies in amount from 8 to 15 kg.[21]

Sclerosing injections of the sacroiliac ligaments (prolotherapy) are occasionally administered. Unfortunately, good literature is not available concerning the results of this form of treatment. On the other hand, there are well-documented examples of instabilities treated by arthrodesis; these are mainly cases of post-traumatic instability.

DISORDERS RELATED TO DECREASED MOBILITY

In order to comprehend dysfunctions in SI movement, theoretically it has to be assumed that the pelvis is perfectly symmetrical and that the mobility of both SI joints is the same. Asymmetrical mobility would then indicate unilateral hypermobility (or instability), decreased mobility (at the other side), or possibly a combination of both. This leads to an asymmetrical pelvis, the so-called pelvic torsion, in positions in which both SI joints are normally symmetrically loaded.

Moreover, in positions in which both SI joints are asymmetrically loaded, either no torsion or an opposite torsion will be found. Symmetry in such a (theoretical) pelvis is expected in standing, sitting, supine, and prone positions, and also in forward flexing and in extending the spinal column both in standing as well as in sitting. If the functional examination in a patient with low back pain is negative, including the SI provocation tests, then the "pelvic torsion" (or asymmetrical pelvis) is of no clinical importance.

Pelvic Torsion

If the pelvis demonstrates the same asymmetry in all examined positions and there are no complaints (which the authors see many times in healthy participants), the asymmetry has no clinical significance.

However, if this asymmetry is found in a patient then this *might* be an indication for an internal derangement of the SI joint on one side, or for a hypermobile or unstable joint at the other side. Usually Vorlauf phenomenon is observed on the painful side in instances of an internal derangement, and on the contralateral side in cases of instability. In both cases the provocation tests are positive.

Pelvic torsion is often found in patients with low back pain for whom the SI joint provocation tests are negative. In these cases, the pelvic torsion is not clinically significant; no one is perfectly symmetrical.

Treatment for an Internal Derangement

As already emphasized in the previous paragraphs a decrease in SI joint motion can be physiological (Tables 3–5 and 3–6).

Radiological examination often shows pelvic asymmetry. In cases of hypermobility and instability, Chamberlain views are well known in which alternating asymmetry is demonstrated when the patient, in standing, alternates loading of the left and right legs. Until now no one has ever published X-ray films of a patient with symptoms whose pelvis became symmetrical after unlocking. Treatment of a long-lasting pelvic torsion may need to be rethought.

In every patient with complaints and an internal derangement, the question remains whether the symptoms are the result or the cause of the disorder. Can these two entities be seen apart from each other? Theoretically

Table 3-5 Factors That Can Limit Nutation and Facilitate Counternutation

- Shortening/hypertonus of the hip flexors (iliacus, tensor fasciae latae, adductor longus, rectus femoris, etc)
- Limitation of hip extension (capsular)
- Left rotation in L5-S1 (nutation limited at the right side)
- Ipsilateral short leg

one assumes that an individual with an internal derangement develops symptoms if one of the joints near the internal derangement becomes disturbed in its normal movement pattern. The mobility of both innominates, sacrum and lower lumbar segments, are mutually dependent to such an extent that when there is a dysfunction in one of these links, the whole chain can become disturbed.

For instance, if an intra-articular derangement of the SI joint causes a counternutated position of the right innominate then the right iliolumbar ligament can pull L5 into a left rotation in relation to S1. It is rather obvious that tension in the iliolumbar ligament can then cause L5 to track incorrectly in relation to S1 with all the possible consequences. Through this phenomenon, the iliolumbar ligament can also become overused .

On the other hand, an internal derangement of L5 in relation to S1 may be a possible cause for a disturbed tracking of the SI joints. The former and the latter are closely related to the mobility of the nonlocked "links" of the chain.

Table 3–6 Factors That Can Limit Counternutation and Facilitate Nutation

- Shortening/hypertonus of the hip extensors (hamstrings, gluteals)
- Flexion limitation of the hip joint (capsular)
- Right rotation in L5-S1 (counternutation limited at the right side)
- Ipsilateral long leg
- Weak sacrotuberous and sacrospinous ligaments

Often the following rule applies: the more mobile the joint, the greater the symptoms. Of course, the demands on the movements play a role as well. A high-level athlete will experience problems from a locked SI joint sooner than a bookkeeper.

All of this reasoning is theoretical, of course, but it indicates that a pelvic torsion, in and of itself, does not necessarily cause problems. At the worst, a pelvic torsion can cause a predisposition for some other disorder. On the other hand, a pelvic torsion may sometimes be observed as a consequence of another disorder in this region, such as a prolapsed disc.

Many extra-articular structures can cause SI locking. In a long-standing locking, more and more of these structures seem to adapt to the situation, and after a while these adaptations will have an influence on the situation.

Besides the extra-articular factors, an intra-articular locking is also possible. As mentioned earlier, in a large number of cases involving men, a bony bridge develops between the sacrum and the ilium. Naturally motion is no longer possible in that joint. The authors have observed this phenomenon in men usually older than 50; however, some of them were just over the age of 30 (see Osteoarthrosis of the SI Joint).

Actual intra-articular internal derangements mostly occur in hypermobile and unstable SI joints. Due to an "insignificant" trauma, a small shift occurs within the joint, which leads to a locking in this position because of forceful contraction of the muscles. A Vorlauf phenomenon on the affected side is the classic finding.

If the clinician decides to initiate treatment, each disturbed biomechanical factor should be restored as much as possible. Factors to consider include compensating leg length differences, restoring shortening/hypertonus of muscles, and influencing the mobility of the hip joints as well as the lumbar spine. In addition, the intra-articular internal derangement of the SI joint has to be restored

manually. Often the locking is due to a "subluxation" because of an instability in the joint. Therefore, it is necessary to direct the treatment on stabilizing the joint in its physiological position after having restored the internal derangement (see Instability).

ANKYLOSING SPONDYLITIS AND RELATED DISORDERS

Introduction

Ankylosing spondylitis (Bekhterev's disease) is a chronic rheumatoid disorder that almost always affects the SI joints. Usually the disease is progressive and can ultimately lead to a full ankylosis of the SI joints (Figure 3–43). Often the process spreads to the thoracic spine and the costovertebral joints as well. Eventually the whole spinal column can become ankylotic.

However, the course can also be mild, particularly in women in whom, over a period of 20 years, almost no progression occurs. In such cases, the disease probably remains undiagnosed.

Other patients, mainly younger ones, experience long-lasting severe exacerbations with severe pain, limitation of motion, and often general malaise. The incidence is one per million and the onset averages around the 25th year. Ten percent of the patients already have symptoms at the age of 15.

Earlier, one assumed that the disease had a higher incidence in men than in women. Now, after closer study, it seems that women present with the disease as often as men but usually in a much less severe form. In family members of patients with ankylosing spondylitis, the disease has an incidence 20 times higher than that in the average population. Often the disease is accompanied by peripheral arthritides (50%), insertion tendopathies (enthesopathies), tendovaginitis, iritis or iridocyclitis (30%), and inflammatory bowel diseases (4%). Complications from aortitis, myocarditis, and amyloidosis seldom occur.

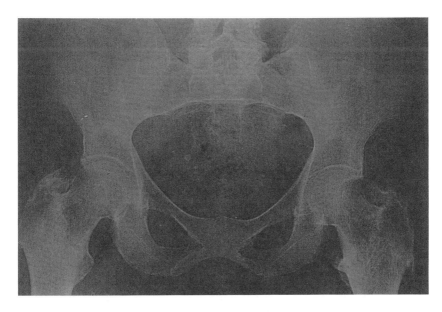

Figure 3–43 Conventional AP X-ray of the pelvis of a patient with ankylosing spondylitis. Visible are the fully ankylotic SI joints as well as periarticular changes of the hip joints (demonstrated as calcifications at the level of the insertions of the muscles).

Clinical Findings

Usually with ankylosing spondylitis there is chronic sacroiliitis with acute exacerbations. Sometimes the disorder starts unilaterally, but during its course both SI joints become affected. The acute exacerbations are usually unilateral and can last months. An inflammatory cause is suspected with the following symptoms and circumstances:

- morning stiffness lasting longer than 30 minutes
- decrease of pain with activity
- symptoms lasting longer than 3 months
- gradual increase in pain over the years
- onset of complaints before the age of 40
- good reaction to nonsteroidal anti-inflammatory drugs (NSAIDs)
- increased ESR

The following are also suggestive: general malaise, weight loss, positive family history, eye disorders such as iritis and iridocyclitis, colitis, peripheral arthritides, and heel pain. A proven sacroiliitis makes the diagnosis of ankylosing spondylitis almost certain.

Functional Examination

In an active sacroiliitis the provocation test of the sacroiliac ligaments is extremely painful. If the lumbar spine is affected, the mobility of the spinal column shows a decrease in all motions. This can be objectified by means of the so-called lumbar flexion index (Schober index): in upright standing the spinous process of L5 is marked, and a mark is placed at a distance 15 cm above. The patient then maximally flexes forward; in healthy young people this distance increases by an average of 6 cm; however, depending on the amount of stiffness, the lumbar flexion index can decrease to 0 cm.

Thoracic stiffness can be objectified by registering the breathing excursion. This is the difference in the rib cage circumference between positions of maximal inhalation and exhalation. In men it is measured at the level of the nipples; in women, just below the breasts. A normal difference is 6 to 9 cm; in most patients with ankylosing spondylitis, the breathing excursion is less than 2.5 cm.[22,23]

During the functional examination, one should pay particular attention to the presence of insertion tendopathies and to signs or residual findings of peripheral arthritis: a capsular pattern of limitation in the large joints; local tenderness or swelling of the sterno-clavicular, manubriosternal, costosternal, and temporomandibular joints; and/or tenderness of the heels and the ischial tuberosities.

Radiological Examination

Principally, the same aberrations are found at the SI joints as described in Table 3–1 (acute sacroiliitis). However, it takes much longer before all stages are experienced. Furthermore, small syndesmophytes can be visible, demonstrating an ossification at the edges of the intervertebral discs. This occurs not only at the site of the posterior and anterior longitudinal ligaments but also along the entire circumference. Later, ossification of all other intervertebral ligaments can occur. The aberrations start mainly in the region of the thoracolumbar junction. Eventually the whole spinal column (also cervical) can become ankylotic, the so-called bamboo spine (Figures 3–44 to 3–47).

Laboratory Tests

There are no specific laboratory tests available for ankylosing spondylitis. The diagnosis is made on the basis of the clinical and radiological findings.

In the acute stage, the ESR is increased (20 to 50 mm). Sometimes there is slight anemia or a slight increase in alkaline phosphates. Eighty-five to ninety-five percent of patients are found to be human leukocyte antigen (HLA)-B27–positive. Meanwhile, only 5% to 9% of the general population is HLA-B27–positive. Carrying this antigen means that the

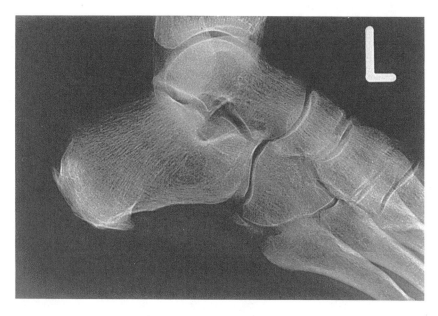

Figure 3–44 Conventional lateral X-ray of the foot in a patient with ankylosing spondylitis. Characteristic changes of the calcaneus are evident.

individual belongs to a "high-risk" group; the chance of getting ankylosing spondylitis is 40 to 100 times larger than in HLA-B27–negative patients. There are indications that the ankylosing spondylitis in HLA-B27–positive patients has a course different from that in HLA-B27–negative patients.

Treatment

NSAIDs and exercise therapy are the foundations of treatment. Earlier, a relatively low dosage of phenylbutazone (Butazolidin) was the drug of choice. Currently the safer NSAIDs are tried. If the use of phenylbutazone is chosen the patient must be monitored for side effects (especially in the beginning), including leukopenia, thrombocytopenia, and gastric ulcers.

The goal of exercise therapy is to maintain the mobility of the affected joints as long as possible and to prevent stiffening of the spine in an unacceptable kyphotic position. One should offer the patient an exercise program in which breathing exercises and exercises for the peripheral joints are included as well. This program must be performed by the patient on a daily basis; from time to time the program should be checked and adapted if necessary.

Prolonged sitting and stooping must be avoided. If possible, these positions should be interrupted regularly by standing or walking. Several times per day, the patient should lie supine for 5 minutes, with the back against the floor.

The peripheral arthritides are mostly transient without residual signs. However, if there is a threat of contractures, those joints should be included in the daily exercise program. When a peripheral arthritis remains for a longer period, a local administration of a corticosteroid should be considered. If the complaints recur too quickly after the injection, this presents a contraindication for a repeated injection.

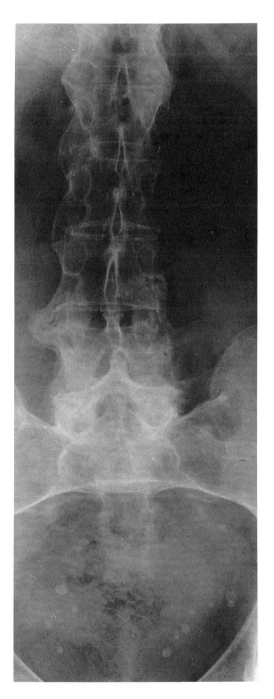

Figure 3–45 Conventional AP X-ray of the lumbar spine of a patient with ankylosing spondylitis. Mainly at the right side a bamboo spine is clearly visible.

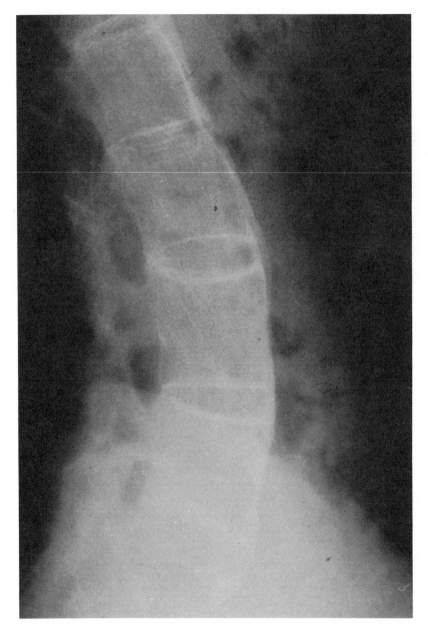

Figure 3–46 Conventional lateral X-ray of the lumbar spine (L2 to L5) in a patient with ankylosing spondylitis. Calcifications of the longitudinal ligaments cause the so-called bamboo spine in the sagittal plane as well.

Due to stiffening of the thorax and rib cage, patients are also increasingly susceptible to respiratory infections. Thus prevention of flu is necessary, as this will almost certainly cause a respiratory infection in these patients.

In the end stages of ankylosing spondylitis, patients can suffer a fracture of the cervical spine if they experience a whiplash trauma. The automobile seat should be adapted to prevent this from occurring.

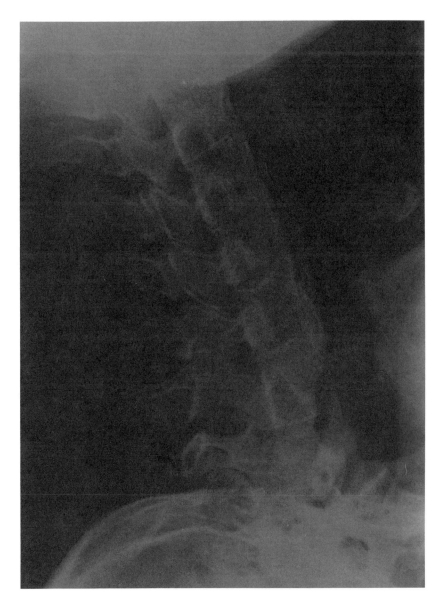

Figure 3–47 Conventional lateral X-ray of the cervical spine in a patient with ankylosing spondylitis. Total ankylosis of the cervical spine is evident, with clearly visible calcification of the anterior longitudinal ligament.

Differential Diagnosis

The following disorders can also cause a sacroiliitis:

- psoriatic arthritis (in 30% of cases)
- Reiter's disease (in 30% of cases)
- Crohn's disease (in 10% of cases)

- ulcerating colitis (in 15% of cases)
- other rare disorders

In a substantial number of these cases, a total ankylosis of the SI joints and a so-called bamboo spine develop. Thus determining the primary cause and its resulting complications can be extremely difficult.

OSTEOARTHROSIS OF THE SI JOINT

Degenerative "disorders" of the SI joint may already be apparent at a relatively young age. In some individuals, microscopic aberrations of the cartilage can be found at the age of 20. These aberrations are almost always present over the age of 30. Macroscopic changes develop 10 to 20 years later. Generally in men osteoarthrosis develops at a much younger age than in women. At the age of 50, approximately 50% of women present with some degree of osteophytes. In men this percentage is already attained at the age of 35. The question is whether the term *osteoarthrosis* is a proper term, because these "aberrations" are actually nothing more than a physiological process.

McDonald and Hunt[24] described four forms of internal derangement of the SI joint. In the first group, the joint surfaces were held together by yellow, sticky, necrotic material. In the cadavers they examined, it was easy to sever these adhesions. The second group demonstrated more fibrous connections. In the third group, there were bridge formations by osteophytes at the edge of the joint, and in the last group intra- and/or para-articular bony bridges were observed. Also, it is important to mention that upon examination of the intact cadaver, no SI joint mobility was found and no radiological aberrations were noted in the first two groups.

Sashin[25] found almost no SI joint movement in cadavers of men over 40 years of age. In 50% of men around 50 years of age, Sashin reported a certain amount of ankylosis. In cadavers of women younger than 60, a small amount of mobility was still noted. In older women, this was rare. In Sashin's examinations the symphysis was removed; thus the true in vivo mobility was probably even smaller in all groups.

Resnick and Niwayama[26] give a clear indication of how to differentiate degenerative changes of the SI joint from ankylosing spondylitis (Table 3–7). Particularly pathognomonic for ankylosing spondylitis are the presence of intra-articular bony bridges and the absence of osteophytes at the edges of the joints. However, sometimes there is only subchondral sclerosis of the ilium without any other signs of degeneration in the SI joint.

In osteoarthrosis of the SI joint there is mostly a mild sclerosis. In radiology, this entity is known as "condensing iliitis." The disorder has a higher incidence in women then in men, especially in women who have had one or more children.

Solonen[27] extensively described 50 patients who were limping for various reasons. In 42 of those 50 patients a unilateral or bilateral condensing iliitis was found. In cases where a unilateral condensing iliitis was present, it was usually found on the nonsymptomatic side. According to Solonen, increased stress on the SI joint during walking was the cause for the radiological aberrations. There was almost no correlation between the radiological findings and the eventual complaints of the patient. In 86 control patients, there was no case of a condensing iliitis.

As in other joints in which the presence of osteoarthrosis does not necessarily cause symptoms, the same is true for the SI joint. On theoretical grounds it could be possible to have a sacroiliitis or an instability along with an osteoarthrosis. In practice, an osteoarthrosis almost always ends up in a hypomobility (capsular limitation) or in an intra-articular locking. In rare cases an instability might develop, particularly if the patient is of a hypermobile morpho-type, is young, and has a disorder whereby the cartilage is destroyed within a short period.

A sacroiliitis might occur because of an overload of the degenerated joint. Of course, this will occur more often when an instability is present and when large forces are placed on the joint, such as in a fall or a manipulation. In very rare cases, calcium pyrophosphate crystals in an osteoarthrosis can cause an arthritis.

Table 3–7 Differential Diagnosis of Arthrosis/Ankylosing Spondylitis According to Resnik and Niwayama[26]

Finding	Arthrosis	Ankylosing Spondylitis
Age	Old	Young
Bony ankylosis	Para-articular	Intra-articular
Sclerosis	Mild, focal	Sometimes extensive
Erosions	None	Sometimes extensive
Ossification of ligaments	Seldom	Often

3.4   TREATMENT: MANUAL MOBILIZATION

In most cases it is impossible to determine whether an SI joint is locked in a nutated or in a counternutated position. The simplest way to deal with this matter is to start with a counternutation mobilization technique. Even though we cannot confirm this assertion, we agree with many of the classic "manual therapists" that the SI joint is usually locked in a nutated position. We have achieved the best results in locked SI joints with these particular counternutation mobilization techniques. However, if pain or an increase in pain occurs during this mobilization, performance of the technique is stopped immediately. The pain probably occurs because, in such a case, the joint is locked in a counternutated position. In these situations one immediately follows with the nutation technique.

Because of the specific characteristic of this type of hypomobility (which is that incongruent ridges in the joint surfaces have locked), the initial mobilization should be performed in a manipulative way. If the collagenous structures around the existing hypomobility have shortened as a result of a prolonged problem, stretching techniques aimed at adapting the collagen are also indicated.

During the manipulation/mobilization a click or similar noise may be heard. One should test the patient again before resuming the treatment. In many cases, the pain will have disappeared. If the locked SI joint was caused through an instability (which is often the case), then the patient should be treated further for this instability. (See section 3.3 Pathology: Instability.)

With all the SI joint manipulation/mobilization techniques described here, the pelvis lies on the horizontal part of the table while the lumbar spine lies on the inclined part. When a manipulation is performed, the desired movement is maximally taken up (optimal pretension) and then a thrust in that direction is applied.

MANIPULATION/MOBILIZATION INTO COUNTERNUTATION TREATMENT TECHNIQUES

4.   Counternutation Mobilization—Provocation Test

Position of the Patient
(Figure 3–48)

The treatment table is brought to a height of the examiner's trochanter. The patient is positioned in sidelying, close to the edge of the table, with the affected side up. In order to localize the manipulation/mobilization as optimally as possible in the SI joint, the lumbar spine is brought into an extended position combined with an axial rotation and sidebending in the direction of the affected side. (In other words, if the left side is af-

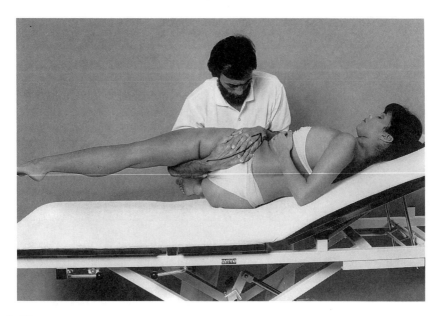

Figure 3–48

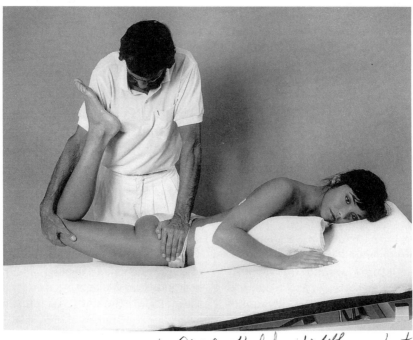

Figure 3–49

pt's Ⓛ LE off bed slightly   but keep
Bk extensio

fected, the patient is positioned in extension with left rotation and left sidebending.) The axial rotation, which is positioned first, remains maximal while the sidebending is added by raising the head of the table. The rotation aids in the stability of the patient during the manipulation/mobilization. The hip of the affected side is then brought into maximal extension, after which the hip of the nonaffected side is flexed without compromising the extension already positioned in the lumbar spine.

Position of the Examiner

The examiner stands in front of the patient at the level of the pelvis, and grasps the patient's top leg from underneath in such a way that the thigh rests on the forearm of the examiner's caudal arm. With clasped hands the top innominate is now grasped at the posterior aspect of the iliac crest; the cranial forearm rests against the more cranial aspect of the iliac crest and the caudal forearm rests against the ischial tuberosity. In order to stabilize the bottom leg of the patient, the examiner places it around his or her trunk with the patient's thigh resting on the examiner's iliac crest.

Performance

The top ilium is now rotated in a ventral direction while, at the same time, the patient's extended leg is brought further into extension by the examiner's upper arm in combination with a rotation of his or her trunk. To increase the effect of the technique, the examiner flexes the hip on the nonaffected side even farther by shifting his or her pelvis in a cranial (in relation to the patient) direction.

ALTERNATIVE MANIPULATION/ MOBILIZATION INTO COUNTERNUTATION

Alternative Test 4

Position of the Patient
(Figure 3–49)

The treatment table is positioned to a height of the examiner's patellas. The patient

lies prone with the nonaffected side close to the edge of the table.

In order to localize the mobilization as much as possible in the SI joint, the lumbar spine is locked in an extended position with an axial rotation and sidebending in the direction of the affected side. (In other words, if the right side is affected then the patient is positioned in extension with right rotation and right sidebending.) The extension is attained by raising the head of the table until movement of the sacrum occurs. The patient is then brought into maximal rotation, and automatically (because of the inclined head of the table) the desired sidebending occurs. This position can be stabilized passively by a pillow.

The hip of the nonaffected side is positioned into flexion by bringing the leg over the edge of the table with the foot resting on the floor.

Position of the Examiner
(Figure 3–50)

The examiner stands next to the patient's nonaffected side at the level of his or her thigh. The examiner places the cranial hand on the PSIS and dorsal aspect of the iliac crest of the patient's affected side. The other hand grasps the anterolateral aspect of the thigh on the patient's affected side just proximal from the knee and brings the hip into extension and slight internal rotation.

At the moment that the sacrum moves ventrally with the ilium, the examiner brings the nonaffected hip into a "maximal" flexion, without losing extension in the spine, by sliding the patient's foot (with the examiner's foot) in a cranial direction. With the cranial (in relation to the patient) foot the examiner fixes the patient's foot on the floor (Figure 3–50).

Performance

The ilium of the affected side is rotated in a ventral direction whereby the cranial hand pushes the ilium ventrally and the caudal hand simultaneously brings the hip even farther into extension (Figure 3–51).

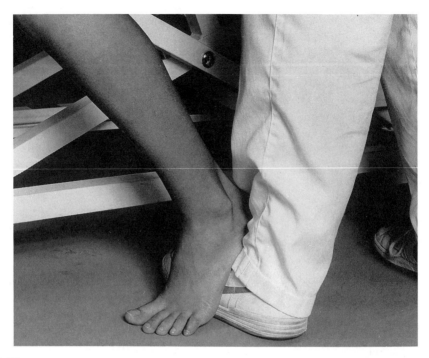

Figure 3–50

MANIPULATION/MOBILIZATION INTO NUTATION

5. Nutation Mobilization—Provocation Test

Position of the Patient
(Figure 3–52)

The treatment table is brought to a height of the examiner's trochanter. The patient is positioned in sidelying with the affected side up.

In order to localize the manipulation/mobilization as much as possible to the SI joint, the lumbar spine is first brought into a flexed position, then rotated in a direction opposite to the affected SI joint. To obtain the most effective locking of the lumbar spine, the spine is now sidebent in the direction of the affected side by raising the head of the table. (In other words, if the left SI joint is affected, the pa-

tient is brought into a right axial rotation and a left sidebend.) The pelvis is positioned on the horizontal part of the table while the lumbar spine lies on the inclined part.

In order to obtain a stable position, the bottom arm is positioned behind the patient's back and the other arm is flexed in a way so that the elbow lies at the level of the patient's head.

Position of the Examiner

The examiner stands in front of the patient at the level of his or her pelvis. The examiner brings the patient's top leg into hip and knee flexion, maintaining this position by one of two possibilities:

1. The examiner can rest the patient's thigh on his or her iliac crest while the lower leg lies against the low back. The thigh is then fixed between the upper

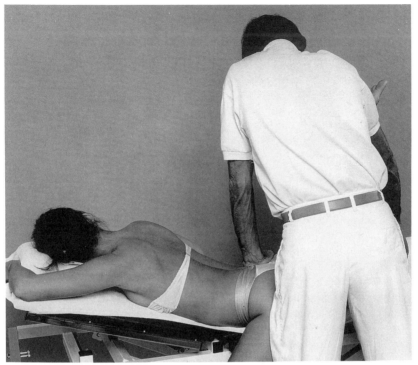

still part
of
counter-nutation

Figure 3–51

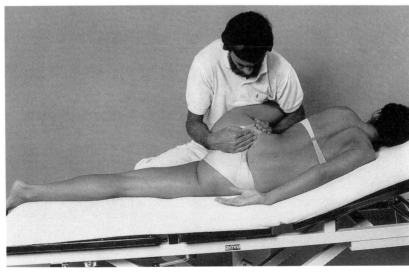

Put PT's (L)
arm under
thigh to ↑
(L) hip ē E R,

Figure 3–52

Non-nutation mob.

arm and the trunk of the examiner (pictured).

2. With his or her cranial arm, the examiner can also grasp the patient's thigh from underneath whereby the thigh is supported on the examiner's proximal forearm. In this way, the patient's hip is allowed to fall into external rotation, which adds to the effectiveness of the technique (not pictured).

Both hands grasp the top innominate, the cranial hand at the anterior superior iliac spine (ASIS) and the caudal hand at the PSIS and PIIS, with the forearm placed against the ischial tuberosity. The ilium is now brought into a position of maximal nutation, directly by the hands and indirectly by moving the patient's hip into more flexion, which the examiner performs with the trunk. The examiner then fixes the patient's bottom leg in extension with the caudal knee. While positioning the patient's bottom leg into extension the examiner must ensure that the pelvis remains vertical and that the top ilium is not pulled ventral, which would cause the lumbar spine to go into extension. The patient's lumbar spine must remain in its flexed position.

Performance

In order to manipulate/mobilize into nutation, the top ilium is rotated dorsally in relation to the fixed sacrum.

ALTERNATIVE MANIPULATION/ MOBILIZATION INTO NUTATION

Alternative Test 5

Position of the Patient
(Figure 3–53)

The treatment table is positioned to a height of the examiner's patellas. The patient lies supine with the nonaffected side close to the edge of the table. The L5-S1 segment lies at the level of the hinge.

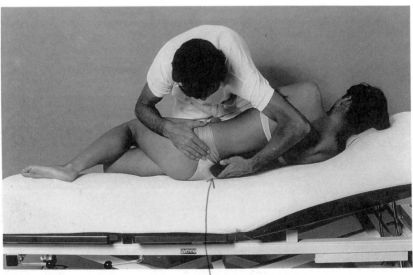

Figure 3–53

In order to perform the manipulation/mobilization as locally as possible, a firm padding is placed underneath the sacrum above the level of S2, directly medial to the PSIS of the innominate on the affected side. This padding should also support the entire lumbar spine.

The lumbar spine of the patient is now brought into a flexed position by raising the head of the table. From this flexed position, an axial rotation of the spine opposite to the affected side is performed. (In other words, if the left side is affected, the spine is axially rotated to the right.) Automatically (because of the inclined table) a sidebending opposite to the axial rotation occurs, thus locking the lumbar spine in an effective way. This rotated position can be maintained either actively by the patient (patient grasps the edge of the table) or passively by means of a pillow.

First the hip of the affected side is brought into maximal flexion and slight external rotation. The hip of the other side is then extended, making sure that the lumbar flexion is maintained, whereby the lower leg of the nonaffected side is off the table and the foot rests on the floor.

Position of the Examiner

The examiner stands at the level of the patient's pelvis, next to the nonaffected side. With both hands, the examiner grasps the ilium of the affected side; the caudal hand is positioned on the patient's ischial tuberosity while the cranial hand has contact with the ventral aspect of the ASIS and iliac crest. The patient's knee and shin of the affected side are supported against the examiner's trunk.

Performance (Figure 3–54)

The ilium is rotated dorsally whereby the cranial hand and the caudal hand work in opposite directions; the cranial hand pushes the patient's ASIS toward the table while the caudal hand pulls the ischial tuberosity away from the table. In order to reinforce the mobilization the examiner can bring the hip into more flexion by moving his or her trunk in a cranial (in relation to the patient) direction.

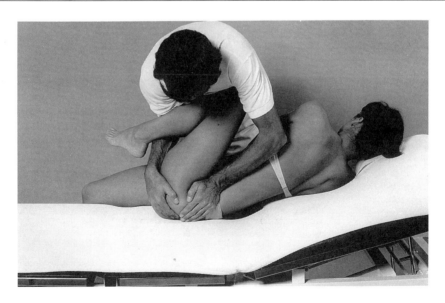

Figure 3–54

REFERENCES

1. Egund N, Olsson TH, Schmid H, Sekvik G. Movements in the sacroiliac joints demonstrated with roentgen stereophotogrammetry. *Acta Radiol Diagn.* 1978;19:833–845.

2. Lavignolle B, Vital JM, Senegas J, et al. An approach to the functional anatomy of the sacroiliac joints in vivo. *Anat Clin.* 1983;5:169–176.

3. Vleeming A. *The Sacro-Iliac Joint.* Rotterdam: Erasmus University; 1990. Dissertation.

4. Bakland O, Hansen JH. The axial sacroiliac joint. *Anat Clin.* 1984;6:29–36.

5. Vleeming A, Stoeckart R, Volkers ACW, Snijders CJ. Relation between form and function in the sacroiliac joint: clinical anatomic aspects. (Part I). *Spine.* 1990;15(2):130–132.

6. Sturesson B, Selvik G, Udén A. Movements of the sacroiliac joints: a roentgen stereophotogrammetric analysis. *Spine.* 1989;14:162–165.

7. Chamberlain WE. The x ray examination of the sacro-iliac joint. *Del State Med J.* 1932;4:195–201.

8. Scholten PJM, Miller JAA, Schultz AB. Biomechanical model studies of sacroiliac joint motions. *Adv Bioeng.* 1984.

9. Scholten PJM, Schultz AB, Luchies CW, Miller JAA. Motions and loads within the human pelvis: a biomechanical model study. *J Orthop Res.* 1988;6(6):840–850.

10. Faraboeuf LH. Sur l'anatomie et la physiologie des ariculations sacro-iliaques avant et apres la symphysectomie. *Ann Gynecol Obstet.* 1984; 41:407–420.

11. Bonnaire E, Bue V. Influence de la position sur la forme et les dimensions du bassin. *Ann Gynecol Obstet.* 1989;52:296.

12. Weisl H. The movements of the sacro-iliac joint. *Acta Anat.* 1995;23:80–91.

13. Kapandji IA. Physiologie articulaire. Paris: Maloine S.A. Editeur; 1982.

14. Lewit K. *Manuele Therapie, Delen I/II.* Lochem: De Tijdstroom; 1981.

15. Haldeman S. Functional and palpatory examination. Presented at the Lumbar Spine Instructional Course, sponsored by the International Society for the Study of the Lumbar Spine; May 11, 1991; Zurich, Switzerland.

16. Cyriax J. Sacroiliac strain. *Br Med J.* 1941;2:847.

17. Rantapää-Dahlquist S, Mordmark LF. HLA-B27 and involvement of sacroiliac joints in rheumatoid arthritis. *J Rheumatol.* 1984;11:27–32.

18. Richter R, Nübling W. Die Tuberkulose der Iliosakralgelenke. *Z Orthop.* 1983;121:564–570.

19. Chamberlain WE. The symphysis publis in the roentgen examination of the sacro-iliac joint. *AJR.* 1930;24:621.

20. Abramson D, Roberts SM, Wilson DD. Relaxation of the pelvic joints in pregnancy. *Surg Gynecol Obstet.* 1934;58:595–613.

21. Snijders CJ, Vleeming A, Volkers AC, Stoeckart R. *Functional Friction in the SI Joints.* 1988.

22. Göhring H. Krankengymnastische Möglichkeiten zur Verbesserung und Erhaltung der Thoraxbeweglichkeit und der Atembewegungen bei Morbus Bechterew. *Krankengymnastik.* 1989;41:47–53.

23. Mieran DR, Cassidy JD. Sacroiliac joint dysfunction and low back pain in school aged children. *J Manipulative Physiol Ther.* 1984;7:81–84.

24. McDonald GR, Hunt TF. Sacro-iliac joints: observations on the gross and histological changes in the various age groups. *Can Med Assoc J.* 1952;66:157–163.

25. Sashin D. A critical analysis of the anatomy and the pathological changes of the sacroiliac joints. *J Bone Joint Surg.* 1930;12:891–910.

26. Resnick D, Niwayama G. Comparison of radiographic abnormalities of the sacroiliac joint in degenerative disease and ankylosing spondylitis. *AJR.* 1977; 128:189.

27. Solonen KA. The sacroiliac joint in the light of anatomical roentgenological and clinical studies. *Acta Orthop Scand.* 1975;27(suppl):1–127.

SUGGESTED READING

Aalam M, Hoffmann P. Beeinträchtigung der Beckenfugen durch einseitige schwere Hüftgelenkleiden. *Arch Orthop Unfall Chir.* 1975;82:257–262.

Abel AL. Sacroiliac strain. *Br Med J.* 1939;1:683–686.

Aberle W, Erlacher PH, Hartwich H, Königswieser A, Stracker O. *Leherbuch der praktischen Orthopädie.* Vienna, Austria: W. Maudrich; 1955.

Alarcon-Segovia D, Cetina JA, Diaz-Jouanez E. Sacroiliac joints in primary gout. *AJR.* 1973;118:438–443.

Albee FJ. A study of the anatomy and the clinical importance of the sacroiliac joint. *JAMA.* 1909;53:1273–1276.

Beal MC. The sacroiliac problem: review of anatomy, mechanics, and diagnosis. *JAMA.* 1982;10:678–684.

Bellamy N, Park W, Rooney JR. What do we know about the sacroiliac joint? *Semin Arthritis Rheum.* 1983;12:282–313.

Bemis T, Daniel M. Validation of the long sitting test on subjects with iliosacral dysfunction. *J Orthop Sports Phys Ther.* 1987;8:336–345.

Bickel WR. True diastasis of the sacroiliac joint with hypermobility. *J Bone Joint Surg [Am].* 1957; 39:1381.

Blower PW, Griffin AJ. Clinical sacroiliac tests in ankylosing spondylitis and other causes of low back pain: two studies. *Ann Rheum Dis.* 1984;43:192–195.

Borell U, Fernstrom I. The movements at the sacroiliac joints and their importance to changes in the pelvic dimensions during parturation. *Acta Obstet Gynecol Scand.* 1957;36:42–57.

Bowen V, Cassidy JD. Macroscopic and microscopic anatomy of the sacroiliac joints from embryonic life until the eighth decade. *Spine.* 1981;6:620–628.

Braam LJ, Keyzer JL, Roon RV. Bewegingsmechanische relaties rondom het sacroiliacale gewricht. *Ned Tijdschr Man Ther.* 1987;87/4,4:64–72.

Braune CW, Fisher O. Bestimmung der Trägheitsmomente des menschlichen Körpers und seiner Glieder. *Abh Math Phys Sächs Ges Wiss.* 1982;18:409.

Brochner JEW. *Die Wirbelsäulenleiden und ihre Differentialdiagnose.* Stuttgart: Georg Thieme Verlag; 1962.

Brook R. The sacroiliac joint. *J Anat Physiol.* 1924; 58:299–305.

Chisin R, Milgrom C. Unilateral sacroiliac overuse syndrome in military recruits. *Br Med J.* 1984;289:590–591.

Cohen AS, McNeil JM, Cilkins E. The normal sacroiliac joint: analysis of 88 roentgenograms. *AJR.* 1967; 100:599–663.

Colachis SC, Worden RE, Bechtol CO, Strohm BR. Movement of the sacroiliac joint in adult male. *Arch Phys Med Rehabil.* 1963;44:490–498.

Coventry MB, Taper EM. Pelvic instability. *J Bone Joint Surg [Am].* 1972;54:83.

Dalphin JC, Mallet H. Gaucher's disease and B27 negative sacroiliitis. *Presse Med.* 1984;13:1278.

Davis P, Lentle BC. Evidence for sacroiliac disease as a common cause of low backache in women. *Lancet.* 1978;2:496–497.

Dejung B. Die Verspannung des M. iliacus als Ursache lumbosacraler Schmerzen. *Man Med.* 1987;25:73–81.

Delbarre F. Pyogenic infection of the sacroiliac joint: report of 13 cases. *J Bone Joint Surg [Br].* 1975;25: 73–81.

Delisle B. Der Kreuzschmerz aus der Sicht des Gynäkologen. *Physikalische Ther.* 1984;5:419–422.

Derry DE. The influence of sex on the position and composition of the human sacrum. *J Anat Physiol.* 1912;46:184–192.

Diemerbroeck I; Salmon W, trans. *The Anatomy of Human Bodies.* London: Brewster; 1989.

Dihlman W. *Gelenke-Wirbelverbindungen, Klinische Radiologie.* Stuttgart: Georg Thieme Verlag; 1982.

Dihlman W. Stadieneinteilung ("grading, staging") bei Spondylitis ankylosans. *Z Rheumatol.* 1983;42:49–57.

Dijkstra PF, van Vugt AC. Alkaptonurie. *Ned Tijdschr Geneeskd.* 1977;121:2069–2073.

Dijkstra PF, Vleeming A, Stoeckart R. Complex motion tomography of the sacroiliac joint: an anatomical and röntgenological study. *ROFO.* 1989;105:635–642.

Drachman DB, Solokoff I. The role of movement in embryonic joint development. *Dev Biol.* 1966;14:401–420.

Duncan JM. The behaviour of the pelvic articulations in the mechanism of parturation. *Dublin Q J Med Sci.* 1854;18:60.

el Ehara A, Khoury GY, Bergman RA. The accessory sacroiliac joint: a common anatomic variant. *AJR.* 1988;150:857–859.

Felmann JL. Les sacro-iliitis infectieuses. *Rev Rheumatol.* 1981;48:83–91.

Felt-Bersma RJF, Bronsveld W. Pijn onder in de rug met koorts. *Ned Tijdschr Geneeskd.* 1985;129:385–387.

Fisher LP, Gonon GP, Carret JP, Dimmet J. *J Biomec Articulaire.* 1976;2:33–36.

Forthergill WF. Walchers position in parturition. *Br Med J.* 1896;2:1290–1292.

Freiber AH, Vinke TH. Sciatica and the sacroiliac joint. *J Bone Joint Surg.* 1934;16:126.

Frigerio NA, Stowe RR, Howe JW. Movement of the sacroiliac joint. *Clin Orthop.* 1974;100:370–377.

Gardner E. Physiology of movable joints. *Physiol Rev.* 1950;30:127.

Goei THS, Cats A, van der Linden S. Isolated lesions of the manubriosternal joint in patients with inflammatory back pain and negative sacroiliac and spinal radiographs. *Rheumatology.* 1986;6:245–249.

Goel VK, Svensson NL. Forces on the pelvis. *J Biomech.* 1977;10:195–200.

Goldenberg DL. Postinfectious arthritis: a new look at an old concept with particular attention to disseminated gonococcal infections. *Am J Med.* 1983;74:925–928.

Goldhwait JE, Osgood RB. A consideration of the pelvic articulations from an anatomical, pathological and clinical standpoint. *Boston Med Surg J.* 1905; 152:593.

Gordon G. Pyogenic sacroiliitis. *Am J Med.* 1980;69: 50–56.

Gray H. Sacroiliac joint pain. Finer anatomy; mobility and axes of rotation; etiology; diagnosis and treatment by manipulation. *Int Clin.* 1938;2:54–96.

Greenfield W. Bone changes in chronic adult Gaucher's disease. *AJR.* 1970;110:800–807.

Grieve FP. *De Wervelkolom.* Lochem: De Tijdstroom; 1984.

Hagen R. Pelvic girdle relaxation from an orthopaedic point of view. *Acta Orthop Scand.* 1974;45:550–563.

Haggart GE. Sciatic pain of unknown origin: an effective method of treatment. *J Bone Joint Surg.* 1938; 20:851–856.

Hakim M. Recherche sur l'articulation sacro-iliaque chez view. *Acta Orthop Scand.* 1974;4:550–563. L'homme et les anthropoides. Paris: 1937. Dissertation.

Halladay HV. *Applied Anatomy of the Spine.* Kirksville, Mo: JF Janisch; 1920.

Harris NH. Lesions of the symphysis pubis in women. *Br Med J.* 1974;4(5938):209–211.

Harris NH. Lesions of the symphysis in athletes. *Br Med J.* 1974;4(5938):211–214.

Heyman J, Lundquist A. The symphysis pubis in pregnancy and parturation. *Acta Obstet Gynecol Scand.* 1932;12:91.

Hisay FL. The influence of the ovary on the resorption of the pubic bones. *J Exp Zool.* 1925;23:661.

Jackson RH. Chronic sacroiliac strain with attendant sciatica. *Am J Surg.* 1934;24:456.

Jajic I. Septic sacro-iliitis: analysis of 14 patients. *Acta Orthop Scand.* 1983;54:210–211.

Jarcho J. Value of Walcher position in contracted pelvis with special reference to its effect on true conjugate diameter. *Surg Gynecol Obstet.* 1929;49:854–858.

Kajava Y; Solonon KA, trans. Ristiluum ja suoliluun toisiinsa luutumisesta. *Duodecim.* 1923;39:425.

Kirkaldy-Willis WH, Hill RJ. A more precise diagnosis for low back pain. *Spine.* 1979;4:102–109.

Klein G. Zur Biomechanik des Iliosacralgelendes. *Z Geburtshilfe Gynaekol.* 1981;21:74–118.

Kneck E, Cronenberg A. Spondylitis ankylosans: Effizienz und Möglichkeiten der krankengymnastischen Behandlung in einer Selbsthilfegruppe. *Krankengymnastik.* 1988;40:821–825.

Konstantinov D. Roentgen picture of the course of purulent sacroiliitis. *ROFO.* 1984;140:195–199.

Kumar MR, Balachandran S. Unilateral septic sacroiliitis: importance of the anterior view of the bone scan. *Clin Nucl Med.* 1983;8:413–415.

Laban MM. Symphyseal and sacro-iliac joint pain associated with pubic symphysis instability. *Arch Phys Med Rehabil.* 1978;59:470.

Lewit K. Beckenverwringung und Iliosakralblockierung. *Man Med.* 1987;25:64–70.

Lifeso RM, Harder E, McCorkell SJ. Spinal brucellosis. *J Bone Joint Surg [Br].* 1985;67:345–351.

Lindner W. Gruppentherapie und Sport mit Bechterew-Patienten. *Krankengymnastik.* 1989;41:14–19.

Lindsey RW, Leggon RE, Wright DG, Nolasco DR. Separation of the symphysis pubis in association with childbearing: a case report. *J Bone Joint Surg [Am].* 1988;70:289–292.

Luhm H. Hilfe zur Selbsthilfe: Die Deutsche Vereinigung Morbus Bechterew e. V. *Krankengymnastik.* 1989;41:12–13.

Lynch FW. The pelvic articulations during pregnancy, labor and puerperium: an X ray study. *Surg Gynecol Obstet.* 1929;30:575.

McCarty DJ. *Arthritis and Allied Conditions.* 9th ed. Boston: Lea & Febiger; 1979.

McMaster MJ. A technique for lumbar spinal osteotomy in ankylosing spondylitis. *J Bone Joint Surg [Br].* 1985;67:204–210.

Meyer CH. Der Mechanismus der Symphysis sacroiliaca. *Arch Anat Physiol.* 1878;1:1–19.

Miehle W. Spondylitis ankylosans mit und ohne periphere Gelenkbeteiligung. *Rheuma Aktuell.* 1985;8,2:2.

Miller JAA, Scholten RJM, Schultz AB, Anderson G. Studies of sacroiliac joint biomechanics. *Trans Orthop Res.* 1984:92–94.

Mixter WJ, Barr JS. Rupture of the intervertebral disc with involvement of the spinal canal. *N Engl J Med.* 1934;211:210.

Moffett BC. The prenatal development of the human temporomandibular joint. *Contrib Embryol Carnegie Inst.* 1957;36:19.

Mohr W. Die morphologischen Veränderungen bei der Spondylitis ankylosans. *Krankengymnastik.* 1989; 41:31–37.

Moll JMH. *Ankylosing Spondylitis.* Edinburgh: Churchill Livingstone; 1980.

Namey TC, Halla JI. Radiographic and nucleographic techniques. In: Schmidt FR, ed. *Infectious Arthritis. Clinics in Rheumatic Diseases.* East Sussex, England: WB Saunders; 1986.

Naveau B. Joint manifestations in sarcoidosis. *Ann Med Intern.* 1984;135:105–108.

Oijen PLM van, Boersema JW. Vertraagde diagnosestelling bij de ziekte van Bechterew. *Ned Tijdschr Geneeskd.* 1982;126:1761–1764.

Oosterhuis WW. *Nekpijn, Buikpijn, Rugpijn. Positieve Aanwijzingen uit Negatieve Bevindingen.* Utrecht: Bunge, 1982.

Pace JB, Nagle D. Piriformis syndrome. *West J Med.* 1976;124:435–439.

Palfrey A. The shape of the sacroiliac joint surface. *J Anat.* 1981;132:457.

Paquin JD, van der Rest M, Marie PJ, et al. Biochemical and morphologic studies of cartilage from the adult human sacroiliac joint. *Arthritis Rheum.* 1983;26:887–894.

Paré A. *The Works of Generation of Man.* London: Cotes and Young; 1634.

Paturet G. *Traité d'Anatomie Humaine.* Paris: Masson; 1951;1:614–623.

Pelkonen P, Byring R, Personen E, Leijala M, Haapasaari J. Rapidly progressive aortic incompetence in juvenile ankylosing spondylitis: a case report. *Arthritis Rheum.* 1984;27,6:698–700.

Pinzani E. *Zentralbl Gynakol.* 1899;23:1057.

Pitkin HC. Orthopaedic causes of pelvic pain. *JAMA.* 1947;134:853–857.

Platt H. Backache: sciatica syndrome and intervertebral disk. *Rheumatism.* 1948;4:218.

Plüss AG. Funktionelles Rückenmuskeltraining bei Morbus Bechterew. *Krankengymnastik.* 1989;41: 38–46.

Porat S, Shapiro M. Brucella arthritis of the sacro-iliac joint. *Infection.* 1984;12:205–207.

Posth M. *Le Sacrum.* Paris: La Sorbonne; 1897. Dissertation.

Rand JA. Anterior sacroiliac arthrodesis for post-traumatic sacroiliac arthritis. *J Bone Joint Surg [Am].* 1985;67:157–158.

Rauber-Kopsch. *Lehrbuch und Atlas der Anatomie des Menschen.* Leipzig: Georg Thieme Verlag; 1940.

Reilly JP, Gross RH, Emans JB, Yngve D. Disorders of the sacroiliac joint in children. *J Bone Joint Surg [Am].* 1988;70:30–40.

Resnick D, Niwayama G, Georgen TG. Degenerative disease of the sacroiliac joint. *Invest Radiol.* 1975;10:608–621.

Ronbergue A, Beauvais P. Acute pyogenic sacroiliac arthritis in children. *Semin Hop Paris.* 1983;59:2541–2545.

Rosenberg D, Baskies AM. Pyogenic sacroiliitis: an absolute indication for computerized scanning. *Clin Orthop.* 1984:128–132.

Saporta L, Simon F. Les osteitis pubiennes en nilieu rheumatologie. *Rev Rheumatol.* 1970;37:451.

Sappey PC. *Traité d'Anatomie Descriptive.* Paris: Delahaye, 1876–1879.

Schaad VB, McCracken GH. Pyogenic arthritis of the sacroiliac joint in pediatric patients. *Pediatrics.* 1980;66:375–379.

Schauer U. Spezifische Mobilisation bei Morbus Bechterew (Manuelle Therapie). *Krankengymnastik.* 1989;41:25–30.

von Schubert E. Röntgenuntersuchungen des knöchernen Bekkens im Profilbild: exakte Messung der Beckenneigung bei Lebenden. *Zentralbl Gynaekol.* 1929;53:1064–1068.

Schumacher EF. *A Guide for the Perplexed.* London: Cape; 1977.

Schuncke GB. The anatomy and development of the sacroiliac joint in man. *Anat Rec.* 1938;72:313–331.

Selvik GA. *Roentgen Stereophotogrammetric Method for the Study of the Kinematics of the Skeletal System.* Lund: Centralen; 1974.

Shanahan MDG, Ackroyd CE. Pyogenic infection of the sacroiliac joint. *J Bone Joint Surg [Br].* 1985;67:605–608.

Shipp FJ, Haggart GE. Further experience in the management of steitis condensans ilii. *J Bone Joint Surg [Am].* 1950;32:841.

Shorter AM, Burrows DA. Is the vacuum sign in the sacroiliac joint a useful radiological sign of chondrocalcinosis? *Diagn Imaging Clin Med.* 1984; 53:141–143.

Simons GW. Iliacus abscess. *Clin Orthop.* 1984:61–63.

Smith GE, Jones FW. *The Archaeological Survey of Nubia: Report for 1907–1908, II.* Cairo: National Printing Department; 1910.

Smith-Peterson MN. Arthrodesis of the sacroiliac joint: a new method of approach. *J Orthop Surg.* 1921;3:400.

Snijders CJ, Snijder JGN, Hoedt HTE. Biomechanische modellen in het besek van rugklachten tijdens zwangerschap. *Tijdschrift Soc Geneeskd.* 1984; 62,4:141–147.

Steiner J, Beck W, Prestel E, Richter D. Symphysenschaden: Klinik, Therapie und Prognose. *Fortschr Med.* 1977;35:2132–2137.

Stewart TD. Pathologic changes in aging sacroiliac joints: a study of dissecting room skeletons. *Clin Orthop.* 1984;183:188–196.

Strachan WF. A study of the mechanics of the sacroiliac joint. *J Am Osteopath Assoc.* 1938;37:576–578.

Strachan WF. Applied anatomy of the pelvis and perineum. *J Am Osteopath Assoc.* 1939;38:359–360.

Strachan WF. Applied anatomy of the pelvis and lower extremities. *J Am Osteopath Assoc.* 1940;40:85–86.

Strasser H. *Lehrbuch der Muskel- und Gelenkmechanik.* Berlin: Springer; 1913.

Suh CH. The fundamentals of computer aided X ray analysis of the spine. *J Biomech.* 1974;7:161–169.

Testut L, Latarjet A. *Traité d'Anatomie Humaine.* Paris, G. Doin & Cie; 1949.

The sacroiliac joint and backache. *Lancet.* 1983;2:1468–1469. Editorial.

Thorp DJ, Fray WE. The pelvic joints during pregnancy and labour. *JAMA.* 1938;111:1162–1166.

Tichauer ER, Miller M, Nathan IM. Lordosimetry: a new technique for the measurement of postural response to materials handling. *Am Ind Hyg Assoc J.* 1973;1: 1–12.

Töndury G. *Andgewandte und topografische Anatomie.* Stuttgart: Georg Thieme Verlag; 1970.

Trotter M. Accessory sacroiliac articulations. *Am J Phys Anthropol.* 1937;22:247–261.

Trotter M. A common anatomical variation in the sacro-iliac region. *J Bone Joint Surg.* 1940;22:291.

van Berkes RJ, Megchelen PJ. Nek- en rugpijn bij gevoelens van agressie en onmacht. *Huisarts Wetenschap.* 1985;28:331–333.

Väsalius A. De corpori humanis fabrica. *Oporini Basileae;* 1543.

Vleeming A, Dijkstra PF, Stoeckart R. Complex motion tomography of the sacroiliac joint. An anatomical and roentgenological study. *ROFO.* 1989;150(6):635–642.

Vleeming A, Snijders CJ, Stoeckart R. The dynamic role of the sacrotuberal ligament. *Clin Biomech.* 1989.

Vleeming A, Snijders CJ, van Wingerden JP, Stoeckart R. Load application to the sacrotuberal ligament, and its effect on displacement in the SI joints. *Clin Biomech.* 1989.

Vleeming A, Snijders CJ, van Wingerden JP, Stoeckart R. A comparative study of sacroiliac joint mobility. *Spine.* 1989;14.

Vleeming A, Stoeckart R, Snijders CJ. The sacrotuberous ligament: a conceptual approach to its dynamic role in stabilizing the sacro-iliac joint. *Clin Biomech.* 1989;4:201–203.

Vleeming A, van Wingerden JP, Snijders CJ, Stoeckart R, Stijnen T. Load application to the sacrotuberous liga-ment: influences on sacro-iliac joint mechanics. *Clin Biomech.* 1989;4:204–209.

Vleeming A, Volkers ACW, Snijders CJ, Stoeckart R. Re-lation between form and function in the sacroiliac joint: clinical anatomic aspects (part II). *Spine.* 1990;15(2):133–136.

Waisbrod H, Lang E, Gerbershagen HU. Die degenerative Erkrangung des Iliosakralgelenkes. *Orthop Prax.* 1985;3:238–242.

Waldeyer A. *Die Anatomie des Menschen.* Berlin: De Gruyter & Co; 1953.

Walheim GG. Stabilization of the pelvis with the Hoffman frame. *Acta Orthop Scand.* 1984;55:319–324.

Walheim G, Olerud S, Ribbe T. Mobility of the pubic sym-physis: measurements by an electromechanical method. *Acta Orthop Scand.* 1984;55:203–208.

Watson-Jones R. *Fractures and Joint Injuries.* Edinburgh: Churchill Livingstone; 1955.

Weisl H. The articular surfaces of the sacroiliac joint and their relation to the movements of the sacrum. *Acta Anat.* 1954;22:1–14.

Wilder DG, Pope MH, Frymoyer JN. The functional to-pography of the sacro-iliac joint. *Spine.* 1980;5:575–579.

Williams PL, Warrick R, Dyson M, Bannister LH, eds. *Gray's Anatomy.* New York: Churchill Livingstone; 1989.

Yeoman W. The relation of the arthritis of the sacroiliac joint to sciatica. *Lancet.* 1928;2:1119–1122.

Zeidler H. Prognose der ankylosierenden Spondylitis. *Rheuma Aktuell.* 1985;8,2:3–4.

Ziedses des Plantes BG. *Planigrafie en subtractie: Röntgenografische differentiaal methodes.* Utrecht: Rijks University; 1934. Dissertation.

4

Lumbar Spine

4.1   FUNCTIONAL ANATOMY

INTRODUCTION

In an upright position, the load from the weight of the body is larger in the lumbar spine than in the thoracic and cervical spines; thus the lumbar spine is the most sturdily built part of the spinal column. The vertebral bodies and the intervertebral discs are relatively large. Although more mobile than the thoracic spine, stability is also a very important feature of the lumbar spine.

FUNCTIONAL OVERVIEW

In the relatively large vertebral body, the transverse diameter is slightly longer than the anterior-posterior (AP) diameter. The pedicles are short. Oriented almost in the horizontal, the spinous process is somewhat rectangular in shape. The dorsal aspect of the spinous process of L5 is usually smaller than the dorsal aspect of the remaining lumbar spinous processes (this is important in surface anatomy). Except for L5, the transverse processes are long and thin. Larger than the thoracic vertebral foramen but smaller than that of the cervical vertebrae, the lumbar vertebral foramen has a triangular form (Figure 4–3).

Large and oval in shape, the intervertebral foramen is located between the pedicles of two adjacent vertebrae. The track of the root running in this foramen is fairly oblique in a caudolateral direction. The angle of inclination averages 30° to the horizontal, becoming steeper the more caudal in the spine.

The fifth lumbar vertebra forms a junction with the sacrum. The most important structures connecting these two bones are the wedge-shaped intervertebral disc, the zygapophyseal joints, and the iliolumbar ligaments.

The cranial aspect of the sacrum forms an angle of approximately 30° to the horizontal (Figure 4–4). When the angle is larger, one speaks of a horizontal or an *acute* sacrum. This manifests itself in the patient with a "hollow back." However, the amount of hyperlordosis can be judged only from inspection. In some patients with a hollow back, the X-ray films show a normal lumbar lordosis. In the same way, patients with a "normal"-appearing lumbar lordosis can have an acute sacrum on radiological examination.

• Combined Motions: not represented. A movement is combined when one of the motions in the coupled movement pattern is changed.

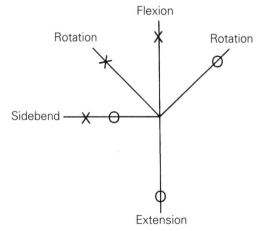

X = Ipsilateral during flexion
O = Contralateral during extension
Figure 4–2 Coupled Motions

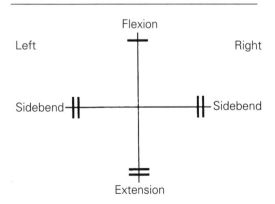

Figure 4–1 Capsular Pattern of the Lumbar Spine

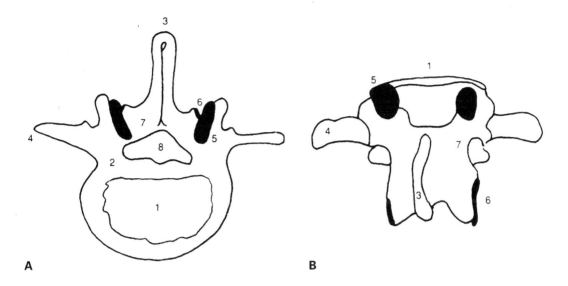

Figure 4–3 A typical lumbar vertebra. **A**, Cranial view; **B**, dorsal view; **1**, vertebral body; **2**, pedicle; **3**, spinous process; **4**, transverse process; **5**, superior articular process; **6**, inferior articular process; **7**, lamina; **8**, vertebral foramen.

Other important radiological angular determinations are the "pelvic tilt" and the lumbosacral angle. The pelvic tilt is the angle formed by one line connecting the ventrocranial corner of the sacrum to the cranial aspect of the pubic symphysis and another line in the horizontal. Normally this angle averages approximately 60°; if this angle is larger, one speaks of an anterior-tilted pelvis; if smaller, a posterior-tilted pelvis (Figure 4–4). The lumbosacral angle is formed by a line that is perpendicular to the middle of the cranial border of the sacrum and a line that connects this latter point with the most dorsal part of the concavity at the ventral aspect of the sacrum (Figure 4–4).

CONNECTIONS

Intervertebral Disc

In the lumbar region the intervertebral disc is relatively large and thick, especially at the L4-5 segment. The fact that the lumbar discs are so large and thick can be related to the large loads that play an important role in the lumbar spine. Unfortunately, the disc is a frequent localization for pathology, especially in the lumbar region.

From the moment that the herniated disc as a pathological entity was diagnosed (and no longer interpreted as a chondroma),[1] the interest in the intervertebral disc as a shock absorber grew. In the years directly after World War II, the mechanical properties of the disc material particularly were the subject of research.[2–5]

A more recent and even greater challenge is to be able to predict the behavior of a disc (normal and degenerated) during different kinds of loading. Therefore, a number of models have been developed by several researchers.

In the study of pathology concerning the herniated disc, it has become obvious that not only the disc should be the subject of study. Junghans[6] describes the so-called *segmentum mobilitatis intervertebrale* in which the zygapophyseal joints are also included in the motion segment.

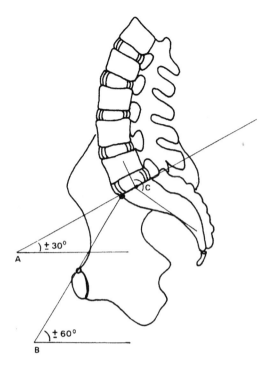

Figure 4–4 Important angles in the lumbosacral region. **A**, Angulation between the cranial border of the sacrum and the horizontal; **B**, pelvic tilt; C, lumbosacral angle.

For the sake of convenience, in the following paragraphs the term *disc* will mean the motion segment without zygapophyseal joints, capsule, ligaments, and muscles. In all other cases, the term *segment* will be used.

Axial Compression

In pure axial compression—always an important component in every load on a motion segment—the transmission of the load onto the zygapophyseal joints is estimated to be about 18% of the total load.[7] The model of Kulak et al[8] studies the behavior of the annulus, nucleus, and end-plate and leaves the zygapophyseal joints out of consideration. From their model, Kulak et al predicted that when a normal disc is subjected to pure axial compression, a certain amount of pressure occurs in the nucleus pulposus: from this aqueous structure the pressure is transferred to the

periphery of the disc in accordance with Pascal's law. In a normal disc, the compression on the disc in the outer annulus fibers results in a tensile stress in several directions:

- parallel to the average inclination of the fibers (approximately 30° to the horizontal)
- axially (from cranial to caudal)
- radially (from the middle to the periphery of the disc)
- tangentially (tangent to the periphery of the disc)

Normally, reaction forces are generated in the inner fibers, but these forces are small and exist only in an axial direction. However, in a degenerated disc, other phenomena are manifested. A tensile stress occurs only in the outer fibers, whereas everywhere else compressive forces are observed[9] (Figure 4–5).

The orientation of the fibers seems to influence different variables. The axial stiffness increases with a decrease of the inclination of the fibers in relation to the horizontal. A decrease of this fiber angle also decreases the amount of bulging.

The model of Shirazi-Adl et al[10] improved on the model from Kulak et al.[8] For instance, they included the construction of the total disc in their model. Earlier, Farfan et al[11] had already distinguished between discs with a flat dorsal aspect and discs with a rounded dorsal aspect. They found that discs with a rounded dorsal aspect were better able to resist torsion forces and were mainly located in the upper lumbar segments. The lower lumbar segments (L4-5, L5-S1) have discs with a more flat dorsal aspect. Based on their calculations, Shirazi-Adl et al concluded that discs with a round posterior aspect bulge more under the influence of pure axial compression. Because Farfan et al and Shirazi-Adl et al used different kinds of load (torsion and pure axial compression, respectively), it is not possible to correlate their findings. Taking into consideration the elasticity in a normal situa-

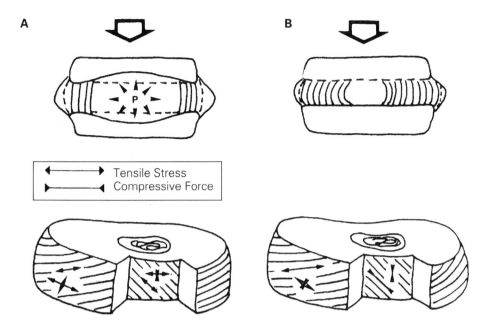

Figure 4–5 Intervertebral disc under axial compression. *A*, Normal disc. The pressure moves in all directions. In the annular fibers this pressure is converted into tensile stress. The size of the arrows depicts the relative magnitude of the forces. *B*, Degenerated disc. The inner fibers undergo only compressive forces, according to White and Panjabi.[9]

tion, the resilience and torsion strength of a normal disc is greater with a round posterior surface than with a flat posterior surface.

Intradiscal pressure and its influence on the behavior of the disc is another important aspect during axial compression. In vitro, the initial intradiscal pressure varies inter-individually. However, the result of calculations on the effect of different initial intradiscal pressures on the behavior of a *normal* disc indicates that this factor is not significant. Another calculation shows that tensile stress occurs in the trabecular bone cranial and caudal from the disc, mainly at the level of the nucleus. The Shirazi-Adl et al[10] disc model was presented with the nucleus totally absent. They determined that the compression force on the cortical bone of the adjacent vertebrae increased by 35%.

Under a compressive influence, the weak spots of a normal disc are the end-plates and the spongy bone at the level of the nucleus.

Only when degenerative changes have occurred is the dorsal aspect of the disc also weakened. In a completely degenerated nucleus, the annulus is the weakest spot.

An attempt to combine compression and torsion in one model was made by Gracovetsky et al.[12] In their model, it is given that the fiber angle is different for the inner and outer annulus layers. They state that the inner fibers form an angle of 37° to the horizontal, and the outer layers form an angle of 24°. Stiffness of the disc is obtained when the annulus fibers become taut through torsion. When the height of the disc decreases (not only due to compression, but also as a result of degenerative changes) the distance over which the fibers have to lengthen before they are taut increases. This mechanism occurs first in the inner annulus layers, where the torsion stiffness decreases. The forces now act almost solely on the outer fibers, which then experience a large load and can become damaged. In this way, a situation can develop in subsequent loads where compression and rotation occur simultaneously; the inner annulus layers relax and therefore are not able to resist torsion forces, while the outer layers become damaged. In this instance, there is only a middle zone that is capable of effectively resisting the torsion forces (Figure 4–6).

According to Shirazi-Adl et al,[10] a more horizontal position of the annulus fibers is more effective in resisting pure axial compression. However, they also warn that a decrease in the fiber angle is detrimental for resisting torsion or a load during sidebending. In pure axial compression, according to the model of Shirazi-Adl et al, the annulus fibers are not very susceptible to damage.

Pure rotation—according to a study by Farfan et al[13]—is damaging to the annular fibers. The amount of rotation necessary to damage the disc is only 10°. This figure is not age related. *For the intervertebral disc, the combination of compression and rotation seems to be a very damaging type of load.*

Finally, the length of time in which the load is applied is of importance. According to Shirazi-Adl et al,[10] stiffness increases with an increased loading, but, according to Gracovetsky et al,[12] this occurs only when the load is applied for more than 4½ seconds. When the load is applied for less than 4½ seconds, the annulus behaves in the manner of a semistiff ring. This is due to the fact that cross-bridges are located between the various annulus layers. These bridges prevent the layers from gliding along each other. The model of Shirazi-Adl et al is applicable only when (after about 4½ seconds) these bridges start to allow movement. The time necessary for the annulus to regain its initial position, including the recovery of the bridges, has not yet been determined.

Difference between Lumbar and Thoracic Discs

From the research of the above-mentioned authors, a number of differences between lumbar and thoracic discs were observed. Summarized, data from this research include the following differences:

- The disc height increases from T5-6 to L4-5, while the disc L5-S1 is narrower. Between T9-10 and L4-5 the increase is larger than that between T5-6 and T9-10.

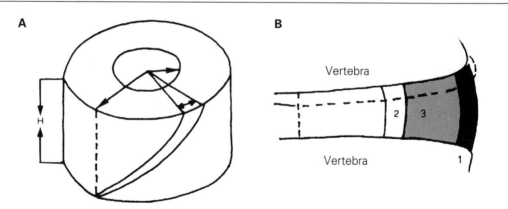

Figure 4–6 A, Normal disc. The fibers at the outer aspect have to cover a greater distance before they become taut, compared with the fibers at the inner aspect of the annulus. **B**, Degenerated disc. After the height of the disc decreases the situation occurs whereby the outer layer (**1**) is damaged, the inner layer (**2**) is relaxed, and only the middle layer (**3**) resists the compressive forces. In this way, the foundation for further degeneration is set.

- The percentage of water in the disc is less in the lower thoracic spine than in the lumbar spine.
- From T8-9 to L4-5 the axial deformation increases.
- A correlation exists between disc height and the amount of axial deformation ($r = 0.86$).
- The ventral bulging of the disc increases from the thoracic region to the lumbar region and also shows a correlation with the height of the disc ($r = 0.84$).
- The lower and midthoracic discs have a more viscous behavior than the lumbar discs. The amount of water cannot serve as an explanation for this, because the lumbar discs contain more water than the thoracic discs; the reason could be due to the different structure of the fibers in the thoracic and lumbar discs.

From the research results mentioned above, it is clearly shown that the mechanical behaviors of the thoracic and lumbar discs are not the same. What is normal for one disc is not automatically normal for the other.

Intradiscal Pressure

Important contributions to the study of load on the spinal column were made by Nachemson.[7] After having first measured the intradiscal pressure of the L3-4 disc in cadavers, Nachemson published the results of a large in vivo study of the pressure in the normal nucleus pulposus of a healthy 35-year-old woman during different positions and activities. Worth noting was that the pressure in an upright position equaled 9.6 kg/cm^2; the pressure increased significantly—up to 15.3 kg/cm^2—in the upright, unsupported, sitting position; and the pressure decreased again when the subject leaned against the chair's backrest.

Although these observations give a good impression of the intradiscal behavior in a normal disc during daily activities, they do not allow one to deduce directly the behavior of a degenerated disc. Merriam[14] published the results of in vivo pressure measurements in degenerated discs. The researchers found a significant variation in the pressure changes. The amounts of pressure in the discs differed greatly from the amounts observed by Nachemson.[7] A correlation with the severity of the degeneration was not established. In lieu of the small consistency in pressure changes in the disc and the absence of a correlation with the severity of the degeneration, one has to conclude that at this point the value of the in vivo pressure measurements is minimal.

Zygapophyseal Joints

In the joint cavity of the zygapophyseal joints, meniscoid structures are found. The capsule is rather loose and does not normally restrict the movements in these joints. The largest joint cavity lies between the inferior articular process of L5 and the superior articular process of the sacrum. The position of the facet on the superior articular process is generally described as being oriented almost in a sagittal plane and directed medially. The facets on the inferior articular process are also usually described as lying almost in the sagittal plane but are directed laterally.However, a very large interindividual as well as an intraindividual variability exists (Figure 4–7).

Remarkable is the large inter- and intraindividual variability in the form of the zygapophyseal joints, the spinal canal, and the dural sac. The position of the zygapophyseal joints can vary from an almost frontal to an almost sagittal orientation. Left-right differences as well as convexity/concavity incongruencies are clearly visible. In Figure 4–7, radiological views of patients with a wide variety of disorders are presented; in no case were the zygapophyseal joints the primary cause for the patients' complaints.

Variations in the diameter of the dural sac can be clinically significant (compare C and D in Figure 4–7). For example, a large disc protrusion or prolapse may not produce symptoms in the presence of a large spinal canal with a small dural sac, whereas a small disc protrusion or the presence of a zygapophyseal joint osteophyte in a spinal canal of small diameter can cause severe pain (Figure 4–7).

Ligaments

In the lumbar spine, the same ligaments are found as in the other parts of the spinal column (with the exception of the upper cervical

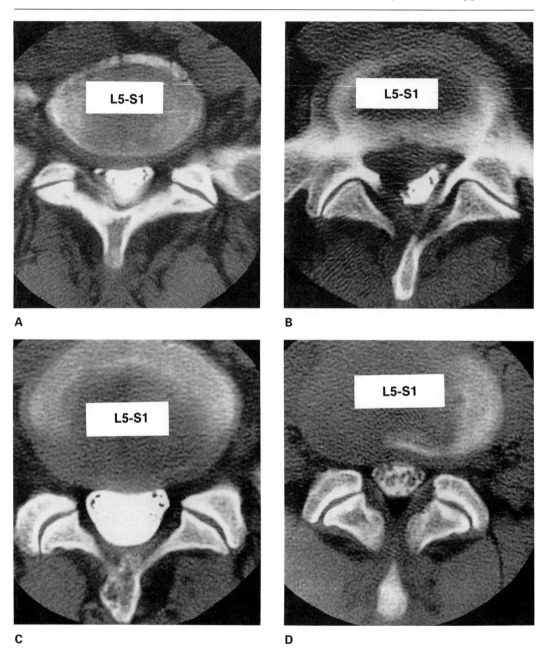

Figure 4–7 Computed tomography (CT) scans of the L5-S1 (**A**, **B**, **C**, **D**), L4-5 (**E**, **F**, **G**), and L3-4 (**H**, **I**, **J**, **K**) segments, in which, along with other structures, the zygapophyseal joints are clearly visible.

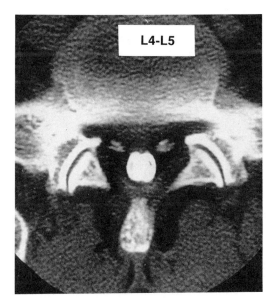

E

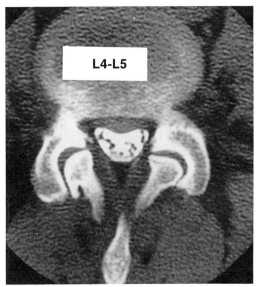

F

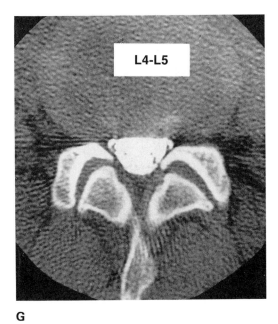

G

Figure 4–7 continued

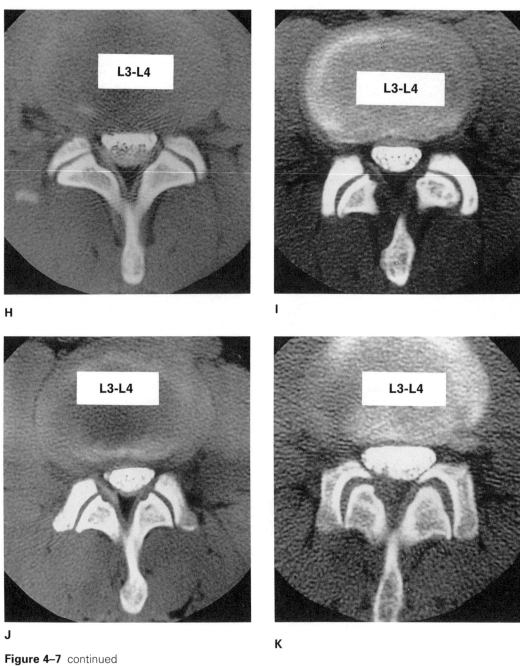

H

I

J

K

Figure 4–7 continued

spine). The posterior longitudinal ligament is significantly narrower in the lumbar region. Therefore, it offers much less resistance against the dorsally acting forces from the intervertebral disc. In this region a high incidence in variation of the vertebrae (for example, hemisacralization or hemilumbarization), the zygapophyseal joints, and the ligaments exists.

In the lumbosacral junction (Figure 4–8) the iliolumbar ligaments are clinically important. The inferior iliolumbar ligament runs from the transverse process of L5 to the mediocranioventral aspect of the iliac crest. This bandlike structure probably plays a less important clinical role than the superior iliolumbar ligament, which also runs from the transverse process of L4 to the iliac crest, and inserts directly dorsolateral to the inferior iliolumbar ligament.   .

KINEMATICS

Taking into consideration the construction of the vertebrae, only a moderate amount of mobility in the sagittal plane is available in the lumbar spine. The construction and position of the zygapophyseal joints allow for only a small degree of sidebending and an even lesser amount of rotation. The range of motion has been studied by White and Panjabi.[9] Table 4–1 illustrates the values established by them.

Worth noticing is the increasing mobility in the sagittal plane from cranial to caudal. The largest mobility in the frontal plane is located at the level of the L3-4 segment. In the sagittal and transverse planes, the motions in the L5-S1 segment are the greatest. These movements are also coupled to each other. Rotation of L5 is accompanied by a flexion of L5 in relation to the sacrum.

Coupled movements occur in the other parts of the lumbar spine, as well. First, there is the coupling of sidebending and flexion, described by Rolander.[15] The axial rotation also appears to be coupled with flexion. Miles and Sullivan[16] described the coupling of sidebending and axial rotation. They indicated that the spinous processes, in contrast to

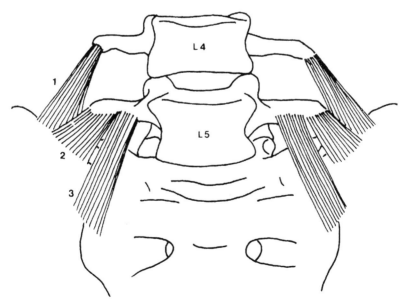

Figure 4–8 The lumbosacral junction. *1*, Superior iliolumbar ligament; *2*, inferior iliolumbar ligament; *3*, lumbosacral ligament.

Table 4–1 Average Values for the Movements around the Three Axes of Rotation in the Lumbar Spine according to White and Panjabi.[9]

Segment	Flexion/ Extension	Sidebending	Axial Rotation
L1-2	12°	6°	2°
L2-3	14°	6°	2°
L3-4	15°	8°	2°
L4-5	17°	6°	2°
L5-S1	20°	3°	5°

what happens in the cervical spine, rotate into the direction of the concavity of the spinal column. In other words, the rotation is opposite to the sidebending. However, this counts only for the normal physiological position (lordosis) and in extension (hyperlordosis). In flexion, the axial rotation is directed ipsilateral to the sidebending.

By establishing the fact that movements in the lumbar spine are always coupled, some remarks may be made about the instantaneous axes of rotation. The concept of "instantaneous axis of rotation," as described by White and Panjabi,[9] is really applicable only to movements that take place in one plane. Therefore, the concept of "helical axis of rotation" actually should be applied. The determination of such an axis in vivo has not yet been achieved.

Based on cadaver studies the instantaneous axes of rotations have been determined for the various movements (for instance, by Rolander[15]). In flexion and extension the axis is located ventrally in the disc. In sidebending the axis is located in the contralateral aspect of the disc. Cosetta et al[17] found an instantaneous axis of rotation in the dorsal part of the disc in axial rotations.

Rather significant changes occur in the locations of the instantaneous axes of rotation in degenerated discs. With a minimal range in variation, the axes of rotation in normal discs are localized in a relatively small area. In degenerated discs this area increases significantly and the range of variation is large.[15]

Function of the Zygapophyseal Joints

In relation to the function of the zygapophyseal joints in lumbar spine movements, the research of Stokes et al[18] indicates that the zygapophyseal joints are involved particularly in restricting the axial rotation, a movement that, in combination with compression, is potentially harmful to the intervertebral disc. Even after removing the dorsal structures of the vertebra (joint facets included), an increase in translation between two adjacent vertebrae is negligible (always less than 1 mm).

In regard to load on the zygapophyseal joints, Nachemson[7] calculated that the zygapophyseal joints account for the transfer of approximately 20% of the vertical load. Adams and Hutton[19] found that in the lordotic lumbar spinal column (in the upright position), 16% of the load is transferred through the zygapophyseal joints.

The mechanism in which the zygapophyseal joint assimilates the load has been studied and described by Yang and King.[20] According to them, the load increases during increasing extension of the spinal column. In relation to the caudal vertebra's superior facet, the cranial vertebra's inferior facet "subluxes" or "seesaws" out of the convexity during extension, termed "bottoming out." When a segment is loaded in extension (compression), the vertebral body translates and tilts somewhat dorsally.[21] This explains the phenomenon of bottoming out.

4.2   EXAMINATION

GENERAL INSPECTION

- How does the patient enter the examination room? Note the following:
  1. Postural deviations
  2. Assistive devices (eg, cane, wheelchair, corset, brace)
- How does the patient sit down? Would he or she rather remain standing?
  1. Is there pain in sitting?
  2. Posture of the patient in sitting (kyphosis, straight back, lordosis, other deviation). Patients with lumbar disc syndromes often sit extremely upright at the edge of the chair or would rather remain standing.
- Notice the facial expression of the patient (exhausted, unhealthy appearing).

HISTORY

Age

Even in the area of the lumbar spine, many disorders are age related. For example, the primary disc-related disorders are predominantly seen in the 35- to 55-year age group, whereas the secondary disc-related disorders occur mostly in people over 60 years of age.

Occupation, Sport, Hobby

People who spend long periods of time either standing or sitting during their work often suffer from postural syndromes. Repeated bending and lifting increase the risk of a disc-related problem. In young gymnasts or athletes in throwing sports, one will occasionally see a spondylolisthesis.

Chief Complaints

Does the patient complain of pain, paresthesia, paresis, or loss of sensation?

Onset

For both diagnosis and treatment, it is important to know whether the problem was of an acute or gradual onset. Also notable is whether or not the problem occurred as a result of a trauma.

Duration

In general the shorter the length of time during which the patient has experienced the symptoms, the better the chance for a successful treatment.

Location of Complaints

Complaints due to a disorder of the sacroiliac (SI) joint are never localized in the midline. Problems in the zygapophyseal joints cause a dull, deep, low back pain that is almost never referred beyond the knee. Most disc-related disorders cause local and/or segmental pain.

Symptoms from the S4 neurological segment such as incontinence, disturbances in sensibility of the perineal area (saddle-block anesthesia), or impotence are generally indications for immediate surgery.

Pain that was initially experienced in the back but has spread to the leg indicates a progression of the disorder.

Factors That Influence Symptoms

The most frequently seen pathology is related to posture or movement. Pain during lifting or bending usually indicates a disc lesion. Complaints with prolonged standing, walking slowly, or prolonged sitting often indicate some type of instability. In cases of constant, increasing pain that is independent of any posture or movement, severe pathology should be suspected.

Pain with Coughing, Sneezing, and Straining

An elevated cerebrospinal pressure can lead to increased pressure on the dura mater, which can cause pain in the back, radiating into the leg.

Prior History

Frequent recurrence of the problem worsens the prognosis. Patients with secondary disc-related disorders often have a prior history of back pain.

Medication

- analgesics
- antiphlogistic (anti-inflammatory) agents (can provide pain relief in some back problems)
- antihypertensive drugs (the exercise program may have to be more closely monitored)
- anticoagulants (all manipulations are contraindicated)
- cytostatic drugs (think of possible metastases)
- antidepressants (of what influence is the patient's psychological status?)

Patient's Reaction to Symptoms

Despite the complaints, does the patient try to continue working? Does the patient need medication, or is the patient completely unable to perform daily activities?

SPECIFIC INSPECTION

The specific inspection is performed from dorsal and ventral aspects and from both sides. The following points may be of significance.

General

- What is the position of the pelvis? Is there a pelvic torsion or asymmetry?
- Is there a leg length difference?

Muscle Atrophy

- Is there atrophy of the gluteal or leg musculature?

Swelling

- Swelling in the lumbar region is rare. After recent trauma, a hematoma may be observed. Lipomas are mostly found in the thoracic area.

Position of the Spine

During the inspection, it is also important to note the presence of the following:

- increased lumbar lordosis
- decreased lumbar lordosis (flat back)
- lumbar kyphosis
- increased thoracic kyphosis
- scoliosis
- deviation (toward or away from the painful side)

PALPATION

If swelling is present, the swelling should be palpated to determine its consistency. Palpation to localize the painful area is performed only after the functional examination is completed.

FUNCTIONAL EXAMINATION

Before the functional examination, it should be determined whether the patient is experiencing symptoms at that specific moment. Note whether the symptoms change per test during the functional examination.

Furthermore, it is imperative always to compare the affected with the nonaffected side. This means that both sides are tested, first the nonaffected side (to have an idea of what is "normal") and then the affected side.

During the examination specific attention is given to the following points:

- *articular signs* (which motions are painful and/or limited, which motions appear hypermobile or unstable?)
- *dural or nerve root signs* (mobility tests for the dura mater; tests for the nerve roots, ie, strength, sensibility, and reflexes)
- *spinal cord signs* (spastic gait, pathological reflexes such as Babinski)
- *in reference to other causes* (SI joint, hip joint, and other lesions of the lower extremities, compression neuropathies)
- *reactions of the patient*[22] (perspiration, facial grimaces, tremors, etc)

The functional examination is performed with the patient in four positions: standing, supine, sidelying, and prone. The examination is divided into a basic examination and a segmental examination. The segmental examination is performed only when a specific diagnosis cannot be made from the information obtained from the basic examination, or when the initial treatment did not produce the desired results. (*Note:* Illustrations with explanations, corresponding to the numbers and tests listed below, can be found in the following pages.)

TESTS FOR BASIC FUNCTIONAL EXAMINATION

In Standing

Active Tests

4.1. Extension

4.2. Left sidebending

4.3. Right sidebending

4.4. Flexion

4.5. Flexion with addition of cervical flexion (Neri test)

4.6. Resisted left sidebending

4.7. Resisted right sidebending

4.8/9. Toe raises: test for triceps surae (S1 and S2 neurological segments)

4.10. Heel raises: test for neurological segments L3 to L5

4.11. Valsalva test

Passive Tests

4.12. Kemp test for the left side

4.13. Kemp test for the right side

4.14. Palpation of the spinous processes in neutral

4.15. Palpation of the spinous processes in extension

4.16. Palpation of the spinous processes in flexion

In Supine

Passive Tests

4.17. Provocation test for the sacroiliac (SI) joint

4.18. Provocation test for the SI joint with support of lumbar lordosis (test performed if test 4.17 is positive)

4.19/20. Straight leg raise test

4.21/22. Bragard test

4.23/24. Neri test

4.25/26. Bragard test in combination with the Neri test

4.27. Slump test (test performed when there is still doubt about a dural irritation)

Quick Tests for the Hip

4.28/29. Passive flexion of the hip

4.30/31. Passive internal rotation of the hip

4.32/33. Passive external rotation of the hip

Neurological Tests

4.34/35. Resisted test for the iliopsoas (L1 to L3)

4.36/37. Resisted test for the tibialis anterior (L3, L4)

4.38/39. Resisted test for the extensor hallucis longus (L4, L5)

4.40/41. Resisted test for the peroneals (L5, S1)

4.42/43. Quadriceps reflex (L3, L4)

4.44/45. Foot sole reflex

4.46. Sensibility tests (L3 to L5 and S1 to S3)

Quick Tests for Vascularization

When suspecting an arterial occlusion or vascular disease (eg, intermittent claudication), the following pulses are tested:

4.47/48. Palpation of the femoral artery

4.49/50. Palpation of the posterior tibial artery

4.51/52. Palpation of the dorsal pedal artery

In Sidelying

4.53/54. Alternative test for SI joint provocation (performed when test 4.17 is negative)

In Prone

4.55/56. Femoral nerve stretch test, roots L1 to L4

Neurological Tests

4.57/58. Achilles tendon reflex (L5 to S2)

4.59/60. Resisted test for the hamstrings (S1, S2)

4.61/62. Resisted test for the rectus femoris (L3, L4)

4.63/64. Resisted test for the gluteus maximus (S1, S2)

Passive Test

4.65. Palpation of the spinous processes

TESTS FOR SEGMENTAL FUNCTIONAL EXAMINATION

The segmental functional examination is indicated in the following circumstances:

- when the symptoms of the patient are not provoked during the basic functional examination
- when the initial treatment series does not produce results
- when the symptoms are not completely eliminated by the general manual mobilization treatment
- when, on the basis of patient history, a form of instability is suspected
- when, despite previous treatments, the symptoms continue to recur

In Sitting

Active General Tests

4.66. Extension

4.67. Left sidebending

4.68. Right sidebending

4.69. Flexion

4.70. Extension with left sidebending and right rotation (coupled movement)

4.71. Extension with left sidebending and left rotation (combined movement)

4.72. Extension with right sidebending and left rotation (coupled movement)

4.73. Extension with right sidebending and right rotation (combined movement)

4.74. Flexion with left sidebending and left rotation (coupled movement)

4.75. Flexion with left sidebending and right rotation (combined movement)

4.76. Flexion with right sidebending and right rotation (coupled movement)

4.77. Flexion with right sidebending and left rotation (combined movement)

Passive General Tests

4.78. Extension

4.79. Left sidebending

4.80. Right sidebending

4.81. Extension with left sidebending and right rotation (coupled movement)

4.82. Extension with right sidebending and right rotation (combined movement)

4.83. Extension with right sidebending and left rotation (coupled movement)

4.84. Extension with left sidebending and left rotation (combined movement)

Coupled and combined motions in flexion are not performed passively as this puts too much load on the intervertebral discs.

Passive Local Mobility Tests

4.85. Extension in weight bearing

4.86. Extension with left sidebending and right rotation in weight bearing (coupled movement)

4.87. Extension with right sidebending and left rotation in weight bearing (coupled movement)

In Prone

Passive Local Mobility Tests

4.88. Segment mobility in ventral translation

4.89. End-feel test in extension

4.90. Test for rotatory hypermobility

In Sidelying

Passive Local Mobility Tests

4.91. Segment mobility in dorsal translation

4.92. Extension in non–weight bearing

4.93. Extension with left sidebending and right rotation in non–weight bearing

4.94. Extension with right sidebending and left rotation in non–weight bearing

SUPPLEMENTARY EXAMINATIONS

In some cases further diagnostics in the form of imaging procedures are necessary. Diagnostic imaging possibilities include conventional X-rays such as functional views and contrast studies, CT scans, and magnetic resonance imaging (MRI). (Refer to Chapter 11 for more detailed information.)

Additional examinations to be considered are as follows:

- electromyography (EMG)
- laboratory tests
- spinal tap
- psychological testing

The functional examination described above gives valuable information in determining the patient's diagnosis. Supplementary examination by a specialist serves as clarification for an unclear diagnosis in order to rule out any malignant pathology.

INTERPRETATION OF THE STRAIGHT LEG RAISE TEST

In 1864, Lasègue originally described flexing the hip and then straightening the knee.[23] The straight leg raise (SLR) test (Figure 4–9) as performed today, flexion of the hip with extended knee, was first performed by his student, J. Forst.

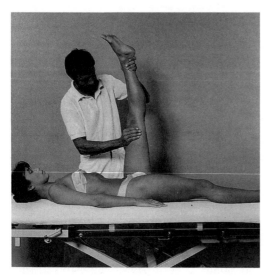

Figure 4–9 SLR test.

During the SLR test, stretch is placed not only on the hamstring muscles but also on the dura mater and the nerve roots from L4 to S2. In a lesion of the muscle group, isometrically resisted knee flexion in combination with resisted hip extension will also be painful. If this is not the case, then the SLR usually indicates a dural irritation or (less often) a disorder of the SI joint.

A positive "crossed" straight leg raise is pathognomonic for disc pathology.

Causes for Pain and/or Limitation of Motion with SLR Test

Disc Lesions

- *SLR test: negative.* This often occurs in cases of aspecific low back pain; nevertheless several authors maintain that the symptoms are caused by a primary disc lesion.[24–26]
- *SLR test: full range of motion, but painful.* This finding can be seen as the result of a smaller disc protrusion. After disc surgery, this test can remain positive for several months.

- *SLR test: negative, but with a painful arc.* This combination is pathognomonic for a disc protrusion.
- *SLR test: limited range of motion and painful, without neurological deficit in the lower extremities.* This can result from a disc protrusion that hinders the mobility of the dura mater and the nerve root but does not compromise the function of the nerve root.
- *SLR test: significant limitation of motion with shooting pain in the lateral or posterior aspect of the leg and possibly severe pain in the back (Lasègue's sign).* Usually, in this situation, neurological deficits are also present. Almost always, this finding indicates a disc protrusion that has compromised both the mobility and the function of the nerve root.
- *SLR test: negative, but with neurological deficits in the lower extremities.* This is an indication of either a massive prolapse with simultaneous ischemia of the nerve root and dural sleeve or a non–disc-related neurological disorder. As a result, the nerve will go numb.
- *SLR test: limited range of motion, but painless.* Most likely there is either an ischemia with adhesions between the dural sleeve and the nerve root or there is a muscle lesion.[24]

Other Disorders

In the following disorders, the SLR test can also be painful and limited:

- intraspinal lesions, such as tumors at the level of or caudal to the L4 vertebra
- osteomyelitis of the ilium or of a proximal part of the femur
- sacrum fractures
- ischiorectal abscess
- ankylosing spondylitis or other disorders of the sacroiliac joint
- hematoma in the hamstrings, usually as a result of a muscle tear

- all disorders that could cause a mechanical irritation of the nerve roots (disc protrusion, a narrowed foramen, etc)

With several of the disorders listed above, passive hip flexion is also painful and limited. Cyriax called this phenomenon "sign of the buttock." When *both* the SLR test and passive hip flexion are painful and limited, often with an "empty" end-feel, more serious pathology (including sacral fractures, osteomyelitis of the ilium or femur, and malignant processes in the buttock region) should be suspected.[24]

Interpretation of Dural Signs

The most significant sign of a dural irritation is increased back pain during coughing, sneezing, or straining. When these lead to increased back pain or referred pain into the leg, then a posterolateral disc prolapse, or at least a protrusion, is present.

Other dural signs, besides the SLR, include neck flexion (Neri test) during trunk flexion, and the SLR in combination with neck flexion (Neri test) and/or dorsiflexion of the foot (Bragard test). The dura mater is maximally stretched during the slump test.

Interpretation of Inappropriate Illness Behavior

Sometimes patients are aware of the meaning of the SLR tests and attempt, either consciously or unconsciously, to influence the results. By use of the already mentioned tests and the following described tests, the examiner has the possibility to objectify the findings. For instance, after performing the SLR test, one can ask the patient to sit up (long sit). If the SLR test were actually positive, then the patient is forced to bend the knee of the affected side when in a long sit position. The flip test is also very useful: the patient sits with the lower legs overhanging the examination table and the examiner straightens the affected leg. If the SLR test were really posi-

tive, then the patient immediately bends (or flips) backward.

Because many patients feign or exaggerate their back pain, it is important, along with help from the history and the clinical examination, to be able to differentiate appropriate versus inappropriate illness behavior. Waddell et al describe six specific findings for obtaining such information[22,27]:

1. complaints of lumbar pain when axial compression is applied at the top of the head.
2. complaints of lumbar pain when rotation of the spine is simulated: rotation is performed through the pelvis, whereby the actual rotation occurs in the joints of the lower extremities.
3. wide-ranging (ie, over many levels) tenderness to pressure on the spinous processes.
4. tenderness over an extensive area when slight pressure is exerted on the skin.
5. complaints of pain during the SLR test that are not confirmed when the test is performed while the patient is distracted (refer to the tests described above).
6. referred pain that does not correspond to anatomical dermatomes; weakness or sensory disturbances that do not correspond to anatomical neurological segments.

DESCRIPTION OF TESTS FOR BASIC FUNCTIONAL EXAMINATION

See Tests for Basic Functional Examination for specific types of tests.

Active Tests: In Standing

4.1 Extension: Views from Behind (4–1A) and from the Side (4–1B)

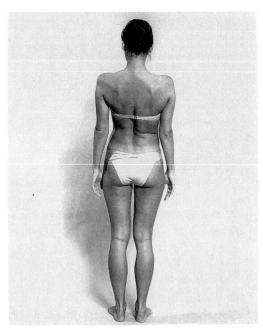

Test 4.1A View from Behind

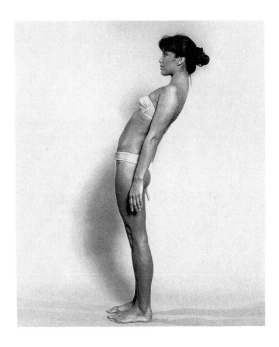

Test 4.1B View from the Side

Position of the Patient

The patient stands with equal weight on each leg and with feet about shoulder width apart.

Position of the Examiner

To assess the motion, the examiner stands first behind the patient and then to the side of the patient.

Performance

The patient is asked to bend backward, keeping the knees straight. The examiner notes the amount of motion, any deviation during the movement, and complaints of pain or other symptoms. The patient should be as precise as possible in localizing the symptoms.

Extension can be limited and/or painful due to numerous disorders, such as disc pathology (especially when the patient has a deviated posture), neurogenic spinal claudication (walking, in particular, elicits the symptoms), and in cases of "kissing spine" or Baastrup syndrome. In nerve root compression syndromes and the various forms of instability, extension is usually the most limited motion. Pathology of the hip can cause extension to be painful as a result of stretch on a superficial anterior structure or compression of a deeper-lying structure.

4.2. Left Sidebending

4.3. Right Sidebending

Position of the Patient

Same as for test 4.1.

Position of the Examiner

Same as for test 4.1.

Performance

The patient is asked to bend the trunk as far as possible to the left, keeping the knees straight and maintaining contact with both feet on the floor. The examiner assesses the

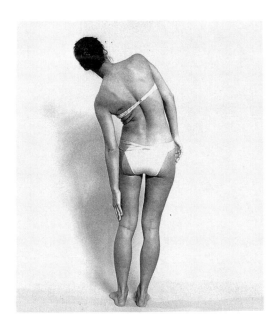

Test 4.2

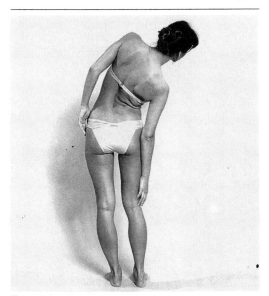

Test 4.3

Complaints of pain or other symptoms are noted. In localizing the symptoms, the patient should be as precise as possible. The distance from fingertips to the floor is a reliable objective parameter.

4.4. Flexion

Position of the Patient

Same as for test 4.1.

Position of the Examiner

Same as for test 4.1.

Performance

The patient is asked to bend forward, keeping the knees straight. The examiner notes the amount of motion (Schober index),[28] any deviation during the movement, and complaints of pain or other symptoms. Not only the lumbar spine, but also the thoracic spine, the sacroiliac joints, and the hip joints are involved in this active motion.

In the forward flexed position one can assess any possible scoliosis. With a scoliosis, a

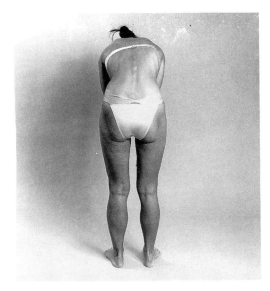

Test 4.4

amount of motion and the direction in which the pelvis moves. Generally during left sidebending the left side of the pelvis moves forward, and in right sidebending the right side of the pelvis moves forward.

distinct difference in the heights of the right and left prominences of the back is noticeable. The sidebend in the scoliosis can induce anatomically an axial rotation that causes a difference in the position of the transverse processes in the transverse plane (bringing the ribs and/or erector spinae with it). However, one cannot deduce the rotational component from the observed sidebend. Because of the morphology, changes in the vertebra itself may result in an inversion of the "normal" physiological coupling patterns in that region.

Usually with primary disc pathology, without a postural deviation, flexion is the most painful motion. In patients with a spondylolitic spondylolisthesis as well as in patients with a segmental instability, the flexion is remarkably mobile. With all forms of instability, the patient moves easily into flexion but usually has difficulty returning to erect standing.

4.5. Flexion with Addition of Cervical Flexion (Neri Test)

Position of the Patient

Same as for test 4.1.

Position of the Examiner

The examiner stands to the side of the patient.

Performance

The test is the same as for test 4.4, but at the end of forward flexion, the patient is asked to bring the cervical spine into maximal flexion (Neri test). This puts a stretch on the entire dura mater. Dural irrigation is indicated when the patient's symptoms increase during neck flexion.

4.6. Resisted Left Sidebending

4.7. Resisted Right Sidebending

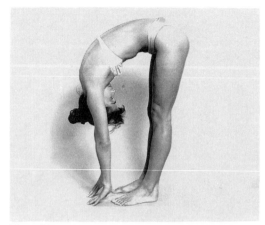

Test 4.5

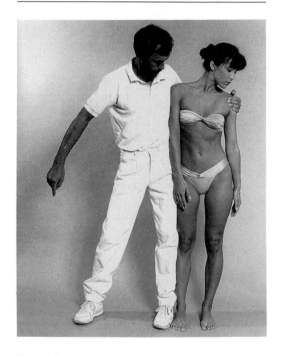

Test 4.6

Position of the Patient

Same as for test 4.1.

Position of the Examiner

The examiner stands next to the patient, facing in the same direction, with the left side

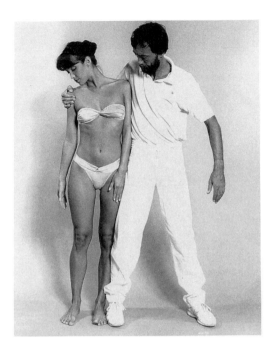

Test 4.7

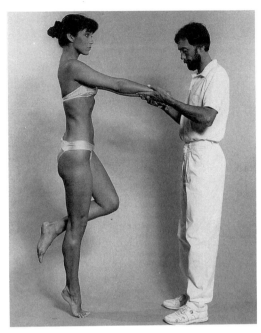

Test 4.8/9

of his or her body against the right side of the patient. The examiner places the left foot next to the patient's right foot and grasps the lateral aspect of the patient's left shoulder with the left hand.

Performance

The patient is asked to hold the position while the examiner exerts isometric resistance against left sidebending. With the examiner against the patient's left side, the test is then repeated for isometric resistance against right sidebending.

The resisted sidebending test is rarely positive. Even when a patient has an acute disc lesion, this test is usually negative or at the most only vaguely positive. Noteworthy in this context, patients with psychosomatic complaints or patients who exaggerate their symptoms often find this test quite painful.

4.8/9. Toe Raises: Test for the Triceps Surae (S1, S2 Neurological Segments)

Position of the Patient

The patient stands on one leg.

Position of the Examiner

The examiner stands in front of the patient and holds the patient's hand(s) in order to give slight balancing support during the test.

Performance

The patient is asked first on one side, and then on the other side, to rise up on the toes 10 times. This tests the strength of the triceps surae, which are innervated by the roots S1 and S2. The patient should be able to rise up on the toes at least 10 times. When there is doubt about the strength, the patient is asked to hop on one foot.

In this test, emphasis is placed on assessing the general strength of the triceps surae; complaints of pain are of little value.

4.10. Heel Raises: Test for Neurological Segments L3 to L5

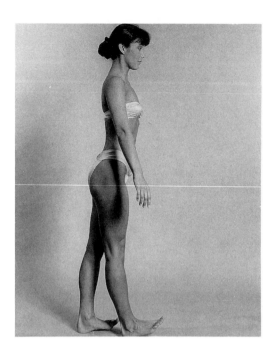

Test 4.10

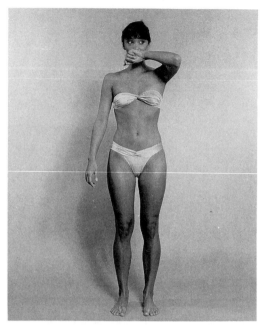

Test 4.11

Position of the Patient

Same as for test 4.1.

Position of the Examiner

The examiner stands in front of the patient.

Performance

The patient is asked to walk on the heels. This tests the function of the nerve roots L3 to L5. The patient should be able to take at least 10 steps; when there is doubt about the strength of the triceps surae, the patient is asked to take more steps. As in the previous test, complaints of pain are of little interest. Whether or not the patient has sufficient strength is noted in particular.

4.11. Valsalva Test

Position of the Patient

Same as for test 4.1.

Position of the Examiner

The examiner stands in front of the patient.

Performance

The patient is asked to exhale vigorously against the back of the hand without letting any air escape. During this test, both the venous pressure and the cerebrospinal fluid pressure are elevated. In an acute nerve root irritation, this test is often positive. Patients with cardiovascular and/or pulmonary problems, as well as those for whom this test is positive, must be very cautious when performing exercises that lead to increased venous or cerebrospinal fluid pressure. Also, when performing the abdominal exercises described in this book, these patients should be reminded constantly to exhale.

Passive Tests: In Standing

4.12. Kemp Test for the Left Side

4.13. Kemp Test for the Right Side

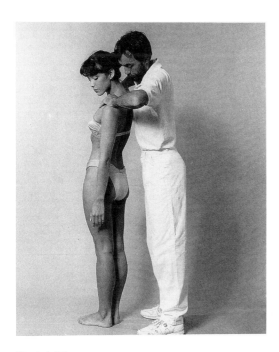

Test 4.12

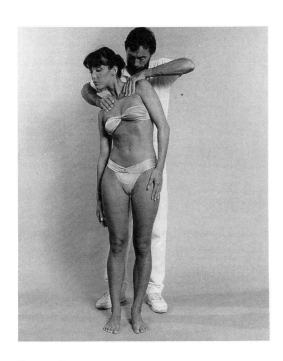

Test 4.13

Position of the Patient

Same as for test 4.1. If the examiner has any doubts about the patient's stability, the patient can be positioned in sitting at the corner of the examination table. The table is positioned at a height to allow for approximately 70° of hip flexion with the feet resting on the floor.

Position of the Examiner

The examiner stands behind the patient and places one hand on each shoulder.

Performance

The examiner brings the patient into the end position of a combined motion of lumbar extension, sidebending, and ipsilateral rotation, then applies abrupt pressure on the shoulders, giving a short axial impulse. The test is performed to the left side and the right side.

The Kemp test is considered positive when the patient's symptoms are provoked in the leg. In this test the intervertebral foramina are narrowed in order to exert pressure on the nerve roots running through them. Keep in mind that the disc can also be compromised in this test.

4.14. Palpation of the Spinous Processes in Neutral

4.15. Palpation of the Spinous Processes in Extension

4.16. Palpation of the Spinous Processes in Flexion

Position of the Patient

Same as for test 4.1.

Position of the Examiner

The examiner stands obliquely behind the patient with the stabilizing hand placed on the patient's abdomen. The testing hand palpates the spinous processes of the lumbar spine.

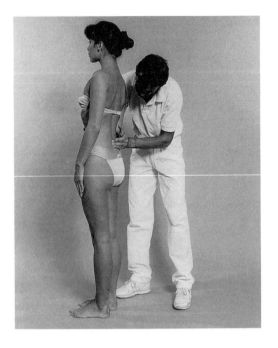

Test 4.14

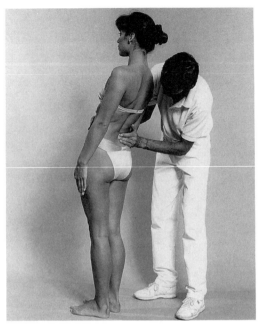

Test 4.15

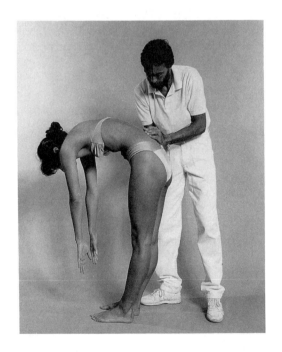

Test 4.16

Performance

In standing, the spinous processes are palpated in the neutral position as well as in extension and flexion. In some cases of instability, an anterolisthesis or (more seldom) a retrolisthesis can be felt.

Passive Tests: In Supine

4.17. Provocation Test for the Sacroiliac (SI) Joint

4.18. Provocation Test for the SI Joint with Support of Lumbar Lordosis

Test 4.18 is performed if test 4.17 is positive.

Position of the Patient

The patient lies supine on the examination table with arms relaxed at the sides. A small

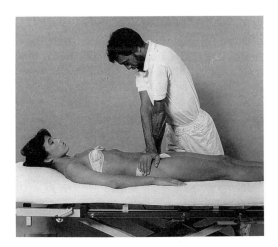

Test 4.17

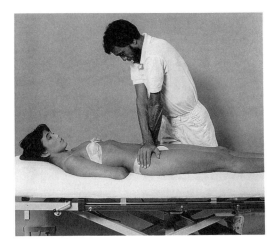

Test 4.18

with arms crossed and elbows extended. The examination table is brought low enough that the examiner can position his or her shoulders directly over the hands. Pressure is applied in a dorsolateral direction and held for about 40 seconds. Then, with the patient relaxed, the examiner exerts a moderate overpressure by abruptly nodding the head (cervical flexion). This puts a stretch on the capsuloligamentous structures of the SI joint (see Chapter 3, section 3.2).

If this test provokes central low back pain, the pain can never be due to a pathology of the SI joint. In this instance, lumbar spine pathology should be suspected. If the patient experiences pain in the paravertebral region during this test, it is repeated with support of the lumbar lordosis (the patient is asked to place a hand/forearm in the small of the back). Pathology of the SI joint is likely if the same pain is again elicited. Further examination of the SI joint is then indicated.

4.19/20. Straight Leg Raise Test

Position of the Patient

The patient lies supine on the examination table with arms relaxed at the sides.

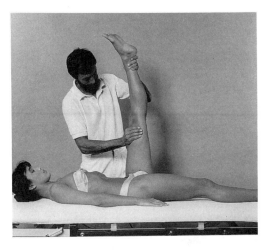

Test 4.19/20

towel roll can be placed under the knees, bringing the hips into about 20° flexion (not shown). This puts the SI joint in a loose-packed position.

Position of the Examiner

The examiner stands next to the patient at the level of the patient's thighs.

Performance

The examiner places his or her hands on the patient's anterior superior iliac spines,

Position of the Examiner

The examiner stands next to the patient at the level of the patient's pelvis.

Performance

The examiner grasps the patient's lower leg from posterior directly above the malleoli. The other hand is placed loosely on the anterior thigh just proximal to the patella. The hip is then brought passively into flexion, keeping the knee extended. The test is performed on each side.

The SLR test can be positive in a variety of disorders. However, the cause is usually due to a compression of the nerve root L5, S1, or S2 as a result of disc pathology (see Interpretation of the Straight Leg Raise Test).

4.21/22. Bragard Test

Position of the Patient

Same as for test 4.19/20.

Position of the Examiner

Same as for test 4.19/20.

Performance

The SLR test can be performed in combination with passive ankle dorsiflexion (Bragard

test). The leg is lifted to the painful level, then lowered slightly and the foot brought into dorsiflexion. The test is performed on each side. This is test is considered to be positive when the patient's symptoms are again provoked. In this instance, dural irrigation is indicated, thereby ruling out tension of the hamstring muscles.

4.23/24. Neri Test

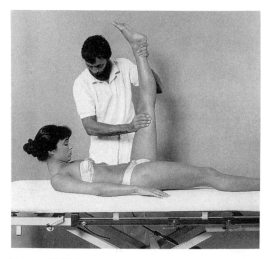

Test 4.23/24

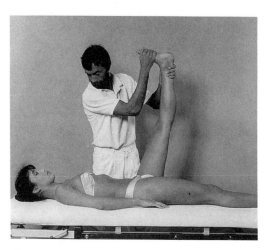

Test 4.21/22

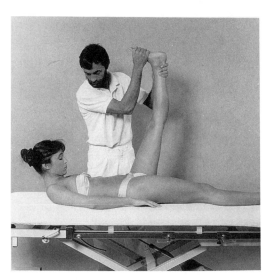

Test 4.25/26

4.25/26. Bragard Test in Combination with the Neri Test

Position of the Patient

Same as for test 4.19/20.

Position of the Examiner

Same as for test 4.19/20.

Performance

Same as for test 4.19/20, only now the patient is asked to bring the chin to the chest.

As in forward flexion in standing, the SLR test can be performed in combination with neck flexion. This puts an additional stretch on the dura mater.

The Bragard test (4.21/22) can also be combined with the Neri test. This brings the dura mater under even more stretch. These tests are performed on both sides.

4.27. Slump Test

When there is still doubt about a dural irritation, the slump test is performed.

Position of the Patient

The patient sits at the edge of the examination table with the legs hanging down.

Position of the Examiner

The examiner stands in front of the patient.

Performance

For maximal stretch of the dura mater, the patient is asked to bring the entire spine into flexion, after which the examiner performs the SLR test.

The patient is instructed to flex the cervical spine first, followed by the thoracic and lumbar spines. Then one leg is brought into an SLR position. If the patient's symptoms are not yet provoked, that leg is returned to its initial position and the other leg is straightened. At this point if the symptoms still are not elicited, both legs are held in an SLR position. Dorsiflexion of the foot (or feet) may also be added. Once the patient's symptoms are elicited, the patient is asked to raise his or her head (extend the cervical spine).

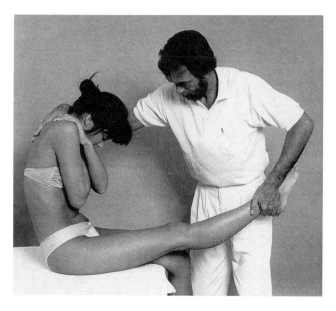

Test 4.27

The slump test is considered positive if the symptoms are alleviated by the cervical extension.

Quick Tests for the Hip: In Supine

4.28/29. Passive Flexion of the Hip

Position of the Patient

Same as for test 4.19/20.

Position of the Examiner

The examiner stands next to the patient at the level of the patient's pelvis.

Performance

With the distal (in relation to the patient) hand, the examiner grasps the patient's distal thigh from posterior just above the knee and brings the hip passively into full flexion. Keep in mind that the lumbar spine is brought into a kyphosis during this test. The test is performed on each side.

Hip pathology can also lead to pain in the back region, and passive hip flexion serves to rule out other causes of low back pain. As mentioned previously, when both passive hip flexion and the SLR test are painful and limited, serious pathology should be suspected (sign of the buttock).[24]

4.30/31. Passive Internal Rotation of the Hip

Position of the Patient

Same as for test 4.19/20.

Position of the Examiner

Same as for test 4.19/20.

With the distal hand, the examiner grasps the posterior aspect of the patient's lower leg just proximal of the malleoli. The other hand supports the medial aspect of the knee at the level of the patella.

Performance

The examiner brings the patient's lower leg, keeping it in the horizontal plane, toward him or her. The test is performed on each side.

Passive internal rotation of the hip is the most limited motion in cases of osteoarthrosis and arthritides of the hip. These patients often have pain in the low back because of the hip pathology. The limitation of motion results in a change in the movement pattern of the entire kinetic chain, from T8 to the foot. Therefore, a loss of motion in the coxofemoral joint often leads to a compensatory hypermobility of the lumbar spine. Differentiating

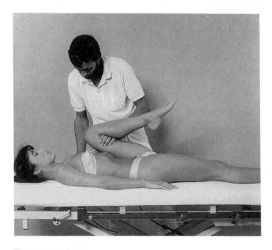

Test 4.28/29

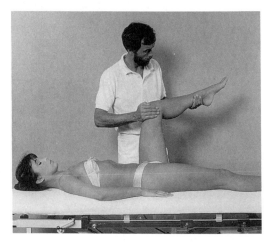

Test 4.30/31

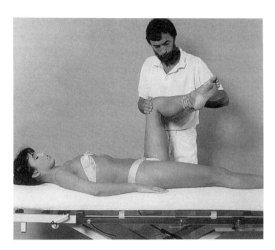

Test 4.32/33

---

between back and hip pathology is not always easy.

Keep in mind that passive internal rotation of the hip will always cause a slight ipsilateral sidebending in the lumbar spine.

4.32/33. Passive External Rotation of the Hip

Position of the Patient

Same as for test 4.19/20.

Position of the Examiner

Same as for test 4.30/31.

Performance

The examiner now moves the lower leg, keeping it in the horizontal plane, away from him or her. The test is repeated on the other side.

Passive hip external rotation is seldom limited (except, for example, in the instance of a loose body). Keep in mind that passive hip external rotation causes a slight contralateral sidebending in the lumbar spine. Differentiation between hip and back disorders is not always easy. When the examiner is unable to rule out involvement of the hip, complete functional examination of the hip should be performed.

Neurological Tests: In Supine

4.34/35. Resisted Test for the Iliopsoas (L1 to L3)

Position of the Patient

Same as for test 4.19/20.

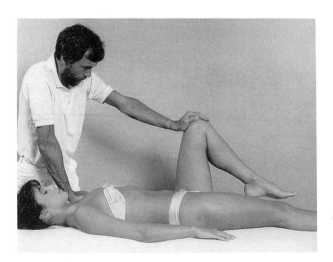

Test 4.34/35

Position of the Examiner

The examiner stands next to the patient at the level of the patient's head. One hand, with arm straight, is placed on the anterior aspect of the patient's knee. The other hand fixes the patient's shoulder.

Performance

The patient is asked, in 90° hip flexion, to push against the examiner's hand.

Against isometric resistance, the strength of the iliopsoas muscle (L1 to L3) is tested. Both sides are examined and compared with each other.

4.36/37. Resisted Test for the Tibialis Anterior (L3, L4)

Position of the Patient

Same as for test 4.19/20.

Position of the Examiner

The examiner stands next to the patient at the level of the patient's lower leg and foot. One hand is placed against the dorsomedial aspect of the patient's foot; the other hand fixes the patient's calcaneus from lateral.

Performance

The patient is asked to bring the foot in the direction of the contralateral knee, while the

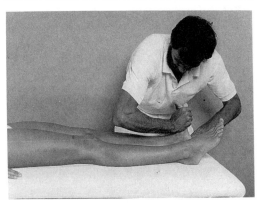

Test 4.36/37

examiner gives isometric resistance. On both sides, the tibialis anterior muscle (extension, adduction, and supination) is tested.

The innervation of this muscle comes mainly from L4. In severe cases, a paresis of the tibialis anterior could warrant surgery.

4.38/39. Resisted Test for the Extensor Hallucis Longus (L4, L5)

Position of the Patient

Same as for test 4.19/20.

Position of the Examiner

The examiner stands next to the patient at the level of the patient's knee and lower leg and places a thumb on the interphalangeal joint of the great toe.

Performance

The patient is asked to bring the great toe into extension while the examiner applies isometric resistance. Both sides are examined and compared with each other. The extensor hallucis longus is innervated by L4 and L5.

4.40/41. Resisted Test for the Peroneals (L5, S1)

Position of the Patient

Same as for test 4.19/20.

Position of the Examiner

The examiner stands next to the patient at the level of the patient's lower leg. One hand is placed on the plantar-lateral aspect of the forefoot, and the other hand fixes the calcaneus from medial.

Performance

The patient is asked to bring the foot in the direction of the examiner's distal elbow, and the examiner applies isometric resistance. On both sides, the peroneals (plantar flexion, abduction, and pronation) are tested and com-

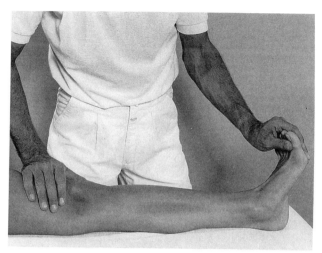

Test 4.38/39

pared with each other. The peroneals are innervated by L5 and S1.

4.42/43. Quadriceps Reflex (L3, L4)

Position of the Patient

Same as for test 4.19/20.

Position of the Examiner

The examiner stands next to the patient at the level of the patient's lower leg. The patient's knee is held in slight flexion.

Performance

The quadriceps reflex (L3, L4) is tested on each side, directly distal from the apex of the patella. The reflex should be tested at least three times in a row. If no reflex is noted, the patient is asked to perform the Jendrassik maneuver. With the fingers of each hand

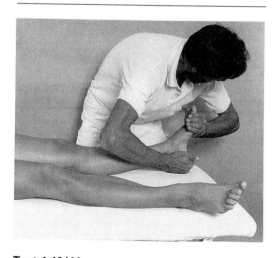

Test 4.40/41

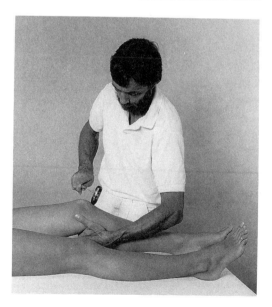

Test 4.42/43

hooked into one another, the patient exerts a force as if pulling the hands apart from each other. This serves to divert the patient's attention to the test and to relax the muscle, thereby facilitating the reflex and making it more evident.

4.44/45. Foot Sole Reflex

Position of the Patient

Same as for test 4.19/20.

Position of the Examiner

The examiner stands at the foot of the examination table.

Performance

The test is performed on each side. The examiner places the pointed end of a reflex hammer on the plantar aspect of the patient's heel. Applying moderate pressure, the examiner sweeps the end of the reflex hammer from the heel, along the lateral aspect of the sole of the foot, and then further medially over the metatarsal heads.

Two responses are possible: one is called Strümpell (normal response) and the other is called Babinski (pathological response). In Babinski, the great toe moves into extension,

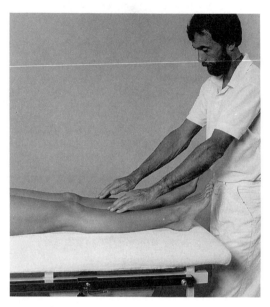

Test 4.46A For L3

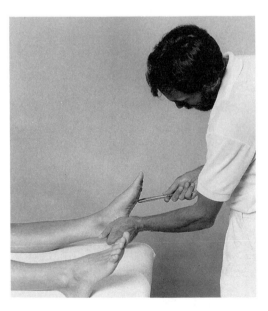

Test 4.44/45

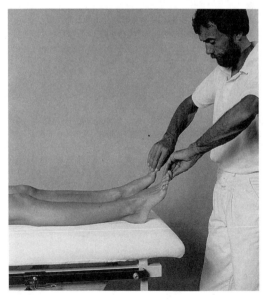

Test 4.46B For L4

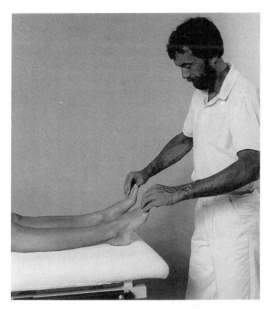

Test 4.46C For L5

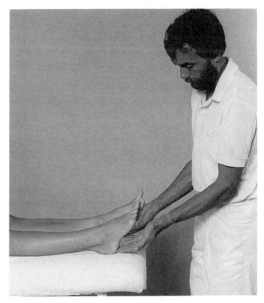

Test 4.46E For S2

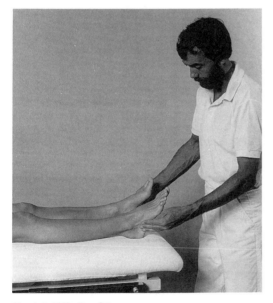

Test 4.46D For S1

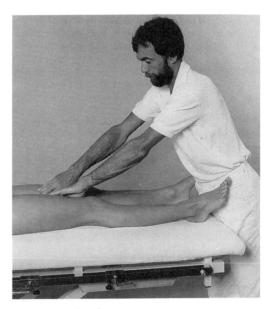

Test 4.46F For S3

the other toes spread and flex, and the knee and hip are pulled into slight flexion. A positive Babinski indicates pathology in the central nervous system.

4.46. Sensibility Tests

Position of the Patient

Same as for test 4.19/20.

Position of the Examiner

The examiner stands at the foot of the examination table.

Performance

The examiner tests the sensibility simultaneously on both sides. In this way, the patient can easily make a judgment as to whether the sensation (to light touch) is more obvious, less obvious, or equal to that of the non-affected side.

Dermatome locations L1 to S4:

L1 groin region

L2 lateral groin to anterior aspect of the thigh

L3 anteromedial aspect of the thigh to just above the malleoli

L4 anterolateral aspect of the thigh and lower leg to the medial aspect of the great toe

L5 lateral aspect of the thigh and lower leg to the lateral aspect of the great toe and the second and third toes

S1 posterior aspect of the thigh and lower leg, the lateral aspect of the foot and the fourth and fifth toes

S2 posterior aspect of the thigh and lower leg to include the plantar aspect of the heel

S3 medial aspect of the thigh

S4 perineum

Quick Tests for Vascularization: In Supine

4.47/48. Palpation of the Femoral Artery (not illustrated)

4.49/50. Palpation of the Posterior Tibial Artery (not illustrated)

4.51/52. Palpation of the Dorsal Pedal Artery (not illustrated)

Position of the Patient

Same as for test 4.19/20.

Position of the Examiner

The examiner stands at the level of the patient's pelvis to test the femoral artery. The examiner stands at the foot of the examination table to test the pulses at the foot.

Performance

One can palpate the pulsations of the femoral artery in the midgroin area, the posterior tibial artery at the level of the tarsal tunnel, and the dorsal pedal pulse between the second and third metatarsals on the dorsal aspect of the foot.

Test: In Sidelying

4.53/54. Alternative Test for SI Joint Provocation

Test is performed when test 4.17 is negative.

Position of the Patient

The patient is in the sidelying position on the painless side, with the hips flexed about 20° and the knees in approximately 90° flexion.

Position of the Examiner

The examiner stands behind the patient and places both hands on the ventrolateral aspect of the above-lying ilium.

Performance

With arms straight, the examiner leans somewhat forward over the patient in order to exert pressure on the patient's pelvis in a contralateral dorsal direction. The position is held for several seconds, followed by an abrupt impulse of increased pressure. One method of performing this impulse is through a quick nod of the head (flexion of the cervical spine). If pain is not provoked, the test is repeated with the patient lying on the other side.

This test emphasizes the dorsal sacroiliac capsuloligamentous structures.

Tests: In Prone

4.55/56. Femoral Nerve Stretch Test, Roots L1 to L4

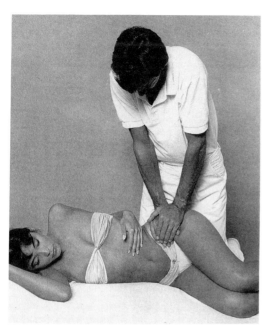

Test 4.53/54

Position of the Examiner

The examiner stands next to the patient at the level of the patient's thighs.

Performance

The examiner places the proximal hand on the patient's ischial tuberosity; the other hand grasps the thigh anteriorly just above the patella so that the patient's lower leg rests against the examiner's forearm. The distal hand brings the patient's thigh into extension, while the proximal hand fixes the ischial tuberosity. At the end range of hip extension, the knee is brought passively into flexion, thereby stretching the femoral nerve. Both sides are tested.

The test is positive when back pain with simultaneous referred pain to the anterolateral thigh is provoked. In lower lumbar pathology, a positive test will indicate dural irritation of the lumbar plexus, particularly L4.

Neurological Tests: In Prone

4.57/58. Achilles Tendon Reflex (L5 to S2)

Position of the Patient

Same as for test 4.55/56.

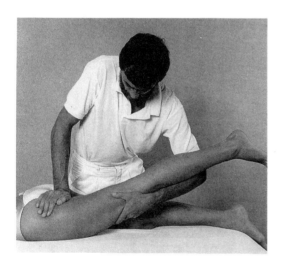

Test 4.55/56A Initial Position

Position of the Patient

The patient lies prone with arms relaxed at the side (Figure 4.55/56A is the initial position and 4.55/56B is the end position).

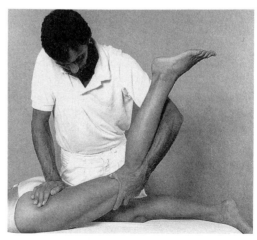

Test 4.55/56B End Position

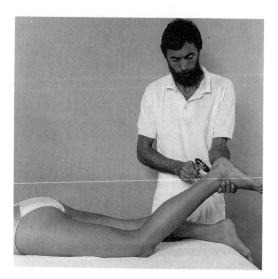

Test 4.57/58

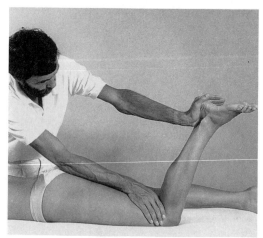

Test 4.59/60

Position of the Examiner

The examiner stands next to the patient at the level of the patient's lower leg.

Performance

With one hand, the examiner grasps the patient's foot from dorsal, whereby the knee is flexed to approximately 30°. The thumb of the same hand holds the foot in extension.

By tapping on the tendon directly proximal from the calcaneus, the reflex is elicited. It is important to repeat this test at least three times.

Comparison is made with each side. When no reflex is seen, the test is repeated using the Jendrassik maneuver (see test 4.42/43).

4.59/60. Resisted Test for the Hamstrings (S1, S2)

Position of the Patient

Same as for test 4.55/56.

Position of the Examiner

The examiner stands next to the patient at the level of the patient's lumbar spine. The examiner places one hand against either the patient's heel or directly proximal to the heel,

with the patient's knee in about 70° flexion. The other hand grasps the thigh just proximal of the knee in order to fix the thigh against the examination table.

Performance

The patient is asked to bring the heel toward the examiner while the examiner gives isometric resistance. Both sides are tested and compared. Innervation of the hamstrings is from the S1 and S2 nerve roots.

4.61/62. Resisted Test for the Rectus Femoris (L3, L4)

Position of the Patient

Same as for test 4.55/56.

Position of the Examiner

Same as for test 4.59/60, but now the hand giving resistance grasps the patient's anterior lower leg as far distally as possible.

Performance

The patient is asked to straighten the knee while the examiner gives isometric resistance. Both sides are tested and compared. Innervation of the quadriceps is from the L3 and L4 nerve roots.

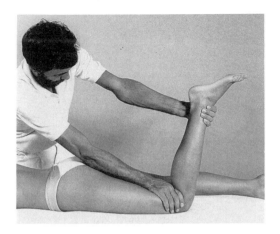

placed on the posterior aspect of the thigh just proximal to the knee. The other hand palpates the gluteus maximus between thumb and fingers.

Performance

The patient is asked to lift the leg, with the knee extended, while the examiner applies isometric resistance. Both sides are tested and compared. In this way, the general strength of the gluteus maximus is examined. Because this muscle quickly atrophies in lesions of the S1 or S2 nerve roots, one should also test the bulk and firmness of the muscle between the thumb and fingers.

4.63/64. Resisted Test for the Gluteus Maximus (L5, S1)

Position of the Patient

Same as for test 4.55/56.

Position of the Examiner

The examiner stands next to the patient at the level of the patient's pelvis. One hand is

Passive Test: In Prone

4.65. Palpation of the Spinous Processes

Position of the Patient

Same as for test 4.55/56.

Position of the Examiner

The examiner stands next to the patient at the level of the patient's lumbar spine.

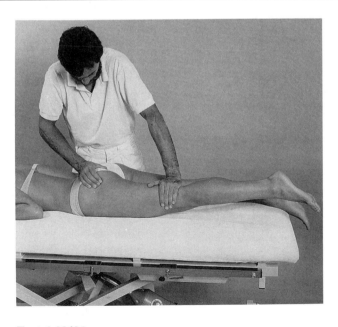

Test 4.63/64

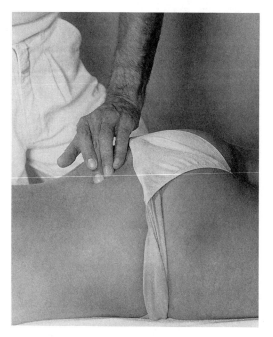

Test 4.65

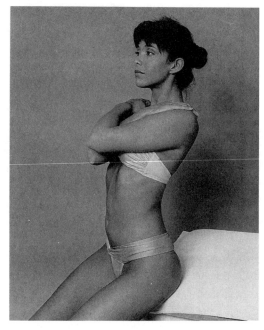

Test 4.66

Performance

The spinous processes are tested both in standing and in prone lying. Palpation of a "step" can be an indication of a spondylolisthesis.

DESCRIPTION OF TESTS FOR SEGMENTAL FUNCTIONAL EXAMINATION

During the active basic tests, provocation of pain is assessed, as well as any local deviation in the lumbar spine curvature in conjunction with a limitation of motion. If a local deviation is noted without provocation of pain, the patient is asked to repeat the movement five times. Usually the deviation disappears.

Active Tests: In sitting

4.66. Extension

Position of the Patient

The patient sits on the corner of the examination table. Table height is adjusted so that the patient sits in about 70° hip flexion. The legs are slightly spread, the lower legs are positioned perpendicular to the floor, and both feet rest fully on the floor. The arms are crossed in front of the body with hands resting on the shoulders. The vertebral spine should be in a physiologically neutral position.

Position of the Examiner

The examiner stands obliquely behind the patient in order to best assess the active movements.

Performance

The patient is asked to extend the lumbar spine actively, whereby the pelvis does not move.

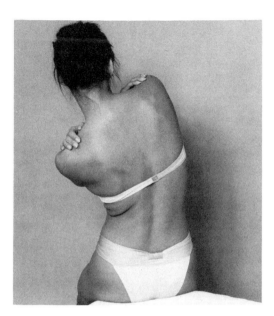

Test 4.67

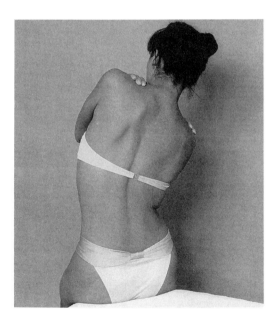

Test 4.68

4.67. Left Sidebending

4.68. Right Sidebending

Position of the Patient

Same as for test 4.66.

Position of the Examiner

The examiner stands behind the patient.

Performance

The patient now performs a sidebending (to the left and to the right) whereby the pelvis does not move and the trunk stays in the frontal plane.

4.69. Flexion

Position of the Patient

Same as for test 4.66.

Position of the Examiner

The examiner stands behind the patient.

Performance

The patient is asked to bend forward, flexing the lumbar spine but without moving the pelvis.

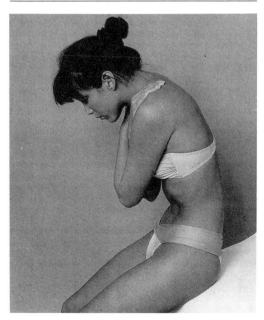

Test 4.69

4.70. Extension with Left Sidebending and Right Rotation (Coupled Movement)

Position of the Patient

Same as for test 4.66.

Position of the Examiner

Same as for test 4.66.

Performance

The patient is asked to bring the lumbar spine *simultaneously* into extension with left sidebending and right rotation (coupled movement).

In the same manner, the patient in turn performs each of the pictured movements (tests 4.71 to 4.77). The trunk, cervical spine, and head are all moved in the same direction.

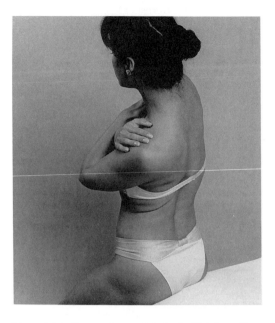

Test 4.71 Extension with Left Sidebending and Left Rotation (Combined Movement)

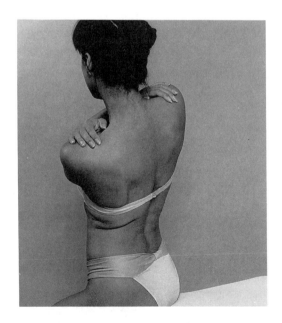

Test 4.70

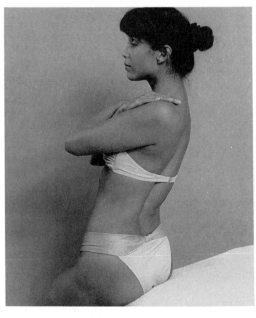

Test 4.72 Extension with Right Sidebending and Left Rotation (Coupled Movement)

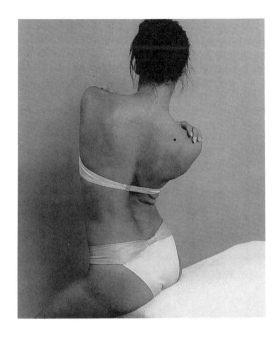

Test 4.73 Extension with Right Sidebending and Right Rotation (Combined Movement)

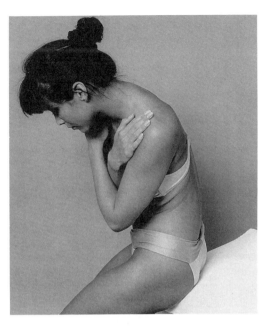

Test 4.74 Flexion with Left Sidebending and Left Rotation (Coupled Movement)

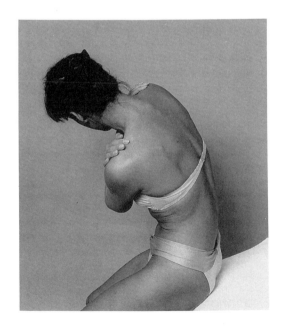

Test 4.75 Flexion with Left Sidebending and Right Rotation (Combined Movement)

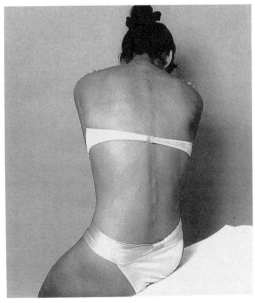

Test 4.76 Flexion with Right Sidebending and Right Rotation (Coupled Movement)

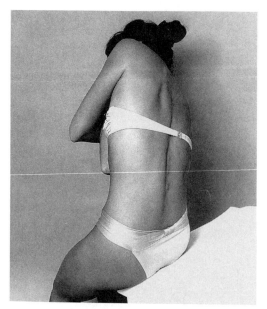

Test 4.77 Flexion with Right Sidebending and Left Rotation (Combined Movement)

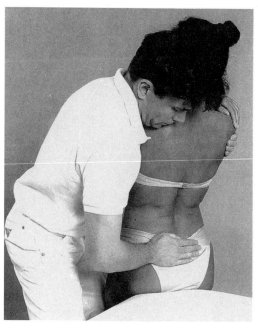

Test 4.78

Passive Tests: In Sitting

4.78. Extension

Position of the Patient

Same as for test 4.66.

Position of the Examiner

The examiner stands with legs apart facing the side of the patient.

Performance

The examiner rests his or her sternum against the lateral aspect of the patient's shoulder. With one hand, the examiner grasps just caudal and dorsal to the patient's opposite shoulder, whereby her or his arm crosses the ventral aspect of the patient's thorax and is positioned underneath the patient's crossed arms. The other hand fixes the sacrum.

Passive extension is now performed in the following way: By shifting weight onto the ventral (in relation to the patient) leg, the examiner brings the patient's thorax, and along with it the center of gravity of the lumbar spine, in a ventral direction. This results in an increase in the patient's lumbar lordosis. Then through a sidebending of the examiner's trunk, the patient's lumbar spine is brought further into extension. At the end of the motion, the examiner exerts gentle overpressure by pushing the patient's thorax in the direction of the sacrum.

4.79. Left Sidebending

4.80. Right Sidebending

Position of the Patient

Same as for test 4.66.

Position of the Examiner

Same as for test 4.78.

Performance

The examiner places his or her shoulder as high as possible against the lateral aspect of the patient's ribs. With an arm coming around

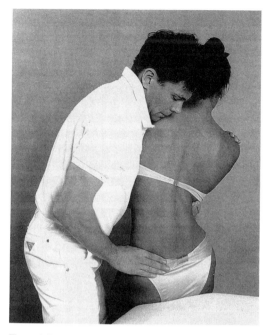

Test 4.80

the patient from ventral, the examiner grasps the patient, whereby the ulnar side of the hand rests against the lateral aspect of the patient's 10th rib on the opposite side. In order to stabilize the pelvis, the other hand is placed on the patient's iliac crest closest to the examiner, and pressure is exerted in a caudomedial direction.

Through a synchronous movement from the examiner's hand and shoulder, the sidebending motion is performed. The examiner pulls the lower ribs toward self while his or her shoulder pushes the patient's upper body away. At the end of the motion, overpressure is exerted. The test is repeated on the other side.

4.81. Extension with Left Sidebending and Right Rotation (Coupled Movement)

or grip her shoulder

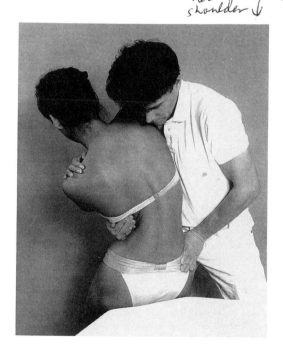

Test 4.79

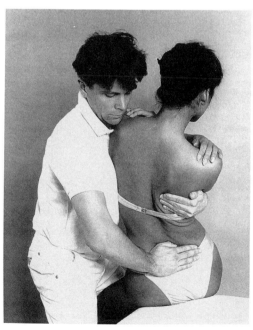

Test 4.81

Position of the Patient

Same as for test 4.66.

Position of the Examiner

Same as for test 4.78. Here the examiner stands on the left side of the patient.

Performance

The examiner grasps the patient in the same manner as in the passive sidebending test (4.80), except in this test, the fixing hand is placed against the patient's sacrum with the fingers pointing away from the examiner. Simultaneously, an extension with left sidebending and right rotation is performed. The rotation movement is performed by a rotation from the examiner's upper body. With the fixing hand continuing to stabilize the pelvis, a slight overpressure is given at the end of the motion.

4.82. Extension with Right Sidebending and Right Rotation (Combined Movement)

4.83. Extension with Right Sidebending and Left Rotation (Coupled Movement)

4.84. Extension with Left Sidebending and Left Rotation (Combined Movement)

Performance

In the same manner, the examiner in turn performs each of the pictured tests (tests 4.82, 4.83, and 4.84). The examiner stands so that the rotation component of the combined and coupled movements is performed away from the examiner (ie, in left rotation he or she stands on the right side of the patient, and vice versa).

For interpretation of these general, coupled, and combined motion tests in the segmental lumbar examination, refer to Appendix B, Algorithms for the Diagnosis and Treatment of Lumbar Spine Pathology.

Passive Local Mobility Tests: In Sitting

All of the following passive local mobility tests in sitting, sidelying, and prone are per-

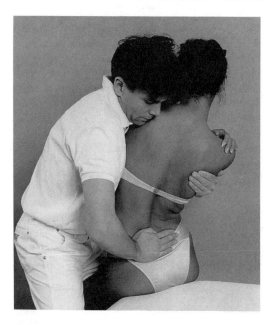

Test 4.82

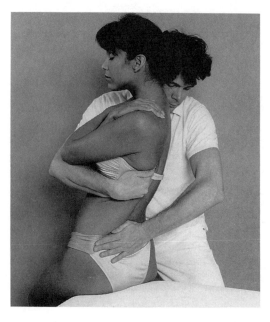

Test 4.83

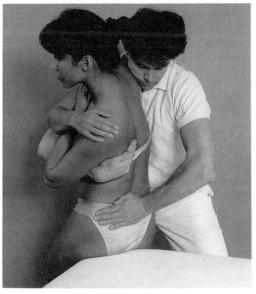

Test 4.84

Test 4.85

formed from segment T10-11 to and including L5-S1.

4.85. Extension in Weight Bearing

Position of the Patient

Same as for test 4.66.

Position of the Examiner

Same as for test 4.78.

Performance

The examiner rests his or her sternum against the lateral aspect of the patient's shoulder. With one hand, the examiner grasps just caudal and dorsal to the patient's opposite shoulder whereby the examiner's arm crosses the ventral aspect of the patient's thorax and is positioned underneath the patient's crossed arms.

The tips of the index and middle fingers of the palpating hand are placed in two adjacent interspinous spaces. Palpation begins between T10-11 and T11-12. The examiner

brings the patient into extension to the point where the segment being tested is involved; this is repeated several times in order to assess the motion, each time returning to the physiologically neutral position. The further caudally one tests, the greater the amplitude of movement the examiner must perform.

The index finger tests the amount of movement in the cranial interspinous space while the middle finger tests the latency time between the beginning of motion in the cranial segment and the respective following movement in the caudal segment.

4.86. Extension with Left Sidebending and Right Rotation in Weight Bearing (Coupled Movement) (A, B)

4.87. Extension with Right Sidebending and Left Rotation in Weight Bearing (Coupled Movement) (A, B)

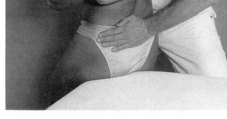

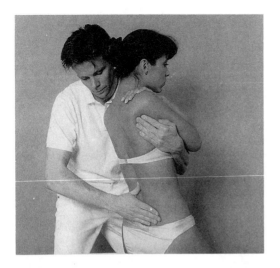

Test 4.86A

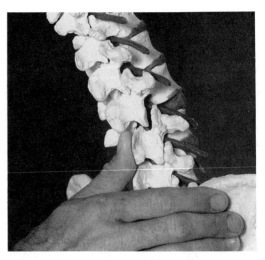

Test 4.86B Skeleton Model

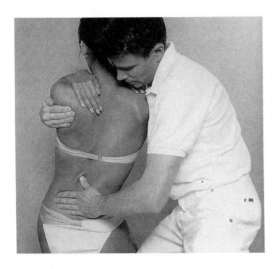

Test 4.87A

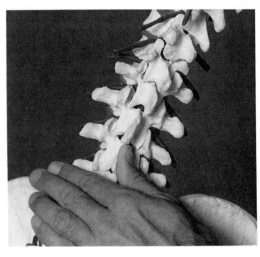

Test 4.87B Skeleton Model

Position of the Patient

Same as for test 4.66.

Position of the Examiner

Same as for test 4.85.

Performance

The performance of these tests follows in the same manner as described for the previ-

ous test, except that here the thumb assesses the segmental movement. Again the examiner begins testing from T10-11 and progresses caudally, in particular noting the amplitude of movement. The thumb is placed in the interspinous space so that the tip just touches the underside of the spinous process of the cranial vertebra. The distal phalanx of the thumb rests against the side of the caudal vertebra's spinous process, opposite to the direction of rotation. In this way, the thumb not only fixes the caudal vertebra but also assesses the amount of movement of the cranial vertebra.

The rotation is always performed away from the examiner, and the stabilizing arm gives counterpressure into extension with simultaneous rotation and contralateral sidebending to the point where the segment being tested is involved; this is repeated several times in order to assess the motion, each time returning to the physiologically neutral position.

Before proceeding to the next segment, the examiner gives slight overpressure at the end of the movement to assess end-feel.

The examiner then stands on the right side of the patient, and in the same way tests extension with simultaneous sidebending right and left rotation.

Passive Local Mobility Tests: In Prone

4.88. Segment Mobility in Ventral Translation (A, B, C) *can skip these*

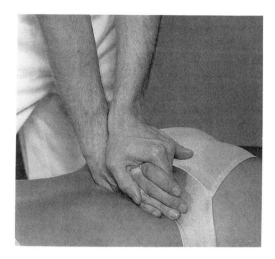

Test 4.88B Mid-Lumbar Segments

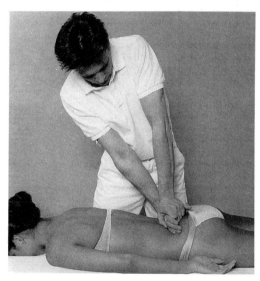

Test 4.88C Lower Lumbar Segments

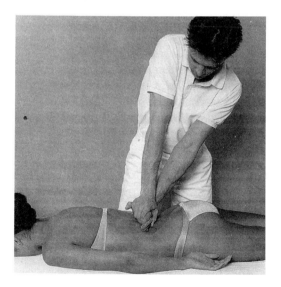

Test 4.88A Lower Thoracic and Upper Lumbar

Position of the Patient

The patient lies prone on the examination table with arms relaxed at the sides. The lumbar spine should rest in a physiologically neutral position. A swayback can be supported in its physiologically neutral position by placing a pillow under the upper body, whereas a flat back can be supported by bringing the head of the table down slightly (into a negative position).

Position of the Examiner

With the table at a height of about midthigh, the examiner stands next to the patient at the level of the patient's lumbar spine.

Performance

The examiner places the ulnar side of the hand (the pisiform has no contact) against the spinous process of the segment being examined. The other hand supports the testing hand, whereby the fingers are placed in the palm of the testing hand between thumb and fingers, and the thumb is placed on the dorsal aspect of the testing hand.

The examiner's elbows remain extended. When testing the upper lumbar segments, the distal (in relation to the patient) hand rests against the spinous process, and when testing the lower lumbar segments the proximal hand is placed on the spinous process. Now with both hands and arms, pressure is applied ventrally in a direction perpendicular to the local curvature of the lordosis.

The amount of movement is assessed through repeated full-ventral movements, whereby the pressure between each interval is completely lifted. During the last ventral movement for that part of the segment, the examiner exerts a slight overpressure at the end of the motion to assess the end-feel.

In this test, each segment is examined starting from cranial and working to caudal.

Assessment

Hypermobility is a subjective concept; it does not necessarily cause problems. On the other hand, a functional instability is distinguished by symptoms in which pain is foremost. When a hypermobility is found with or without symptoms, treatment to prevent a functional instability is indicated.

Segmental mobilization is indicated when decreased mobility of the segment is noted and is determined to be responsible for the patient's symptoms.

Summary

A hypermobility with or without symptoms is an indication for stabilization through an exercise program. However, treatment with use of mobilization techniques is performed only for a hypomobility *with* accompanying symptoms.

4.89. End-Feel Test in Extension (A, B)

Position of the Patient

Same as for test 4.88.

Position of the Examiner

Same as for test 4.88.

Performance

The performance of this test is similar to that for test 4.88, except that here the above-lying segment is first brought into full extension. With the index and middle fingers of one hand, the examiner tests the interspinal spaces of two adjacent segments. The index finger palpates the extension in the cranial segment, while the middle finger palpates to ensure that no extension takes place in the caudal segment.

Various methods can be used to achieve the extension:

- by gradual lifting of the adjustable part of the examination table, with the patient positioned so that L1 lies over the hinge,
- whereby the patient actively, with assistance from the examiner, pushes the trunk up with both hands, or
- whereby the examiner lifts the patient's trunk when testing the upper lumbar segments (4.89A) and then lifts the patient's legs when testing the lower segments (4.89B).

The examiner's hand lies on the cranial spinous process of the segment being tested.

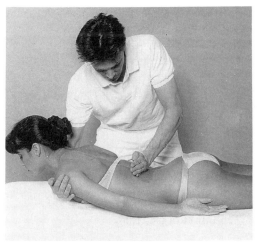

Test 4.89A Upper Lumbar Spine

m. Pronson elbows

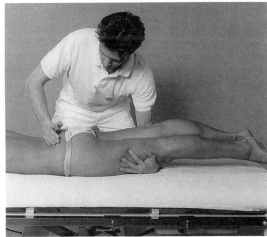

Test 4.89B Lower Lumbar Spine

The examiner exerts a ventral pressure with the ulnar side of the hand against the segment's cranial spinous process in a direction perpendicular to the local curvature of the lumbar lordosis.

For the most part, this test offers a further possibility for provocation of pain.

4.90. Test for Rotatory Hypermobility (A, B)

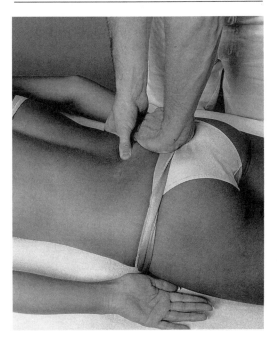

Test 4.90A L5–S1 Segment

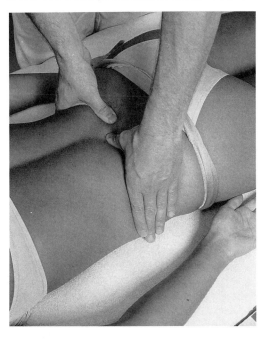

Test 4.90B L4–5 to T10–11

Position of the Patient

Same as for test 4.88.

Position of the Examiner

The examiner stands next to the patient at the level of the patient's pelvis.

Performance

Testing the L5-S1 Segment (4.90A). The examiner places the hypothenar eminence of the caudal hand on the base of the sacrum just medial of the posterior superior iliac spine. The tip of the thumb of the other hand rests against the L5 spinous process on the same side. The examiner then exerts pressure with the tip of the thumb in a medial direction while the other hand fixes the sacrum. The test is repeated, with the appropriate corresponding hand position, in the other direction.

Testing the L4–5 to T10-11 Segments (4.90B). In these segments, the test is performed with the tip of each thumb. The thumbs are placed on opposite sides of the spinous process of two adjacent vertebrae. While the caudal thumb fixes, the cranial thumb performs a rotation by exerting pressure against the spinous process. In the same way, the opposite direction is tested by alternating the position of each thumb.

The examiner assesses the amount of movement and the end-feel. Provocation of pain is of less importance. However, in the presence of a retrolisthesis, this test may be extremely painful.

Passive Local Mobility Tests: In Sidelying

4.91. Segment Mobility in Dorsal Translation (A, B)

Position of the Patient

The patient lies in a stable position on one side, facing the edge of the table. He or she should be positioned as close to the edge of the examination table as possible. In order to maintain a physiologically neutral position in the spinal column, a pillow or a small towel roll is placed under the head and, when appropriate, at the waist. Initially, the hips are flexed to approximately 70° with the knees flexed to a degree that is comfortable for the patient.

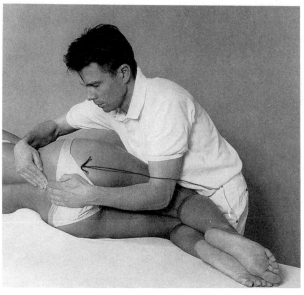

Test 4.91A Lower Lumbar Segments

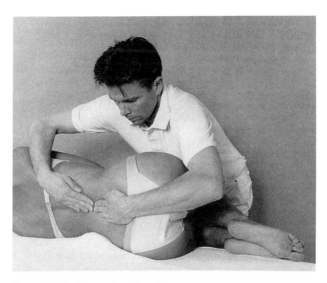

Test 4.91B Upper Lumbar Segments

Position of the Examiner

The examiner stands next to the patient at the level of the patient's pelvis and brings the examination table to a height even with the hips.

Performance

Both knees of the patient are supported between the examiner's proximal thighs, pelvis, and lower abdomen. The examiner places his or her caudal hand flat against the patient's sacrum with fingers pointing in a cranial direction. The fingertips rest against the upper edge of the spinous process of the caudal vertebra in the segment to be tested. For instance, in testing the segment L5-S1, the fingertips rest against the upper edge of the sacral base. The index and middle fingers of the other hand are placed on the spinous process of the segment's cranial vertebra, whereby the index finger rests in the interspinal space in order to assess possible motion. The motion segment to be assessed remains in a neutral position.

With his or her trunk, the examiner exerts an axial force through the patient's femurs so that a dorsal translation occurs in the particular segment. The cranial hand fixes. At the end of the dorsal translation, the caudal vertebra and everything that lies below it are brought as a unit back to the starting position. Per segment, this movement is repeated several times.

Each segment is assessed in this manner, beginning with L5-S1 and working upward. After one segment is tested, it is brought into flexion by bringing the patient's hips further in flexion. This helps to fix that segment while the above-lying segment, which is now being tested, remains in a neutral position. The index finger of the cranial hand assesses the amount of motion.

4.92 Extension in Non–Weight Bearing

Position of the Patient

Same as for test 4.91.

Position of the Examiner

The examiner stands next to the patient at the level of his or her pelvis, with the table at a height of the examiner's midthigh.

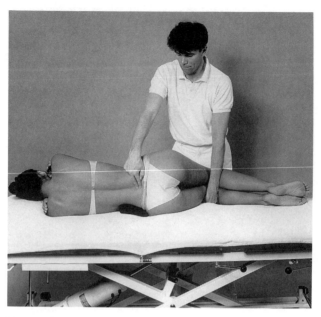

Test 4.92

Performance

The examiner holds the patient's posterior thighs just above the knees, between the examiner's caudal arm and either the thigh, pelvis, or trunk. The index and middle fingers of the other hand palpate the interspinal spaces of the two adjacent segments to be tested. The examiner brings the patient's legs in a backward direction and simultaneously exerts axial pressure in a proximal direction through the patient's legs. In this way a segmental lumbar extension can be achieved even in the higher segments without requiring much hip extension.

Because the movement is induced from a caudal direction, first the L5-S1 segment is tested, then the examiner tests progressively upward until T10-11 is reached. The index finger assesses the movement in the caudal segment, while the middle finger monitors that no movement occurs in the cranial segment.

4.93. Extension with Left Sidebending and Right Rotation in Non–Weight Bearing

Position of the Patient

Same as for test 4.91, whereby the patient lies on the left side in the middle of the examination table. In instances where the patient is very mobile, the sidebending can be supported by placing a larger pillow at the waist or by raising the middle of an adjustable table (as pictured).

Position of the Examiner

Same as for test 4.91.

Performance

The examiner places his or her cranial hand on the ventrolateral aspect of the patient's ribs, at approximately midthorax. If necessary, the patient's hand can be placed between the examiner's hand and the ribs. The fingers of the other hand are placed at the

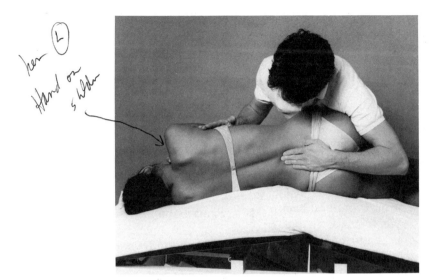

her (L)
Hand on
shoulder

Test 4.93

segment to be tested, with the hand and arm supporting all that lies caudal of that segment. The middle finger, which can be reinforced by the index finger, is placed against the lateral aspect (on the table side) of the caudal vertebra's spinous process. The tip of the middle finger rests in the interspinous space in order to palpate, while the other fingers stabilize. With the cranial hand the examiner then exerts pressure against the ribs in a dorsal and contralateral direction. In so doing, a three-dimensional movement is induced: extension, left sidebending, and right rotation. In order for the motion to occur only down to the segment being tested, the examiner begins by testing from cranial with a small amount of movement and ends caudal with a somewhat greater amplitude of movement. The patient remains relaxed and allows the head to follow the rotation of the trunk.

The middle finger of the caudal hand assesses the amount of motion in the segment.

4.94. Extension with Right Sidebending and Left Rotation in Non–Weight Bearing (not pictured)

Position of the Patient

Same as for test 4.93, except that now the patient lies on the right side.

Position of the Examiner

Same as for test 4.93.

Performance

Same as for test 4.93, except that extension, right sidebending, and left rotation are now performed.

4.3 PATHOLOGY

PRIMARY DISC-RELATED DISORDERS

Primary disc-related disorders are the direct result of "degenerative" changes in the lumbar intervertebral discs. A good 60% of all disc pathology occurs in the lumbar spine.[25] The symptomatology is quite variable and can include local central or paravertebral back pain and/or radiating symptoms via the buttock region into the groin or into the leg down to the toes. Possible neurological deficits consist of paresthesia, paresis, sensory deficits, and/or reflex deficits.

Most patients are between the ages of 30 and 45, although disc prolapses can also be seen in children and in patients over 70.

The lumbosacral motion segment represents a point of least resistance (a weak link in the chain) in the vertebral column. Compared with discs of all the other lumbar segments, the disc here is the most obviously wedge shaped, and there is the greatest amount of flexion-extension at this level. In addition, the L5-S1 intervertebral foramen is the smallest; thus the exiting L5 nerve root comes rather quickly into contact with a protruding or prolapsed disc. By far, the lower two lumbar segments are the most often affected in terms of disc protrusions or prolapses.

Prolapses of the upper lumbar discs are rare. In the authors' experience, they are most often seen in patients between the ages of 40 and 55. Upper lumbar disc problems can be extremely painful. Initially, symptoms from an upper lumbar motion segment should be considered as coming from serious pathology until it is proved otherwise. In many cases, what appears to be a disc prolapse turns out to be a tumor (Figure 4–10).

Static deviations, such as differences in the level of each side of the pelvis and anomalies of the lumbosacral junction, were overemphasized in the past. Recent studies indicate that they are of little clinical significance. When problems do occur, they are generally not found at the level of the anomaly, but instead (particularly with the various forms of sacralization) at the segment directly above.

Disc Protrusion

Acute Lumbago from a Posterocentral Disc Protrusion Due to a Massive Intradiscal Nucleus Displacement in Children and Adolescents

Juvenile protrusion or prolapse of the lumbar intervertebral disc is seldom seen in children and adolescents. It is assumed that complaints are caused by an irritation of the posterior longitudinal ligament and the dura mater. The severity of the symptoms is not always dependent on the size of the protrusion or prolapse. In children and adolescents with a disc prolapse, the absence of severe symptoms is frequently a significant phenomenon. The neurological signs often dominate the symptoms. Sometimes the patients complain only of a stiff back and a "pulling" feeling in the back and/or one or both legs; they have fewer symptoms than signs.

Clinical Findings

- The symptoms can be located in the back and/or leg(s). The pain is usually moderate. In some cases, there is no pain in the back but only in one or both legs. Sometimes the pain is localized solely to the back of the knee. For instance, the authors saw two 14-year-old patients with a diagnosis of Baker's cyst. The functional examination of the knee was

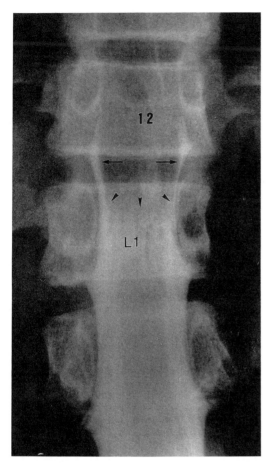

Figure 4–10 Myelogram of the T12-L1 segment in a patient with, at first, a T12-L1 root compression syndrome, which quickly expanded into a medullary compression. A complete stoppage of the contrast medium at L1 by a fast-growing intramedullary tumor is seen (*arrowheads*).

hyperesthesia, and minimal changes in the reflexes.

- The most extreme form of juvenile disc protrusion or prolapse is the hip-waist extension stiffness phenomenon. In such cases, during the SLR test the other leg and the entire back move immediately with the tested leg. Bending forward is entirely impossible, as is neck flexion. These children walk with a shuffling gai,t whereby the hip and knee joints are slightly flexed.

- Myelography, CT scan, or MRI can indicate a disc protrusion or prolapse. It is important in instances of the hip-waist extension stiffness phenomenon to differentiate between a protrusion/prolapse, tumors, or inflammatory process of the spinal column.

Treatment

In the first instance, treatment is conservative. Information about the lesion, whereby the parents or caretakers must be involved, generally takes away a significant amount of anxiety. Very cautious manual mobilization of the spine in combination with muscle-stretching techniques gives only very gradual improvement. If there is no improvement after 6 to 8 weeks, surgery should be considered.

Because of the relatively late ossification of the growth centers of the vertebral body, manipulation (particularly rotatory manipulation) and traction in children (under 16 years of age) is absolutely contraindicated.

Sometimes, in cases of the hip-waist extension stiffness phenomenon, extreme stiffness remains even after surgery. This is probably due to adhesions of the nerve root within the dural sleeve.

After the mobility in the lumbar spine normalizes, the patient should perform the entire exercise program described in Appendix 4–A.

completely negative. Forward bending of the trunk was absolutely impossible; the entire spine was as stiff as a board. If most of the pain is felt in the leg, one speaks of a *posterolateral* or *lateral* disc protrusion or prolapse.

- The SLR test is always very painful.
- Slight neurological signs are generally present: slight muscle weakness, mild

Acute Lumbago from a Posterocentral Disc Protrusion Due to a Massive Intradiscal Nucleus Displacement in Adults

The mechanism of onset of the symptoms is the same for adults as it is for children, described previously. This syndrome is most often seen in people younger than 30 years of age.

Clinical Findings

- The patient complains of acute pain in the low back, usually after (too much) activity. Generally there is vague pseudoradicular, extrasegmental radiating pain in one or both legs.
- Coughing, sneezing, and straining increase the back pain.
- Sometimes there is an antalgic posture; often the patient stands with a flattened lumbar spine, and in severe cases with a lumbar kyphosis.
- The motions of the lumbar spine are limited and painful in a noncapsular pattern. Usually, extension is the most limited and painful motion.
- There are no neurological deficits.
- Myelography, CT scan, or MRI can confirm the disc protrusion (Figures 4–11 and 4–12).

Treatment

Generally, in adults, manipulation is the most indicated treatment for symptoms with an acute onset (sudden sharp pain in the back). On the other hand, traction is best utilized for patients who had a gradual onset of back pain several hours or one day after performing (heavy) activity, although in such cases it is worthwhile to try treating first with mobilization/manipulation.

Usually, a long lever rotation manipulation is very effective. If the patient is unable to tolerate the technique because of pain, soft tissue techniques and oscillations and/or vibrations can be used to reduce the pain. Strong analgesics or, better yet, a sacral epidural anesthetic can be administered if these techniques do not provide pain relief. Generally, 1 or 2 days after an injection it is possible to begin treatment with manual mobilization/manipulation techniques. For a description of the mobilization/manipulation techniques, refer to section 4.4, Treatment.

As with the other primary discogenic disorders, a thorough explanation of the problem, followed by postural instruction, is an important part of the treatment. An abdominal- and back-strengthening exercise program is initiated only after the lumbar motions have returned to normal. The exercises will have a negative effect if they are performed when a painful limitation of motion is still present.

For a description of the exercise program, refer to Appendix 4–A.

Acute Lumbago from a Posterolateral Disc Protrusion Due to a Massive Intradiscal Nucleus Displacement

As with the posterocentral disc protrusion, a posterolateral disc protrusion can also be seen in children, adolescents, and young adults (to approximately 30 years of age).

The symptoms are caused by an irritation of the innervated dorsal aspect of the disc, (part of) the posterior longitudinal ligament, and the well (nociceptive)-innervated ventral part of the dural sleeve. Often these patients have had previous incidences of acute back pain such as described for posterocentral disc protrusion in children, adolescents, and adults.

Clinical Findings

- This lesion differs from the posterocentral disc protrusion in that, besides the severe low back pain, pain is felt largely in a segmental distribution in the leg.
- Coughing, sneezing, and straining increase pain in the back and/or leg.

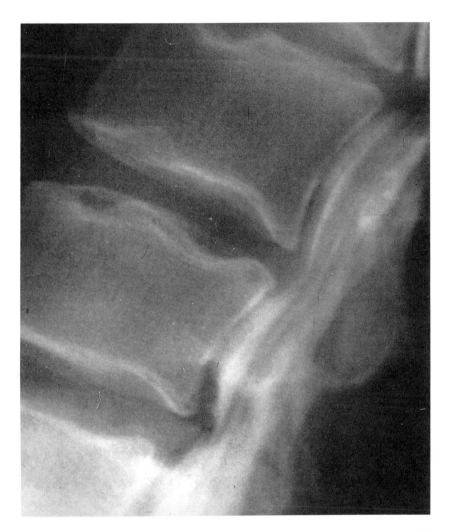

Figure 4–11 Lateral-view myelogram at the lumbar spine level (L2 to L5) in a 36-year-old man with back pain. At the level of segments L2-3 to L3-4 and L4-5, a bulging of the intervertebral disc is visible. Clinically, the patient had an acute lumbago due to a posterocentral L4-5 disc protrusion. The other protrusions seen on the X-ray are not of clinical importance. At the same time, "wavy" irregularities (Schmorl's nodules) are seen in the end-plates of several vertebral bodies, characteristic of a lumbar affliction due to Scheuermann's disease.

- Depending on the size and localization of the protrusion, there may be a deviation of the lumbar spine. This deviation is characterized by a horizontal position of the pelvis and a shift of the entire trunk to one side without obvious compensation, such as in an idiopathic scoliosis. The deviation often disappears in lying (and sometimes also when hanging, such as from a doorsill). Generally, the deviation remains when standing on the ipsilateral (painful) leg and disappears when standing on the contralateral leg.
- A deviation always indicates a disc protrusion. Some authors suggest that a deviation seldom occurs as a result of a disc

R   L

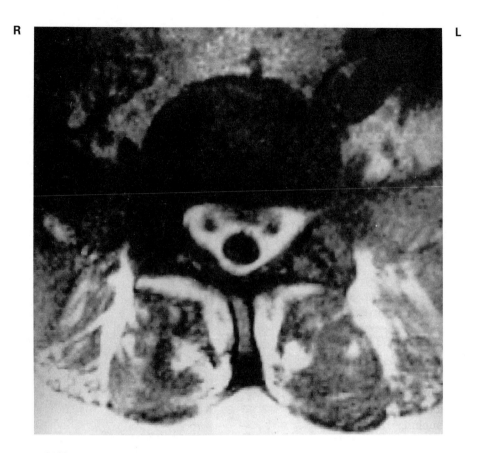

Figure 4–12 MRI view at the level of the lumbosacral junction in a 33-year-old woman with a disc protrusion at L5-S1. The disc protrusion is visible as a hypointense (darker) zone between both of the strongly hypointense (black) roots of S1. The epidural fatty tissue has a high signal intensity (white) in this view.

protrusion at the L5-S1 level because of the strong iliolumbar ligaments. However, this does not correspond to surgical findings. For instance, Porter[26] documents that in 100 patients with a deviation, in which 20 underwent surgery, 12 had protrusions at the L5-S1 level, 6 at the L4-5 level, and 2 at the L3-4 level.

- Deviations to the left are seen twice as often as to the right. Porter and Miller[29] suggest that this is due to a dominant reflex. Some patients present with an alternating deviation. White and Panjabi[9] present the following theory, which is very useful in practice: When the disc protrusion exerts pressure on the shoulder of the nerve root, the patient shifts (deviates) away from the painful side. With pressure exerted in the axilla of the nerve root, the patient shifts toward the painful side (Figure 4–13).

- The lumbar spine motions are limited in painful, noncapsular proportions. Extension is often significantly limited, as well as sidebending away from the deviated side.

- The SLR test, in combination with neck flexion (Neri test) and in combination with ankle extension (Bragard test), is usually positive. Neurological deficits are not (yet) present.

Diagnosis of which particular nerve root is affected is not easy. Symptoms radiating into a specific dermatome make this possible. However, one is still not able to determine the level of the disc lesion. A lesion of the L4-5 disc can cause symptoms from the L4, L5, or S1 nerve roots. An L5-S1 disc lesion can result in L5, S1, or S2 root symptoms.

Treatment

The treatment is the same as described for posterocentral disc protrusion in children, adolescents, and adults. However, continuous traction is never performed in patients with a deviation. The traction should be well tolerated by the patient and should even be considered comfortable. Sometimes in releasing the traction severe pain occurs, even when the patient has no deviation in lying. In this instance, a possible alternative is cautious manual or mechanical traction, whereby the pull is given in the direction of the deviation.

Differential Diagnosis

One must always bear in mind that benign or innocent-appearing back symptoms can also be due to tumors or inflammatory processes or from an extravertebral cause such as gynecological, urological, or other internal disorders. Furthermore, one should differentiate between a disc protrusion and the other pathological conditions described later in this chapter.

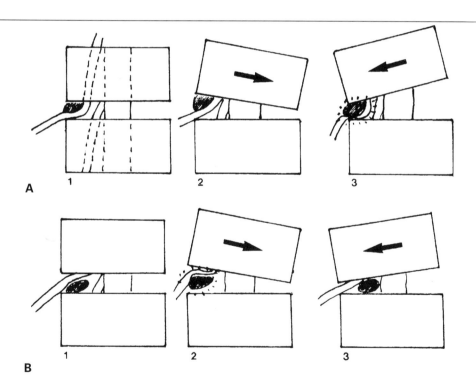

Figure 4–13 A, Shoulder compression; **1,** normal standing; **2,** no pain during sidebending away from the painful side; **3,** pain during sidebendingtoward the painful side. **B,** Axilla compression; **1,** normal standing; **2,** pain during sidebending away from the painful side; **3,** no pain during sidebending toward the painful side.

see workbook p. 68½, 69.

Often, a meticulously performed functional examination can detect tumors or inflammatory processes of the various spinal structures even before they are visible on X-ray. Tumors usually cause symptoms that are experienced independent of position or movement. This is an important indication in the patient's history. In addition, there is often (but not always) local tenderness to tapping (percussion) and pain when falling back onto the heels from a tiptoe position. Tumors, as well as inflammatory processes, can cause a limitation of motion in a capsular pattern. In particular, sidebending is severely and symmetrically limited.

Disc Prolapse

To a certain extent, a disc prolapse differs from a disc protrusion in that the annulus fibrosus, through which the nucleus pulposus now protrudes, is no longer intact.

Acute Lumbago from a Posterolateral Disc Prolapse with Radicular Symptoms

Clinically, it is difficult to differentiate a large disc protrusion from a prolapse. The S1 nerve root is the most frequently affected. Krämer[30] reports the following numbers: 54% involve the S1 nerve root and 44% the L5 nerve root. The other roots are seldom affected. Although occasionally seen in children and adolescents, the age span in which this disorder mainly appears is between 30 and 45 years.

Monoradicular

Clinical Findings

- Acute or gradual onset of pain occurs in the low back and in one leg. The leg pain is felt in one dermatome.
- Coughing, sneezing, and straining are almost always painful, not only in the back, but also in the leg.

- Most patients exhibit a deviation of the lumbar spine. The direction of the deviation depends on the factors described for posterolateral disc protrusion (Figure 4–13).
- The lumbar motions are painful and limited in noncapsular proportions; flexion and/or extension, as well as sidebending away from the shifted direction, are usually the most limited motions.
- The SLR, Neri, and Bragard tests can be painful.
- Neurological signs
  1. With slight pressure on the nerve root, first a *hyperesthesia* often occurs in the affected dermatome.
  2. With increasing pressure a *paresthesia* occurs, followed by a *hypoesthesia*, and finally ending with an *anesthesia*.
  3. Strength of the muscles belonging to the affected nerve root decreases.
  4. Reflex changes can vary from hyperreflexia to areflexia.
- Usually the X-rays do not show any specific findings, or are—as Porter[26] says—"positively unhelpful." Radiological findings such as "degenerative changes" are worthless when they are interpreted separately from the history and the functional examination. In most cases, a CT scan or an MRI clearly shows the size and the form of the disc lesion (Figures 4–14 to 4–16). Occasionally a CT scan in combination with myelography is necessary.

Treatment

Provision of extensive information to the patient, followed by instruction in proper posture, is an important part of the treatment. The most significant effect of instruction is actually to reassure and calm the patient.

As long as there are no neurological deficits, mobilization, as well as traction, can be a

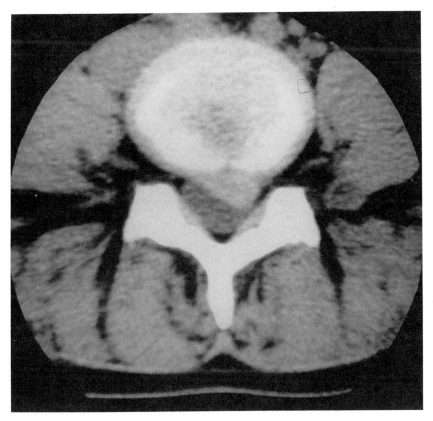

Figure 4–14 CT scan at the level of L4-5 in a 32-year-old man with complaints of back pain and an L5 radicular syndrome. There is a massive left lateral disc prolapse.

successful form of treatment. However, if neurological deficits are exhibited, a sacral epidural anesthesia or bed rest (no more than 2 to 3 days), or a combination of both, is indicated.

In orthopaedic medicine, one question remains under constant discussion: When does one decide to operate on a patient with a disc prolapse?

The American Academy of Orthopaedic Surgeons recommends surgery for disc herniation when

- there is functionally incapacitating pain in the leg, extending below the knee within a nerve root distribution;
- there are nerve root tension signs (for instance, a positive SLR), with or with-

out neurological abnormalities, fitting the radiculopathy;
- there is failure of clinical improvement after 4 to 8 weeks of conservative treatment; or
- there is a confirming imaging study, such as an abnormal myelogram, CT scan, or MRI, *correlating with the physical signs and distribution of the pain.*

The term *bulging disc* should not be used in radiological terminology or as an indication for surgery. Clinical symptoms and findings remain the most important basis for diagnosis.[31]

In the authors' opinion, 4 to 8 weeks is too short a period for conservative treatment un-

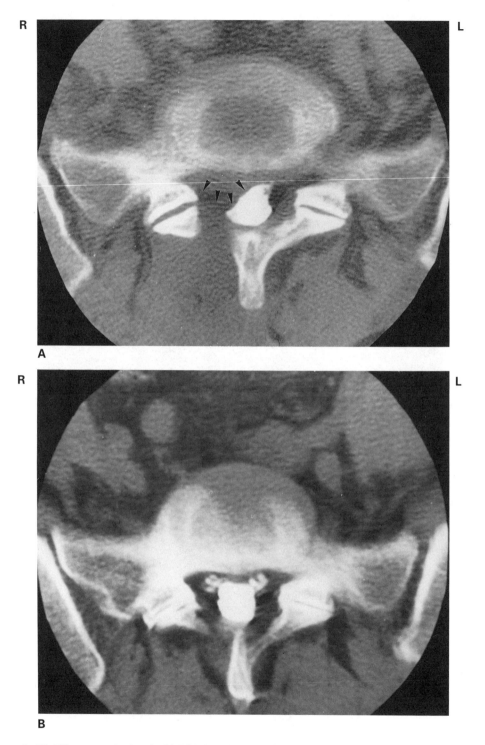

Figure 4–15 CT scan at the level of L5-S1 in a 30-year-old woman with a severe S1 and S2 radicular syndrome. **A**, Large posterolateral disc prolapse; **B**, the same patient, but the view is 3 mm lower. The disc is normal; the roots of S1 are clearly visible on each side.

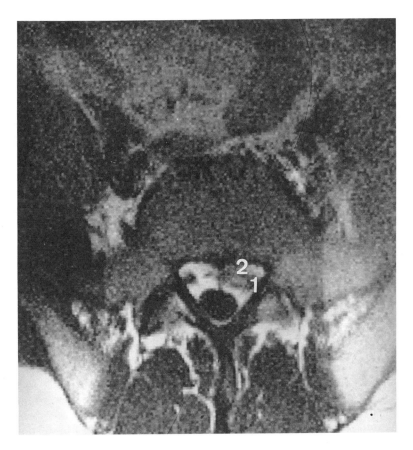

Figure 4–16 Axial MRI view of a patient with severe neurological deficits from the S1 nerve root. The left S1 root (*1*) is displaced by the prolapsed disc (*2*).

less there are two or more roots involved (paresis) or there are S4 signs and symptoms. The last case is an indication for immediate surgery. Otherwise the patient should be observed for at least 2 to 3 months before a final therapeutic decision regarding surgery is made. This is also one of the most important conclusions from Weber's study in 1983.[32]

Differential Diagnosis

Differential diagnosis possibilities are the same as for the other primary disc-related disorders. One should also consider peripheral vascular disturbances, aneurysm, and meralgia paresthetica.

With atypical symptomatology, the erythrocyte sedimentation rate (ESR) should be tested. An increased rate indicates an inflammatory process, which of course can also be caused by a nonrelated inflammation. If there is suspicion of bone pathology, additional blood tests should be performed. In most cases, CT scan and MRI are diagnostic.

EMG can be helpful in differentiating a peripheral compression neuropathy such as meralgia paresthetica. In root irritation, the EMG can be negative; however, this does not rule out root pathology.

Polyradicular

In the monoradicular syndrome, either a protrusion or a prolapse can be the cause of the symptoms. The polyradicular syndrome is almost always caused by a (posterolateral) disc prolapse. Here, too, the L5 and S1 nerve roots are the most frequently affected. Normally the patients are between 30 and 45 years old.

Clinical Findings

- The clinical findings are the same as those mentioned for the monoradicular syndrome, but now the radicular pain is the chief complaint. The pain in the leg is experienced in different dermatomes.

Treatment

See monoradicular syndrome. In this disorder, the chance that mobilization and/or traction brings improvement is extremely small.

Primary Posterolateral Disc Prolapse

The term *primary* indicates that the disc prolapse is not initially directed more posterocentrally, but immediately directed so far laterally that there is only an irritation of the dural sleeve (covering the nerve root), resulting in radiating pain down the leg with minimal to no back pain.

This disorder is mainly seen in young adults between the ages of 18 and 35 years.

The primary posterolateral disc protrusion/prolapse is different from the "normal" posterolateral disc protrusion/prolapse in that the affected disc compresses the exiting nerve root of the same level. In "normal" cases, the same disc compresses the nerve root exiting one level lower. However, a frequent clinical observation in primary posterolateral disc protrusion/prolapse is that not only L4 and L5 syndromes but also S1 syndromes occur (S1 exits at the S1-2 level). This means that at the level of L5-S1, the S1 root is compressed from lateral. If the S1 root is compressed from medial, the patient will experiences more back pain (and this would be considered a "normal" posterolateral protrusion/prolapse).

Clinical Findings

- Radicular pain in one leg, usually in one dermatome (mostly in L5 or S1), is elic-

ited during prolonged disc loading, such as prolonged standing, sitting, walking, etc.
- Flexion of the lumbar spine is severely limited and painful; the patient bends the painful leg in order to be able to perform more flexion. Sometimes a deviation is observed during flexion.
- The SLR, Neri, and Bragard tests are positive. Neurological deficits are not common.
- Conventional X-rays are negative; therefore, a CT scan is indicated (see Figure 4–17).

Treatment

Again, provision of information about the disorder, postural instruction, and exercises (as described in Appendix 4–A) are an important part of the treatment program.

If the duration of the disorder is less than 3 months, continuous traction is usually very effective (see section 4.4, Treatment: Lumbar Traction). The traction is given on a daily basis and the SLR is tested before each session of traction. As long as there is improvement of the SLR, the traction treatment is continued. When the SLR remains constant, a (sacral) epidural anesthesia is indicated and is almost always very effective.

Cauda Equina Syndrome

The cauda equina syndrome is a result of a massive disc prolapse in which the posterior longitudinal ligament ruptures. The syndrome can be described as a bilateral polyradicular root syndrome and occurs mainly at the L3-4 or L4-5 level. This disorder can be seen at almost any age between 10 and 65 years.

Clinical Findings

- Acute or gradually increasing pain is felt in both the back and the legs (bilateral sciatica). In severe cases, the so-called saddle anesthesia occurs, as well as impotence and loss of bowel and bladder control.

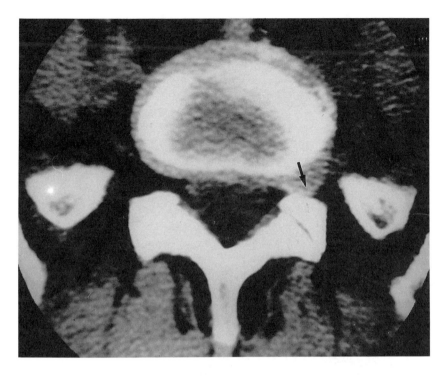

Figure 4–17 CT scan at the level of L5-S1 in a 27-year-old man with L5 radicular pain but without back pain. There is an extreme left lateral disc prolapse in which the intervertebral foramen is completely obstructed, resulting in compression of the L5 root.

- Usually a kyphotic deviation of the lumbar spine is present, sometimes in combination with a lateral shift.
- The motions of the lumbar spine are painful and limited in noncapsular proportions. Extension is the most limited and painful motion.
- The SLR, Neri, and Bragard tests are positive.
- Usually a bilateral areflexia of both Achilles tendons is present, as well as weakness of the calf muscles. In most cases, as soon as significant neurological deficits occur, the back pain disappears.
- A CT scan, an MRI, or a myelogram indicates the prolapse (Figures 4–18 and 4–19).

Treatment

The cauda equina syndrome is one of the few disorders of the lumbar spine in which immediate surgery is required. Symptoms that have been present for only a few hours, such as incontinence, can remain irreversible.

Differential Diagnosis

An important differential diagnosis to consider in the cauda equina syndrome is compression of the cauda equina by another source: tumors. Various types of tumors found in this area include neurinomas, meningiomas, gliomas, epidermoids, caudal ependymomas, and metastases from other primary tumors. Generally, the cauda equina syndrome caused by tumors has a very gradual onset with progressing symptoms.

In primary disc-related disorders, congenital anomalies of the lumbar roots can give rise to suspicion of a large disc prolapse or even a cauda syndrome. For instance, it is possible that two nerve roots run together in a common recess and then exit through the

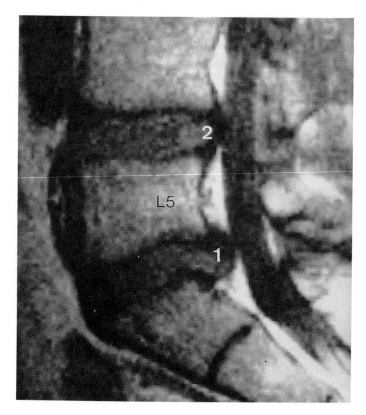

Figure 4–18 MRI view of the lumbosacral junction in a patient with a cauda equina syndrome. There is a massive L5-S1 disc prolapse (*1*) and a less severe protrusion at L4-5 (*2*).

same intervertebral foramen. If a disc protrusion causes a root compression, a radicular syndrome of two roots can occur. The so-called conjoined roots are more frequently found in people with a hemisacralization or other anomalies at the lumbosacral junction. Such variations are detectable by means of a myelogram or a myelo-CT scan (Figures 4–20 and 4–21).

NONSPECIFIC LOW BACK PAIN

General Concept

Nonspecific low back pain, as we understand it, concerns complaints of frequently recurring back pain that is clearly related to posture and movement and usually does not lead to an inability to continue working. This is a common form of back pain and is seen most often in work that involves sitting or standing primarily (eg, secretaries, teachers, assembly-line workers).

During the course of puberty and adolescence, there is a surprising increase in non-acute back pain. In 1977, Grantham[33] examined schoolchildren between the ages of 12 and 16. In boys, the incidence of low back pain was three times higher than in girls.

In regard to nonspecific low back pain, the various schools are in considerable disagreement. Particularly within manual medicine, the possible causes of nonspecific low back pain are vehemently debated. In the 1970s it was assumed that the cause lay in a dysfunction of the SI joint. Already in the 1940s,

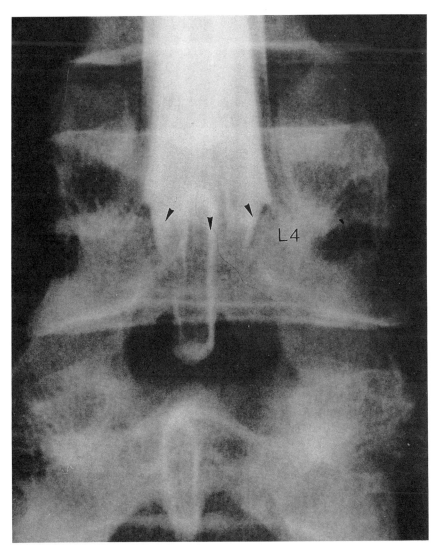

Figure 4–19 Myelogram, AP view, of the lower lumbar spine in a patient with a cauda equina syndrome. There is complete interruption of the contrast medium (*arrowheads*) just cranial to the L4-5 disc due to a massive disc prolapse.

James Cyriax referred to an involvement of the intervertebral disc.[24] Later, the role of the SI joint, particularly for manual therapists, was quickly replaced by the small intervertebral joints, the so-called "facet joints." Still others make a causative connection with the ligaments and have described nonspecific low back pain as a dysfunction of the ligamentous structures, in other words, a functional instability.

In our opinion, the *segment* plays the main role; that is to say that there is an interplay of all the structures composing the motion segment. In addition to the intervertebral disc at the center of the segment, other structures include the zygapophyseal joints with their

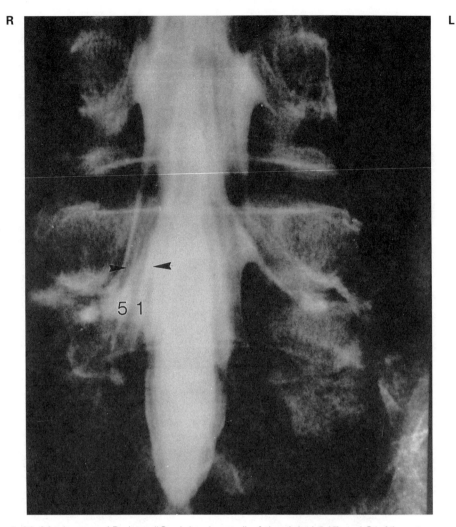

Figure 4–20 Myelogram: AP view. "Conjoined roots" of the right L5 (**5**) and S1 (**1**) roots.

capsuloligamentous structures, the dura mater, and the blood vessels and nerve supply. We are convinced that the physiological conditions of the disc can lead to nonspecific low back pain. However, whether or not the symptoms are caused by the capsular structures, the zygapophyseal joints, or the ligaments is not yet clear.

In several adults with nonspecific low back pain, we performed a CT scan at a time when their symptoms were severe. In every case, an unequivocal disc protrusion was evident, usually in combination with degenerative changes (which are almost always present).

When the history and functional examination indicate a disc lesion, but this is not confirmed by conventional X-rays or CT scans, a myelogram in standing should be performed. In many cases, an unstable disc protrusion becomes very apparent. Unfortunately, in such instances when X-rays and/or MRIs are negative, the false diagnosis of nonspecific low

R   L

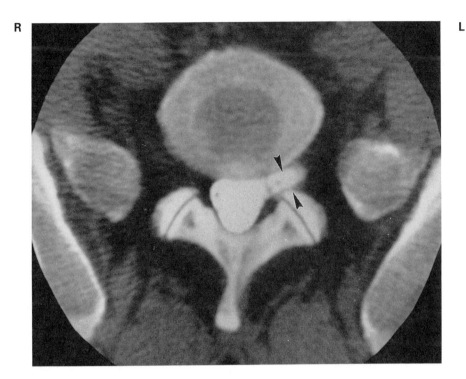

Figure 4–21 Myelo-CT scan at the L5-S1 level. The roots of L5 and S1 run in a common recess at the left side.

back pain is determined (Figures 4–22 to 4–24).

Clinical Findings

- In nonspecific low back pain, the patient history is of critical importance because the functional examination is often negative. The patient complains of a vague, difficult-to-localize pain either midline or paravertebral in the lower lumbar area. The pain is almost always provoked by prolonged sitting, prolonged standing, prolonged lying, prolonged "strolling about" (such as window shopping, visiting museums, etc), or prolonged stooping (such as during vacuum cleaning). With these complaints, one must also consider lumbar or SI instability as a differential diagnosis.

- Usually, the functional examination is either negative or too vague to afford a diagnosis. In other words, several motions are painful and others not.

- The SLR test is never positive.

- Coughing, sneezing, and straining never provoke the symptoms, and there are no neurological deficits in the lower extremities.

- The radiological examination is usually negative or gives misleading information. In other words, sometimes minimal arthrotic changes and/or a minor discopathy is visible. The older the patient, the more notable are the degenerative changes. An interesting observation is that the most pronounced arthrotic changes often occur in the zygapophyseal joints that lie more in the sagittal plane (Figure 4–25).

Treatment

SI instab c̄ vage LBP

Probably the most important step in treatment is a thorough explanation to the patient regarding the problem. Posture should be corrected, and a program of isometric abdominal exercises, strengthening of the back musculature (particularly in the thoracic region), and quadriceps strengthening should be performed daily at first. (In our opinion, the patient should actually devote more attention to the abdominal muscles than to the back muscles.) The exercises are described in Appendix 4–A. In referring back to Chapters 2 and 3, it is clear from the available literature on nonspecific back pain that, although (secondary) prevention may not be possible in many cases, the patients are better able to cope with their back problems if extensive information and appropriate management are given.

The abdominal exercises must be performed in such a way that optimal activity of the various abdominal muscles is achieved

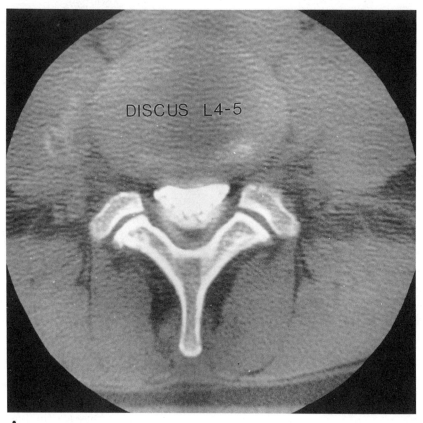

DISCUS L4-5

A

Figure 4–22 Myelogram and myelo-CT scan from a patient with severe low back pain accompanied by minor radiating symptoms. From the conventional X-rays a discopathy of L5-S1 was visible. Several months later, a myelo-CT scan of both the L5-S1 and the L4-5 levels showed no protrusion or prolapse. Because of continued complaints, a few months later a myelo-CT scan and a myelogram were performed. This time views were taken not only in lying but also in standing. Although the imaging in lying was negative, in standing a large protrusion was noted. **A**, Myelo-CT scan in supine, at the level of the L4-5 disc. Minimal disc bulging is noted.

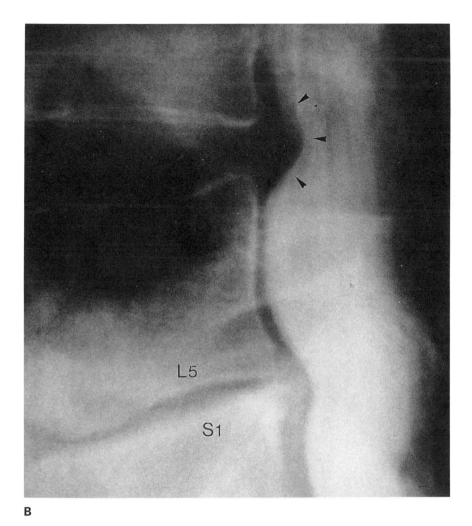

B

Figure 4–22 B, Myelogram of the lower lumbar spine in standing. Large disc protrusion at L4-5. The L5-S1 disc has practically disappeared.

while the iliopsoas activity remains as low as possible. Too much activity of the iliopsoas muscle has a lordosing effect on the lumbar spine and also increases intradiscal pressure. Contraction of the abdominal musculature increases the intra-abdominal pressure, which leads to a decrease in the intradiscal pressure, as long as the patient exhales in a steady and relaxed way. If this does not occur, the opposite happens: the intradiscal pressure increases, which results in an increase in the symptoms. Therefore, it is imperative to instruct the patient thoroughly and to check regularly how the patient is performing the exercises.

Abdominal exercises should be initiated when the patient is able to perform the lumbar motions without pain and when the prior limitations of motion have improved. These basic requirements can be achieved through manual therapy.

For the most part, manual mobilization is most effective when the patient has had symptoms for less than 1 year. The best-

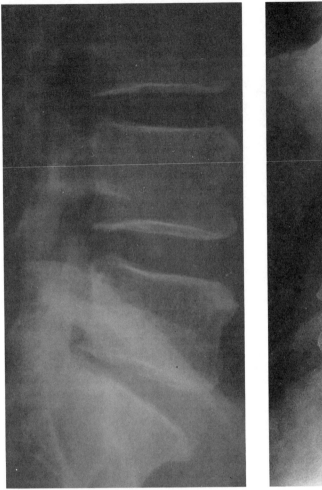
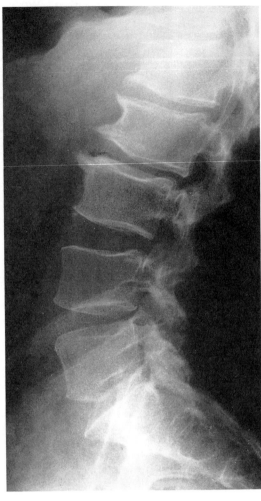

A   **B**

Figure 4–23 X-rays of two lumbar spines with pathological changes. However, the complaints of the patients were not due to these changes. **A**, Disc narrowing, L5-S1. **B**, Spondylosis, L1, L2, and L3.

researched technique is the long lever rotation manipulation. (For performance of this technique, refer to section 4.4, Treatment: General Manual Mobilization for the Lumbar Spine.) If this technique proves ineffective, local segmental mobilization or manipulation will be needed in order to reach the desired treatment goals.

Note: In many cases, nonspecific low back pain ultimately "develops" into a disc syndrome. The border between nonspecific low back pain and disc problems is very vague. Thus, credit can be given to the argument that there is a primary discogenic cause for nonspecific low back pain.

Stages of Nonspecific Low Back Pain

As mentioned earlier, degeneration of one or more discs can lead to low back pain; the

R   B

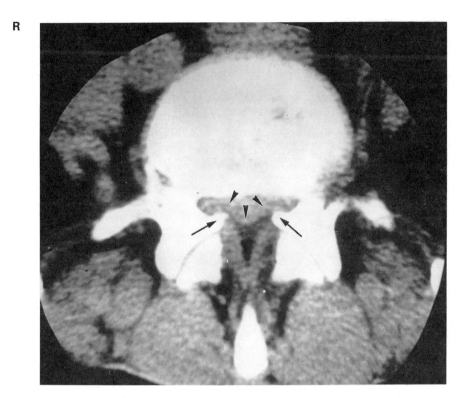

Figure 4–24 CT scan of L4-5 from a 34-year-old woman with nonspecific low back pain. At the time this was taken, the patient was experiencing severe symptoms. A small central disc prolapse is seen (*arrowheads*). At the same time, osteoarthrosis of the L4-5 zygapophyseal joints is evident: joint space is significantly reduced, and ventromedial osteophytes (*arrows*) all lead to a narrowing of the lateral recesses.

nature of the pain and its course are dependent on the stage of the degeneration (discosis). Although gradual transitions exist between the various forms of disc-related low back pain, it is still possible to make specific classifications. Often, the patient's history includes a period of nonspecific low back pain that ultimately progresses into a disc syndrome.

Three clinical stages can be differentiated.

Stage 1: Pseudospondylolisthesis

Because of a gradual diminishing of the volume and elasticity of the disc, the affected segment first experiences a hypermobility and later an instability (pseudospondylolisthesis). As a result, the zygapophyseal joints are overloaded, and little by little arthrotic changes occur. The ligaments are abnormally loaded, which leads to muscle hypertrophy.

Clinical Findings

- Symptoms in this stage consist of pain in the back, sometimes with radiating symptoms via the buttock region into the groin or into one leg. Some patients have a "referred" coccygodynia. The pain usually comes on during activities and increases as the day goes on. Lying down relieves the symptoms.

- Coughing, sneezing, and straining sometimes increase the pain in the back or leg.

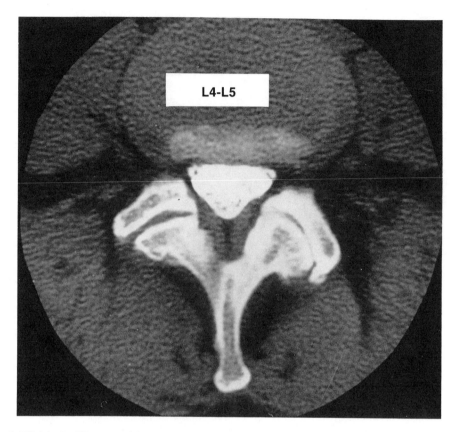

Figure 4–25 Myelo-CT scan of L4-5 in a patient with a clinically diagnosed disc prolapse at L5-S1 (confirmed by CT scan, view not shown). Osteoarthrosis is evident in the left zygapophyseal joint with a distinct lengthening of its edges. It is interesting to note that, compared with the opposite side, the affected joint lies significantly more in the sagittal plane.

- Some of the lumbar spine motions are slightly limited and/or painful in a noncapsular pattern. The motions most often involved are flexion and extension.
- The X-rays indicate either no changes or a beginning disc degeneration with spondylolitic reaction. Osteophytes develop at a short distance from the vertebral end-plate. Sometimes a pseudo-spondylolisthesis (spondylolisthesis without spondylolysis) is visible on functional X-rays. However, the findings from the X-rays often give misleading information. In many cases, a visible narrowing of the intervertebral disc is not at the level that is causing the (clinical) symptoms. Through utilization of a CT scan or an MRI, additional relevant information can be obtained. Nowadays myelography is often applied in combination with a CT scan or an MRI.
- Disc protrusions are often seen at the level with Scheuermann's disease. The further dorsal a Schmorl's nodule is located in a vertebral body, the greater the chance that the obviously weakened disc can protrude dorsally (Figures 4–26 and 4–27).
- Occasionally in disc degeneration, the so-called vacuum phenomenon occurs. This is indicated on X-ray by a radiolucent zone (black line) in the in-

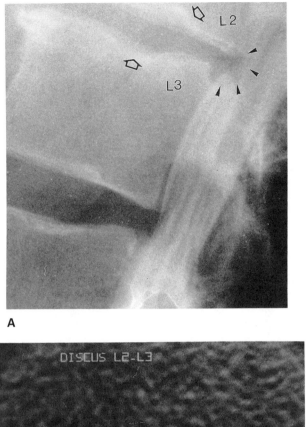

A

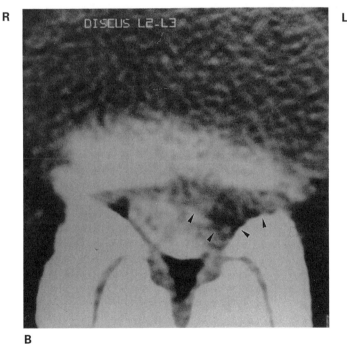

B

Figure 4–26 Myelogram and myelo-CT scan of a 24-year-old patient with upper lumbar complaints (L2). **A**, Myelogram at the level of L2 to L4. Shown are a Schmorl's nodule (*open arrows*) and a disc prolapse L2-3 (*arrowheads*). **B**, Myelo-CT scan at the level of the L2-3 disc. A large posterolateral disc prolapse is seen, left. Also apparent are sagittally directed zygapophyseal joints.

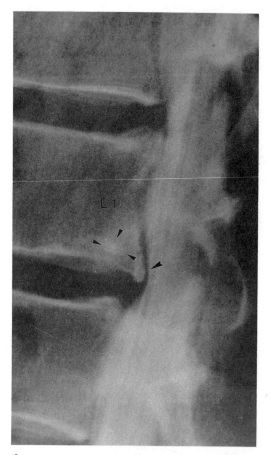

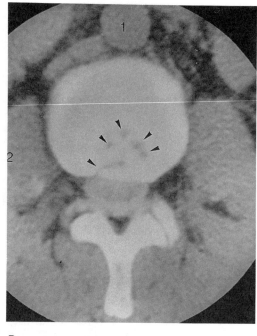

Figure 4–27 Myelogram and myelo-CT views of a 28-year-old patient with upper lumbar symptoms. **A**, Myelogram at the level of T11 to L1. Local calcification in the L1 vertebral body (*small arrowheads*) and an osteophyte (*large arrowhead*). **B**, Myelo-CT scan at the level of the T12-L1 disc. Scheuermann's disease (*arrowheads*) with fragmentation, resulting in slight compression of the posterior longitudinal ligament and the dural sac. **1**, Aorta; **2**, iliopsoas muscle.

tervertebral joint space. On the CT scan, the phenomenon can be seen as a concentric (black) radiolucency. Like the initial contents of the disc, the position of this vacuum can change, which can be seen on functional X-rays (Figures 4–28 and 4–29).

• Frequently an anomaly of the lumbosacral junction is also seen. As mentioned earlier, these congenital aberrations do not necessarily cause symptoms; however, sometimes there is an overload on the segment just cranial to the anomaly. Usually, such anomalies concern a (hemi)sacralization: one side of the fifth lumbar vertebra is fused or has an "articulation" with the sacrum and sometimes also with the ilium. The disc from the L5-S1 segment is then generally severely narrowed and can sometimes be a source of symptoms. The joint between the transverse process of L5 and the sacrum (and/or ilium) can also cause symptoms. In a (hemi)lumbarization, the same situ-

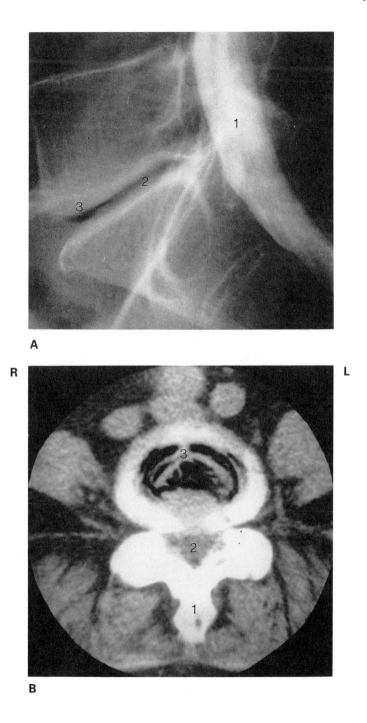

A

R   L

B

Figure 4–28 Vacuum phenomenon due to L5-S1 disc degeneration in two patients with complaints of back pain. **A**, Myelogram, lateral view. **1**, Contrast-filled dural sac; **2**, narrowed L5-S1 disc; **3**, vacuum phenomenon (visible as a line-shaped radiolucent zone in the intervertebral disc). **B**, CT scan. **1**, L5 spinous process; **2**, spinal canal; **3**, vacuum phenomenon (visible as concentric radiolucent zones).

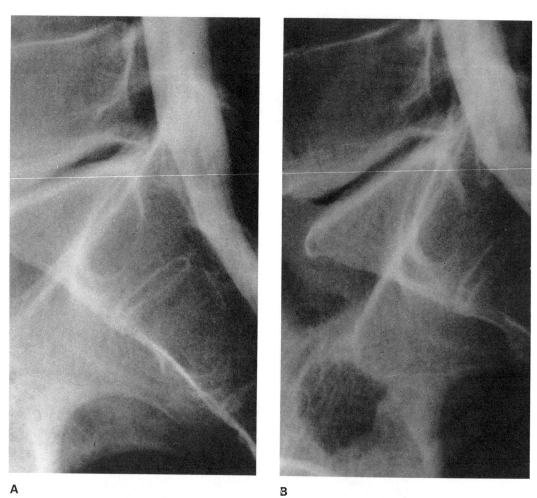

A   **B**

Figure 4–29 Conventional lateral X-rays of the upper lumbar spine with a vacuum phenomenon in the L5-S1 disc. *A*, Flexion: the vacuum shifts dorsally; *B*, extension: the vacuum shifts ventrally.

ation can arise, with the understanding that there is now a disc between S1 and S2. In such cases, the L5-S1 disc is usually the "weak spot" (Figure 4–30).

Treatment

First, information is given about the lesion, as well as instruction in proper posture. Isometric abdominal exercises are added to the treatment program when, for instance, after mobilization/manipulation of the lumbar spine, the patient's normal range of motion is again possible. When correctly performed, isometric contraction of the abdominal muscles can decrease the intradiscal pressure by approximately 30%.[7]

Manual mobilization/manipulation is best performed with a long lever rotation technique. (See section 4.4, General Manual Mobilization for the Lumbar Spine, and the literature review in Chapter 14.) For further progression in the exercise program, see Appendix 4–A. If no improvement is achieved with this treatment, continuous traction can be tried. If traction also is not effective, segmental mobilization or manipulation may be indicated. (See section 4.4, Local Manual Mobilization.)

Stage 2: Segmental Laxity

With further progression of the degenerative process of the disc and the other structures in the segment, the instability of the segment at first increases. Complaints usually begin at approximately 35 years of age.

Clinical Findings

- Pain in the back and/or in one leg is experienced not only during activities but also at rest. The patient often has pain in lying, particularly prone. The pain is worse in the early morning.

- As in stage 1, coughing, sneezing, and straining sometimes cause pain in the back and/or leg.

- Initially, pain was the main complaint; now it is particularly a painful limitation of motion that was initially in noncapsular proportions and has slowly progressed into a capsular pattern.(See Segmental Instability.)

- In comparison to stage 1, on the X-rays one sees an increase in the spondylosis. The zygapophyseal joints exhibit arthrotic changes. Degenerative changes of the

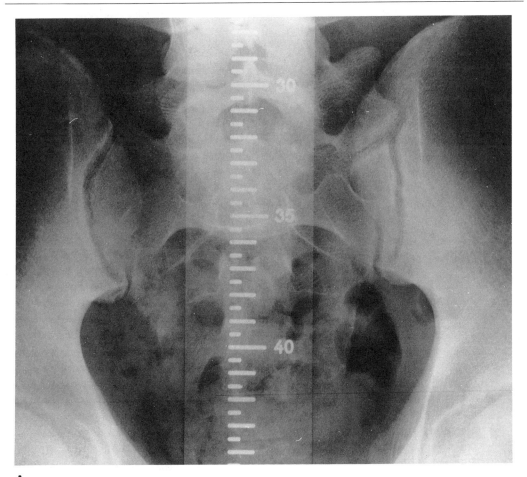

A

Figure 4–30 Lumbosacral junction and the sacroiliac joints of a 22-year-old man with complaints of back pain and radicular pain, right, from the L5 and S1 nerve roots. **A**, Conventional X-ray, AP view. Hemisacralization on the left with a joint between the L5 transverse process and not only the sacrum but also the ilium.

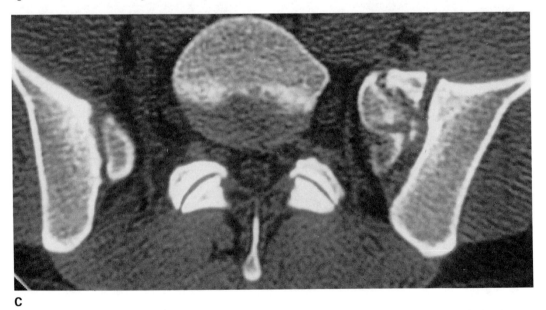

R   L

B

Figure 4–30 B, CT scan, L4-5. Wide posterior disc protrusion (*arrowheads*) and thickening of the flaval ligament (*arrows*), causing a narrowing in the diameter of the spinal canal.

C

Figure 4–30 C, CT scan, L5-S1. The plane of view runs through the joint between the sacrum and the L5 transverse process. It also shows an articulation between the transverse process and the ilium.

zygapophyseal joints (spondylarthrosis) and the vertebral bodies (deforming spondylosis) are almost always visible on conventional X-rays. Usually there is a discrepancy between the level where the degenerative changes are found and the clinically affected level (Figures 4–31 and 4–32). Here, too, CT scan and MRI examinations make further differentiation possible.

Treatment

As in stage 1, information about the problem, instruction in proper posture and body mechanics, and an appropriate exercise program are an important part of the treatment.

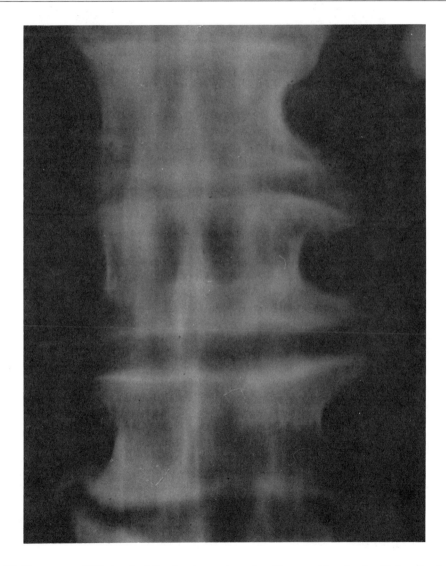

Figure 4–31 Tomogram (AP view) of the lumbar spine of a 45-year-old patient with low back pain. Although the tomogram shows severe spondylarthrosis at several levels, clinically the patient has an L5-S1 disc protrusion.

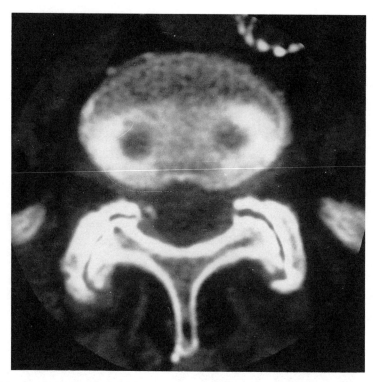

Figure 4–32 CT scan at the level of the L4-5 zygapophyseal joint in a 48-year-old patient with complaints of back pain. From interpreting only the CT scan, one might diagnose a severe arthrosis of the zygapophyseal joints: the joint space is narrowed, the contours of the joint spaces are markedly irregular, and osteophytes are visible. However, clinically, there is actually an L5-S1 disc protrusion.

The symptoms have likely been present for longer than 1 year, and manual mobilization and traction are usually not as successful as in stage 1 when the pain was activity related. Epidural anesthesia is a good alternative treatment. (See section 4.4, Treatment: Therapeutic Nerve Blocks.)

Stage 3: Segmental Remodeling

In general, the disc degeneration ends with a decrease in the instability and leads to an immobility of the motion segment. Usually, in this stage the symptoms decrease.

Clinical Findings

If the symptoms do not, or only temporarily, improve, one of the following disorders, or a combination of these, may be involved:

- nerve root compression syndrome
- neurogenic claudication
- degenerative spondylolisthesis
- retrolisthesis

Each of the above disorders is described later in this chapter.

Treatment

See the recommended treatment discussed under the previous stages.

SECONDARY DISC-RELATED DISORDERS

Secondary discogenic disorders are seen in patients who have already experienced primary discogenic pathology. These disorders mostly include forms of instability, nerve root compression, or cauda compression as a result of degenerative changes in which narrowing of the spinal canal, the lateral recess, or the intervertebral foramen occurs.

Because of changes in the length of the spinal canal and its adjacent structures, at the intervertebral disc level, the spinal canal is widest in a kyphotic position and narrowest in a lordotic position. In a lordotic position the dorsal parts of the vertebral bodies approach each other and the interposed discs and ligamenta flava bulge in the direction of the spinal canal. In a kyphotic position the opposite occurs, resulting in a widening of the spinal canal.[34] Therefore, when symptoms arise during activities such as walking, patients with spinal claudication (due to spinal stenosis) exhibit kyphosis of the lumbar spine.

The phenomenon of a narrowed spinal canal in lordosis can also create significant problems for patients with a postsurgical syndrome. Patients in this group develop radicular symptoms after having undergone a (hemi)laminectomy. Although these symptoms could be caused by a disc protrusion at a different level, they are sometimes a result of adhesions of the dura mater with one or more nerve roots (Figure 4–33).

Segmental Instability

Segmental instability is seen almost exclusively in people older than 35 years of age. The disorder affects slightly more women than men.

Most patients have a long history of discogenic back pain. Because of the changed

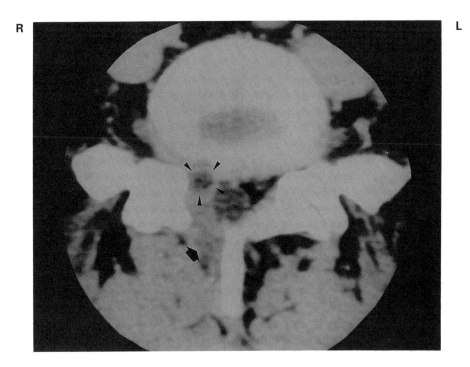

R   L

Figure 4–33 CT scan after intravenous injection of a contrast medium in a patient with postsurgical epidural fibrosis at the level of the lumbosacral junction. Note interruption of the lamina (status post hemilaminectomy) (*arrow*) and epidural fibrosis, which completely surrounds the S1 nerve root (*arrowheads*).

symptomatology it is now possible to make the diagnosis of "segmental instability."

Often patients have a congenital disorder of the shape of their vertebral bodies, such as platyspondylitic or platydystrophic vertebrae. The vertebrae are wide and flat with average to poor disc material, and the spinal canal is narrow (Figure 4–34). Segmental instability can eventually develop.

Clinical Findings

- The patient usually complains of back pain with or without radiating pain into the pelvic region and into the posterior aspect of one or both legs. The pain increases during prolonged walking, especially strolling about (shopping, visiting museums), and prolonged standing. In lying the symptoms disappear completely. Pregnancy and obesity increase the symptoms.

- Pain is provoked when returning to upright standing from a slumped or bent-forward position, as well as in standing up from a chair. The patient comes up by supporting himself or herself with both

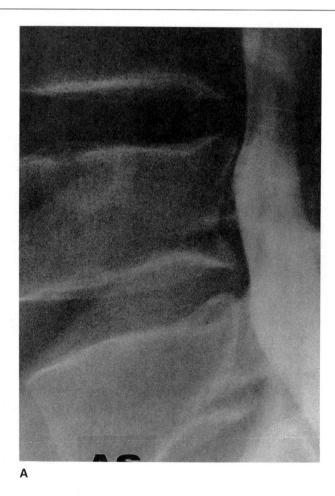

A

Figure 4–34 Conventional X-rays and myelogram of the lower lumbar spine in a 40-year-old man with a segmental instability. Very wide, flat vertebrae (platyspondylisis) are evident. *A*, Lateral view;

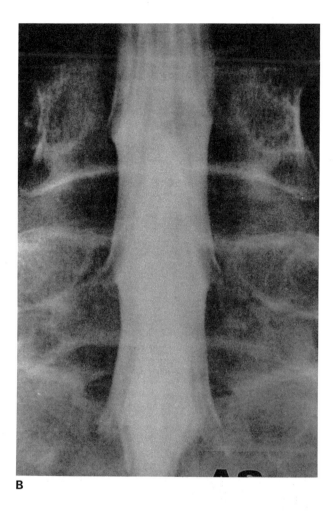

B

Figure 4–34 *B*, AP view.

hands on the thighs ("climbing up the legs").[26]

- In the functional examination, a striking observation is the mobility in flexion; the patient is able to bend forward through a large range of motion without pain, but he or she is forced to "climb up the legs" with both hands in order to return to the upright position. Sidebending is symmetrically limited and sometimes slightly painful. For experienced examiners, the instability is detectable in the local segmental examination. The level most often affected is L4-5; L5-S1 is less often affected.

- Usually the X-rays show a distinct narrowing of the disc space with traction osteophytes at both adjacent vertebral bodies. Objectifying the instability is possible in some cases by means of functional X-rays; however, significant disagreement exists concerning this issue. Some authors state that a segmental subluxation larger than 2 mm indicates a segmental instability, and others judge this as arbitrary because measurement utilizing X-rays is not fully reliable.

- Often the amount of instability does not correspond with the degree of symptoms. In other words, some patients have significant symptoms, but a small instability; others have almost no symptoms with a large instability (confirmed by X-rays and local segmental examination).

Thus, the diagnosis of segmental instability is based chiefly on the history and the functional examination.

Treatment

Reassuring the patient by explaining the problem as much as possible is of great importance in this disorder. In instances of obesity it may be helpful for the patient to lose weight so that the exercise program can be more eas-ily performed. The exercise program as described in Appendix 4–A is useful in this disorder. Sometimes a lumbosacral support (corset) can aid in diminishing the symptoms, particularly when worn during heavy labor or during prolonged activities.

Usually the prognosis is good and the symptoms decrease to an acceptable level for the patient. In some cases, the pain disappears completely. Surgical stabilization is rarely necessary.

Nerve Root Compression Syndrome

Compression of the nerve root produces a clinical syndrome that is different from an acute disc lesion. In a nerve root compression syndrome, the root usually becomes compressed by bony and soft tissue structures within the root canal (lateral recess) and only seldom within the central spinal canal (Figure 4–35). In contrast, an acute lesion com-

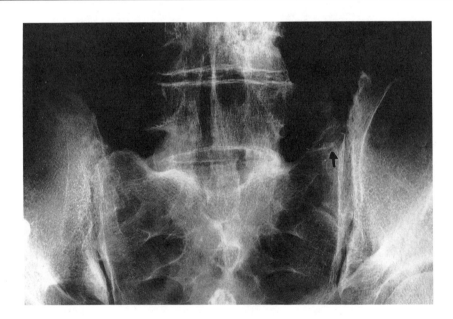

Figure 4–35 Conventional AP X-ray of the lumbosacral junction and the SI joints of a 65-year-old patient with unilateral radicular L4 pain. A hemisacralization, left, can be seen; L5 is partly fused with the sacrum, and in this case there is still a rudimentary joint between the transverse process of L5 and the sacrum. There is L4-5 disc degeneration (severe narrowing). In this patient, only the L4-5 disc lesion is of clinical importance; the patient has an L4 nerve root compression syndrome.

presses the root in the central spinal canal and seldom within the nerve root canal. Both disorders cause leg pain, but the symptoms and treatment are not the same.

The most often affected root is L5. Probably this is due to the frequently occurring degenerative changes at the L5-S1 level as well as the long nerve root canal caudal to the broad pedicle. The nerve roots of L4 and L3 are seldom compressed within the root canal. In the central spinal canal the L5 root can be affected because of degenerative changes at the L4-5 disc level; the root of S1 is most often compressed just ventral of the cranial lip of the upper sacral lamina.

The form of the root canal varies interindividually; the smaller the diameter the larger the chance of compression of the root by osteophytes from the zygapophyseal joints or by a ridge at the caudolateral aspect of the vertebra due to degenerative changes. Besides the radiologically visible bony protrusions, soft tissue swelling also usually occurs. This is a result of the reorganization of annular tissue after a disc prolapse or a sequestered nucleus. The posterior longitudinal ligament and the ligamentum flavum, as well as the capsule of the zygapophyseal joints, can thicken.

The root canal (lateral recess) never becomes totally occluded; thus the root is never totally compressed. The root actually remains somewhat mobile. The normal lumbar nerve root excursion amounts to only a few millimeters. However, in the presence of a "hostile surrounding," the root becomes thicker, harder, and less elastic due to perineural fibrosis with a resulting decrease in its mobility.

In most cases the history includes a previous incident of symptoms from a primary disc pathology.

In the nerve root compression syndrome, the symptoms can vary greatly. Although most patients complain of radicular pain, some patients describe only back pain. Even years postlaminectomy or chemonucleolysis, there is still a chance for the development of a nerve root compression syndrome.

EMG and radiculography are not very sensitive in indicating a nerve root compression syndrome. A CT scan usually confirms the diagnosis.

Clinical Findings

- The patient usually complains of severe pain in the L5 or S1 (seldom L3 or L4) dermatomes that is present day and night. The pain at night often forces the patient to get out of bed and walk around. For some patients, sitting is uncomfortable and driving a car is almost impossible. Other patients mainly have problems during standing or walking. There is no typical course for this disorder; sometimes the pain slowly arises over weeks, months, or even years and can even disappear or decrease in the same gradual way. In other patients, however, the pain is very progressive and surgery is required.

- Coughing, sneezing, and straining do not exacerbate the pain.

- Rotation and extension are the most painful motions. In most cases, the SLR test and flexion of the lumbar spine are not limited.

- Reflexes, sensibility, and strength are normal in over 80% of all cases.

- Conventional X-rays reveal disc narrowing. CT scans show the root compression (Figure 4–36).

Treatment

First, very thorough information must be given to the patient regarding the cause of the symptoms. Movements aggravating the symptoms should be avoided as much as possible (extension and rotation). If prolonged standing or sitting increases the complaints, the patient should change positions regularly.

It is important for the patient to understand that in most instances the symptoms will gradually decrease without any surgical intervention. In patients with severe pain, an epidural injection is the treatment of choice.[26]

Some patients ultimately require surgical decompression.

Differential Diagnosis

In the differential diagnosis, primary lateral disc protrusion and disc prolapse (mostly young patients) should be considered.

Neurogenic Claudication

Neurogenic or spinal claudication occurs mostly in male patients over 50 years of age

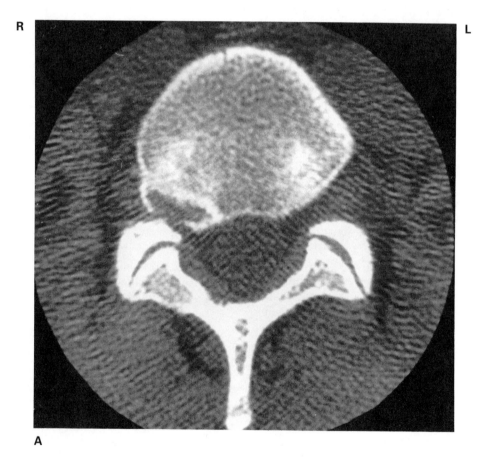

R   **L**

A

Figure 4–36 *A* and *B*, CT scan at the level of L4 in a 19-year-old patient with a nerve root compression syndrome. The difference in the level between view *A* and view *B* is 3 mm. A prolapsed Schmorl's nodule (Scheuermann's disease) is localized within the right dorsolateral aspect of the vertebral body.

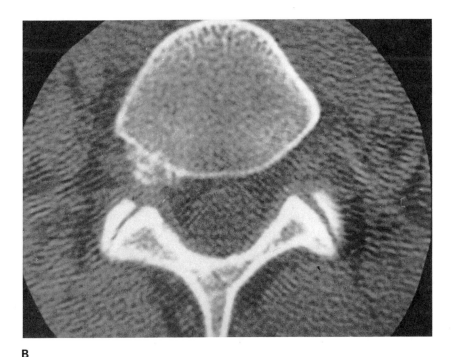

B

Figure 4–36 B, The difference in the level between view **A** and view **B** is 3 mm.

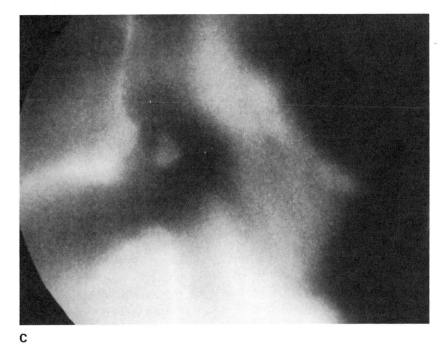

C

Figure 4–36 C, Lateral tomogram at the L4-5 level in the same patient. This view clearly shows that a fragment of the vertebral body is now located within the intervertebral foramen.

whose work activities include heavy labor. The symptoms start during movement, especially walking, and disappear in rest and/or when the lumbar spine is in a kyphotic position.

Verbiest[35] found that neurogenic claudication was associated with a narrow spinal canal, "spinal stenosis." However, "spinal stenosis" is not a synonym for neurogenic claudication. Spinal stenosis is only *one* of the factors in this syndrome. Many people have a congenitally narrow canal but never experience symptoms of claudication.

Heavy physical labor generally results in a higher incidence of degenerative changes in the lumbar spine, including either a ventral or a dorsal slipping of one vertebra but without a lysis. This so-called degenerative spondylolisthesis effectively reduces the diameter of the vertebral canal.[36] Patients can have either a degenerative anterolisthesis or a degenerative retrolisthesis. In approximately 50% of all patients with neurogenic claudication, a degenerative anterolisthesis is present.[37] Sometimes neurogenic claudication also occurs in combination with a nerve root compression syndrome.

The mechanism causing the symptoms is purely speculative. An arterial ischemia or venous swelling may be the cause of inadequate nerve function during movement, but still allows for adequate function at rest.

Various factors contribute to the phenomenon that the symptoms typically occur while walking. First, during walking a segmental rotation occurs (especially in the presence of a segmental instability) that decreases the space in an already narrow vertebral canal. Many patients with neurogenic claudication have a stenosis at the L3-4 level (Figure 4–37). In the lower levels, the cauda equina has more space. However, it is also possible that a large L5-S1 disc prolapse or severe degenerative changes at that level can cause the same symptoms (Figure 4–38). Second, swelling of the veins occurs as a result of walking. Third, the blood supply of the cauda equina may be disturbed if the space is compromised. Nutri-

ents are unable to reach the nerve roots, and waste products (metabolites) are inadequately transported away, resulting in disturbed function. It is not yet clear how important a role the cerebrospinal fluid plays in the proper function of the cauda equina. There are indications that if there is not enough cerebrospinal fluid surrounding the cauda equina (due to the vertebral canal stenosis), the metabolic function of the cerebrospinal fluid as well as the function of the cauda equina and the nerve roots is compromised.

Clinical Findings

- Patients are usually men and over 50 years of age. They complain about an uncomfortable feeling in the legs during walking. Both legs generally are equally involved. The patient describes a "heavy" or "tired" feeling, especially in the thighs, the calves, and the feet. Usually the symptoms occur after walking a certain distance, forcing the patient to stop. This distance can vary from day to day. Sometimes, after a taking a short rest, it is possible for the patient to walk a longer distance. Often, the patient starts to stoop forward gradually during walking until he or she has to stop. The patient then leans forward or sits down with a kyphotic lumbar spine; generally the symptoms disappear within minutes. As the pathology increases, the walking distance finally decreases to an average of approximately 20 yards.

  Because of the kyphotic position of the lumbar spine, climbing up a hill or stairs is easier than going down. In severe cases, extending the spine from an upright position provokes the symptoms. Biking is very well tolerated, which is of great importance in making the differential diagnosis with intermittent claudication.

- At night the patient complains of "restless legs" and cramps in the legs. Getting up and walking is often the only remedy.

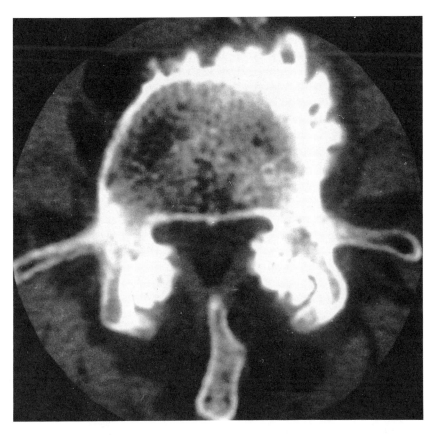

Figure 4–37 CT scan at the L4 level in a 56-year-old patient with neurogenic claudication. Severe, destructive zygapophyseal joint arthrosis narrows the spinal canal. A severe spondylosis is apparent at the left ventral aspect of the vertebral body.

- Back pain often occurs in combination with the claudication symptoms. Usually there is a long history of back pain and even years of claudication symptoms before medical help is sought.
- In the functional examination, flexion of the lumbar spine is normally possible; extension, on the contrary, is very limited. Some patients are unable to stand totally straight. They assume the so-called ape posture ("simian stance")[38] in which their hips and knees are held in slight flexion.
- Generally, the SLR test is negative, and there are no sensory, reflex, or motor disturbances.

- Objectifying the walking distance can be evaluated by using a treadmill; this is especially important in order to validate the response to treatment.
- X-rays indicate degenerative changes in the lumbar spine. Approximately 50% of the time there is a degenerative spondylolisthesis. MRI and/or CT scans are diagnostic. A CT scan reveals the decreased midsagittal diameter of the vertebral canal.

Treatment

Either the patient has to learn to cope with the symptoms (in some cases medication has a positive influence on the symptoms) or a

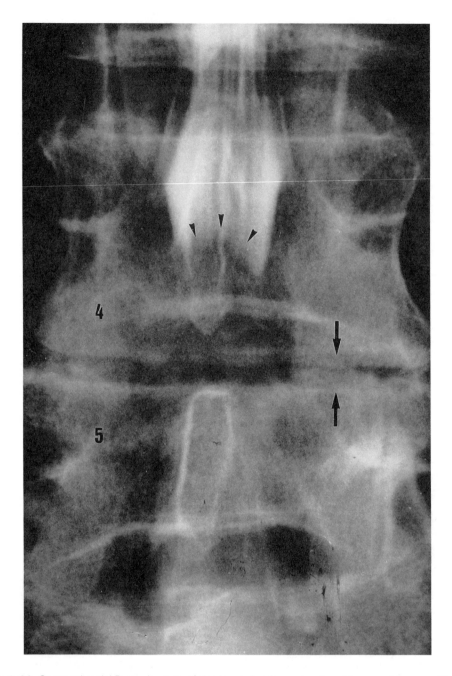

Figure 4–38 Conventional AP myelogram of the lower lumbar spine in a 61-year-old man with severe spinal claudication. The view is made in a forced upright position. This patient could stand only with the lumbar spine in a slight kyphosis. Note the severely degenerated L4-5 disc (*arrows*) and the complete stop of the contrast medium just cranial to the L4-5 disc (*arrowheads*).

surgical decompression is indicated. When the symptoms are not too severe, the patient should try to limit those activities that cause the complaints.

Johnsson et al[39] studied the natural progression of lumbar spinal stenosis and compared the course of nonsurgical patients with that of patients who underwent surgical decompression. After 4 years, the majority of the nonsurgical patients with spinal stenosis remained unchanged; severe deterioration was not found. Thus, observation seems to be a good alternative to surgery. Immediate surgery should be advised only if the pain is intolerable, and/or in the rarer instance that neurological symptoms develop.

Porter[26] reports good results using calcitonin. He administers an injection of 100 U of calcitonin, intramuscularly, four times per week for 4 weeks. If the walking distance does not increase after 4 weeks, the treatment is discontinued. If improvement is noted, the treatment is continued for another 4 weeks. Porter and Hibbert[37] use the calcitonin treatment as a selection method for surgical indication.

Differential Diagnosis

Intermittent Claudication.[40] The typical stooped posture in neurogenic claudication is not observed in an intermittent claudication. Walking uphill or upstairs is worse than going downhill or downstairs, and the patient with intermittent claudication can neither walk nor bike.

The "bicycle test"[41] offers a good possibility in making the differentiation. The patient performs the bicycle test on a stationary bicycle, first with the lumbar spine in extension and then in flexion. There will be no difference in distance in patients with intermittent claudication, while the neurogenic claudication patient performs better and longer in flexion.

In intermittent claudication, one leg can be more affected than the other; sometimes only the calves are involved. Peripheral pulsations are usually not palpable.

In some cases, both disorders occur at the same time.[39]

Sciatic Claudication.[42] Ischemia of the sciatic nerve can arise due to an insufficiency of the inferior gluteal artery. Symptoms from the claudication are limited to the S1 and S2 dermatomes. Examination of the spine and results of a CT scan and/or MRI are negative. The treatment is surgical: an endarterectomy of the aortic-iliac segments.

Referred Pain. Referred pain from the lumbar spine, as a result of a disc protrusion, can increase during walking. Venner and Crock[43] found that 18% of their disc patients complained of an increase in pain and/or paresthesia in one leg when walking distances greater than 500 yards.

Nerve Root Compression Syndrome. Some patients with a nerve root compression syndrome have pain chiefly in one leg during walking. However, sitting is usually also painful.

Aortic Occlusion. Symptoms accompanying this disorder consist mainly of upper lumbar pain with referred pain in both legs. When the symptoms arise during walking, the patient is forced to stop and rest.

Degenerative Spondylolisthesis

The term *degenerative spondylolisthesis* indicates a ventral subluxation (slipping) of a cranial vertebra in relation to the adjacent caudal vertebra without the presence of a spondylolysis.[44]

The disorder is seen more often in women, usually around 60 years of age, and is generally localized between L4 and L5. This is in contrast with spondylolytic spondylolisthesis, which occurs more often in men and in most cases is located at the level of L5-S1.

Some patients have a nerve root compression syndrome as well, usually of the L4 or L5 nerve root. In men, neurogenic claudication can also be present; this is much less common in women.

A study by Rosenberg[36] showed that degenerative spondylolisthesis occurs 10 times more often at the level of L4-5 than at the level of L5-S1 or L3-4. The incidence is six times higher in women than in men. In addition, the incidence of sacralization is four times higher in people with a degenerative spondylolisthesis than in the general population. Degenerative spondylolisthesis affects black women three times more often than white women.

Because of degenerative changes in the zygapophyseal joints, ventral slipping is possible. Cranial and caudal grooves are formed, creating an S-shape that is very well detectable on an oblique-view X-ray (Figure 4–39) Usually the amount of subluxation in degenerative spondylolisthesis does not exceed 15%.[28] In spondylolytic anterolisthesis, on the other hand, percentages of more than 30% subluxation are not uncommon (Figure 4–40).

Clinical Findings

- The patient complains of acute pain when rising from a flexed or forward-bent position or when getting up out of a chair. All sudden and unexpected movements cause back pain. Turning in bed is often painful. Standing and walking cause back pain and posterior upper thigh pain.

- As in segmental instability, the patient with a degenerative spondylolisthesis is very mobile in flexion. Returning to upright standing from a flexed position can only be performed by supporting the hands on the upper thighs ("climbing up the legs"; see Segmental Instability). Extension is painful and very often severely limited.

- The SLR test is negative and there is an absence of neurological signs.

- On X-ray the degenerated L4-5 disc and the anterolisthesis of L4 are demonstrated (Figure 4–41). In instances of degenerative spondylolisthesis in combination with neurogenic claudication, a CT scan is indicated.

Treatment

The prognosis is usually good. The patient should receive extensive information about the disorder and its prognosis. Instruction concerning posture and body mechanics is very important, as well as the exercise program described in Appendix 4–A.

Spondylosyndesis (fusion) is rarely indicated. When the disorder is present in combination with neurogenic claudication and/or a nerve root compression syndrome, surgical treatment is more often indicated.

Retrolisthesis

The term *retrolisthesis* indicates a dorsal subluxation of a vertebra in relation to an adjacent caudal vertebra. Retrolisthesis is usually the result of disc degeneration and is common at the levels of L3-4 or L4-5. There is no lysis. The disorder mainly involves middle-aged men with a history of several years of discogenic back pain.

Clinical Findings

- The patient complains of back pain. In many cases the patient also experiences pain in one leg, usually in the L3, L4, or L5 dermatome. (Porter[26] reports that 42% of patients have leg pain with involvement of one dermatome.)

- Extension of the lumbar spine is painful with a severe limitation of motion and is sometimes even impossible to perform. Baastrup's syndrome can occur at the same time. In this instance, the patient also complains about local central pain during extension (Figure 4–42). Often one rotation is also painful. Segmental rotation, performed in the prone position, can cause severe local and/or radiating pain ("doorbell sign"[26]).

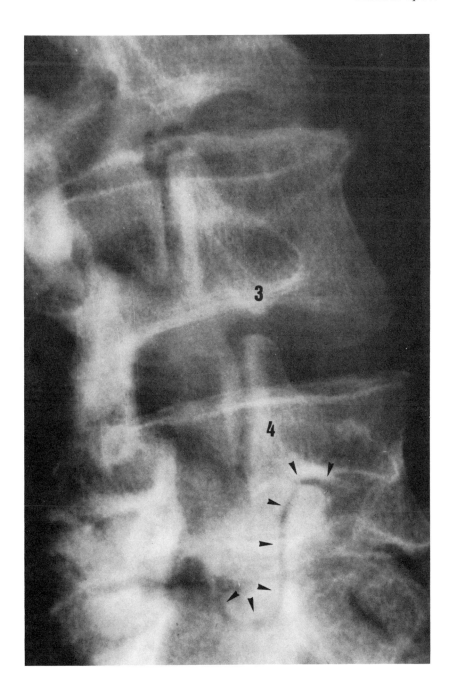

Figure 4–39 Conventional oblique-view X-ray of the lumbar spine. A narrowing of the joint line at L4-5 is visible, along with a reactive sclerosis of the adjacent bone. Because of the "rounder" features of the zygapophyseal joints (S-form), ventral slipping is possible.

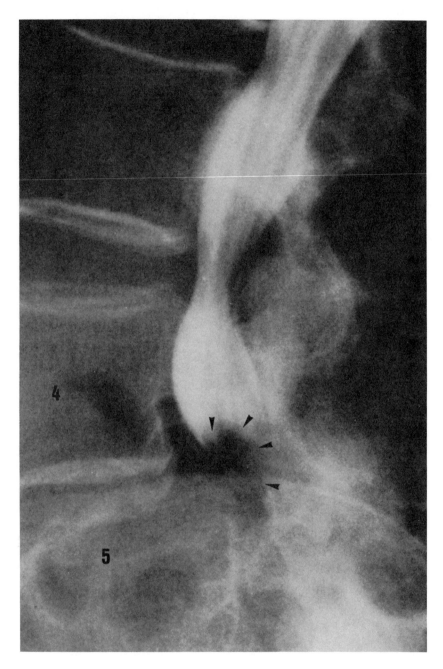

Figure 4–40 Myelogram, lateral view, in a 58-year-old woman with degenerative spondylolisthesis of L4-5. This obvious anterolisthesis causes cauda equina compression (*arrowheads*).

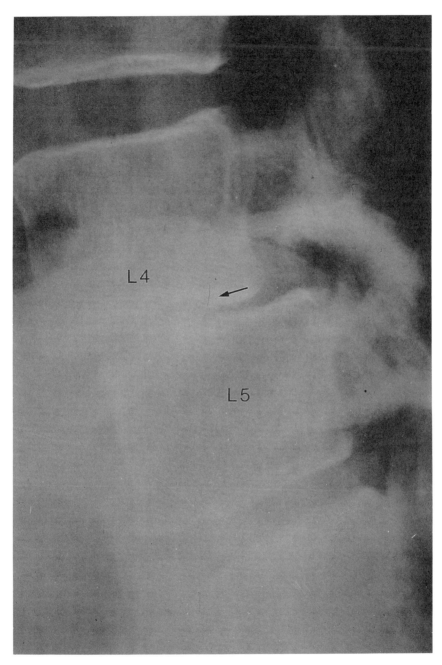

Figure 4–41 Conventional X-ray, lateral view, in a 55-year-old man with spinal claudication based on degenerative spondylolisthesis of L4-5.

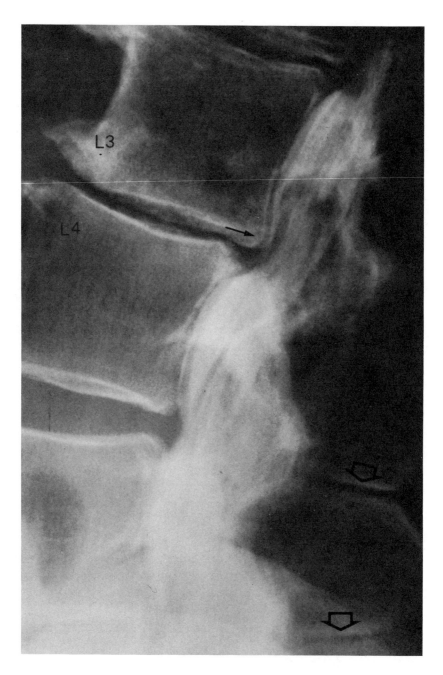

Figure 4–42 Myelogram, lateral view, at the level of L3 to L5 in a 49-year-old man with back pain and L3 radicular pain. In addition, this patient complains of local central pain during lumbar spine extension. Retrolisthesis is evident at L3-4 (*small arrow*). At the same time, Baastrup's syndrome ("kissing spine") can be seen at the level of the spinous processes of L3-4 (not visible here), L4-5, and L5-S1 (*open arrows*). This explains the local pain during extension.

- The X-ray reveals retrolisthesis at the L3-4 or L4-5 segment (Figure 4–43). Often a rotatory subluxation exists at the same level. In some cases, osteophytes are visible on both sides of the disc degeneration at the level of the retrolisthesis.

Treatment

Information about the disorder, instruction concerning posture and body mechanics, and an appropriate exercise program usually enable the patient to manage the problem (see Appendix 4–A). Epidural injections are indi-

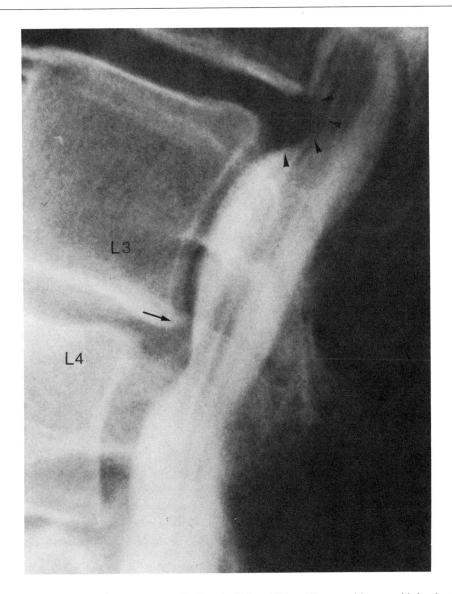

Figure 4–43 Myelogram, lateral view, at the level of L2 to L5 in a 58-year-old man with back pain and L2 and L3 radicular pain. Retrolisthesis L3-4 (*arrow*) is demonstrated along with a disc prolapse at L2-3 (*arrowheads*), a rare combination.

cated in patients with severe root pain. Surgery is seldom indicated.

SPONDYLOLYTIC SPONDYLOLISTHESIS

The term *spondylolisthesis*, the slipping of one vertebra in relation to the underlying vertebra, is derived from the Greek words *spondyl* (vertebra) and *olisthanein* (to slip). Spondylolytic spondylolisthesis is a ventrally subluxed vertebra due to a bilateral spondylolysis, a fracture of the interarticular part of the neural arch.

It is assumed that this disorder has a traumatic etiology; however, some authors still advocate the congenital hypothesis. In support for the "congenital" hypotheses, some children with a (severe) spondylolisthesis have no history of participation in sports and never experienced a relevant trauma (Figures 4–44 and 4–45).

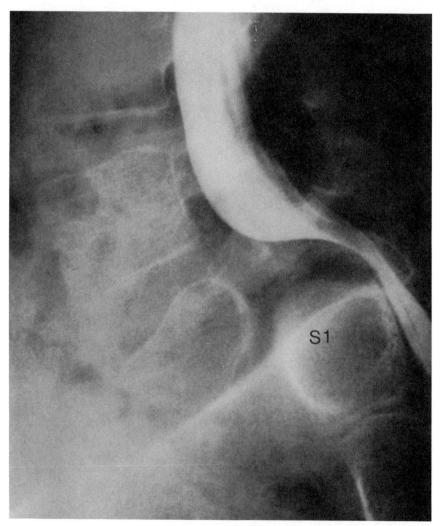

Figure 4–44 Myelogram, lateral view, of a 12-year-old child with a grade 4 (very severe) spondylolytic spondylolisthesis. L5 is situated ventral to S1. S1 has a rounded appearance at its ventrocranial aspect, which is also apparent at the dorsocaudal aspect of L5.

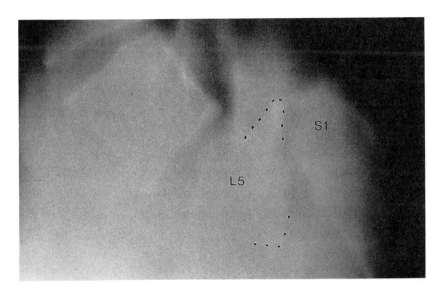

Figure 4–45 Lateral tomogram of a 10-year-old child with a grade 4 spondylolytic spondylolisthesis. L5 lies in front of S1. L5 is totally misformed at its dorsal aspect (the dorsal and ventral borders of the L5 vertebra are partially highlighted by black dots).

Whether or not the lysis of the interarticular element (pars interarticularis = isthmus = component of the neural arch at the junction of the two articular processes), with or without a listhesis, plays any role in the symptoms is still heatedly debated. This disorder occurs fairly often, is often asymptomatic, and is seen more frequently in men than in women (ratio of 3:1).

In gymnasts and ballet dancers, as well as in athletes who perform frequent flexion and extension movements (eg, javelin throwers), the incidence of this disorder is 5% to 21%,[45,46] often without any symptoms.

Lysis of the interarticular element is most often seen at L5 (L5-S1) and in the second instance at L4 (L4-5) (Figures 4–46 and 4–47). Rarely does a lysis occur in the more cranial segments. When the lysis is present at the level of L4-5, there is a slightly greater chance for an instability than when the lysis is at the L5-S1 level.

Although this is not always the case, the lysis can cause a ventral subluxation (Figure 4–48). Often a lysis is detected without any listhesis (slipping). If an anterolisthesis occurs, this listhesis can be larger than a 30% slip (compare with Degenerative Spondylolisthesis).

During childhood, the subluxation can progress, but it usually remains stable from adolescence on. Some adolescents with a severe anterolisthesis of L5 develop acute severe symptoms in the back as well as in the legs.

Clinical Findings

- The often-young patient usually already has a long history of back pain, often with radiating pain in both legs (generally the posterior aspect). In a large number of cases, (ex-)athletes are concerned (Figure 4–49). One of four patients is able to recall a relevant traumatic event.

- The pain usually occurs during sports activities, prolonged standing, and prolonged walking (especially strolling). In lying, the symptoms are relieved.

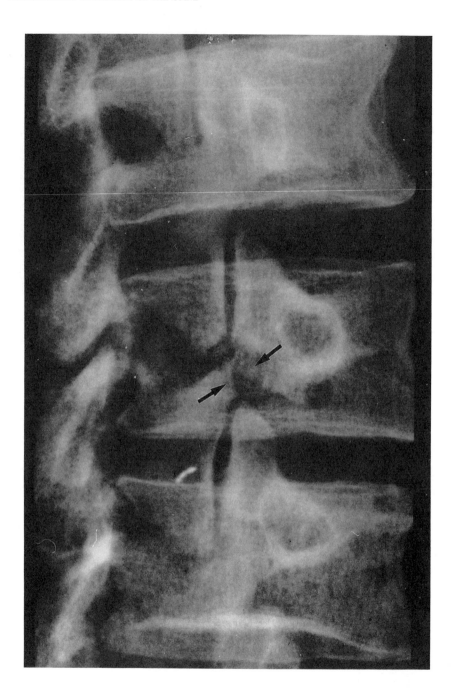

Figure 4–46 Conventional oblique X-ray of the lumbar spine in an adult patient with back pain. A spondylolysis of L4 is shown. The "collar" of the "Scottie dog" is clearly visible (*arrows*).

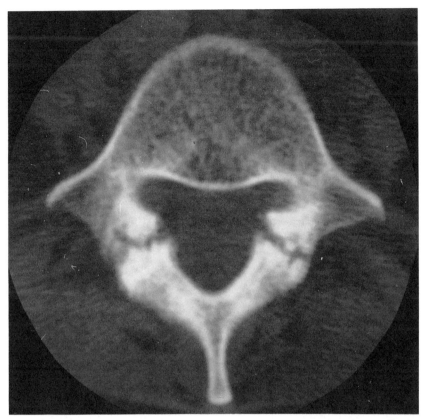

Figure 4–47 CT scan of a bilateral spondylolysis of L4. Bilateral discontinuation of the interarticular part of the vertebra's neural arch is clearly demonstrated.

- Many patients report that they hear or feel a click.
- Approximately 20% of all female patients indicate that the symptoms came on during or after pregnancy.
- On inspection, a deep groove between the long erector spinae muscles is frequently noted, especially in children ("the midline hollow").
- Flexion of the lumbar spine is remarkably good; the patient is often able to place the hands flat on the floor with the legs straight. Extension of the lumbar spine is limited and often painful.

- The SLR test is negative and there are no neurological signs.
- In some cases one can detect an unstable spondylolisthesis by palpation: during palpation between two spinous processes a little "step" is felt. In an unstable spondylolisthesis this step can increase or decrease in bending forward or backward.

The unstable spondylolisthesis may also be palpated as follows: with the patient in sidelying, the examiner positions the tips of the middle three fingers on the three caudal spinous processes. The

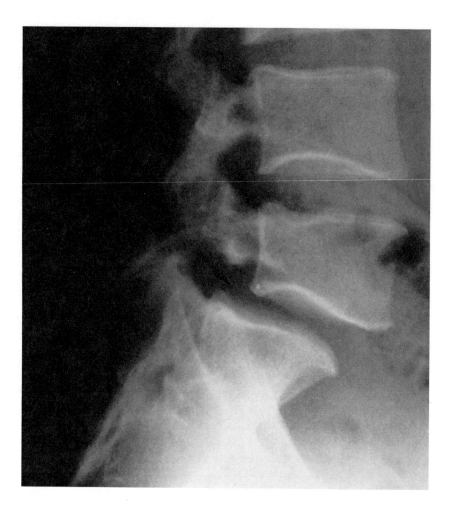

Figure 4–48 Conventional X-ray of the lower lumbar spine in an adult patient with back pain radiating down both legs. The patient has a spondylolytic spondylolisthesis of L5. The ventral slipping of L5 in relation to the sacrum is clearly demonstrated.

patient is then passively rotated. In an intact spine, this results in movement of all of the spinous processes. With an unstable bilateral lysis of L5, the spinous process of L5 does not move with the L4 spinous process during the rotation.

- During local segmental examination, the mobility in dorsoventral translation is increased. (This can be easily assessed in a relaxed patient.)

- In many patients a unilateral or bilateral shortening of the psoas muscle is observed.

- Despite the fact that the disc cranial of the vertebra with the lysis is often degenerated (indicated on X-ray), it is rare to find classic disc symptoms in patients with spondylolytic spondylolisthesis. The X-ray shows the lysis most clearly in the oblique view. The Scottie dog, which

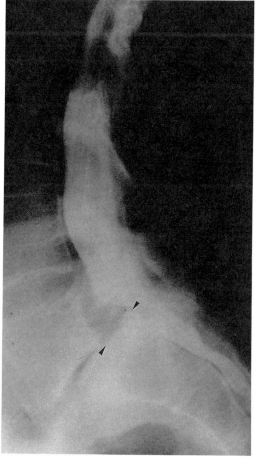

A

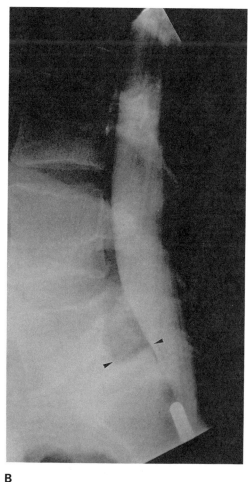

B

Figure 4–49 Myelogram, lateral view, of a 24-year-old man with back pain and pain in both legs during sports activities. There is a grade 3 (approximately 40% ventral subluxation) spondylolytic spondylolisthesis. **A**, View in flexion; **B**, view in extension. During flexion and extension, L5 does not shift in relation to the sacrum. The findings of the clinical examination were hereby confirmed.

is clearly visible in this view, wears a collar (Figure 4–46).

- As a complication, a nerve root compression syndrome can develop. Neurogenic claudication is a rare complication.

Treatment

Reassuring the patient with a thorough explanation regarding the disorder is very important. Every form of traumatic sports activity (contact sports and sports requiring explosive movements of the spine) should be avoided. Young women should be aware that abdominal exercises before and during pregnancy are of great importance, because otherwise the chance for an instability is considerable. Patients must try to avoid becoming overweight. Carrying heavy loads must be avoided.

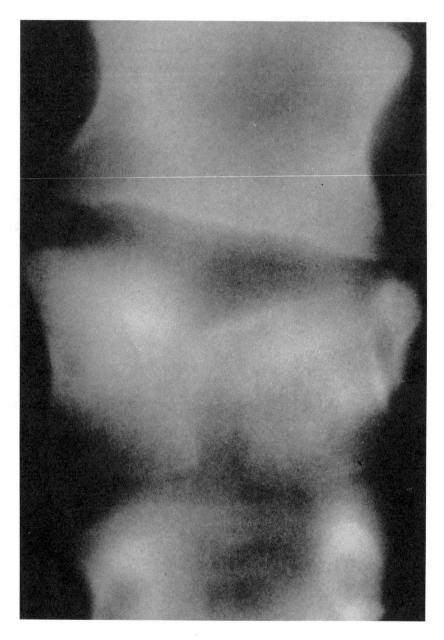

Figure 4–50 Tomogram at the level of L1 to L3 in a patient who sustained a severe flexion trauma. There is an unstable burst fracture of L2.

Instruction in proper posture and ergonomics, as well as strengthening exercises for the abdominal muscles and (careful) stretching of the iliopsoas, is indicated. In some resistant cases, an epidural anesthesia is a further treatment possibility. Generally the prognosis is good. In only a very small number of instances is surgical stabilization indicated.

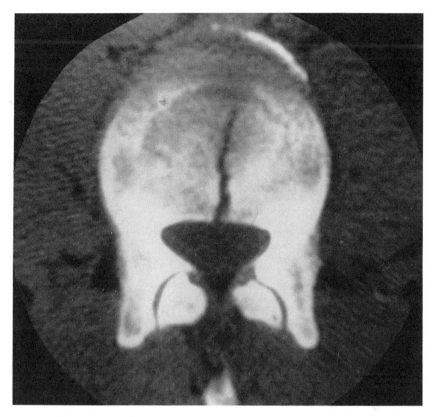

Figure 4–51 CT scan at the level of L3 in a patient who was injured in a severe traffic accident. There is a splitting fracture of the L3 vertebral body.

Differential Diagnosis

A traumatic spondylolisthesis (an acute fracture) or a spondylolisthesis due to bone pathology (tumor) are two disorders that should be considered in the differential diagnosis.

FRACTURES

Traumatic Compression Fractures

Traumatic compression fractures of thoracic or lumbar vertebral bodies are almost always the result of a vertical compressive force. Usually it involves either a fall from a great height or a large weight that falls upon the shoulders or upper back (Figures 4–50 to 4–54). In recent years, an increase in vertebral body fractures has been observed, especially in the various winter sports.

T12, L1, and L2 are the most frequently fractured vertebral bodies. Fractures above or below these levels are rare.[47] The traumatic compression fracture of the vertebral body is not related to age. Sometimes two or more vertebral bodies, not necessarily adjacent to each other, are fractured. In these instances (severe) disc damage can also occur. Although frequently undiagnosed, persisting symptoms in the low back can be an indication of accompanying disc problems.[26]

Clinical Findings

- The acute complaints are not related to the severity of the compression fracture;

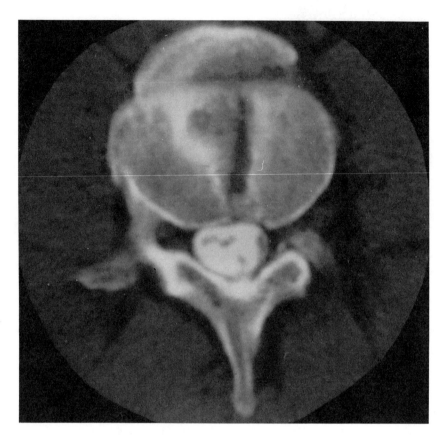

Figure 4–52 Myelo-CT scan at the L4 level in a patient who experienced a compression trauma of the spinal column. There is a burst fracture of the L4 vertebral body.

in other words, very severe fractures can cause relatively few symptoms, and vice versa. Most patients complain of severe pain in the back at the level of the fracture. The pain is often exacerbated by bleeding in the retroperitoneum and mediastinum.

- There is local tenderness to palpation, percussion pain, and pain when falling onto the heels from a tiptoe position. Some patients with acute symptoms experience tenderness to palpation at a level other than the level where the compression fracture (according to the radiological examination) is localized. In such cases the fracture is a "fossil" of an earlier sustained trauma.[26]

- All positions and motions are painful in the acute stage. The X-ray indicates the fracture; the CT scan shows the severity of the fracture.

Treatment

Initially the best treatment consists of bed rest, until the complaints have diminished to the degree where self-mobilization is possible. This can vary from days to weeks. The patient is encouraged to swim and walk during the recovery period. The prognosis is usually good, and most patients are eventually rid of their symptoms. In some cases the symptoms persist, but they are intermittent and not severe.

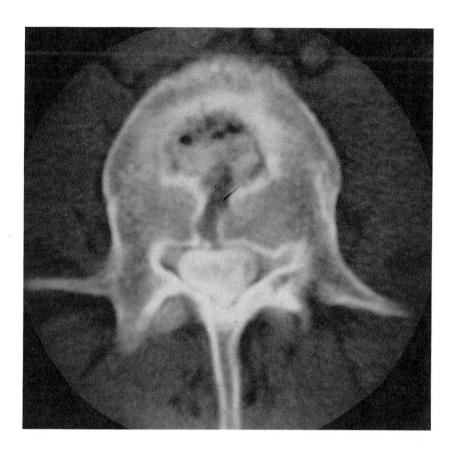

Figure 4–53 Myelo-CT scan at the level of L4 in a patient who sustained a flexion trauma of the spinal column. There is a burst fracture of the L4 vertebral body. The dark spots in the vertebral body are caused by the vacuum phenomenon within the disc. Because of the compression, the disc penetrated through the end-plate and burst in the vertebral body.

Spontaneous Compression Fractures

Nordin et al[48] indicate that approximately 2.5% of all women over the age of 60 and 7.5% of all women over the age of 80 develop one or more spontaneous compression fractures of the thoracolumbar spinal column. The disorder seldom occurs in men.

Osteoporosis is the most frequent cause of a spontaneous compression fracture. Age, gender, and especially menopause are important factors in the development of osteoporosis. Other possible causes include a long period of immobilization, the use of corticosteroids, hyperparathyroidism, Cushing's syndrome, hypogonadism, and reticuloen-dothelial disorders. Therefore, these disorders must be ruled out as a possible cause before one can assume that the compression fracture is the result of an age-related osteoporosis. Also, osteomalacia, which can occur in combination with osteoporosis, should be excluded. For further information, see Chapter 5, Thoracic Spine, section 5.3, Pathology.

Clinical Findings

- One or more vertebral bodies can either gradually or suddenly collapse. The acute fracture causes severe back pain that may persist for several weeks.

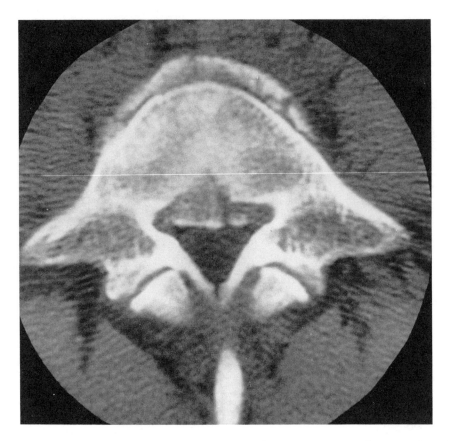

Figure 4–54 CT scan at the L5 level in a patient who fell from a great height. There is a burst fracture of the L5 vertebral body with displacement of the posterior wall, resulting in severe compression of the cauda equina.

In most patients, however, the fractures occur very gradually, resulting in chronic back pain. Eventually an obvious thoracolumbar hyperkyphosis develops.

- Many patients complain about symptoms that are the result of an increased compensatory cervical and/or lower lumbar lordosis. The symptoms resulting from the lower lumbar lordosis are usually due to compression between the spinous processes of the three caudal lumbar vertebrae (see Baastrup's Syndrome [Kissing Spine]).

- Due to the decrease in height, a possible complication occurs: the lower ribs rub against the iliac crest ("costoiliac impingement syndrome"). In this compression syndrome, the patient also experiences pain at the side or in the back at level of the 12th or 11th rib. The pain can be constant or intermittent.

- Sitting on a low chair, rotation, and sidebending of the trunk, as well as walking, increase the symptoms. There is local tenderness to palpation below the 12th rib, especially in sidebending toward the affected side.

- The radiological examination confirms the diagnosis: the thoracic vertebral bodies have collapsed at their ventral aspect, causing a hyperkyphosis. Be-

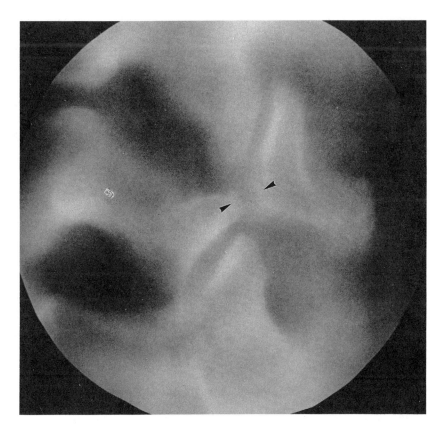

Figure 4–55 Tomogram (oblique view) of L3. Shown is a classic stress fracture (arrowheads) of the interarticular part (isthmus).

cause of the microfractures here, the discs protrude into the adjacent vertebral bodies, resulting in the typical so-called codfish vertebrae. In an earlier stage, the vertebral bodies can give the impression of increased translucency on the X-ray (ghost vertebrae).

Treatment

When there is an acute onset, a few days of bed rest are recommended. However, because inactivity causes an increase in the osteoporosis, the bed rest should be kept to a minimum. Thus, early movement and activation of the patient is encouraged. Activity (exercise therapy) is probably the best way to decrease the demineralization in the

osteoporosis.[26] Corsets are often prescribed; however, they sometimes increase the discomfort. Furthermore, a corset cannot prevent the vertebrae from further collapse.

Mobilization techniques (manual therapy) are contraindicated.

Medication therapy with calcium, vitamin D, fluoride, anabolic steroids, and calcitonin can have a positive influence on demineralization. However, it has not yet been proved that the occurrence of the fractures can be prevented.[49,50]

In the costoiliac impingement syndrome, conservative treatment is ineffective. If the patient has persistent complaints, surgical removal of the 12th and sometimes the 11th rib is indicated.

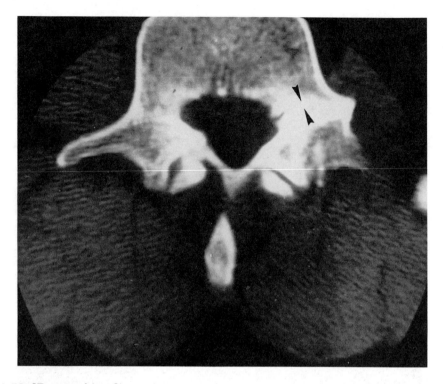

Figure 4–56 CT scan of L4. Shown is a stress fracture (arrowheads) of the left pedicle. There is reactive sclerosis at both sides of the fracture line due to minute shifting occurring during movements of the spine under heavy loads. Plasticity of the bone allows for movement in the pedicle.

"Jogger's Fracture" and Other Stress Fractures

The dorsal halves of the lower lumbar vertebrae are susceptible to stress fractures. They can occur in the interarticular part of the neural arch (Figure 4–55), in the pedicle (Figure 4–56), in the articular process (Figure 4–57), and in the lamina (Figure 4–58). Typically, a sports injury is involved. Stress fractures of the lamina occur particularly in long-distance runners. The other stress fractures are seen more often in ballet dancers and in athletes participating in various throwing sports. Often in these athletes the stress fracture is not well consolidated.

Clinical Findings

- The patient, usually young, complains of chronic low back pain, especially during activity. The pain is localized and is deep and unilateral. In only a few cases there is a vague radiation of symptoms into the gluteal region, sometimes in the form of a mild sciatica. Repeated extension of the lumbar spine is thought to play a role in the mechanism of injury.[51]
- Radiological examination is usually negative; in some cases, a tomogram or CT scan is positive.

Treatment

Besides reassuring the patient and providing adequate information concerning the disorder, no other appropriate treatment is possible. Usually the pain is well tolerated, which allows the patient to continue with the sport. Only in rare cases is it necessary to stop or diminish the sports activities.

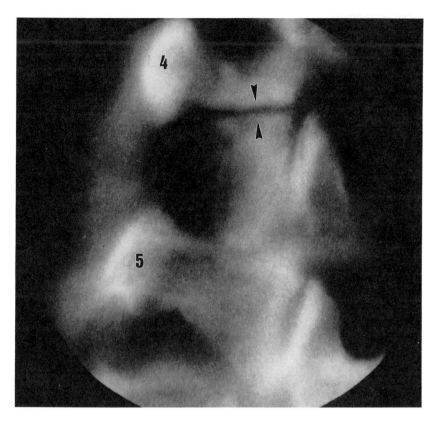

Figure 4–57 Tomogram (oblique view) of L4-5. There is an interruption at the base of the L4 inferior articular process (arrowheads).

BAASTRUP'S SYNDROME (KISSING SPINE)

Baastrup's syndrome concerns the so-called kissing spine, a compression syndrome of the lumbar spinous processes. In almost every case, Baastrup's syndrome is an extra finding caused by other disorders, such as the following:

- spontaneous compression fractures in osteoporosis,
- degenerative changes of mainly the intervertebral disc, causing an approximation of the vertebral bodies
- retrolisthesis
- Paget's disease (osteitis deformans) (This disorder is not described in this book; kissing spine rarely occurs in this disease.)

Some people have congenitally large spinous processes, flattened vertebral bodies, or both. As a result, irritation of the interspinous ligament can occur; in chronic cases a bursa can develop between the spinous processes. In the congenital type it is even possible that joints with capsuloligamentous structures develop.

Generally in athletes, particularly in acrobats, gymnasts, and ballet dancers, an isolated extension trauma of the lumbar spine can cause Baastrup's syndrome.

Clinical Findings

- The patient complains of midline back pain.

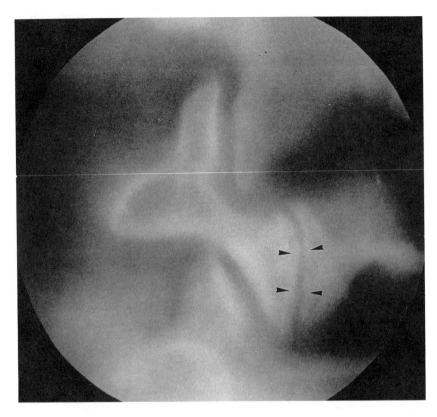

Figure 4–58 Tomogram (oblique view) of L3-4. There is an interruption of the lamina of L4 (arrowheads).

- In the functional examination, extension is usually the most limited and painful motion. Occasionally, sidebending also causes some discomfort. Flexion usually is not painful; however, because of a stretch on the affected structures, slight discomfort may be elicited.

Treatment

Treatment depends on the cause of the complaints. Refer also to the sections discussing spontaneous compression fracture and retrolisthesis (Figure 4–42).

When the complaints are the result of an isolated trauma, an injection with a corticosteroid at the most painful site of the affected spinous process is usually very effective. If the disorder is the result of chronic microtraumas, two to four injections are often required. The injection is given once every 2 weeks. During treatment with the injections, the patient should avoid extension movements of the lumbar spine. In therapy-resistant cases, surgery is sometimes indicated.

COCCYGODYNIA

The term *coccygodynia* indicates that there is pain at the level of the coccyx. The cause can be traumatic, for instance, in a fall on the buttocks causing a ventral and/or lateral subluxation of the coccyx. Coccygodynia can also be caused by referred pain from the lumbar spine, usually as a result of a central disc protrusion of L4-5 or L5-S1.

Clinical Findings

Referred Coccygodynia

- The patient usually complains of pain not only in the coccygeal region but also in the lower lumbar region and often in both gluteal regions.
- Sitting is sometimes painful.
- Coughing, sneezing, and straining sometimes exacerbate the pain.
- The SLR test can be positive.

Local Coccygodynia

- Pain is caused by a sprain of the ligamentous structures between the coccyx and the sacrum and by irritation of the periosteum.
- Sitting, especially with poor posture (slouched in a kyphosis), causes the symptoms. All movements involving contraction of the gluteal musculature can provoke pain, especially walking and climbing upstairs. Some patients hear or feel a click when getting up (or rising) from a sitting position.
- Pressure on the coccyx in a ventral direction is very painful. Lateral movements of the coccyx (performed through the rectum) are also painful.

Treatment

In referred coccygodynia, treatment is primarily aimed at the cause of the complaints. (See Disc Protrusion.)

Local coccygodynia can be treated in several ways. A ventral or lateral subluxation can be repositioned manually (via the rectum), after which the patient is instructed to sit on an inflatable ring and to avoid sitting with a lumbar kyphosis.

In a nonsubluxated coccyx, the ligamentous structures can be injected with a corticosteroid. Usually this injection has to be repeated 2 weeks later. Follow-up is the same as for reposition treatment.

STRAIN/RUPTURE OF THE ERECTOR SPINAE

Strain or rupture of the erector spinae muscles rarely occurs. Typically it is the result of a sports injury, and is seen almost solely in athletes participating in throwing or racket sports, in gymnasts, soccer players, Olympic handball players, and ballet dancers. Generally it is caused by a sudden active change in an already ongoing motion (Figure 4–59). Such maneuvers are performed often by soccer and Olympic handball goalies; the goalie is forced to make an abrupt turn because of a change in the direction of the ball.

Clinical Findings

- The patient complains of local paravertebral pain in the back, usually in the upper lumbar area.
- Deep inspiration is often painful. In the acute stage, the first 2 to 3 days, turning in bed is painful. Walking and sitting do not usually provoke the symptoms.
- All active motions can be painful due to either contraction or stretch. Resisted extension and ipsilateral sidebending are very painful.

Treatment

Friction massage and careful stretching are very helpful forms of treatment. The patient usually has symptoms for 7 to 10 days. During the treatment period, all strenuous sports activities should be discontinued. Generally, running can be continued to maintain the athlete's physical condition.

Differential Diagnosis

Stress fracture of one of the dorsal parts of the vertebrae and an acute disc lesion should be ruled out in these patients.

R   L

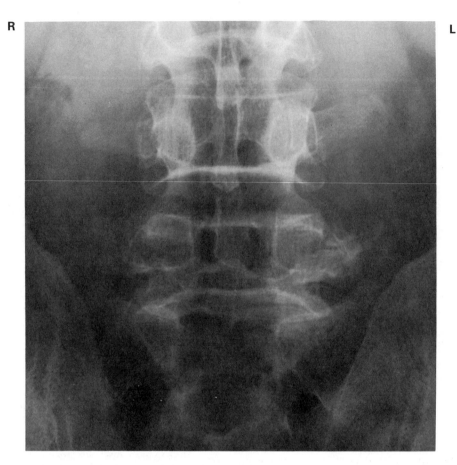

Figure 4–59 Conventional AP view of the lumbosacral junction in a young adult man with an acute onset of back pain as a result of a sudden twist during tennis. Hemisacralization, left, can be seen between the transverse process of L5 and the sacrum. Clinically, a muscle sprain of the erector spinae was determined. The anomaly is not clinically relevant.

SPRAIN OF THE SUPERIOR ILIOLUMBAR LIGAMENT

Sprain of the iliolumbar ligament is similar to the lesion of the erector spinae, a typical sports injury. Usually it is caused by a forced lumbar flexion movement with a simultaneous contralateral sidebending.

Clinical Findings

- The patient complains of local pain that, depending on the severity of the disorder, can also be present at rest.

- In the functional examination, flexion and sidebending away from the painful side elicit the symptoms.

Treatment

This disorder responds quite well (and quickly) to a treatment of transverse friction massage and careful stretching. Usually only three to five treatments are necessary.

DIFFERENTIAL DIAGNOSIS

Not described in this book are many other disorders that can cause back pain, groin pain, buttock pain, or leg pain. In the general practitioners' or physical therapists' clinics, these disorders are seldom encountered. However, they do exist. Therefore, it is extremely important, early on, to differentiate these disorders from the more frequently occurring back problems. Unfortunately, valuable time is too often lost when such disorders are first diagnosed (and thereafter unsuccessfully treated) as a spondylosis or disc syndrome. In many cases the underlying cause is recognized too late. Even with modern examination methods it is often impossible to recognize a malignancy in its early stage. However, the functional examination almost always shows an atypical pattern.

Below are some clinical indications by which malignancies or systemic diseases, in an early stage, can be differentiated from the more frequently occurring disorders (or at least suspected).

During the clinical examination, disorders of the lumbar spine and SI joint almost always show a classic pattern, which is described extensively in this book. The history is of extreme importance: age, onset, and course of the symptoms; postural and movement dependency; and symptomatology. The smallest aberration in the history and functional examination should immediately catch the examiner's attention. "To be able to recognize a sparrow on the street means that one will not confuse the sparrow for a hummingbird" (personal conversation with Dr. P Hirschfeld, orthopaedic physician in Bremen, Germany).

The most often occurring of these rare conditions include the following:

- neoplasm
- lumbar neurinoma
- afebrile osteomyelitis
- aortic occlusion

Particularly in people from the Arabic and African countries, tuberculosis of the spinal column (Pott's disease) should always be considered (Figure 4–60). Post-trauma fractures should be ruled out through a radiological examination.

Neoplasms and Inflammations

Neoplasms in the spinal column are almost always metastases (Figures 4–61 to 4–63). An exception to this last statement is multiple myeloma (Kahler's disease). A remarkable finding is the very high ESR—more than 100 mm within the first hour. Usually, neurological deficits are the most apparent signs, and pain is relatively insignificant. There is almost always an insidious onset of this disorder—in other words, no trauma.

Typical symptoms and signs that should make the examiner suspicious of malignant tumors or inflammations include the following:

- progressively increasing back pain and/or neurological deficits
- symptoms that are often not related to posture or movements
- pain often only at night
- pain radiating into both legs without a clear segmental relation
- hyperlordotic posture of the lumbar spine (in contrast to the discogenic kyphotic lumbar spine)
- (large) symmetrical limitation of sidebending. In younger people, this is usually an indication of spondyodiscitis (Figures 4–64 and 4–65); in older patients, malignancy
- paresis of the psoas muscle, especially bilateral (always an indication of severe pathology)
- pain on percussion
- pain when falling back onto the heels from a tiptoe position

In instances of upper lumbar symptoms or pain in the first or second lumbar dermatome, the clinician should always rule out non-discogenic disorders first.

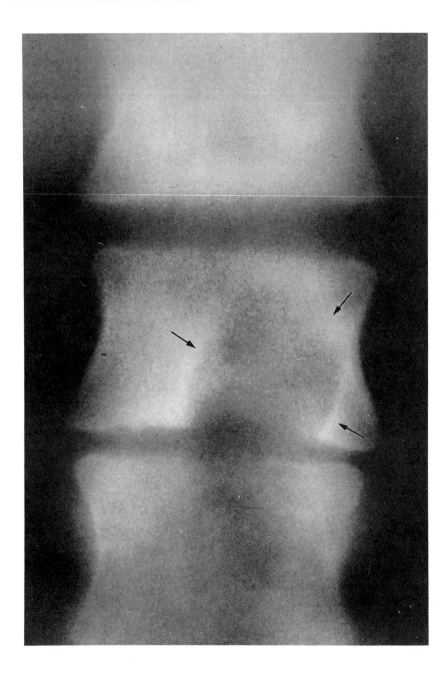

Figure 4–60 Tomogram of the lumbar spine in a patient with low back pain. In an earlier examination the cause could not be determined. A radiolucent zone (arrows) is visible on the tomogram (an osteolytic zone). After further examination Pott's disease (tuberculosis of the spine) was diagnosed.

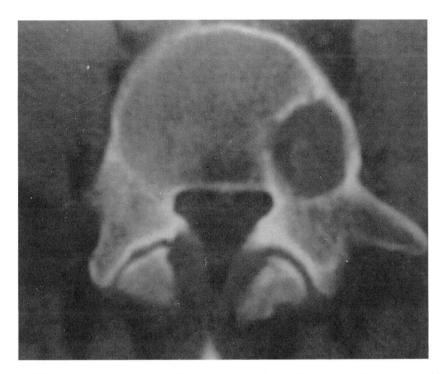

Figure 4–61 CT scan at the level of the L5 vertebral body in a patient with initially obscure back pain. The osteolytic zone (dark spot) is a metastasis from an unknown primary tumor.

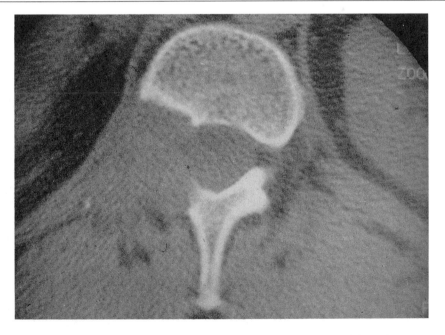

Figure 4–62 CT scan at the level of the L3 vertebral body in a patient with an L2 root syndrome initially, which rapidly progressed into a severe cauda syndrome. The vertebral body, the right neural arch, and the cauda are severely affected due to the metastasis from a kidney tumor.

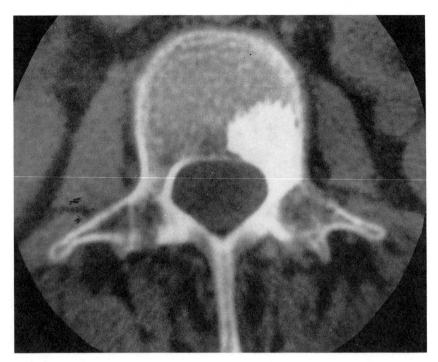

Figure 4–63 CT scan at the level of the L4 vertebral body in a 36-year-old patient with initially obscure low back pain. A benign osteoma (white zone) is present within the vertebral body.

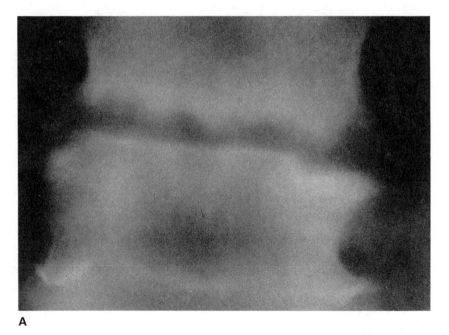

A

Figure 4–64 Tomogram at the L4-5 level in a 26-year-old patient with severe back pain and a large limitation of motion in a capsular pattern (sidebending is especially limited). **A**, AP view.

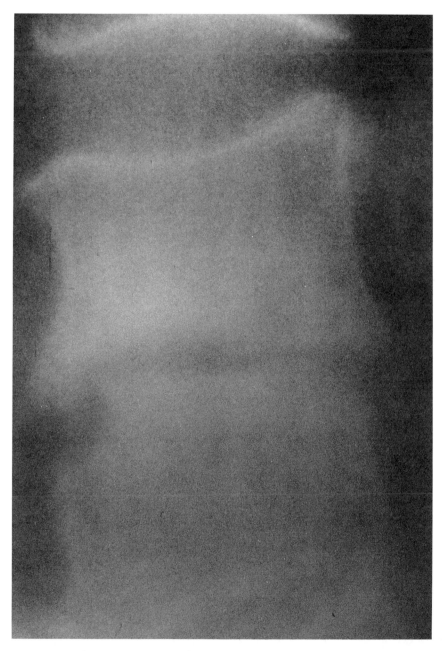

B

Figure 4–64 *B*, Lateral view. Classic findings of a spondylodiscitis are evident: The disc is severely narrowed, the end-plates are irregular, and there are zones of increased density within the vertebral body (in this case particularly of L4).

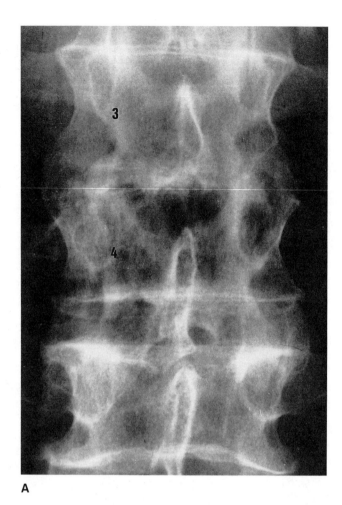

A

Figure 4–65 Conventional X-rays of a patient status postspondylodiscitis of L3-4. **A**, AP view.

Neurinoma

Neurinomas occur at a higher incidence in the cervical and thoracic regions than in the lumbar region. Usually they are frequently seen in patients with neurofibromatosis (von Recklinghausen's disease) (Figures 4–66 and 4–67). In principle, one should keep in mind that this disorder concerns severe pathology until the opposite is proved.

Afebrile Osteomyelitis

Initially, afebrile osteomyelitis has the same appearance as a disc syndrome of gradual onset. Within a week, however, severe limitations of motion develop, along with severe pain. It is significant to note that there is a total absence of dural signs. Coughing, sneezing, and straining do not cause pain. Usually the ESR amounts to 40 to 60 mm within the first hour.

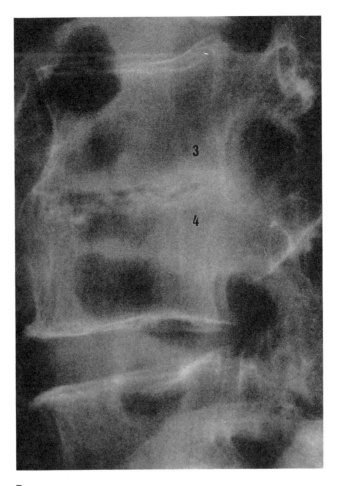

B

Figure 4–65 *B*, Lateral view. Due to destruction of the disc there is an almost complete fusion. The patient has no complaints.

Aortic Occlusion

Back pain due to an occlusion of the aorta is almost always localized in the upper lumbar spine. Discogenic disorders rarely occur in this area. In this disorder, claudication-like symptoms are experienced; the patient is forced to stop when the symptoms arise during activities.

For a quick overview of the common pathologies of the lumbar spine, refer to Appendix B, Algorithms for the Diagnosis and Treatment of Lumbar Spine Pathology.

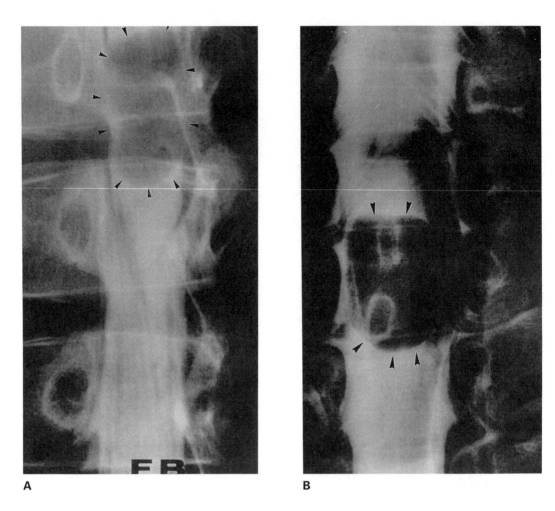

A   **B**

Figure 4–66 Myelogram of a 31-year-old patient with von Recklinghausen's disease (neuro-fibromatosis) and severe lumbar and cervical neurological deficits. **A**, Lumbar spine, AP view. A large neurinoma is visible as a zone of decreased density within the contrast medium (*arrowheads*). **B**, Cervical spine, AP view. A large neurinoma is visible as a zone of decreased density within the contrast medium (*arrowheads*).

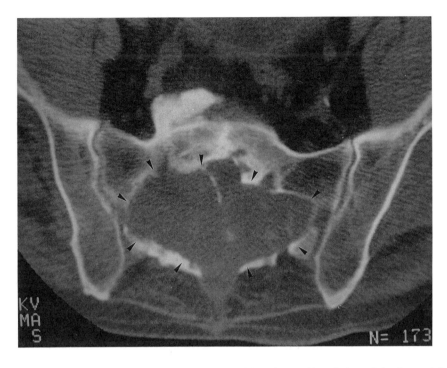

Figure 4–67 CT scan at the level of S2 in a 38-year-old patient with a "sign of the buttock" (severe pain in the gluteal region, strongly limited SLR, and a painful and severely limited hip flexion). Neurofibromatosis was diagnosed. The patient had significant destruction of the sacrum by a neurinoma arising from different sacral roots (arrowheads).

4.4 TREATMENT

MANUAL TREATMENT TECHNIQUES

Patient Information

After the clinical examination, the patient should be given a thorough explanation about his or her back problem. Specific information on this topic is detailed in Appendix 4–A.

Ergonomics

Instruction in proper posture and body mechanics for such daily activities as sitting, standing, lying, getting up from lying, bending, and lifting is also extremely important. Chapter 12, Prevention of Back and Neck Pain by Improving Posture, and Appendix 4–A, Patient Handbook, discuss these matters in detail.

Mobilization

Mobilization and manipulation of the lumbar spine may be indicated in primary disc-related lesions, which are sometimes accompanied by dural signs (positive SLR test, Bragard test, and/or Neri test). Mobilization should be performed very carefully and only by experienced therapists. Zygapophyseal joint pathology, without involvement of the disc, can be treated manually. Pain-relieving techniques of transverse friction or transverse stretching (with or without movement) are usually performed before the mobilization of the lumbar spine.

The techniques for mobilization and manipulation that we use consist of the following:

- axial separation with rotation
- repositioning technique without axial separation
- segmental rotation techniques with slight axial separation

Rotation techniques with axial separation are most often described in the literature. In patients with acute primary disc-related pathology, these techniques are applied in a particular sequence.

Indications

The best results with mobilization and manipulation are achieved when (apart from flexion and extension) sidebending away from the painful side provokes the symptoms. Cyriax and Russel[52] described a hard versus a soft protrusion. The former case corresponds with an annular protrusion and the latter with a nuclear protrusion or prolapse.

White and Panjabi[9] offer a further theoretical explanation. If the protrusion lies more below the nerve root (comparable to lying in the "axilla"), then sidebending to the opposite side is the most painful motion. By sidebending to the affected side, tension on the nerve root is released. This kind of protrusion responds very well to mobilization or manipulation. On the other hand, if the disc presses on the nerve root more from above (on the so-called shoulder of the root), then sidebending toward the affected side will be the most painful motion. This localization responds best to treatment with traction. Established empirically, these facts can be brought into good accordance with the theories of Cyriax and Russel.[52]

However, mobilization and manipulation should never be the only method of treat-

ment. Before the first treatment is administered, every patient should be given a thorough explanation as to the characteristics of the pathology. In addition, the patient should be instructed in proper posture and body mechanics pertaining to everyday positions and activities. After treatment, it must be determined whether isometric abdominal exercises and/or other exercises are indicated.

In patients with a deviated posture, the technique of repositioning without axial separation is performed.

Local segmental mobilization and manipulations are used in patients in whom the limitation of motion is not due to a primary disc-related problem. There is still no conclusive research as to the effectiveness of these techniques.

The sequence of treatment techniques is dependent upon various factors, including size and weight of the patient as well as of the therapist. Duration and onset of the symptoms along with the findings in the clinical examination also play a determining role.

Contraindications

Contraindications for manual treatment techniques include the following:

- Patients with symptoms from nerve roots S3 to S5 absolutely should not be treated with these techniques.
- In general, all pathology other than primary disc-related pathology or zygapophyseal joint pathology is a contraindication for joint mobilization. The most important exception is the patient with nonspecific low back pain of which the etiology is still unclear. The intervertebral disc almost always plays a role in this "segmental" problem, however. Also, when the patient's complaints are not elicited at any time during the examination (at least at that time), the problem should be interpreted as being

of a nonprimary disc or zygapophyseal origin and is therefore a contraindication for mobilization/manipulation.

- The techniques should not be performed when there is bilateral sciatica from the same segment.
- The techniques should not be performed if there is suspicion of psychosomatic back pain in neurotic patients.
- The techniques should not be performed in children with back pain.
- The techniques should not be performed in the last months of pregnancy.
- Patients taking anticoagulant medications should not undergo this treatment.
- The techniques should not be performed when there is radiologically visible calcification of the abdominal aorta or when there is an aortal prosthesis.
- Treatment should not be given under anesthesia.

Precautions

- Acute disc prolapse
- Onset or increase of radicular pain in sidebending to the affected side
- Pronounced osteoporosis

MANUAL SOFT TISSUE TECHNIQUES

Manual soft tissue techniques have two goals: (1) they work as a strong analgesic and (2) they are a good preparation for every type of manual mobilization for the spine. Some of these techniques can also be applied before performing the segmental functional examination to relax the back musculature and allow for better palpation.

Transverse Friction Massage

Even when no muscle lesion is present, transverse friction is an effective pain-relieving technique that can be used before performing manual mobilization. Usually tenderness in the musculature or ligaments belonging to the pathological segment can be treated.

Transverse Friction Massage of the Interspinous Ligament (Figure 4–68)

Position of the Patient

The patient lies prone with the arms resting at the sides; the head is either in a neutral position or rotated to one side. If necessary, a small pillow can be placed under the abdomen in order to increase the space between the spinous processes.

Position of the Therapist

The therapist stands next to the patient at the level of the lumbar spine.

Performance

First, the most tender spot at the caudal aspect of the affected segment's spinous process is localized. Here transverse friction massage is performed with the index finger reinforced by the middle finger. Pressure is exerted in a cranial direction against the caudal aspect of the spinous process, and the action phase of the transverse friction is toward the therapist. About 5 minutes is required to obtain pain relief.

Transverse Friction Massage at the Insertion of the Deep Rotatory Muscles (Figure 4–69)

Position of the Patient

See previous technique.

Position of the Therapist

The therapist stands next to the patient, opposite the side to be treated, at the level of the pelvis or upper legs.

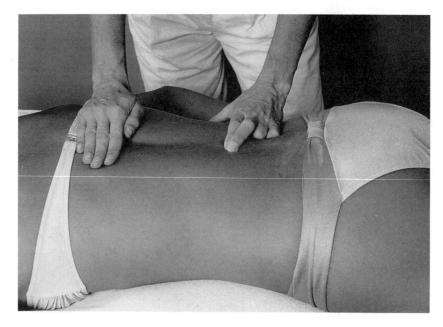

Figure 4–68 Transverse friction massage of the interspinous ligament at the caudal aspect of a spinous process.

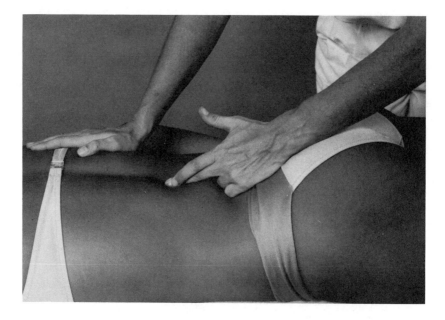

Figure 4–69 Transverse friction massage of the deep rotatory muscles at their insertion on the lateral aspect of the base of the spinous process.

Performance

The therapist places the tip of the middle finger on the tender spot at the lateral aspect of the spinous process. The index finger reinforces the middle finger. During the transverse friction, the action phase consists of a supination of the forearm. The technique is performed for approximately 5 minutes.

Transverse Friction Massage of the Multifidus Muscles (Figure 4–70)

Position of the Patient

The patient lies prone with the arms resting at the sides; the head is either in a neutral position or rotated to one side.

Position of the Therapist

The therapist stands next to the patient, opposite the side to be treated, at the level of the musculature to be treated.

Performance

The multifidus muscles run in an oblique, craniomedial to caudolateral, direction. Both thumbs of the therapist are placed on the muscle parallel to the running of the fibers. The tip of one thumb is placed over the tip of the other thumb and both are kept in line with each other. By simultaneously supinating both forearms and keeping the thumbs in line with each other, the transverse friction massage is performed. The action phase consists of a movement away from the spine, in other words, in a craniolateral direction.

Transverse Friction Massage for the Superior Iliolumbar Ligament (Figure 4–71)

Position of the Patient

The patient lies prone with arms resting at the sides.

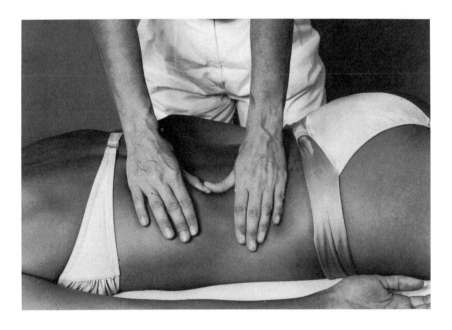

Figure 4–70 Transverse friction massage of the multifidus muscles.

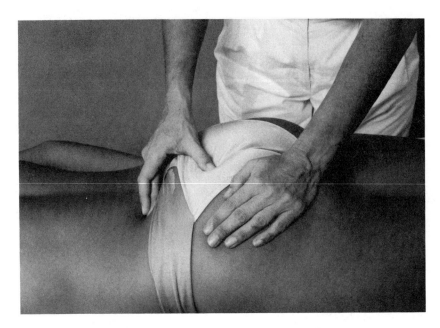

Figure 4–71 Transverse friction massage for the superior iliolumbar ligament.

Position of the Therapist

The therapist stands next to the patient, opposite the side to be treated, at the level of the pelvis.

Performance

On the cranial aspect of the posterior superior iliac spine (PSIS), at the transition of the iliac crest into the PSIS, the most tender spot is located. The transverse friction massage is performed with either the index finger or the middle finger, whereby the nonfrictioning finger reinforces the frictioning finger. It is performed in a lateral to medial direction, in which pressure is exerted lateral of the ligament and then the finger is moved medially over the ligament. The therapist performs this movement by simply extending the wrist. During the relaxation phase of the transverse friction, the therapist's hand with the patient's skin returns to the lateral starting position.

Ten minutes is a sufficient length of time for this treatment. Afterward the patient is instructed in cautious stretching of this ligament in which he or she slowly performs a contralateral sidebend from a slightly forward-flexed position. The stretching exercise should be performed several times daily. Usually, the number of treatments of transverse friction massage varies between two and six times in order to reach the desired results.

Transverse Stretching of the Paravertebral Musculature without Movement of the Lumbar Spine
(Figures 4–72 and 4–73)

Position of the Patient

The patient lies prone with the arms resting at the sides. The head is either in a neutral position or rotated to one side.

Position of the Therapist

The therapist stands next to the patient, opposite the side to be treated, at the level of the musculature to be treated.

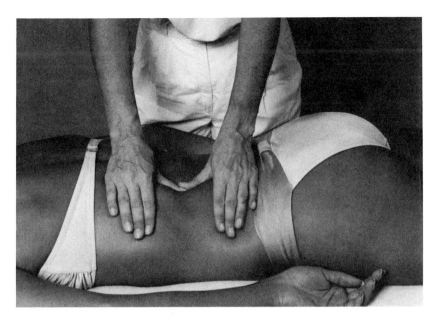

Figure 4–72 Transverse stretch of the paravertebral musculature: starting position (thumbs are in line with each other).

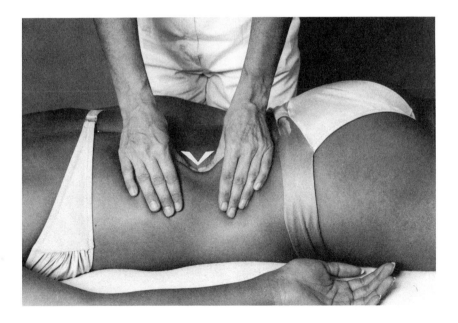

Figure 4–73 Transverse stretch of the paravertebral musculature: end position (thumbs are at an angle to each other).

Performance

The tips of both thumbs are placed end to end and in line with each other at the medial aspect of the paravertebral musculature of the segment to be treated. Both thumbs are now moved laterally against the musculature without sliding over the skin and muscles. By slightly supinating the forearms, a transverse stretch of the local musculature (particularly the iliocostal and longissimus muscles) is performed.

The stretching is performed in a rhythmic manner and within the limitations of pain. Duration of the treatment varies from about 10 seconds to 1 minute.

In the same way the musculature can also be stretched from lateral to medial. In principle, the technique is the same except that now the therapist stands next to the patient on the same side to be treated.

Usually the paravertebral muscles on both sides are treated.

Transverse Stretching of the Paravertebral Musculature with Movement of the Lumbar Spine (Figure 4–74)

Position of the Patient

The patient lies prone with the arms resting at the sides. The head is either in a neutral position or rotated to one side. To emphasize the stretching component of this technique, the patient's pelvis can be positioned closer to the edge of the treatment table (the side at

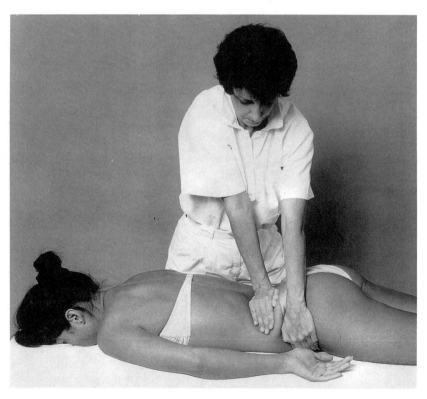

Figure 4–74 Transverse stretching of the lower lumbar paravertebral musculature with coupled sidebending and (contralateral) rotation during extension of the lumbar spine.

which the therapist is standing) in order to bring about a slight sidebending toward the affected side. To emphasize the movement component more as a warming-up technique, the patient lies in a neutral position.

Position of the Therapist

The therapist stands next to the patient opposite of the side to be treated at the level of the convexity of the patient's now slightly sidebent lumbar spine.

Performance

With his or her caudal hand, the therapist grasps the patient's anterior superior iliac spine (ASIS) of the affected side and the other hand is placed at the medial aspect of the musculature to be treated. In so doing, both arms of the therapist are extended.

While the caudal hand moves the pelvis in a dorsal direction, the cranial hand (particularly the hypothenar eminence) pushes the musculature ventrally and laterally. Note that the hand does not slide over the musculature.

This technique is best suited for the lower lumbar segments. In the middle and upper lumbar segments, the thumb of the therapist's cranial hand is used to stretch the musculature.

The technique is performed in a rhythmic manner in which, after each stretch, the patient is brought back to the starting position before further stretching is performed.

Transverse Stretching of the Paravertebral Musculature with Simultaneous Sidebending
(Figure 4–75)

Position of the Patient

The patient lies in a stable position on the side, near the edge of the treatment table. The head is supported by a pillow.

Position of the Therapist

The therapist stands in front of the patient at the level of the patient's lumbar spine.

Performance

The therapist places the fingertips of both hands at the level of the affected segment just medial to the paravertebral musculature of the side closest to the therapist. The therapist's forearms lie against the patient's thorax and pelvis.

With the fingertips, the musculature is now pulled laterally. At the same time, the therapist moves the patient's thorax cranially and the pelvis caudally with the forearms. In so doing, a stretching of the musculature and a sidebending of the lumbar spine occur simultaneously.

In order to increase the sidebending component of this technique, the patient's top leg can be placed in adduction.

The technique is performed in a rhythmic manner in which, after each stretch, the patient is brought back to the starting position before further stretching is performed.

Transverse Stretching of the Paravertebral Musculature with Coupled Sidebending and Contralateral Rotation during Extension of the Lumbar Spine
(Figure 4–76)

Position of the Patient

The patient lies in a stable position on the side, with the head supported on a pillow. To emphasize the stretching component of this technique, a pillow is placed at the patient's waist to bring in a slight sidebend in the direction of the table. To emphasize the movement component more in warming up, a small pillow is used at the waist only if necessary to maintain the lumbar spine in a neutral position.

Position of the Therapist

The therapist stands in front of the patient at the level of the lumbar spine.

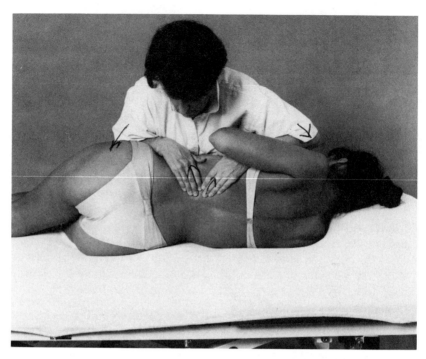

Figure 4–75 Transverse stretching of the paravertebral musculature with simultaneous sidebending.

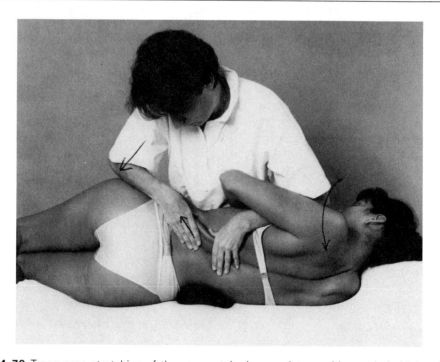

Figure 4–76 Transverse stretching of the paravertebral musculature with coupled sidebending and contralateral rotation during extension of the lumbar spine.

Flex RSB (R) Rot

Performance

The therapist places the fingertips of the caudal hand at the medial aspect of the paravertebral musculature. At the same time, the forearm lies against the dorsolateral aspect of the pelvis.

The thumb of the other hand is placed on the lateral aspect of the paravertebral musculature cranial to the caudal hand's fingertips. The forearm of the cranial hand lies against the ventrolateral aspect of the thorax.

In order to bring about a transversely running torsion in the musculature, the fingers of the caudal hand and the thumb of the cranial hand are moved in opposite directions. Simultaneously, the cranial forearm pushes the patient's thorax in a dorsal and cranial direction while the caudal forearm pulls the pelvis in a ventral and caudal direction.

The technique is performed rhythmically, whereby, after each stretch, the patient is returned to the neutral position before repeating the procedure. By moving both hands caudally or cranially and continuing with the same maneuver, neighboring segments can also be treated.

SEGMENT-SPECIFIC PAIN RELIEF TECHNIQUES

Besides the techniques for soft tissue, there are also segment-specific techniques for pain relief. They consist of rhythmic movements called oscillations and vibrations that are performed within the limits of the translatory range of motion.

Segmental Vibration and Oscillation (Ventral) (Figures 4–77A,B)

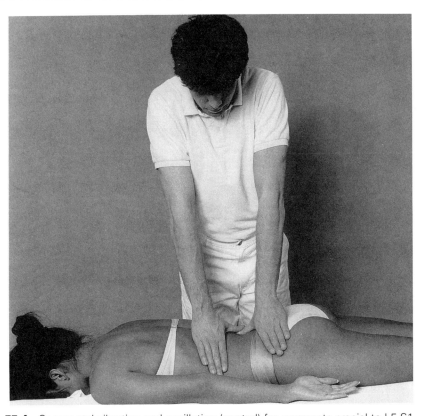

Figure 4–77 A, Segmental vibration and oscillation (ventral) for segments cranial to L5-S1.

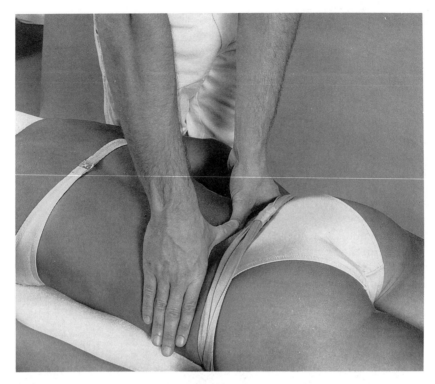

Figure 4–77 B, Segmental vibration and oscillation (ventral) for the L5-S1 segment.

Position of the Patient

The patient lies prone with the arms resting at the sides. The head is either in a neutral position or rotated to one side. The table is brought to a height of about midthigh to the therapist.

Position of the Therapist

The therapist stands next to the patient at the level of the lumbar spine.

Performance

The therapist places the tip of one thumb, reinforced by the other thumb, on the dorsal aspect of the affected segment's spinous process. The remaining fingers of both hands rest gently on the patient's back. Both arms are extended and positioned perpendicular to the local curvature of the spine.

Vibration is now performed locally in a ventral direction during which transitions can be made into oscillations, and the therapist can alternate between the two. Gradually the therapist can change from an oscillation into a cautious mobilization. This treatment should last for several minutes.

Because the spinous process of L5 is generally very small, when performing oscillations or vibrations with the L5 spinous process, the therapist places the thumbs in such a way to allow both hands to rest at either side of the trunk. In this instance, the therapist stands facing the foot of the table.

Segmental Vibrations and Oscillations (Caudal) (Figure 4–78)

Position of the Patient

The patient lies in a stable position on the side, as close as possible to the edge of the table. Pillows support the head and, if neces-

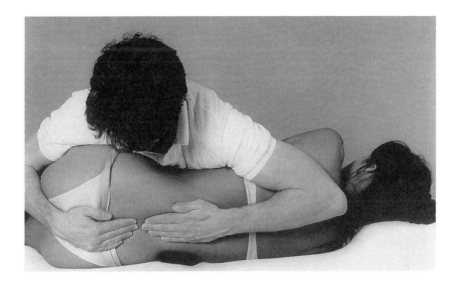

Figure 4–78 Segmental vibrations and oscillations (caudal).

sary, the waist in order to support the spine in a neutral position.

Position of the Therapist

The therapist stands in front of the patient at the level of the segment to be treated. The table is brought to a height of the therapist's iliac crests.

Performance

The caudal hand's middle finger is placed on the cranial aspect of the affected segment's caudal spinous process. The middle finger of the other hand is placed at the caudal aspect of the same segment's cranial spinous process. To ensure that the skin does not restrict caudal movement, the skin is pushed together between the tips of each middle finger. Both hands lie flat against the back, while the forearms have as much contact as possible with the patient's body.

The therapist then places the ventrolateral aspect of his or her trunk against the patient's pelvis and anterior aspect of the upper legs. By firmly grasping the patient's pelvis and upper legs between the forearm and trunk, the therapist and patient move as one unit.

Now by moving the trunk sideways, the therapist's forearm and the patient's pelvis are brought in a caudal direction. At the same time, the cranial hand and forearm stabilize.This slight movement is performed in oscillations.

GENERAL MANUAL MOBILIZATION FOR THE LUMBAR SPINE

Axial Separation in Extension
(Figures 4–79A–F)

Position of the Patient

The patient is in sidelying with the affected side up. The top leg is in approximately 45° of hip flexion with the forefoot hooked behind the bottom leg. The head can be rotated as far as is comfortably possible in the direction of the trunk rotation. If the position of the patient is correct, the therapist should be able to visualize a straight line from the heel to the head whereby the physiological curves in the spine are preserved.

The patient's top arm is placed in a relaxed position with the forearm resting against the

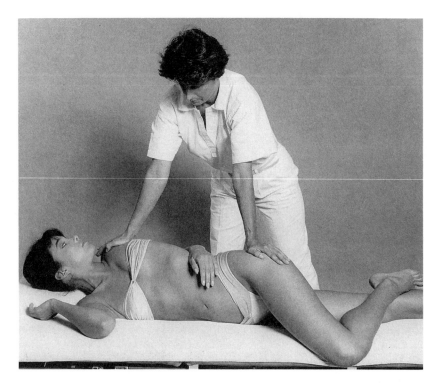

Figure 4–79 A, Starting position.

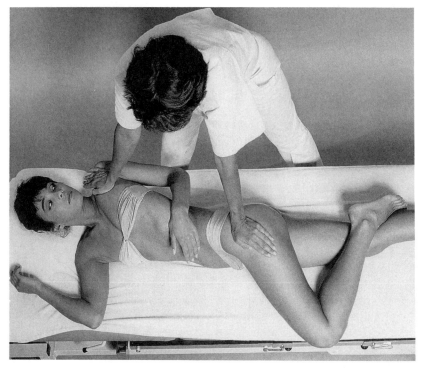

Figure 4–79 B, View from above.

side. The bottom arm also lies in a relaxed position, in front of the patient.

The treatment table is positioned as low as possible.

Position of the Therapist

The therapist stands behind the patient at the level of the lumbar spine, with the thenar and hypothenar eminences of the caudal hand placed directly proximal of the greater trochanter. The fingers point in an anterior and distal direction while the long axis of the hand makes a 30° angle to an imaginary line through the patient's body.

The cranial hand rests against the pectoralis major of the top shoulder, and the fingers

point posteriorly and superiorly; this hand also makes an angle of approximately 30° to the patient.

Performance

The therapist now leans over, bringing the shoulders perpendicular above the 30° diagonal formed by the hands. In so doing, the patient's entire spine is brought into extension. At the same time a slight sidebend toward the table and a contralateral rotation occur. In this way the lumbar spine remains in its normal physiological lordosis. The patient is instructed to continue breathing in a relaxed manner.

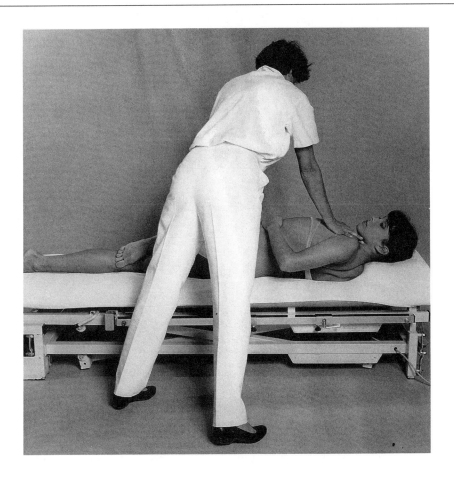

Figure 4–79 C, View from behind.

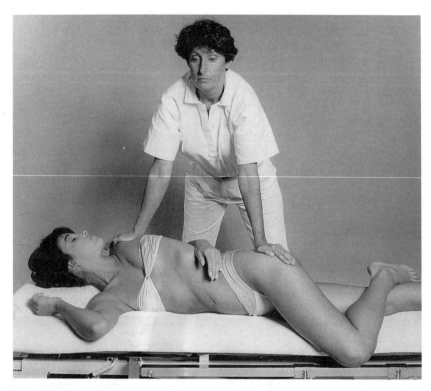

Figure 4–79 D, Optimal pre-tension directly before the end of the patient's exhalation.

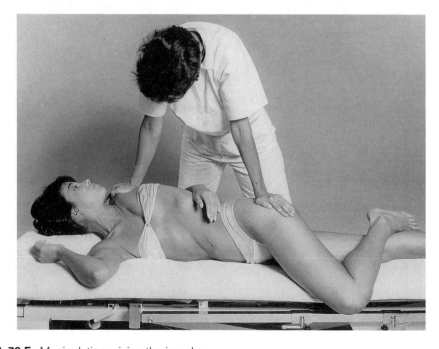

Figure 4–79 E, Manipulation: giving the impulse.

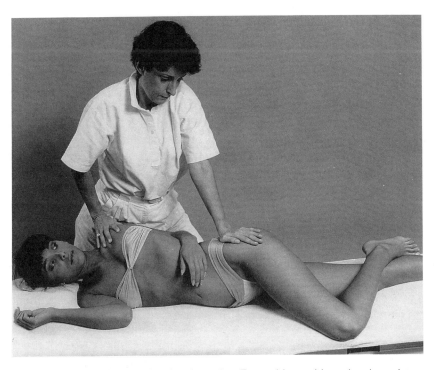

Figure 4–79 F, Alternative position for the therapist. From this position, the therapist exerts force exclusively through the caudal hand.

Depending on the pathology, the therapist has several possible ways of performing this technique. If a "hard protrusion"[52] is not confirmed, better results are usually achieved with a continuous axial separation than with a manipulative axial separation. If the symptoms are of an acute onset, a manipulation is preferred. In cases of doubt, the therapist can perform a combination of both.

Manipulative axial separation is performed as follows: As the patient exhales, the therapist extends his or her thorax whereby the head and trunk are in the same plane. Directly after the end of the patient's exhalation, the therapist gives a manipulative impulse through a short, quick nod of the head. This impulse causes both of the therapist's hands to move away from each other. In this way, the two most caudal segments of the patient's lumbar spine are the most influenced.

If the SLR test was positive before the treatment, then after the manipulation it is checked again. When improvement is noted, the manipulation is repeated. The technique can be performed up to three times in a row.

If the SLR test was negative before the treatment, the patient is again examined in standing. In so doing, it is imperative that the patient move correctly from lying to sitting and then to standing. Both knees are pulled up and, while tightening the abdominal muscles, the lower legs are brought over the edge of the table. Then, using both hands, the patient pushes himself or herself up into a sitting position. Further manipulations can be performed if the tests in standing indicate an improvement. Lying down is performed in the reverse sequence.

The main force of the manipulation is given through the caudal hand. In order to increase the caudal influence, the therapist can stand at the level of the patient's head. Now the cranial hand stabilizes only, while the entire force is administered through the caudal hand.

Axial Separation in Extension with Rotation (Figures 4–80A, B)

This technique can be used when axial separation in extension offers no further improvement.

Position of the Patient

The patient lies in the same position as described under Axial Separation in Extension. The treatment table is positioned as low as possible.

Position of the Therapist

The therapist stands behind the patient. The base of the caudal hand lies directly behind the major trochanter with the fingers pointing forward. The other hand rests on the pectoralis major of the same shoulder with the fingers pointing in a cranial direction.

Performance

The therapist shifts his or her body weight so far forward that the shoulders lie over an imaginary line between the two hands. While the patient breathes in a relaxed manner, the therapist exerts substantial axial separation. The patient is then instructed to take a deep breath whereby the separation is maintained. During exhalation, the therapist extends the spine, lifting the head, and shifts weight to the caudal hand. Directly before the end of the patient's exhalation, the therapist performs a manipulation by a quick nod of the head and further shifting of the body weight. In every manipulation technique, the pre-tension phase is critical. The trunk rotation, performed after pre-tension, should be of minimal amplitude and maximal velocity.

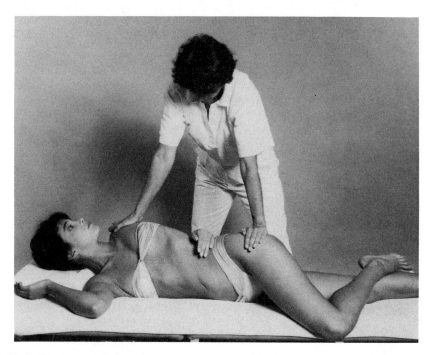

Figure 4–80 A, Starting position.

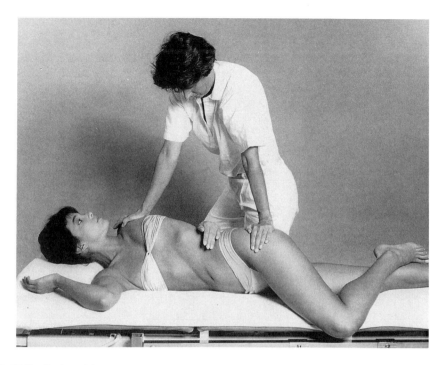

Figure 4–80 B, End position.

After the manipulation the therapist proceeds as described under Axial Separation in Extension.

Axial Separation in Flexion (Figures 4–81A–C)

This mobilization technique can be used when the previously described techniques offer no further improvement or are impossible to apply because of pain. As with the previous techniques, this technique can be applied with emphasis on axial separation, with emphasis on rotation, or with a combination of the two.

Position of the Patient

The patient lies on the side with the affected side up. The bottom arm lies in a relaxed position behind the back and the other arm lies on the table at the level of the head. The bottom hip is flexed at least 45° and the top leg is extended.

If the patient is positioned correctly, a straight line can be visualized from the heel of the patient's top leg to the head.

The treatment table is brought to a height of the therapist's knees.

Position of the Therapist

The therapist stands behind the patient and places the caudal hand on the ventral aspect of the patient's ASIS. The cranial hand rests against the patient's thorax at the midthoracic level.

Performance

Depending on the position of the caudal elbow, the therapist can determine the amount of rotation. If the therapist's elbow faces more in the direction of the patient's head, the axial separation is emphasized. If the elbow faces more in a ventral direction, more rotation occurs.

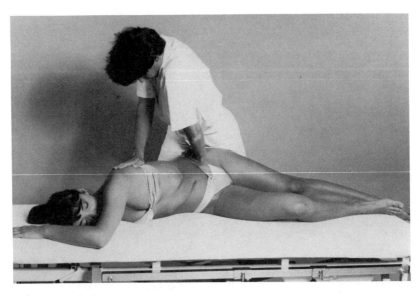

Figure 4–81 A, Axial separation in flexion.

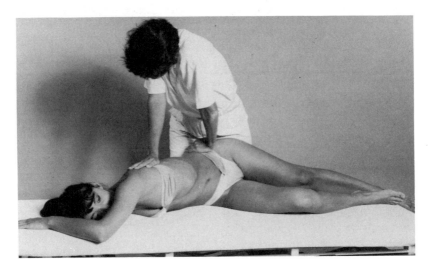

Figure 4–81 B, Axial separation in flexion: emphasis on the rotation.

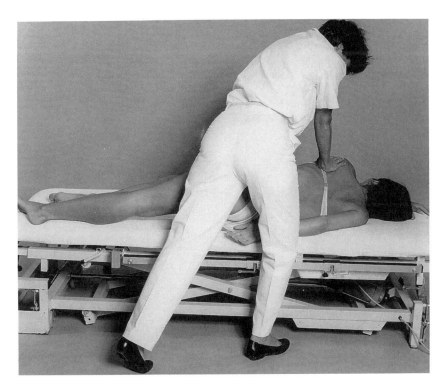

Figure 4–81 C, Axial separation in flexion: view from behind.

The pre-tension is taken up during the patient's exhalation; the manipulation is performed immediately after the end of the exhalation.

As with the other techniques, the therapist applies pre-tension not through the patient alone but also by extending his or her own spine. Again the manipulation is performed through an abrupt nod of the head.

Following each mobilization/manipulation technique, a quick assessment should be performed before deciding to continue with the treatment.

Long Lever Axial Separation in Extension with Rotation
(Figures 4–82A–D)

This technique is most indicated in instances when the therapist is significantly smaller than the patient. It can also be used when axial separation in extension offers no further improvement.

Position of the Patient

The patient lies supine with the legs straight, the head supported on a pillow, and the arms relaxed either alongside the body or under the head.

The table is positioned at the level of the therapist's knees.

Position of the Therapist

The therapist stands next to the patient on the nonaffected side.

Performance

With both hands, the therapist grasps the patient's knee (on the affected side) and brings the hip into 90° flexion, allowing the knee to flex also. From this position, the leg is pulled upward (toward the ceiling) until rota-

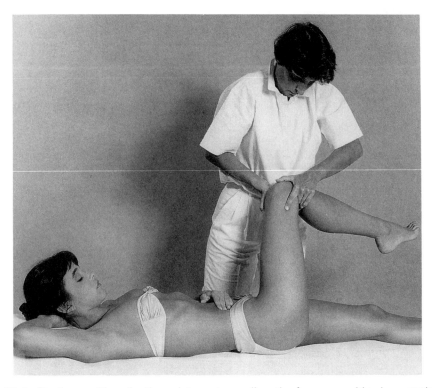

Figure 4–82 A, Starting position: the therapist exerts a pull on the femur, resulting in a rotation in the lumbar spine.

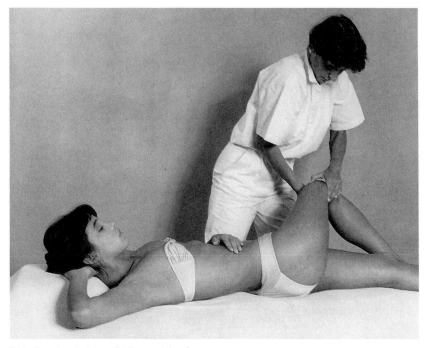

Figure 4–82 B, The leg is brought into adduction.

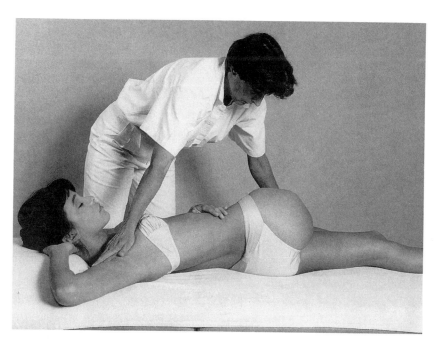

Figure 4–82 C, End position: view from in front of the therapist.

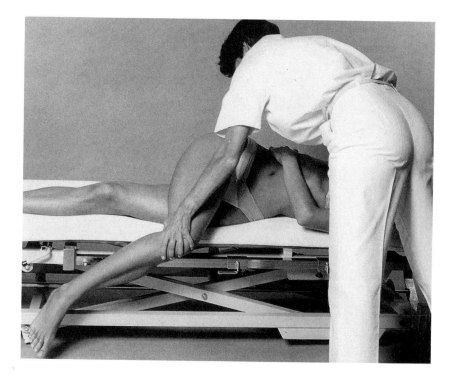

Figure 4–82 D, End position: view from behind the therapist.

tion in the lumbar spine is observed; the leg is then slowly adducted and brought into approximately 45° of hip flexion.

The therapist places the cranial hand on the anterior aspect of the patient's shoulder in order to stabilize the patient's upper body. The caudal hand grasps the lateral aspect of the patient's knee. An imaginary line running between both hands of the therapist should form an angle of 30° to 40° to the long axis of the patient. The therapist positions himself or herself parallel to this diagonal.

In order to emphasize the axial separation, the direction of the force is more in line with the patient's top leg.

To emphasize the rotational aspect of this technique, the force exerted on the leg is primarily toward the floor.

Pre-tension is achieved through rotation of the patient's trunk. During exhalation, the therapist extends his or her spine and per-

forms a manipulation by using an abrupt nod of the head directly after the end of the patient's exhalation. After the manipulation the therapist proceeds as described under Axial Separation in Extension.

Repositioning Technique without Axial Separation (Figures 4–83A–H)

The technique described below is indicated for patients who present with a deviated lumbar spine due to a disc protrusion. It can also be used as a technique primarily for pain relief. This technique should *never* be applied as a manipulation.

Position of the Patient

The patient lies supine with the arms relaxed at the side or under the head. Because it is usually impossible for the patient to lie fully straight, the legs are slightly bent. A pillow supports the head.

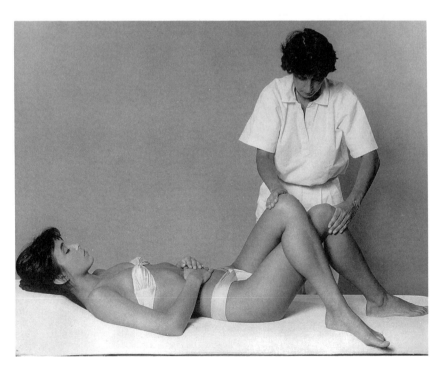

Figure 4–83 A, Starting position.

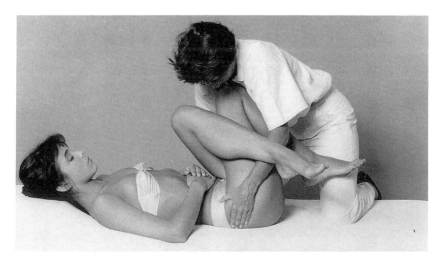

Figure 4–83 B, The pelvis is rotated, resulting in a sidebending of the lumbar spine, opening the painful side.

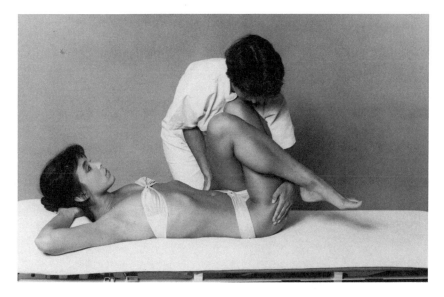

Figure 4–83 C, End position of the lumbar spine in a sidebent position.

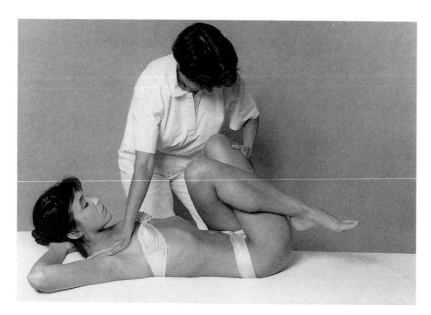

Figure 4–83 D, Fixing the patient's trunk.

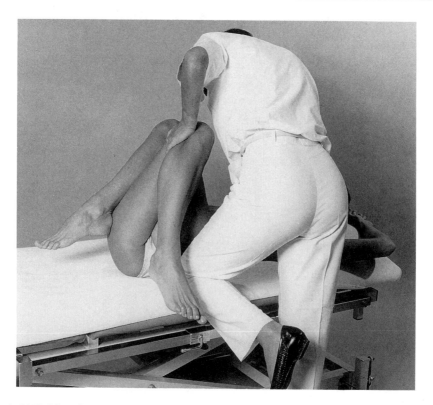

Figure 4–83 E, View from behind: the therapist places the knee against the patient's ischial tuberosity and grasps the lateral aspect of the patient's knee with fingers placed in the popliteal fossa.

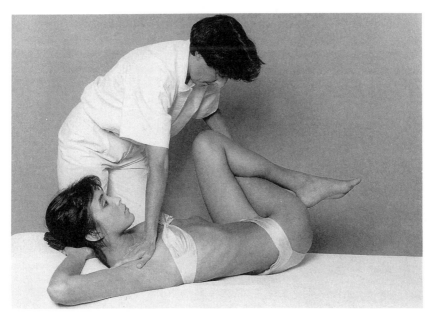

Figure 4–83 F, Rotation of the trunk: view from in front of the therapist.

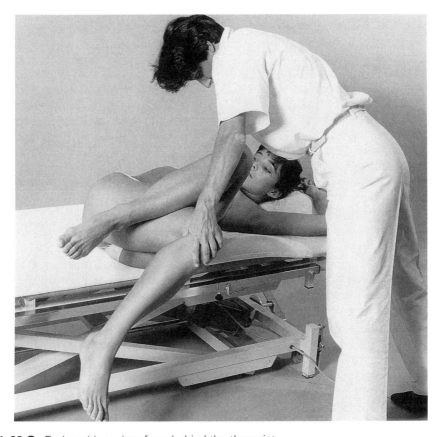

Figure 4–83 G, End position: view from behind the therapist.

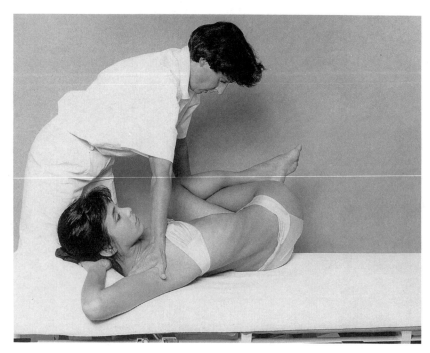

Figure 4–83 H, End position: view from the side.

The treatment table is positioned at a level just above the therapist's knees.

Position of the Therapist

If this technique is performed mainly for pain relief, the therapist stands at the patient's nonaffected side at the level of the legs. If this technique is used primarily for improving a deviation, the therapist stands at the patient's convex side (of the deviation).

Performance

The therapist takes the patient's leg closest to him or her and crosses it over the other leg. While respecting pain and muscle splinting, the therapist brings both of the patient's hips into about 90° of flexion. The therapist then grasps the patient's pelvis with both hands whereby the knee of the patient's affected side rests against the therapist's sternum. The pelvis is very carefully rotated away from the affected side, resulting in a sidebending of the trunk, opening the painful side. (When performed to correct a deviation, this move-

ment results in a sidebending of the trunk opposite to the patient's deviation.)

Each motion during this technique must be performed very cautiously, and as soon as a motion provokes pain, it is brought back slightly.

The therapist places his or her knee against the ischial tuberosity lying closest to the edge of the table (this maintains the sidebent position of the patient's trunk) and fixes the patient's shoulder against the treatment table with the cranial hand. With the caudal hand, the therapist grasps the lateral side of the knee closest to him or her (the knee from the affected side), whereby the fingers lie in the popliteal fossa.

Now rotation of the trunk is performed slowly until either the normal end-feel is reached or until provocation of pain prevents the therapist from going further into the range of motion. The patient is held for several seconds or even minutes in this *painless* position before being slowly and carefully returned to the starting position. If the therapist is unable to reach the end-range of motion with the patient, the patient's legs are supported against the therapist's thighs while the therapist holds the patient in the painless position.

As mentioned above, often at first the patient has difficulty lying with the legs extended. This fact can be taken into consideration as a measure of improvement. The patient is then assessed in standing.

If the deviation is corrected, there are two possibilities for further treatment:

1. Continue treatment with the previously described axial separation techniques. As the patient improves, rotation can be added.

2. Apply the McKenzie technique.[53] Here also it is essential to give the patient a thorough explanation about the cause of the problem and instruction in proper posture and body mechanics. The home exercises are supplemented with the McKenzie technique.

Correcting the Deviated Posture (McKenzie Technique)
(Figures 4–84A–C)

Correction of the deviated posture is the goal of this McKenzie technique. For details refer to his publications.[54]

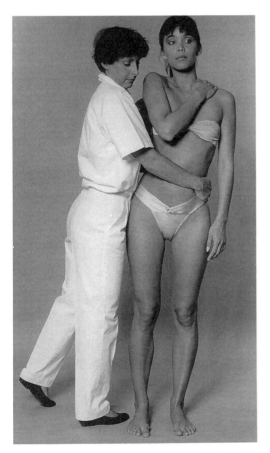

Figure 4–84 A, Correcting the deviated posture.

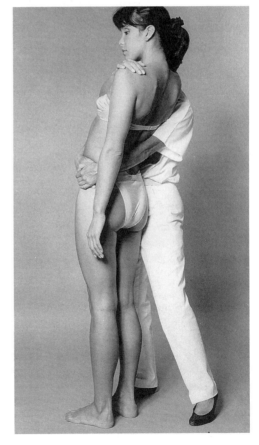

Figure 4–84 B, Extension in the corrected position.

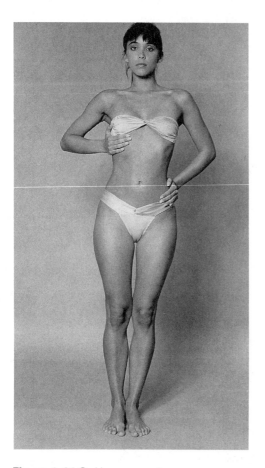

Figure 4–84 C, Home exercise.

Position of the Patient

The patient stands. The hand of the side to which the patient's shoulders are shifted rests on the opposite shoulder.

Position of the Therapist

The therapist stands next to the patient, on the side to which the patient's shoulders are shifted. With a pillow between his or her sternum and the lateral aspect of the patient's trunk, the therapist grasps the patient's pelvis on the opposite side.

Performance

With the thorax, the therapist pushes the patient's trunk to the opposite side. Simulta-

neously, the patient's pelvis is pulled toward the therapist.

While the therapist maintains this corrected position, the patient performs an active extension in the lumbar spine, assisted by the therapist.

By applying pressure to the pelvis and the thorax, the patient can perform this exercise at home. In this case, it is best to do the exercise while standing in front of a mirror. The exercise should be performed several times daily.

LOCAL MANUAL MOBILIZATION

These techniques are especially beneficial in cases where the symptoms are caused mainly by one or more zygapophyseal joints. The following techniques can be used from T10-11 to L5-S1.

After both open and microsurgery for a disc protrusion, the load in the segment changes, which can cause problems particularly in the zygapophyseal joints. In these instances, the local manual mobilization techniques can also be applied.

Technique for Pain Relief: Traction, with Locking in Extension, Sidebend, and Coupled (Contralateral) Rotation (Figures 4–85A, B)

Position of the Patient

The patient lies on the side with the painful side up and the head supported by a pillow. The bottom leg is extended; the top leg is flexed at the hip and knee. The hip should not be flexed more than approximately 70°. The treatment table is positioned at the level of the therapist's trochanter.

Position of the Therapist

The therapist stands in front of the patient at the level of the lumbar spine.

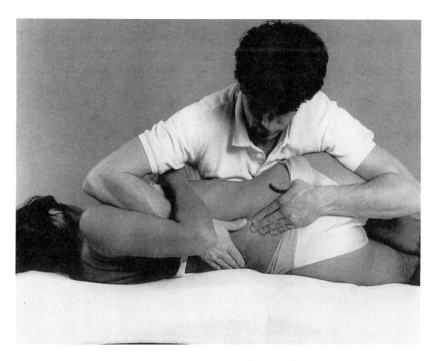

Figure 4–85 A, Traction in the upper-lying L4-5 zygapophyseal joint.

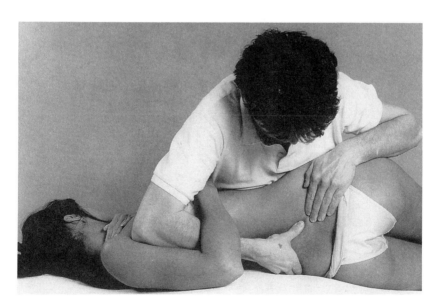

Figure 4–85 B, Traction in the upper-lying L5-S1 zygapophyseal joint.

Performance

The therapist localizes the spinous processes of the affected segment. In so doing, the index finger of the caudal hand palpates the segment's caudal spinous process, and the index finger of the cranial hand palpates the segment's cranial spinous process. With the caudal hand, the therapist raises the middle of the adustable treatment table so that a sidebending in the lumbar spine occurs, reaching no further than the segment cranial to the segment being treated. If the table is not adjustable, the sidebending can also be positioned by use of a pillow under the lower thoracic spine.

Next the therapist rests the ventral aspect of the forearm against the patient's pectoral area. In order to stabilize the structures lying caudal to the affected segment, the caudal forearm and hand are placed against the patient's ischial tuberosity, sacrum, and the lumbar segments up to the segment to be treated. With the tip of either the index finger or middle finger of the caudal hand, the segment's caudal spinous process is fixed from the side.

Using the cranial forearm to push the top shoulder in a dorsal direction, the therapist now rotates the patient's trunk in a direction opposite to the sidebending. The trunk rotation is brought only to the point where the segment cranial to the affected segment has been reached. The therapist places the thumb on the upper lateral aspect of the cranial spinous process.

While the caudal hand and forearm stabilize, the cranial hand and forearm perform a rhythmic movement into the rotatation. This combined motion results in a diagonal, dorsal, medial, and cranial direction. During the oscillatory movement, both hands, although still remaining in alignment, move away from each other along this diagonal. In this way a slight intermittent local traction occurs in the upper-lying zygapophyseal joint.

To treat the upper L5-S1 zygapophyseal joint, the therapist fixes the spine in extension, sidebending, and contralateral rotation down to and including the segment just cranial to the affected segment. Oscillatory movements are then performed in a traction direction (now ventral, lateral, and caudal), with the caudal hand and forearm against the patient's sacrum and pelvis.

The application of these techniques can vary from about 10 seconds to several minutes.

Technique for Pain Relief: Gliding, with Locking in Extension, Sidebend, and Coupled (Contralateral) Rotation
(Figures 4–85C and D)

Position of the Patient

Same as the previous technique.

Position of the Therapist

Same as the previous technique.

Performance

The performance of this technique is similar to that of the previous technique; however, here the thumb of the caudal hand is placed against the lower lateral aspect of the segment's caudal spinous process.

Through the cranial forearm the therapist now induces a movement in a dorsal, medial, and *caudal* direction. The thumb on the cranial spinous process assists the motion while the caudal thumb fixes the caudal spinous process. As opposed to the previous technique, during this diagonal movement both hands move toward each other.

In order to treat the L5-S1 segment the caudal hand grasps the patient's ilium from posterior. In this case, the cranial thumb fixes the cranial spinous process from the upper lateral aspect. The caudal hand brings the pelvis in a ventral, lateral, and *cranial* direction.

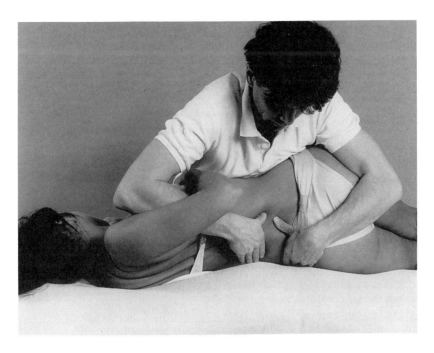

Figure 4–85 C, Oscillatory gliding of the L4-5 segment.

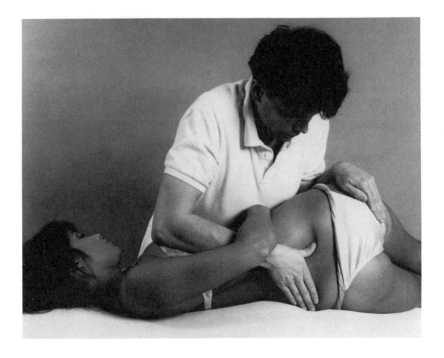

Figure 4–85 D, Oscillatory gliding of the L5-S1 segment.

Traction Mobilization with Locking in Extension, Sidebend, and Coupled (Contralateral) Rotation

Position of the Patient

Same as for Technique for Pain Relief: Traction. . . .

Position of the Therapist

Same as for Technique for Pain Relief: Traction. . . .

Performance

The therapist places the hands in the same position as for Technique for Pain Relief: Traction. The performance of this technique is essentially the same, as well. Here, the sidebend and rotation are now pre-positioned in the affected segment. Instead of perform-

ing oscillations, the therapist brings the zygapophyseal joint in the traction direction and holds this end position for 10 to 40 seconds.

Gliding Mobilization with Locking in Extension, Sidebend, and Coupled (Contralateral) Rotation

Position of the Patient

Same as for Technique for Pain Relief: Gliding. . . .

Position of the Therapist

Same as for Technique for Pain Relief: Gliding. . . .

Performance

This technique is similar to Technique for Pain Relief: Gliding, in terms of hand place-

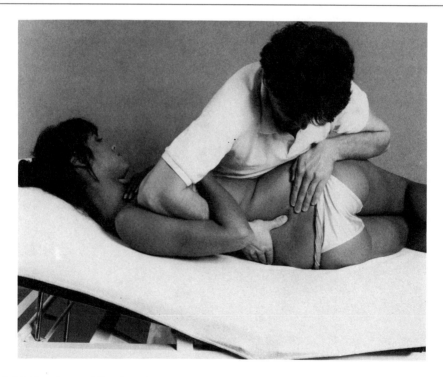

Figure 4–86 Traction mobilization of the L5-S1 segment with the lumbar spine locked in a combined position through L4-5.

ment and performance. As with the previous mobilization technique, the sidebend and rotation are now pre-positioned in the affected segment. The therapist brings the zygapophyseal joint in the glide direction and holds this end position for 10 to 40 seconds.

* * * *

Note: Locking the spine in a coupled position is sometimes painful for the patient in an area that is not being treated (for instance, thoracic spine). In these cases, the spine can be locked in a combined position, which results in less total range of motion, and a firmer fixation of the segments not being treated. In addition, due to the combined locking of the spine, the cranial and caudal fingers now require much less pressure against the spinous processes in order to fix or to mobilize.

Traction Mobilization with Locking in Extension, Sidebend, and Combined (Ipsilateral) Rotation (Figure 4–86)

Position of the Patient

The patient lies on the side with the painful side up. A pillow supports the head. The legs are flexed at the hips and knees whereby the amount of hip flexion is not greater than 70°.

The treatment table is positioned to a height of the therapist's trochanter.

Position of the Therapist

The therapist stands in front of the patient at the level of the lumbar spine.

Performance

With the middle and index fingers of the caudal hand, the therapist palpates the

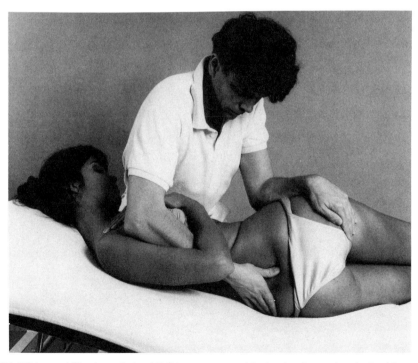

Figure 4–87 Glide mobilization of the L5-S1 segment with the lumbar spine locked in a combined position through L4-5.

interspinous spaces of the affected segment and the segment directly above it, respectively. He or she then lifts the head of the table as far as necessary to produce a sidebending in the spine, reaching no further than the segment cranial to the segment being treated.

Now the therapist rests the cranial forearm against the patient's pectoralis region and the thumb at the segment's cranial spinous process. The other hand and arm lie against the patient's sacrum, pelvis, and lateral upper thigh with the fingers at the segment's caudal spinous process.

By using the cranial forearm to push the patient's shoulder in a dorsal direction, the therapist now rotates the patient's trunk in the same direction as the sidebending. This induced rotation is opposite to the automatic coupling and results in a firmer locking of the lumbar segments cranial to the affected segment. Because the affected segment was not pre-positioned in a sidebending, the rotation is allowed to reach this segment as well.

For all of the lumbar segments except L5-S1, the thumb lying against the upper lateral aspect of the cranial spinous process creates the movement in the segment. The thumb, index finger, or middle finger of the other hand stabilizes the caudal spinous process from its lower lateral aspect. The cranial hand performs the traction in a dorsal, medial, and cranial direction.

To treat the L5-S1 segment, the cranial thumb fixes L5 while the fingers of the caudal hand perform the traction in the upper-lying L5-S1 zygapophyseal joint. In so doing, the sacrum and pelvis are pulled in a ventral, lateral, and caudal direction.

Gliding Mobilization with Locking in Extension, Sidebending, and Combined (Ipsilateral) Rotation
(Figure 4–87)

Position of the Patient

Same as the previous technique.

Position of the Therapist

Same as the previous technique.

Performance

For mobilization of the lumbar segments cranial to the L5-S1 segment, the hand placement remains the same as for the previous technique. Now the direction of movement with the cranial thumb is dorsal, medial, and caudal.

In mobilization of the L5-S1 segment, the thumb fixes the cranial spinous process, while the caudal hand moves the sacrum and the pelvis in a ventral, lateral, and cranial direction.

Due to the locking of the lumbar spine in a combined position, the cranial thumb now requires much less pressure against the spinous process in order to fix L5 (and all of the segments cranial to L5-S1).

LUMBAR TRACTION

Indications

Theoretically, traction as a treatment (Figure 4–88) is indicated in all primary discogenic pathology that has a gradual onset and in which there is no deviation of the spine. The presence of neurological deficits are generally considered to be a contraindication.

In almost all cases, the therapist can conclude that unloading the spine will be the treatment of choice when the patient indicates that bed rest diminishes the symptoms and/or that hanging on a doorsill or pull-up bar is also helpful. Bed rest normally means a loss of time at work and is therefore not very cost effective. In addition, it has been proved that bed rest for longer than 2 days is obsolete.[55] The decrease in intradiscal pressure achieved by diminishing gravity—lying down—can be improved by traction.

By means of epidurography, Matthews proved that disc protrusions "disappeared" during treatment with traction. During traction the space between the vertebrae in-

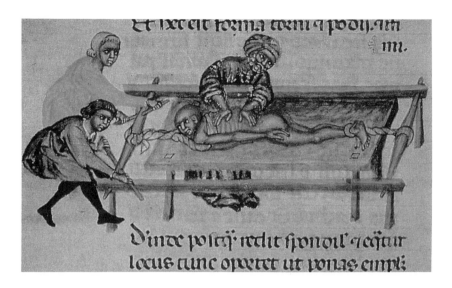

Figure 4–88 Traction treatment according to Hippocrates.[57]

creases. The posterior longitudinal ligament becomes more taut and a negative pressure is created in the disc, along with a centripetal force, that causes the disappearance of the protrusion (Figure 4–89).[56] The same author demonstrated that after 4 minutes of sustained traction a decrease of the protrusion was visible; after 20 minutes the protrusion even disappeared completely in most cases. After conclusion of the traction treatment, the protrusion increased slightly but remained clearly less than before the treatment.

Matthews' X-rays showed an increase in the distance of the vertebral bodies by 2 mm per segment. With 69 kg (approximately 152 lb) of tensile force, not only did the disc protrusion resolve, but the contrast medium also was partially sucked into the intervertebral space.

White and Panjabi[9] mention that when the disc protrusion compresses the shoulder of the nerve root, the patient demonstrates a particularly painful ipsilateral sidebending; this situation is a good indication for traction treatment (Figure 4–90).

The relation between the decrease or disappearance of the protrusion and the decrease or disappearance of the symptoms, however, has never been demonstrated.[55,58] (See Chapter 15.) In instances of an upper lumbar disc protrusion, manipulation is a relative contraindication. Even with locally performed segmental mobilizations, complaints due to an upper lumbar disc protrusion tend to increase. Therefore, traction is indicated and often provides a very beneficial result. Traction can also be a beneficial treatment in patients with a recurrence of symptoms postlaminectomy. An excellent indication for traction treatment is primary posterolateral disc protrusion or prolapse within the first 3 months of its onset.

Contraindications

- Traction is contraindicated for all nondiscogenic lesions; most secondary discogenic problems are considered to be contraindications.

- Traction is contraindicated for very acute disc protrusions, with or without a

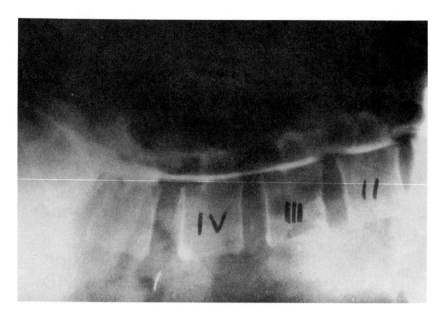

Figure 4–89 Epidurography in a patient with an upper lumbar disc problem, L1-2 and L2-3.[56] **A,** Disc protrusion is clearly visible at the level of L1-2 and L2-3.

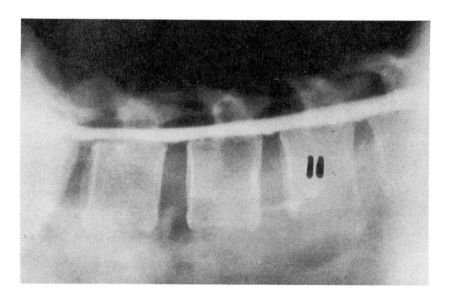

Figure 4–89 B, After 30 minutes of sustained traction, the protrusions have disappeared, and "dimples" are even visible as a result of the centripetal force occurring during traction.

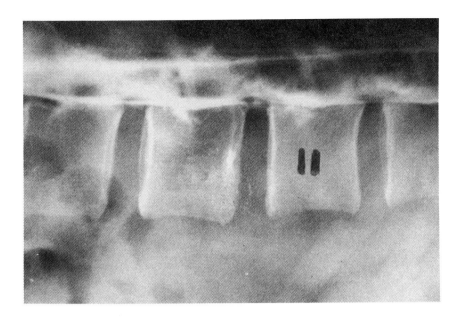

Figure 4–89 C, Same patient, 20 days after the traction treatment. After a fall, the symptoms recurred. Epidurography showed the same situation as in **A.**

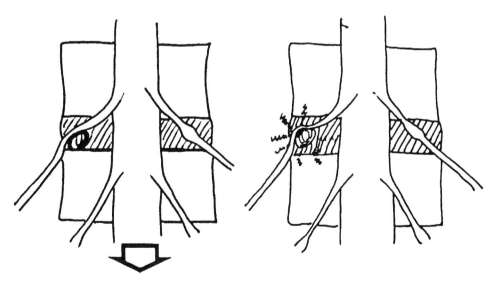

Figure 4–90 With compression in the axilla of the nerve root, pain increases during traction. In the functional examination, sidebending away from the painful side is the most painful motion. This is usually a good indication for manual mobilization, according to White and Panjabi.[9]

deviation, in which the patient experiences severe "twinges" with even the most minimal movement.

- Sustained axial traction is contraindicated in patients who are deviated in standing as well as in supine. If the patient is not deviated (anymore) in lying, traction may be applied cautiously.
- Traction is contraindicated for primary discogenic lesions with neurological deficits.
- Traction is contraindicated for radicular pain existing for more than 6 months.
- Traction is contraindicated for primary discogenic lesions in patients over 60 years of age.

Precautions

- Primary discogenic lesions with an acute onset (in these instances mobilization/manipulation is generally the treatment of choice)
- Primary posterolateral protrusion or disc prolapse that has been present for more than 3 months
- If, during the traction treatment, radiating pain occurs or the existing radiating pain increases
- When, during traction, there is an increase of local pain
- Directly after mobilizing or manipulating
- In the last 5 months of pregnancy
- When the patient suffers from a cold or bronchial infection (coughing and sneezing during the traction treatment can result in a worsening of the symptoms)

Requirements

Traction is considered the proper treatment when the appropriate indications are met (see above) and the patient feels comfortable during the treatment. Traction is applied continuously with the highest possible pulling force whereby the patient is still able to relax (the force can vary from 80 to 180 lb).

Material

Generally, in orthopaedic medicine, *continuous* traction is applied. On the treatment tables used by the authors, axial traction is the only possible kind of traction. However, there are traction tables available in which different parts of the table can be positioned in such a way that a deviated patient can also be treated. The fixation belts must be very sturdy, and no shifting of the belts should be possible during the treatment. A thick layer of firm foam (1 in) can be placed between the belts and the patient. In order to be able to evaluate the treatment in terms of the applied force, a scale is positioned between the winch and the caudal belt. The winch should be manually adjustable to allow the force to be increased very gradually. The fixation point for the cranial belt should be adaptable in height. Additional items that may be necessary for proper traction treatment include a roll to support the knees, a pillow to support the head, and an adjustable (in height) stool to support the lower legs (Figure 4–91).

Electric traction tables are also available. The disadvantage here is that the traction force, as well as the increase and decrease of the traction force, cannot be applied in exact doses. The above-described equipment consists of either a complete traction table or separate pieces of equipment that can be attached to a normal treatment table.

Initial Positions

The initial position of the patient depends on the functional examination. If the patient cannot lie supine, the initial position will be prone. If the patient prefers to lie supine and, for instance, extension of the lumbar spine is possible, the initial position can be supine (Figure 4–92). The different positions are

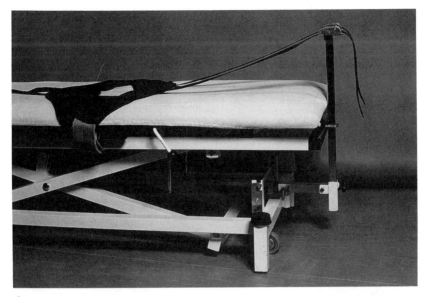

A

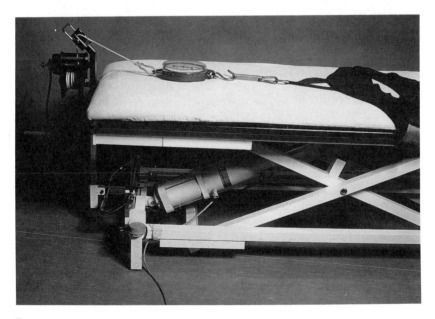

B

Figure 4–91 Traction table. **A**, Cranial fixation belt with attachment; **B**, winch, scale, and caudal fixation belt.

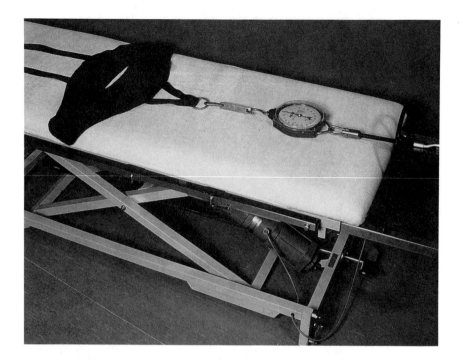

Figure 4–91C, Winch, scale, and caudal fixation belt.

demonstrated in the following drawings and pictures.

Application of Traction

- The first traction treatment lasts about 15 minutes and is increased daily up to 30 to 45 minutes.
- The traction treatment preferably is given on a daily basis (5 days in a row, followed by a 2-day break).
- Different initial positions usually have to be tried in order to find the most comfortable position for the patient.
- Attachment and detachment of the fixation belts are executed carefully. Sudden movements must be avoided.
- The pull force should be increased gradually and released slowly. After the traction the patient should remain in the initial position (with the belts released) for approximately 15 minutes.

- The patient receives as many treatments as necessary for a full cessation of the symptoms (usually 2 to 3 weeks).
- The traction never stands alone as a treatment. Further management involves giving the patient extensive information about the lesion, as well as postural and ergonomic advice, as described in Appendix 4–A.
- An exercise program can be initiated when the patient is able to perform the exercises without pain and there is no increase in pain afterward. This is tested daily, prior to the traction treatment. (Here the isometric abdominal exercises are of most importance.)
- Always examine the patient before the traction treatment and never afterward.
- If, after four treatments, no improvement is noted, the therapist should try a different initial position. If after 2 weeks

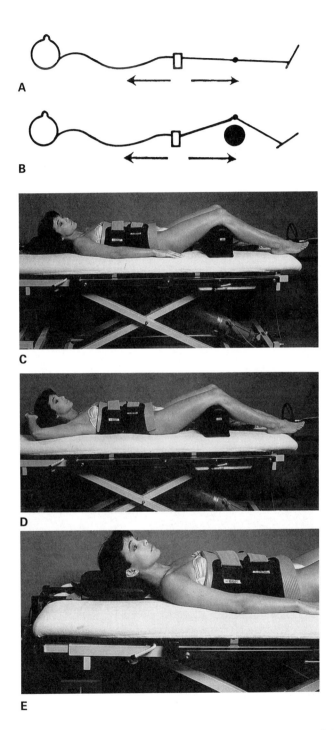

Figure 4–92 *A*, The patient prefers the supine position. Extension is not very painful or limited. Flexion provokes the symptoms. This is the initial position for the patient who presents with a deviation in standing but not in lying. *B*, A roll supports the knees for greater relaxation. See accompanying photographs, *C* to *F*.

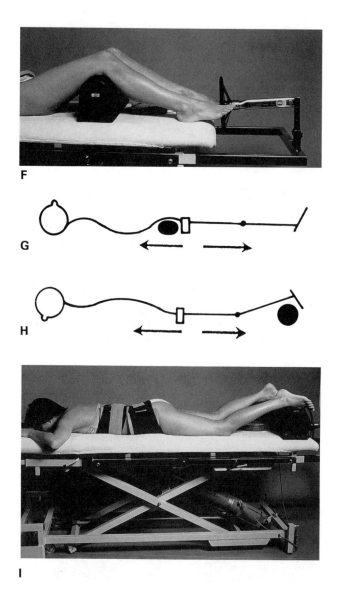

Figure 4–92 *G*, Initial position for a patient with minimal S3-5 symptoms: minimal pull and short duration (eg, 80 lb for 20 minutes). *H*, The patient prefers the prone position. Extension is not very limited. Flexion provokes the symptoms. See accompanying photograph, *I*.

there is still no change in symptoms, the treatment should be discontinued.

The transition from the supine to the sitting position is performed as follows: The patient brings both knees up with the feet still in contact with the treatment table. The patient then contracts the abdominal muscles, turns on one side (keeping the painful side up), and with both hands and arms pushes the upper body into the sitting position. At the same time, both legs are brought over the edge of the table.

As already mentioned, it is of utmost importance to perform a thorough examination

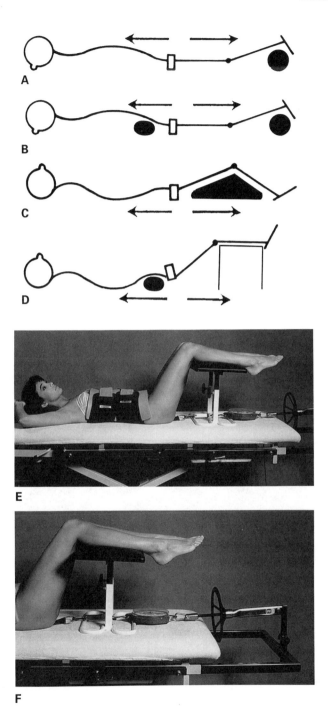

Figure 4–93 **A**, The patient prefers the prone position. Extension provokes the symptoms. Flexion is slightly limited. **B**, Adding a pillow under the abdomen can increase the degree of relaxation. **C**, The patient prefers the supine position. Extension provokes the symptoms. Flexion is slightly limited. *Note:* **B** and **C** are very effective in L3 root pain (with a strong pull and duration of 40 minutes). **D**, The patient prefers the supine position. Extension is painful and limited. In this position the intradiscal pressure is the lowest. See accompanying photographs, **E** and **F**.

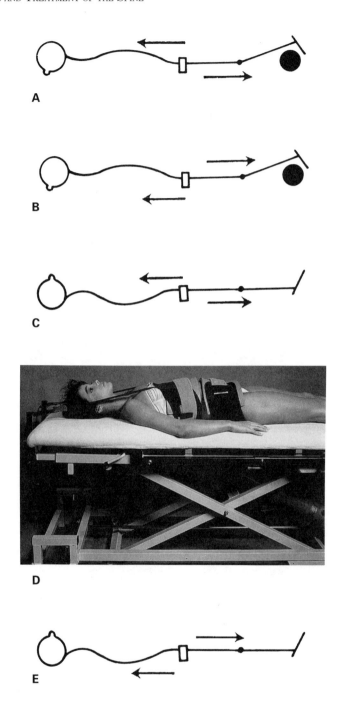

Figure 4–94 *A*, The patient prefers the prone position. Both flexion and extension provoke the symptoms. ***B*,** The patient prefers the prone position. Both flexion and extension provoke the symptoms. ***C*,** The patient prefers the supine position. Both flexion and extension provoke the symptoms. See accompanying photograph, ***D*. *E*,** The patient prefers the supine position. Both flexion and extension provoke the symptoms.

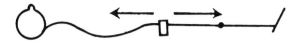

Figure 4–95 The patient prefers the supine position and has no pain in extension. Flexion provokes the symptoms. This position is seldom used.

---

before instituting the treatment. Proper instructions to the patient are imperative. Instructions should emphasize clearly that the treatment absolutely must not be painful and therefore the patient must notify the therapist immediately if pain arises. If the therapist cannot be present during the traction treatment, then the patient must have the means, for instance by bell, to notify the therapist. The patient should also try to avoid coughing or sneezing while receiving the traction.

Before the first treatment the patient should receive all the necessary information concerning his or her problem. By means of a functional examination performed at the beginning of each treatment, the therapist can determine whether it is possible to begin an exercise program. In this case, the exercises should be performed or tried before the traction treatment. The patient continues with the exercises at home.

THERAPEUTIC NERVE BLOCKS

Introduction

With nerve blocks in and around the spinal column, one has to realize that the nervous system is not a simple "wiring system." Almost every therapist is familiar with the "law of specific sensory organ energy," as formulated by Muller in 1826.[59] Perception does not depend upon the type of stimulus, but rather upon the particular sensory organ triggered and its corresponding neuronal connections. The body consists of a number of "wiring systems" that transport information (ie, pain). For instance, pain in the foot provoked by fire is transmitted via the foot to the spinal cord

and then further on to the central nervous system (Figure 4–96). Although such pathways exist in the nervous system, the situation is actually much more complicated than just described. Some manifestations such as causalgia, neuralgia, and especially phantom pain cannot be explained or therapeutically blocked.

Around 1950 the "specificity theory" was gradually replaced by the "pattern theory," which states that the pattern of the afferent impulses determines the reaction of the nerve cell. If all incoming stimuli are equal and normal, the cell "declares" that this is not pain; if one fourth of the stimulus is normal, one fourth is too weak, one fourth is too strong, and one fourth is missing, the cell interprets this as pain. Noordenbos[60] defended this concept in his dissertation, postulating that pain is a quantity. Phantom pain would then be based on the missing of a normal afferent stimulus from the missing body part; this is also called deafferentation pain.

Elements of both of these theories can be found in the "gate" theory proposed by Melzack and Wall,[61] which was further developed later by Melzack.[62] The main concept of the gate theory is that sensory input of pain occurs via thick and thin fibers, in which the thicker fibers have a lower threshold and a faster conduction than the thinner fibers (Figure 4–97). These fibers converge in the spinal cord (Rexed's lamina V), where a modulation takes place in the substantia gelatinosa (Rexed's lamina II).[63] Superimposed on this system is a central control from the brain. For example, when a soccer player is kicked in the shin, he or she will forcefully rub the shin, which creates such a domination

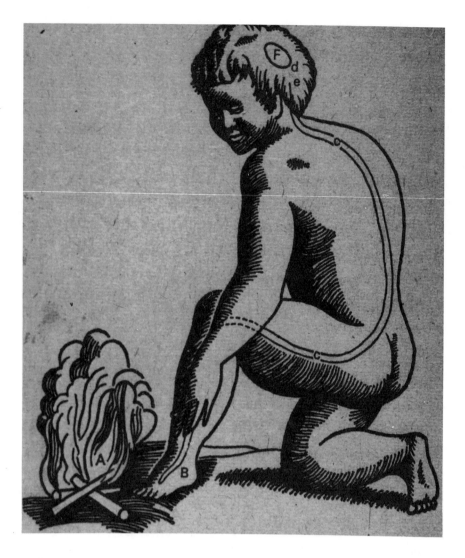

Figure 4–96 The pain sensations are transmitted through the spinal cord to the central nervous system, according to Muller.[59]

of the thick, fast-conducting fibers that the deep pain of the slower-conducting, thin fibers will be perceived as less; the gate closes to the pain. In addition, if the referee awards a penalty kick, the victim will probably jump up cheerfully and continue to play—central control of the stimulus.

Besides the various theories concerning the *conduction* of a pain stimulus, the *nature* of the pain stimulus also needs to be taken into account. Therapists sometimes

have the tendency to think in a mechanical way: a disc prolapse causes pain due to compression on sensitive structures. This is certainly possible, but there are generally more factors to consider.

After tissue damage, substances such as bradykinin, histamine, and prostaglandin are released, which can cause an increased sensitivity to a stimulus; even normal stimuli are experienced as painful. As a result of these chemical changes, a change in the pH value of

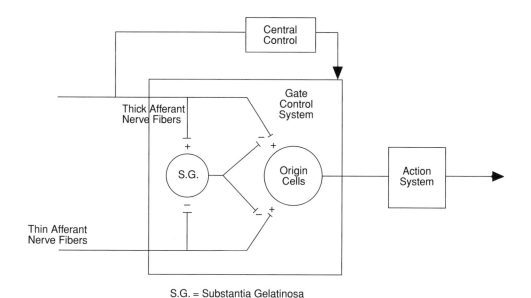

S.G. = Substantia Gelatinosa

Figure 4–97 Diagram of the gate theory.

the tissue occurs, which in turn can cause a long-lasting disturbance of the normal balance.[64,65] Secondary changes in muscles and fasciae can arise and limit motion, and can even become "trigger points" for pain.[66]

Just as the brain is able to exert central control over the pain stimulus, there are factors other than neurophysiological pathways that can also conduct a signal. To demonstrate this fact, Loeser and Fordyce[67] use four concentric circles (Figure 4–98) The innermost circle represents nociception: the pain stimulation. Next comes the pain sensation: the stimulation is recognized as pain. The third circle is the experience of pain, in other words, how the individual interprets the pain sensation. Finally, the outer circle represents the pain behavior. For instance, if someone is scratched by a cat (pain trigger), he or she has a sensation of pain (feeling the pain in the hand). The person then pulls the hand away and gives the cat a slap (pain behavior).

In chronic pain, the outer two circles can become enormous in proportion to the two inner circles, which are almost nonexistent. Generally, this is true for all pain, but it is es-

pecially true for pain originating in the musculoskeletal system. Obviously this form of pain cannot simply be quelled by a block of the structure originally triggering the pain: the pain has started to live a life of its own. Prevention in such situations is best, since treatment at this stage is sometimes impossible.

Procedures

Once the decision has been made to block a nerve, a *diagnostic* block using a local anesthetic (lidocaine with a concentration of 0.25% to 1.0%) is almost always performed first. Afterward a judgment can be made as to whether or not it is worthwhile to anesthetize the concerned structures. If the symptoms are indeed relieved, then the following options are available to the physician to perform a *therapeutic* block.

Repetition of the Block with a Local Anesthetic (Lidocaine or Bupivacaine Hydrochloride) with or without Corticosteroids. In this method, by interrupting the vicious cycle a certain number of times, one hopes

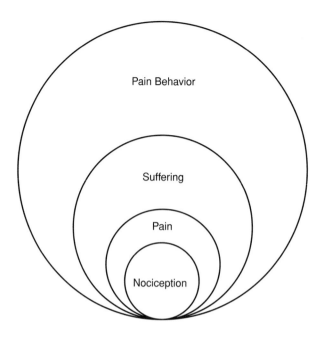

Figure 4–98 The four concentric circles of Loeser and Fordyce.[67]

that the normal physiological circumstances and reactions will again take the upper hand. If this vicious cycle—muscle tension, change in posture, pain—can be interrupted and the pathological trigger pattern of the sensory neuron is temporarily shut down, then a long-lasting or even permanent improvement can occur despite the limited time that the local anesthetic has an effect.

Chemical Neurolysis. Chemical neurolysis is the elimination of a nerve with the help of a chemical substance, usually alcohol or phenol. Because of the inability to keep the injected substance localized, this technique is of importance only in special blocks when a diffuse effect is desired, for example, a block of the coeliac ganglion.

Physical Neurolysis. This method uses cold (cryolesion) or heat (radiofrequency or RF lesion) to damage the nerve.

Cryolesion. Cryolesion[68] has some technical problems. Restoration of the nerve function is sometimes undesirably fast.

Heat Lesion (RF Lesion). This method is the technique of choice as a result of technical developments over the last years. Special equipment has been developed in which Teflon-coated needles are used. Only the tip of the needle makes electric contact with the tissue. Through sensory and motor stimulation one determines the precise position of the tip of the needle in relation to the nerve before proceeding with the neurolysis.[65]

Because of the techniques described above, the need for surgery in order to perform nerve blocks has decreased significantly. The choice of therapeutic options depends on the type of nerve, the kinds of symptoms, the condition of the patient, and many other factors. In general, greater risks are taken in the treatment of malignant diseases than, for instance, in the treatment of nonspecific low back pain. To the same extent, in surgery on the autonomic nervous system one will decide to proceed more quickly with a neurolysis than in other cases in which important motor pathways could be endangered.

Conclusion. In summary, the following considerations are of importance when performing a nerve block:

- Pain is not a "pipeline."
- Triggers can be mechanical and/or chemical.
- A pain stimulus is not equal to pain sensation.
- A therapeutic block does not equal a neurolysis.

Anatomy

The spinal cord and the emerging roots lie well protected in a wrapping of cerebrospinal fluid, dura mater, arteries, ligaments, and bony structures. (See also Chapter 8.) The spinal cord consists of the well-known H-shaped structure, along with ascending and descending pathways consisting of a network of mutual linking and recurrent linking (feedback) systems. Much is still unknown about these networks.

Of the structures that envelop the spinal cord, the dura mater is of special interest because several block techniques are performed just outside the dura (epidural or peridural) or just through the dura (subarachnoidal or spinal) into the cerebrospinal fluid.

The emerging nerve divides into different branches. The most important are the following:

- Anterior ramus, lying in front. This ramus is usually the largest branch, with sensory, motor, and sympathetic components. All the anterior rami are responsible to a great degree for the sensory and motor innervation of the body.
- Posterior ramus, lying in back. This ramus is usually rather small, except in the upper cervical region. For therapists this branch is significant because the articular branch of this nerve is responsible for the innervation of the zygapophyseal joint capsule.

In studying the motion segment of Junghans,[6] it is demonstrated that every zygapophyseal joint receives its innervation from the upper, as well as the lower, posterior ramus (Figure 4–99).

Sympathetic nerves run within the spinal nerves, but synapse with each other in the first sympathetic (paravertebral) ganglion just outside the intervertebral foramen. All the sympathetic centers of synapsing form the sympathetic chain, which is located either lateral or ventrolateral to the spinal column. Therapeutically this is important because at this site the sympathetic fibers (axons) run separately from the sensory and motor axons,

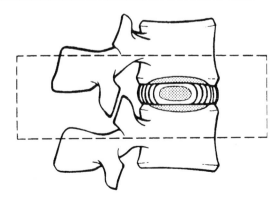

Figure 4–99 Motion segment of Junghans.[6]

which allows for separate blocks. The sympathetic chain condenses at several sites:

- the stellate ganglion, at the level of the cervicothoracic junction
- the celiac ganglion, ventrolateral to the first lumbar vertebra
- the lumbar sympathetic nerve, at the level of the second to the fifth lumbar vertebrae

Nerve Block

In order to define clearly the situations and structures that can benefit from a nerve block, it is necessary to exclude those techniques that fall outside the direct scope of orthopaedic medicine:

- Interruption of pathways within the spinal cord, for example, the spinothalamic tract. This procedure is considered only in cases of malignancy.
- Epidural and spinal use of neurolytics. This is a fascinating technique in which one makes use of opiate receptors within the spinal cord. This technique is considered only in cases of malignancy; often an epidural block is performed instead.
- Epidural stimulation with electrodes. This is a relatively new procedure; it is very experimental, very expensive, and, for the time being, reserved for untreatable peripheral vascular diseases and some forms of spasticity.
- Subarachnoid (spinal) local anesthesia and/or corticosteroid injections. Through the opening in the dura, cerebrospinal fluid leakage can occur and corticosteroids within the cerebrospinal fluid give rise to the danger of permanent neurological damage.[69]
- Neurolysis of peripheral nerves. Perineural local anesthesia with or without the use of corticosteroids in peripheral compression neuropathies. This technique usually causes too much motor

deficit and has too many side effects, the most common one being neuritis.

Within the framework of orthopaedic medicine the following four techniques are of importance:

1. *epidural block* with a local anesthetic, with or without corticosteroids
2. *facet block* with a local anesthetic or neurolysis with an RF lesion
3. *block of the dorsal root ganglion* with a local anesthetic or partial lesion with RF neurolysis
4. *block of the sympathetic chain* with a local anesthetic or chemical, if not physical neurolysis

Epidural Block

Indications for an epidural block primarily concern chronic low back pain with or without involvement of the lower extremities, without surgical indication and resistive to adequate physical and/or manual therapy. The principle of the epidural block for this syndrome is based on local anesthesia with, for instance, 0.25% lidocaine (a kind of anesthesiological "dishwater") that causes a very temporary numbing of the adjacent structures such as the irritated dura mater or the posterior longitudinal ligament.

From the pattern theory of pain, the effects of this procedure can be explained as follows: For a short period of time the chronic pathological pattern of incoming information is interrupted, without notable loss of sensory or motor function. In the instance of inflammation or secondary swelling a corticosteroid may be added.

The method is already very old. Initially cocaine was used, later procaine. In more recent times, the technique is performed using a local anesthetic of the amide type (for instance, lidocaine); the pharmacological effect is predictable with a minimal chance of allergic side effects. The addition of corticosteroids has been propagated since the 1950s.

Sehgal and Gardner[70] report that for an epidural injection of corticosteroids, it is best to use a suspension of methylprednisolone acetate (Depo-Medrol). This substance gives a long-lasting effect with few side effects; the suspension is slowly resorbed from the epidural space, and a 40-mg dose of this substance gives a therapeutic concentration for approximately 2 to 3 weeks. For an entry point, one chooses between a caudal injection through the sacral hiatus (Figure 4–100) or the median approach between the spinous processes of the lumbar spine (Figure 4–101).

Research concerning this method of treating chronic low back pain, with or without sciatica, indicates results of varying success.[71] However, one should also keep in mind that such disorders tend to recur. This treatment method, which offers a smooth recovery with less pain and greater mobility, can be extremely beneficial for the patient because it is possible to repeat this block.

The research mentioned above was limited to the treatment of chronic back pain, with or without referred pain. Besides being used for chronic pain, the epidural treatment lends itself very well to an acute situation in this region, particularly in instances of acute lumbago. Unfortunately, for this temporary but very handicapping problem, the advice usually given by the physician is bed rest in combination with oral analgesics. However, in the authors' experience, one epidural injection followed by manual therapy the next day accomplishes a much faster recovery.

Another indication for use of this technique is acute herpes zoster. Acute herpes zoster almost always improves after a single epidural administration of a suspension of methylprednisolone acetate. The effect is likely based on a decrease in the edema of the dorsal root ganglion, by which a better vascularization arises, thus inhibiting the herpesvirus. Therefore, this method of treatment is not appropriate for a postherpetic neuralgia. (For further information, see Herpes Zoster in Chapter 5, Thoracic Spine.)

The indications for epidural anesthesia in orthopaedic medicine can be divided into two categories: diagnostic and therapeutic.

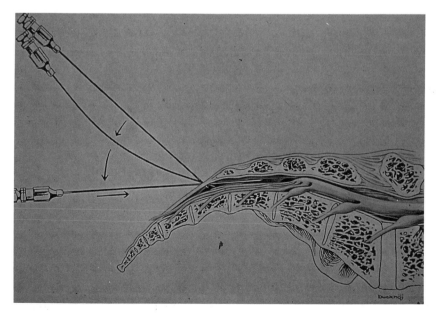

Figure 4–100 Caudal injection via the sacral hiatus.

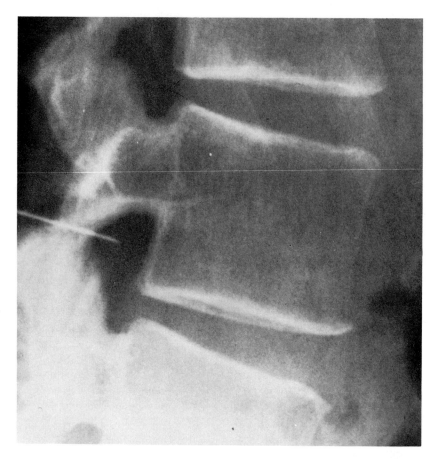

Figure 4–101 Median-approach injection between the spinous processes of the lumbar spine.

Diagnostic Indications

- Nonspecific low back pain: for differentiating discogenic disorders from non-discogenic disorders
- Leg pain without back pain: for instance, to differentiate primary posterolateral disc protrusion or prolapse from peripheral compression neuropathies
- Groin pain: to differentiate a local or sacroiliac cause from a lumbar cause
- Pain in the lower abdomen: to differentiate a local or sacroiliac cause from a lumbar cause
- Coccygodynia: to differentiate a local cause from a lumbar cause
- Conflicting diagnoses: for instance, for medicolegal purposes (libel suits) or psychosomatic disorders (let the patient judge the effect of the anesthesia)

Therapeutic Indications

- Hyperacute lumbago
- Primary disc-related lesions that are resistant to mobilization and/or traction and/or exercise therapy
- Primary disc-related lesions with neurological deficit
- Primary disc-related lesions in which sidebending to the painful side causes or increases the radicular pain

- Primary disc-related lesions existing longer than 1 year
- Primary posterolateral disc protrusions or prolapses after 4 months from the onset (in the first 3 months continuous traction is the treatment of choice)
- Pain at night and/or early in the morning in patients who have minimal to no symptoms during the day
- Disc-related back pain during pregnancy
- Nocturnal radicular pain or cramps in the calves after a disc syndrome
- Persisting radicular pain after laminectomy, chemonucleolysis, or percutaneous discectomy
- Secondary disc-related lesions, especially the nerve root compression syndrome; less effective in degenerative spondylolisthesis

Contraindications

- Oversensitivity or allergy to local anesthetics
- Local irritation or inflammation of the skin at the level of the sacral hiatus
- General sepsis
- After spinal inflammations, for instance, meningitis
- Shortly after myelography
- Under total anesthesia

Block of the Intervertebral Joints: Facet Block

"Anterior" and "posterior" pain syndromes can be differentiated by noting whether the spinal nerve is approached at the dorsal root ganglion (anterior pain) or whether the posterior ramus is blocked (posterior pain). Exactly what role the zygapophyseal joints play in lumbar pain syndromes is not totally clear. In many imaging examinations, significant changes in the zygapophyseal joints are found, even though a different structure is responsible for the symptoms. (See also Chapter 2, section 2–1, Functional Anatomy.)

Still, pain relief can be achieved in various lumbar lesions of mechanical origin via local "elimination" of the zygapophyseal joint. Whether or not this will be an effective treatment can be confirmed by a trial injection of the median branch of the posterior ramus at the transverse process, at the base of the zygapophyseal joint. Because of the overlapping innervation of the zygapophyseal joints, a facet block should always be performed on at least two (preferably three) levels.

After a positive trial block, the choice between a definite RF lesion of this nerve branch or destruction of the zygapophyseal joint by chemical neurolysis is made. Because of the danger of leakage of the neurolytic substance in a damaged joint capsule and because of the possibility of problems secondary to the joint destruction, the authors' treatment of choice is physical neurolysis with an RF lesion (Figure 4–102).

Denervation has been described by Reese,[69] further modified into a percutaneous technique by Shealy,[72] and, with a more sensitive method, improved by Sluijter and Mehta.[73] This method can be performed in the cervical spine as well as the lumbar spine.

Positive results of this treatment vary from 10% to 50%, depending on the technique, indication, and follow-up. Although these results do not seem impressive, with modern techniques this procedure can be performed with almost no risks and minimal stress for the patient who has already undergone many conservative treatments.

Partial Block of the Dorsal Root Ganglion

This procedure is considered for patients in whom neither conservative methods nor the above-described techniques were successful. Through a series of diagnostic paravertebral blocks, the nerve responsible for the pain is determined; for example, only L5 is positive and blocks of L3, L4, and S1 are negative. If the trial block is positive at different levels or negative for every level, the patient is not suited for this denervation.

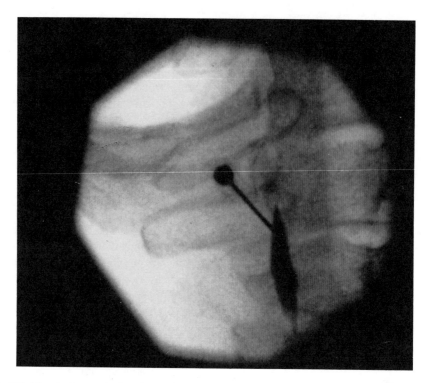

Figure 4–102 Physical neurolysis with an RF lesion.

Uematsu[74] first described this procedure. The aims in a partial block are to significantly decrease pain, without occurrence of motor deficit, and with minimal to no occurrence of hypoesthesia. Sluijter and Mehta[73] report good results in 40% and some improvement in another 27% of their patients.

Block of the Sympathetic Chain

As already mentioned, the sympathetic chain "condenses" at three levels: cervicothoracic, upper lumbar, and lower lumbar. Blocking of the upper lumbar celiac ganglion is not described in this book. However, it is an eminent tool in the treatment of pain due to malignancies of the upper abdomen. In that sense it has no relativity to orthopaedic medicine.

Block of the Cervicothoracic Sympathetic System ("Stellate Ganglion")

Indications for this procedure include the suspicion of a sympathetic component in vascular or neurological disturbances in the upper quadrant of the body. Vascular disturbances can be involved in a wide variety of clinical disorders, from angina pectoris to Raynaud's syndrome. In neurological disturbances, disorders such as the "shoulder-hand" syndrome and other forms of reflex sympathetic dystrophy can benefit from this technique. The rule here also is that a trial block is considered only when less-aggressive treatment methods have provided unsatisfactory results.

A diagnostic block is simple to perform by injecting lidocaine ventral to the transverse process of C6, C7, or T1.[75] When the diagnostic block is well placed, a disturbance in the sympathetic supply of the ipsilateral eye (Horner's syndrome) is observed: miosis, enophthalmos, and ptosis (Figure 4–103).

With positive trial results, block of the stellate ganglion can be repeated several times with a local anesthetic. In the authors' opinion, chemical neurolysis is not performed because of long-lasting side effects (eye symptoms and difficulty swallowing).

Regional physical neurolysis, on the other hand, is possible using an RF lesion. One can choose between an RF lesion medial to the transverse processes of C6, C7, and T1 or a lesion of the thoracic sympathetic chain lateral to the vertebral bodies of T1 and T2. The first technique is still in an experimental stage; the thoracic percutaneous block of the sympathetic chain is more common. Besides the above-mentioned procedures, there is also the possibility of a cervicothoracic sympathectomy.

Block of the Lumbar Sympathetic System

Indications for this procedure are similar to those mentioned for the cervicothoracic sympathetic system: vascular and neurological disturbances of the lower extremity. In practice, inoperable disturbances in vascularization of the leg are the most important indications. Again a block of the sympathetic chain is a treatment of second choice; improvement of the vascularization by conservative methods or vascular reconstruction are always considered first.

The lumbar sympathetic nervous system is located ventrolateral to the vertebral bodies of L2, L3, and L4; a trial block using lidocaine is not extremely stressful for the patient.

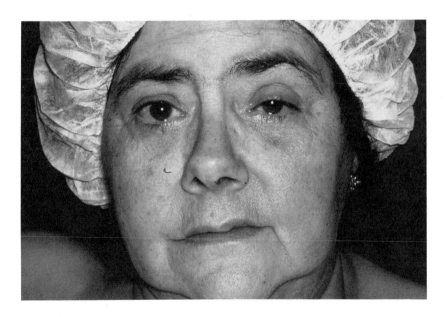

Figure 4–103 Horner's syndrome.

Chemical neurolysis is possible here and is usually performed using a 6.5% solution of phenol in water. Surgical sympathectomy is also possible.

Unfortunately, the results of a chemical sympathectomy, as well as those of a surgical sympathectomy, are often poor. However, at this stage of the disease, an amputation is the only alternative. Thus, a more conservative treatment method is worth consideration.

Technique

Many of the above-described blocks require a highly specified set of instruments. With all forms of block in and around the spinal column, resuscitation equipment should be available. Just as important, physicians should know how to use it.

In nerve blocks, the use of needles with a short and somewhat dull point (short bevel) are generally preferred in order to prevent direct mechanical damage to the peripheral nerves. For exact positioning, usually a form of nerve stimulation is required.

Epidural blocks fall mostly within the competence of the anesthesiologist because of the danger of penetration of the needle through the dura into the cerebrospinal fluid. If this false position of the needle is not noticed and the block takes place, severe hemodynamic and respiratory complications can arise, demanding immediate treatment.

Caudal epidural injections can also be technically difficult because of the highly interindividual anatomical variations in this region. The chance of penetration of the dural sac is much smaller (but indeed possible). When all the necessary precautions are taken, the chance of complications is minimal and the treatment can be performed on an outpatient basis.

In chemical neurolysis of the lumbar sympathetic nervous system and RF lesions of the zygapophyseal joints, block of the dorsal root ganglion or the cervicothoracic sympathetic nervous system should be performed with the use of nerve stimulation—neurophysiological control. Direct radiological imaging—anatomical control—should also be used. In particular, the RF lesions require highly specialized equipment, a lesion generator and injection needles especially developed for this method. In practice, these blocks should only be performed in specialty centers where enough technical experience has been acquired.

For the time being, it is debatable whether various forms of blocks should be performed by a surgical procedure or by percutaneous neurolysis using a needle. The superiority of one technique over the other will be difficult to prove with concrete evidence. However, controlled-effect studies are necessary. For the patient, percutaneous neurolysis is almost always a less stressful procedure than surgery. Surgery can always be considered in instances of unsatisfactory results with percutaneous neurolysis.

Summary

For each of the above-described block techniques, the considerations mentioned in the introduction should always be kept in mind. In the treatment of musculoskeletal soft tissue lesions, nerve blocks add support to the total package of possible measures (physical therapy, manual therapy, occupational therapy, psychological support, etc) and cannot be seen as a separate entity. In this context, the nerve block techniques can be considered a valuable tool in dealing with certain handicapping acute and chronic syndromes of the lumbar spine.

SCLEROSING INJECTIONS FOR INSTABILITY IN THE LOWER LUMBAR SPINE

In the realm of orthopaedic medicine, the treatment method of sclerosing ligaments and capsules of the lumbar zygapophyseal joints is not frequently applied. In this procedure, an irritating substance is injected into the structures contributing to the passive stability of the lumbar spinal column. The sclerosing substance, a phenol-dextrose-glycerin solution, causes a local inflammation resulting in a permanent contraction of the injected structures. At the same time, destruction of the local nociceptive innervation occurs.

Indications

- Frequent recurrent disc protrusions
- Ligamentous instability
- Traumatic ligamentous sprain without instability
- Unstable spondylolytic spondylolisthesis
- Unstable SI joint

In instances of a recurring disc protrusion, the patient should be treated first by means of manual mobilization or traction in order to alleviate any deviated position of the lumbar spine and to allow for full and painless range of motion.

Composition of the injected substance is as follows:

- phenol, 2.0% to 2.5%
- dextrose, 20% to 25%
- glycerin, 20% to 25%
- pyrogen-free water, up to 100%, mixed in a ratio of 5:1 with a local anesthetic (2% solution)

Injection Technique

The patient lies supine on the treatment table with a small pillow under the abdomen in order to position the lumbar spine in slight kyphosis. The cranial and caudal borders of the spinous processes of S1, L5, and L4 are localized.

First Treatment

A 10-mL syringe and a 6-cm long, thin needle are used for this injection. The needle is inserted between the spinous processes of L5 and S1. First, the supraspinous collagenous connections are injected, dropletwise, at their insertions on the spinous processes of L5 and S1, as well as in their midportions. At each location (at the insertions as well as intraligamentous), 0.5 mL of the sclerosing solution is injected. The insertions are reached, and subsequently injected, only when the needle touches bone after piercing through the sturdy collagenous resistance.

Next, injection of the interspinous ligament is performed. Here, too, both the intraligamentous portion and the insertions are injected. The ligaments between L4 and L5 are then treated in a similar way.

Finally, both superior iliolumbar ligaments are treated, by which only the insertion at the iliac crest is injected. First the spinous process of L5 and then the iliac crest at the same level are located. At the iliac crest, the needle is inserted in a ventrolateral direction until the ilium is reached. Upon reaching the ligamento-osseous junction of the superior iliolumbar ligament, 0.5 mL is injected (Figure 4–104).

Second Treatment

One week after the first treatment, the second treatment takes place. During this session, the zygapophyseal joints of L4-5 and L5-S1 are injected. The goal of this treatment is not only to facilitate contracture but also to "desensitize" the capsule.

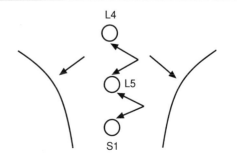

Figure 4–104 Injection sites for the first treatment.

Upon locating the spinous processes of L5 and S1, a needle is inserted perpendicularly, 2 cm lateral to the midpoint of a line connecting both spinous processes. If correctly located, the firm resistance of the zygapophyseal joint capsule is felt before contacting bone. At that point, 1 mL of the solution is injected. The procedure is repeated on the other side.

Next, the needle is inserted perpendicularly, 1.5 cm lateral to the midpoint of a line connecting both spinous processes of L4 and L5 (Figure 4–105, line *a*) The zygapophyseal joints between L4 and L5 are injected in a similar manner (Figure 4–106).

Third Treatment

The third treatment is a repetition of the first procedure and is given 1 week after the second treatment.

Because the final contraction of the scar generally occurs 3 weeks later, the patient should try to maintain a normal lumbar lordosis as much as possible during this period. After the injection, the patient experiences pain for only a short while—generally about 1 minute—but complains mostly of a hypersensitive back the entire day after the injections.

SURGICAL TREATMENTS

Surgery for Herniated Nucleus Pulposus

Most herniations are found in the lower two lumbar segments. In 1934, for the first time, Mixter and Barr described the intervertebral disc prolapse as a possible cause for low back pain.[1]

Examination Methods

A patient with symptoms indicating a lumbar disc prolapse should undergo radiological examination of the lumbar spine, sacrum, and pelvis in order to ascertain the architecture of the spinal column and also to exclude other

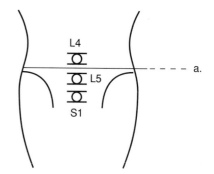

Figure 4–105 Localization of the zygapophyseal joints of L4-5 and L5-S1.

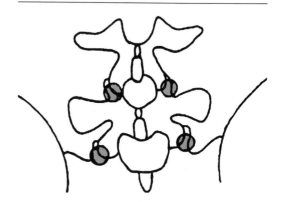

Figure 4–106 Injection sites for the second treatment.

possible disorders. Although not always necessary for the diagnosis of a prolapsed disc, a myelogram is important in preparing for the surgical treatment.

Computed tomography (CT), with or without contrast medium, can be of great help in the preparation for surgery because not only the disc prolapse but also a spinal stenosis can be causing the radicular syndrome. A lateral recess stenosis is better demonstrated on a CT scan than with a classic myelogram.

Indications

Everyone agrees that delicate treatment of the tissue structures during surgery is necessary for a good final result. However, the exact indication for the surgery is more important than the operative method itself. One can distinguish between absolute and relative indications for surgical treatment of the lumbar disc prolapse.

Absolute indications are as follows:

- large central protrusion, resulting in severe and sudden paresis or paralysis of the extremities or bladder
- increasing neurological deficit

In these cases, immediate surgical intervention generally is required. However, in most cases the indications are not quite as clear. A gray zone of relative indications may be encountered, such as

- absence of or inadequate reaction to the appropriate conservative treatment
- recurrent sciatica, causing a severe negative influence on the life and work activities of the patient

Among surgeons there is not a consensus as to what constitutes adequate conservative treatment. Fair surgical results are mainly found in the less–well-defined area of relative indications. The success of disc surgery depends not only on a good nerve root decompression but also on an actual prolapse, which should be confirmed during surgery.

Nachemson and Rydevik[76] state that international and national (Sweden) comparisons of frequencies of surgery for disc herniations may indicate that surgery is performed two to four times too often in the United States.[77] This means a substantial cost to society, which is further increased by the number of so-called failed backs. Again, international comparisons demonstrate a failed-back rate of approximately 15% in North America, but of no more than 5% in some Western European societies.[78]

No studies demonstrate a particular superiority among the present commonly used surgical interventions[31]; on the contrary, one published study[79] found no difference. Nor is there any support for performing a fusion along with an ordinary discectomy for a herniation in the lumbar spine.

All the new methods, such as percutaneous laser disc surgery, lumbar microdiscectomy, and automated percutaneous discectomy, have been supported only by short-term biased follow-ups of small patient groups for a limited period. At the present time none of these methods can be recommended.[31]

Surgical Procedure

As mentioned above, along with the proper indication for surgery, the surgical technique is also important for the final result. For clarification, a few surgical terms are defined below.

Laminectomy entails the removal of the bone between the base of the spinous process and an area approximately 1 cm medial to the zygapophyseal joint (Figure 4–107 C). The pars interarticularis remains. When a bilateral laminectomy is performed, the laminae at both sides are removed, including the spinous process (Figure 4-107A).

If a laminectomy is combined with a *facetectomy*, the lamina is removed at the base of the spinous process, including the articular process and a part of the superior articular process of the caudally adjacent vertebra (Figure 4–107B). In this way, a complete unilateral decompression is obtained, and two spinal nerves are fully "deroofed."

When a laminectomy is combined with a *foraminotomy*, less bone is removed. In a foraminotomy, besides the laminectomy, the pars interarticularis and only a part of the articular process are removed.

Laminotomy entails the removal of a *part* of one lamina. In classic disc surgery, bone from the two adjacent laminae is removed; it is actually more appropriate to use the term *bilaminotomy*. (Figure 4–107D).

Recently there has been a clear trend to remove as little bone as possible in disc surgery. This technique often uses the so-called mini-approach. The surgeon uses a magnifying glass or a surgical microscope. Postoperative recovery time is much less after surgery through the mini-approach. In keeping the

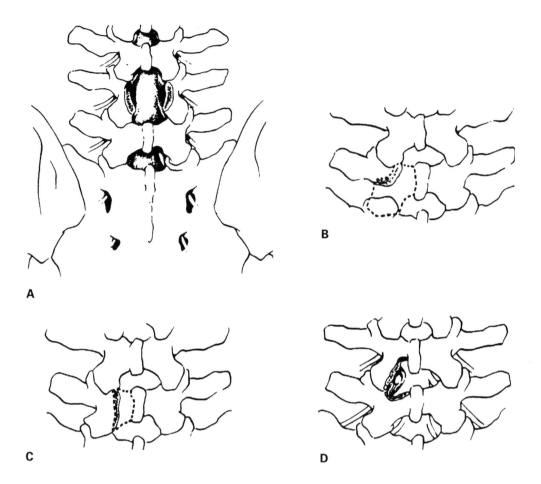

Figure 4–107 *A*, Bilaminectomy; *B*, laminectomy combined with facetectomy; *C*, laminectomy; *D*, bilaminotomy for a classic discectomy.

soft tissue traumatization and bleeding to a minimum, the postoperative immobilization period can also be shortened.

When applying the mini-approach, it is extremely important to mark radiologically the affected level preoperatively. Poor results from surgery are often related to an approach at the wrong level.

Technique

The position of the patient on the operation table, either in prone or in sidelying, is of significance in relation to the occurrence of bleeding. The sidelying position bears an im-

portant advantage in that less hematogenic stasis will occur. On the other hand, the prone position offers a better overview of the surgical field. Flexing the spinal column brings the spinous processes and the laminae away from each other. Pressure on the abdomen and chest can be decreased by using one of the frames available on the market in different variations. The knee-chest position is obsolete because of the high incidence of vascular damage in this position.

In a laminotomy, the skin incision is made midline over the spinous processes. If only the affected side is operated on, the fascia is cut in the same direction approximately 1 to 2 cm lateral to the spinous process. For the most part, the ligamentum flavum is removed. At the affected level, the epidural fat has usually disappeared or has been transformed into stiff connective tissue. In order to reach the disc material, the nerve root is held aside medially. In rare cases, disc material is found at the medial side of the nerve root as well. In this instance, it is often necessary first to remove a part of this material before moving the nerve root aside. Strong muscle contractions frequently occur even if the nerve root is handled with extreme care. In cases of a disc prolapse, the root often demonstrates signs of irritation: it is red and swollen. However, this is not always the case, particularly if the compression has already existed for a long period.

Surgeons have not reached a consensus regarding how much disc material should be removed. Some surgeons limit themselves to removing only the prolapsed part itself, while others excise as much of the disc as possible.

Caution is recommended when inserting the instruments into the disc space, in order to avoid damaging important vascular structures at the ventral part of the spinal column (the abdominal aorta or common iliac arteries).

If a prolapse is not encountered, but instead only a diffuse "bulging" at the affected level, no disc material should be removed. Empirically it has been found to be related to poor final results.

The wound is closed with the spinal column in a flexed position. When the fascia is closed with the spine in a straight position, rigidity results and the patient is unable to bend forward for weeks to months. Incision of the fascia a few centimeters lateral to the spinous process and closure of the wound with the spine flexed allow for less pain in the patient's back and less mechanical stress on the wound as well. After the operation, the patient should remain in a supine position for 24 hours.

Surgery for Spinal Stenosis

In 1954, Verbiest[80] described the case histories of seven male patients with a radicular syndrome. During surgery, he encountered general narrowing of the spinal canal, which he determined probably occurred during the individual's development. He termed this type of narrowing "developmental stenosis." These patients experienced an onset of their symptoms at adult age; the caudal equina was almost always involved. The normal lumbar spinal canal has the form of a pentagon with the largest diameter between the pedicles; these patients demonstrated a normal interpedicular space, but there was a narrowing apparent in the sagittal direction.

Other authors have reported a compression of the nerve root in the lateral recess of a spinal canal with normal dimensions. In these cases, pathological changes were found, especially at the zygapophyseal joints. Decompression resulted in decreased symptoms.

As an individual ages a certain amount of narrowing of the spinal canal is not unusual. Therefore, older people may experience some discomfort when lying prone. This could be due to a combination of a small narrowing of the spinal canal and the position of hyperextension. An uncomfortable feeling is created by slight pressure on the nerve roots. Only when this discomfort occurs more regularly in normal daily life do patients seek help from the physician.

Diagnosis

Classic symptoms indicating a spinal stenosis include the following:

- Pain occurs in the low back with claudication- or sciatic-like symptoms in one or both legs.
- The pain occurs chiefly in standing, decreases to a certain degree in lying, and is even less in sitting.
- There is a gradual decrease in symptom-free walking distance.

- Cramps occur in the calves when walking even short distances.
- There is onset of paresthesia and numbness in the legs if the walking is continued.
- Walking uphill is easier and accompanied with milder symptoms than walking downhill.
- The gait pattern becomes hesitant.
- A minimal hyperextension of the lumbar spine causes pain and is sometimes impossible to perform.
- In general, the patient is older than 50 years of age.

In diagnosing spinal stenosis, the case history and radiological examination by means of a CT scan (with or without contrast medium) are important. The primary goal of surgery is to decrease pressure on the neural elements within the central canal or lateral recess. As a result of such decompression surgery, a decrease in the nerve root pain occurs. In other words, the pain or the cramps experienced in the legs will decrease or disappear. The effect on the back pain in such a procedure is less predictable. Often the back pain remains.

Indications

Compression of a nerve root within the central canal or lateral recess can be due to degenerative changes usually involving several levels. In this instance, however, the surgical treatment is only directed at freeing the nerve root.

Thus, in order to prevent disappointment postsurgically, it is extremely important to explain to the patient preoperatively that the decompression surgery is exclusively directed at decompressing the nerve root and decreasing the leg complaints. Decrease of the back problems should be interpreted as a possible bonus. Surgery is *not* advisable if the back pain is the patient's chief complaint.

After failure of conservative treatment the main indication for performing decompression surgery in patients with back pain due to narrowing of the central canal or lateral recess resulting from degenerative changes is the presence of continuous or intermittent radiating pain in one or both legs distal from the knee that is accompanied by obvious functional disturbances and/or progressive neurological deficit.

Technique

Many techniques for a facetectomy[81-85] are described. Getty et al[86] describe a new technique in order to perform a decompression with preservation of spinal stability (Figure 4–108).

The spinal canal is opened through a laminotomy at the level of the root compression, as determined through clinical and radiological examination. If other changes are found within the spinal canal, these are dealt with at the same time. With the help of a dissector, a bone dimple at the medial aspect of the pars interarticularis is localized and then removed. Now the roof over the root canal (lateral recess) is opened. The nerve root is then identified and the direction of the root canal determined. The origin of the nerve root from the dural sac has to be identified as well.

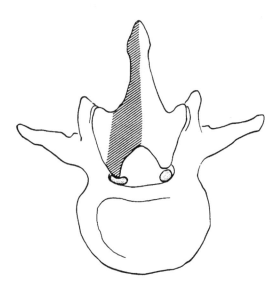

Figure 4–108 A form of spinal stenosis. The shaded area is removed for decompression.

For this purpose, it is sometimes necessary to remove more bone from the lamina.

The lateral recess is then decompressed using an osteotome. The osteotome is oriented in a slightly oblique direction, approximately in line with the nerve. This is more or less parallel to the longitudinal axis of the spinal canal. After the osteotome reaches the plane of the superior articular process (in front of the inferior articular process), the osteomed fragment is detached by a slight turn and then removed with a rongeur. Next, a part of the superior articular process is removed in the same manner; this part is also removed with a rongeur.

In order to obtain a total decompression it is sometimes necessary to remove osteophytes originating from the vertebral body at the ventral aspect of the nerve root. Although not a simple procedure, it is possible through this approach.

After the operation the patient should remain in the supine position for 24 hours.

Lumbar Spinal Fusion (Spondylosyndesis)

In recent years, the significance of spondylosyndesis in the treatment of degenerative changes in the spinal column has been the subject of critical scrutiny.[87] For years, it was assumed that a well-performed spondylosyndesis automatically meant relief of back pain symptoms. If the pain was persistent, a re-exploration and, if necessary, a re-arthrodesis were performed. In children or young adults with spondylolisthesis, spinal fusion generally has good clinical results. This is also true for a fracture of a vertebra or in cases of tuberculosis. However, the value of the spondylosyndesis in patients with degenerative changes in which pain is the primary complaint is limited.

Spondylolisthesis

The term *spondylolisthesis*, the ventral slipping of one vertebra in relation to the other, is derived from the Greek words *spondyl* (vertebra) and *olisthanein* (to slip). The spondylolisthesis can be classified into five types[44]:

1. the *dysplastic* type, a congenital abnormality in the upper part of the sacrum or the arch of L5.
2. the *isthmic* type, a lesion of the interarticular part (pars interarticularis); this type of spondylolisthesis can be classified further into three subgroups:
   (a) a lytic fatigue fracture of the pars interarticularis
   (b) an elongation of the intact pars interarticularis
   (c) an acute fracture of the pars interarticularis
3. the *degenerative* type, caused by a long-standing intersegmental instability
4. the *traumatic* type, a bony fracture at parts other than the pars interarticularis.
5. the *pathological* type, caused by a general or local bone disease

In people younger than 40 years of age, the isthmic spondylolisthesis of the lytic subtype is the most often occurring form of spondylolisthesis. The onset of slipping seldom occurs after age 20 and usually takes place between the ages of 9 and 15. The disorder can be confirmed on plain X-rays: AP, lateral, and oblique views.

In children as well as in adults, the spondylolisthesis generally can be treated conservatively; however, if complaints persist, surgical treatment should be considered.

In deciding to perform surgery, there are some critical differences to consider concerning a child versus an adult. In a child, the spondylolisthesis can worsen; this in itself can be a reason for performing surgery even without evidence of pain. Because the slipping in spondylolisthesis almost never increases after the age of 20, this indication does not apply for an adult. Another important difference between a child and an adult is that an adult is more easily able to adapt his or her activities to the pain tolerance. A child cannot do this; thus, despite adequate conservative therapy, if complaints of pain persist, this can be an appropriate reason to perform an earlier spondylosyndesis.

Dorsal Spondylosyndesis

One of the most commonly used techniques by which to fuse one or two segments is posterolateral spondylosyndesis (Figure 4–109).

Technique. The position on the operating table is similar to that for a laminectomy: it is performed with the patient either in prone or in sidelying. The incision in the skin can be performed at the midline over the spinous processes or bilaterally paraspinal, approximately 4.5 cm lateral to the spinous processes.

The main advantage to the lateral approach is that the tip of the transverse process can be approached more easily. Some surgeons perform the skin incision at the midline and then at the subcutaneous level penetrate bilaterally through the fascia and the underlying muscles at a distance of 4.5 cm. For this purpose the skin incision has to be lengthened, both caudally and cranially. The muscles are shifted, subperiostally, from the spinous processes and laminae, and the capsule is removed from the zygapophyseal joints. At this point the transverse processes can be palpated.

The transverse process is localized at a level between both articular processes; in other words, the transverse process of L5 is localized just caudal to the superior articular process of L5. After the transverse process is found, it is stripped of its soft tissues. Fracturing the transverse process must be avoided. Next, approximately two thirds of the facet joint is excised and an avivement (roughening) is performed on the lamina. Corticospongious bone grafts are taken from the ilium and are placed on the roughened areas.

The patient should be monitored closely for 24 hours postoperatively. After a few days the patient may begin activities while wearing an immobilizing corset.

When the procedure is performed on one segment, posterolateral spondylosyndesis offers a success rate of about 94% regarding the bony fusion. An 83% success rate is achieved when two segments are fused using this procedure.[88] This particular fusion technique is not recommended for more than two levels. Without application of an internal fixation system, an undesirably high percentage of pseudoarthrosis will occur.

Ventral Spondylosyndesis

Approaching the spinal column from the ventral aspect can be indicated for several

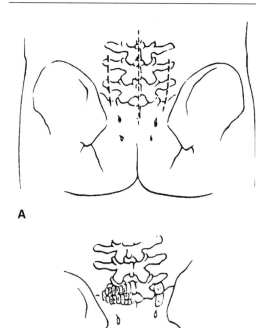

A

B

Figure 4–109 A, Posterolateral spondylosyndesis. If desired, one can perform the skin incision at the midline and then, after opening the skin and the subcutaneous tissue, incise the paramedian fascia. **B**, Placement of the bone graft.

reasons, including performing a ventral decompression of the spinal canal for injury due to a fracture, tumor, or inflammatory mass whereby a spondylosyndesis is performed simultaneously.

For disc pathology or spondylolisthesis, the anterior fusion of two vertebral bodies is generally not accepted. In these instances, the success rate in obtaining a solid fusion is lower than it is in a dorsal approach, especially in inexperienced hands.

Also, the possibility of eventual complications is higher with this approach than with the dorsal procedure. One of the more serious complications is impotence, reported in almost all studies dealing with anterior interbody (corporal) fusion. In most cases it is a temporary phenomenon; complete recovery is generally seen after 1 or 2 years. Nevertheless, the chance of such a complication should be discussed preoperatively with the patient.

Technique. The ventral aspect of the spinal column can be approached transperitoneally or retroperitoneally. For the *transperitoneal approach*, the patient is positioned supine with the lumbar spine hyperextended. This can be done by lowering the ends of an adjustable table or by placing an inflatable pillow in the lumbar region. A longitudinal incision along the midline of the lower abdomen, or a transverse incision, is made. After identifying the rectus sheath, this is opened as well. Directly underneath the rectus sheath the peritoneum is localized and opened very carefully. Through palpation, the abdominal aorta and the common iliac arteries are located, and the peritoneum is then opened posteriorly. The spinal column is now visible.

A ventral spondylosyndesis of the lumbar spine can also be performed through a *retroperitoneal left flank approach*. For this purpose, the patient is in sidelying in a decubitus position. The incision is made along the midaxillary line in the direction of the rectus sheath; the level depends on the segment of the spinal column to be operated upon. In this approach the spondylosyndesis can easily be performed between the levels of T12 and L5.

After the spinal column is made visible through one of the approaches described above, the prominences of the discs appear like small hills, and the lumbar artery and vein are found at the valley of the vertebral body.

At the level of the fusion, the lumbar artery and vein are ligated and cut. After this the disc is excised whereby close attention is given in order not to cut the posterior longitudinal ligament. The end-plates of the vertebral bodies at both sides are then removed with an osteotome. The disc space is now filled from ventral or dorsal with bone graft (Figure 4–110). Some surgeons use bone from the iliac crest; others prefer to take bone chips from the fibula.

After closing the wound the patient is monitored in a supine position. Depending on the status of the patient, activities (with the support of a corset) are begun after a few days. Until a solid fusion is confirmed radiographically, the corset should be worn.

Considerations

Turner et al[88] undertook a systematic literature synthesis concerning the outcomes of lumbar spinal fusion. The most remarkable finding of this review was the wide range of successful outcomes (ranging from 16% to 95%). It is unclear whether this represents true differences in clinical success rates or simply differences in study design.

Turner and his colleagues list several conclusions from their meta-analysis of the results of lumbar spine fusion, including the following:

- The indications for lumbar spondylosyndesis are not scientifically established.

- There is a wide range of satisfactory outcomes. Because of study design flaws and the possibility of publication bias, the average success rate of 68% may

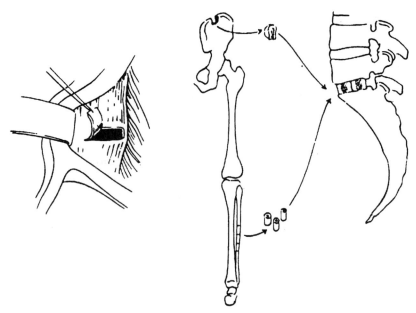

Figure 4–110 Intercorporal (interbody) spondylosyndesis. Both the ilium and the fibula can serve as donor sites.

overestimate the actual clinical results.
- There is little support for one fusion technique over the others.
- Randomized controlled trials are necessary to compare fusion with other surgical and nonsurgical approaches to the various lumbar spine disorders.

Reposition of a Spondylolisthesis

Many have attempted to reposition a severe spondylolisthesis.[89] However, the main problem is in maintaining the obtained repositioning. Thanks to modern internal fixation systems, this has become more and more possible. Repositioning is indicated only in cases of severe slipping, greater than 50%.

In performing the repositioning, it is indisputable that a better cosmetic result will be obtained. However, the important question remains whether this reposition will be safe and therefore worthwhile. If the main problem is only that the hamstrings are too tight, a spondylosyndesis in situ is sufficient. In the

following weeks and months the shortening will disappear on its own. Of course, the trunk remains shortened.

The greatest danger in attempting a reposition is development of a neurological complication. Therefore, the patient should weigh whether a cosmetic improvement is worth the risk of a possible neurological complication.

Repositioning a spondylolisthesis can be performed in various ways. Scaglietti et al[84] described a cast reduction technique: after establishing the reposition, a stabilizing procedure was performed as shown in Figure 4–111.

The reposition can also be obtained during the stabilizing surgery. In this case, a dorsal approach can be used. First a form of decompression is performed in order to offer the nerve roots at the involved level enough space, then repositioning and fixation are carried out.

The surgeon can also choose to combine the ventral and dorsal approach. By excising the disc and necessary bone, space is created to achieve the reposition. Fixation from the

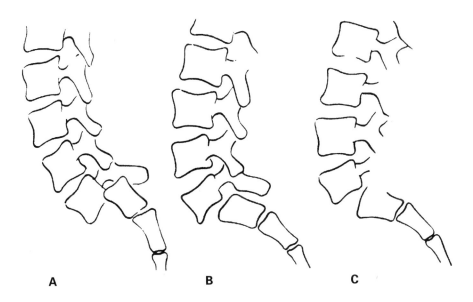

A   **B**   **C**

Figure 4–111 *A*, Severe spondylolisthesis, L5-S1I; *B*, reposition according to cast method of Scaglietti et al[84]; *C*, fixation with a Harrington system.

dorsal aspect follows. The obtained reposition must be maintained; for that reason, use of an internal fixation system is of utmost importance.

Different options also exist for internal fixation. The Harrington fixation system is well known. One can also use the Luque system. Pedicle screws and plates have recently become available in order to obtain a good internal fixation.

Degenerative Spondylolisthesis

In a degenerative spondylolisthesis, also called pseudospondylolisthesis, there is no lysis in the neural arch but rather widespread degenerative changes in the zygapophyseal joints and the disc. A study by Rosenberg[36] showed that degenerative spondylolisthesis is seen 10 times more often at the L4-5 level than at L5-S1 or L3-4. The incidence is approximately six times higher in women than in men. Sacralization is four times more common in people with degenerative spondylolisthesis than in the general population. Furthermore, there is a three times higher incidence of degenerative spondylolisthesis in black women than in white women.

In cases of degenerative spondylolisthesis, the surgical treatment is directed toward decompression of the neural elements, as described under Spinal Stenosis. The danger for further slipping exists only if an extensive decompression is performed with a complete facetectomy or if, during the decompression, the disc is excised as well. In these instances the decompression should be combined with a spondylosyndesis. Thus one may choose to perform a posterolateral fusion of one or two segments or, in some cases, a fusion of several segments using an internal fixation system. An anterior intercorporal spondylosyndesis can also be performed. (See Ventral Spondylosyndesis for more information.)

CHEMONUCLEOLYSIS

Introduction

Chymopapain (Discase, Chymodiactin) is a protein-dissolving enzyme originating from the latex of the tropical melon tree (*Carica papaya*). If chymopapain is injected into the core of the lumbar intervertebral disc (nucleus pulposus lumbalis), it causes a fast depolymerization of the noncollagen basic substance, which consists mainly of proteoglycans. The water-binding capacity of the nucleus decreases, resulting in a decrease in intradiscal pressure and volume.

Smith,[90] in 1964, was the first to publish findings regarding the use of chymopapain in patients with herniated discs. If the term *hernia nuclei pulposi lumbalis* is interpreted literally, it is clear that complaints of this disorder are caused by nuclear material. Due to degeneration of the annulus fibrosus, a weakening develops, causing an unequal distribution of the pressure arising from normal physiological loads. This can lead to a very local overload, resulting in an asymmetrical protrusion of the annulus. In instances of a total rupture of the annulus, the nucleus prolapses outward. If it is possible to dissolve the nucleus chemically, then this should be the logical treatment.

This approach had been propagated by Barr, who is well known as one of the discoverers of the lumbar herniation. During a lecture in San Diego, California, in May 1961, Barr stated:

> Now that we can bring a needle within the intervertebral disc, it has to be possible to remove part of the collagenous tissue biochemically. I won't be surprised that one day surgery for the lumbar HNP [herniated nucleus pulposus] is totally or almost totally obsolete. The intervertebral disc consists of 90% water; why should we have to remove this surgically? As a matter of fact, I think it is a little bit ridiculous. I don't know how we are going to do it, but it has to be possible.

Smith[90] called the enzymatic dissolution of the nucleus pulposus "chemonucleolysis." Af-

ter Smith's first publications, chemonucleolysis was performed in the United States on more than 15,000 patients until 1974, when the enzyme was temporarily taken off the market. Large scientific, and especially political, discussions arose about the effectiveness of this treatment. In a double-blind study, there were no significant differences in results after treatment with Discase or placebo.

Since then the discussion between those favoring and those opposing chemonucleolysis continued. Then, in 1982, a new-generation chymopapain (Chymodiactin) was approved for use in the United States. Chymodiactin is thermostable, in contrast to Discase.

In a very precise double-blind study, the results of treatment with Chymodiactin proved to be significantly better than results of treatment with placebo. Keep in mind that the effect of the placebo treatment is similar to the percentage of patients who demonstrate minimal to no complaints 6 months after onset, because of a spontaneous recovery.[91]

Chemonucleolysis can now be considered an accepted treatment method. Still, the discussion between convinced advocates and opponents persists.

Effect of Chymopapain; Toxicity

Chymopapain is a substance with a positive charge, causing an interaction with the negatively charged acid mucopolysaccharide of the disc. The result is that the chymopapain is immediately bound. Because of the resulting depolymerization of the basic substance, for the most part consisting of proteoglycans (acid mucopolysaccharides bound with polypeptides), the water-binding capacity of the nucleus decreases. In animals, the nucleus seems to disappear shortly after an injection of chymopapain. The annulus is not affected, unless an overdose is injected.

In a human when the injected disc was explored after chemonucleolysis, it proved to be empty. Electron microscopic examination of removed disc material no longer revealed any basic substance.[15] In the past, an inactive enzyme appeared to be the reason that some nucleus material was still found. The decreasing water-binding capacity of the nucleus can be nicely demonstrated through MRI. After chemonucleolysis, the signal of the nucleus pulposus gradually decreases until it has completely disappeared, after about 6 weeks.[92]

The action of chymopapain is fast and limited. The effect on the intervertebral disc is related to the dosage. Otherwise, a small amount of enzyme would have the same effect as a larger amount. The working action of the enzyme seems to be of short duration, because only in the first 3 days is there a fair increase in the secretion of acid mucopolysaccharides in the urine.

Recently, this was once again demonstrated by means of the enzyme-linked immunosorbent assay (ELISA) technique: keratan sulfate is a glycosaminoglycan, occurring only in the proteoglycan of cartilage, discs, and the cornea. Degeneration of proteoglycans led to demonstrable amounts of keratan sulfate in the serum. After 3 to 4 weeks, the amount of keratan sulfate normalized, again proof that the effect of chymopapain is fast and of short duration.[91]

Dolan et al[93] demonstrated that when chymopapain was injected into the intervertebral disc of human cadavers, the magnitude of prolapsed nuclear material decreased by 24% after 1 hour, and by 80% after 48 hours.

Obviously, with the decreased volume of the intervertebral disc, the disc narrows. Although in animal studies it was demonstrated that the nucleus disappeared quickly (in young animals a disc narrowing was radiographically visible after only a few days), it appears that narrowing of the disc in the treated human occurs 2 to 3 weeks after the injection. Thus, the disc is very vulnerable in the first weeks after treatment. The average narrowing in the human amounts to 30% after 6 weeks and to 35% after 3 months.[94]

In canine experiments, Bradford et al[95] demonstrated that after chemonucleolysis, the height of the intervertebral disc increased again after a certain period of time, to include a regeneration of normal disc material. Experiments with rabbits demonstrated that 6 months after injection with chymopapain, the intervertebral disc again contained proteoglycans with the same characteristics as the normal, nontreated intervertebral disc.

Regeneration of the intervertebral disc can also be observed in the treated human. It is visible on X-ray by an increase in disc space (re-expansion) (Figure 4–112). Biomechanically seen, the effect of chymopapain on the disc is obviously reversible. In the first instance, the disc becomes substantially less stiff, whereby particularly the resistance against torsion decreases. After 3 months, however, the biomechanical properties return to the same level as before the injection.[96]

Chymopapain does not have any influence on collagen unless it is administered in a very high concentration. In vivo, chymopapain does not have any influence on the structures surrounding the nucleus, such as the annulus fibrosus, the end-plates, and the dura mater. However, chymopapain is indeed toxic if it comes into contact with the subarachnoid space. In animal experiments, intrathecal injection of chymopapain caused bleeding that ultimately appeared to be lethal due to an increase in pressure of the cerebrospinal fluid. By normalizing this pressure, death could be prevented. The animals that survived did not demonstrate any neuropathological aberrations afterward. Arachnoiditis, in particular, was never found.

After approval of the enzyme in the United States, severe complications were reported, presumably in relation to needle trauma or injection of the chymopapain into the cerebrospinal fluid, causing bleeding within the central nervous system. Paraplegia, paraparesis, and other neurological reactions arose several hours to days after the

A

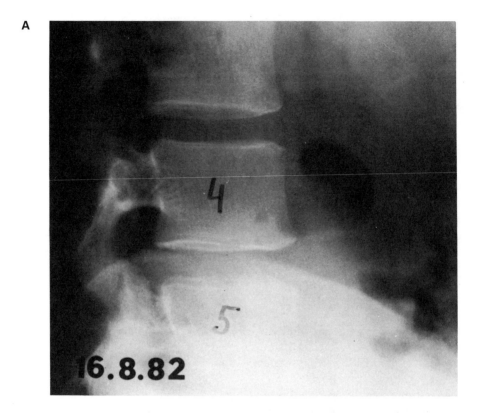

B

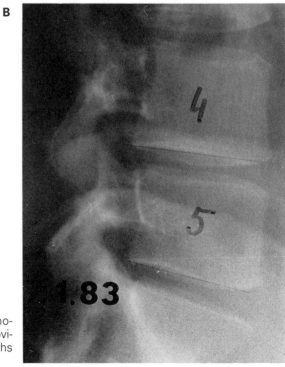

Figure 4–112 *A*, Disc height before chemonucleolysis, L4-5, in a 30-year-old man; ***B*,** obvious narrowing of the L4-5 disc space 3 months after chemonucleolysis.

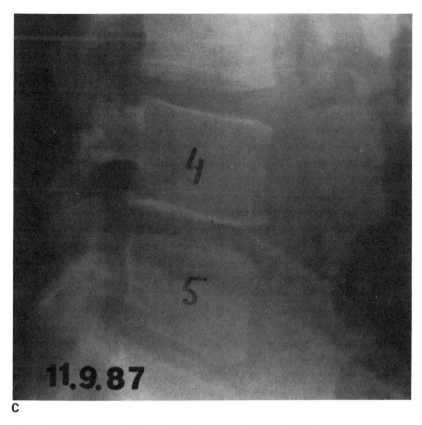

C

Figure 4–112 *C*, Re-expansion of the L4-5 disc 5 years after chemonucleolysis.

---

chemonucleolysis, in a ratio of approximately 1:2000.[97]

Since these severe complications and the presumable causes are generally known, they are no longer reported. In chimpanzees such complications were only encountered if the enzyme together with a contrast medium came into close contact with the cerebrospinal fluid. Afterward somewhat of a panic reaction led to the advice to discontinue performance of discography. Based on animal experiments and extensive clinical experience, when the technique is performed precisely, there is a significant difference between therapeutic and toxic doses; thus the chance for complications is extremely small.

Although chymopapain is a relatively weak antigen, it can give rise to acute life-threatening anaphylactic reactions. Initially, these anaphylactic reactions were reported in about 1% of the treated cases; of late this frequency has decreased. The incidence of such a response decreased from 1% to 0.5% in the United States, while the frequency in Europe amounts to 0.2%. In recent years, the mortality related to such a reaction has decreased from 1 in 5,000 to 1 in 30,000. The merit of skin testing and determining specific immunoglobulins before treatment is not clear.

In evaluating the complications described above, one has to realize that complications related to surgical treatment are seen in a much higher incidence, in relation to their severity as well as in the amount.

Indications

Chemonucleolysis is indicated in instances of a herniated nucleus pulposus (HNP). Certain criteria must be met in the diagnosis of the lumbar HNP in order for it to be an indication for chemonucleolysis:

- The leg (and buttock) pain is more dominant than the back pain.
- Neurological symptoms (paresthesia) are localized to a dermatome.
- There is a positive Lasègue sign. The SLR is limited because of provocation of the radicular pain.
- A contralateral Lasègue sign can also exist (provocation of pain in the symptomatic leg with SLR in the other leg).
- The often-described bowstring phenomenon is also typical of a lumbar HNP. In this test, at the point in the range of motion during the SLR test that pain is provoked, the knee is bent, resulting in a disappearance of the pain. While maintaining this position, the radiating pain reoccurs when pressure is exerted on the tibial nerve in the popliteal fossa. The test is negative if the patient indicates only local pain in the popliteal fossa.
- At least two of the following four neurological signs are apparent:
  1. atrophy of the affected leg
  2. weakness (especially of the extensor hallucis longus, L5 root)
  3. decreased sensation
  4. decreased reflex activity (especially of the Achilles tendon reflex, S1 root)
- There are changes on the myelogram, CT scan, or MRI confirming the clinical diagnosis.

Contraindications

An absolute contraindication for chemonucleolysis is the relatively rare cauda equina syndrome, which gives rise to disturbances of bowel and bladder functions. At the same time some reservation is appropriate in patients with the following conditions:

- a severe spondylolisthesis
- severe spinal stenosis
- diffuse degeneration of the disc without any symptoms of radicular irritation
- pregnancy
- arachnoiditis
- a proven segmental instability

Although different opinions exist concerning the application of chemonucleolysis in paresis and/or the suspicion of a loose fragment (sequestration), until now this has not been a contraindication for surgeons.

Until very recently, a previous application of chemonucleolysis was considered a contraindication for a second injection with chymopapain. However, in such cases the administration of histamine blockers before the procedure offers good protection, thus making a second chemonucleolysis treatment no longer a contraindication.

Chemonucleolysis treatment in regions other than the lumbar spine is still not sufficiently studied; therefore the treatment is still contraindicated in disorders of the thoracic and cervical spines.

Treatment

In deciding to perform a chemonucleolysis, patient education is very important. Patients must be aware that the treatment is more than just an "injection." They have to be prepared for a recovery period of 6 to 12 weeks. The effect of the treatment is in part immediate, but for full recovery the intervertebral disc, and with it the whole motion segment, needs several weeks to adapt to the new situation.

Chemonucleolysis is a treatment with a setup similar to that for surgery; this mainly counts for the sterile field. Furthermore, every precaution must be taken to prevent or to deal with an anaphylactic reaction. Therefore, the presence of an anesthesiologist is mandatory.

Chemonucleolysis has been performed in our clinic since 1980. The procedure has always been done with the patient under general anesthesia and endotracheal intubation. To prevent a possible anaphylactic reaction, the patient is premedicated with promethazine hydrochloride (25 mg) and then during treatment is given an infusion of glucose, saline, and hydrocortisone (200 mg/L). Although many surgeons prefer to perform the treatment with a form of local anesthesia, we have not yet changed our protocol. Because the patient is fully immobile under anesthesia, the surgeon can concentrate completely on the precise technique.

The technique itself is simple: The patient is positioned in sidelying. Through a lateral approach, 8 cm from the midline, an 18-gauge needle is inserted into the disc. With this approach the spinal canal is protected by the zygapophyseal joints (Figure 4–113). The position of the point of the needle is controlled in two directions. If the position of the needle is correct, discography is performed using a nonionizing contrast medium (iopamidol [Jopamiro]). With the injection of the contrast medium, a videotape is used that allows for repeated study of the discography. Furthermore, the discogram is recorded using the so-called subtraction technique (Figure 4–114).

When it is certain that the contrast medium arrived at the site of the bulging disc, chymopapain (Chymodiactin) is injected very slowly into the disc. It is important to perform the injection slowly, offering the opportunity for the enzyme to bind directly to the negatively charged acid mucopolysaccharides of the nucleus. During the injection of the enzyme, the chance for an anaphylactic reaction is the greatest. A few minutes after the injection, the intubation is removed, and the patient is placed under observation in the recovery room.

The organization of the procedure will differ from hospital to hospital. Whether the procedure is performed in the surgical department or the radiography department can be a

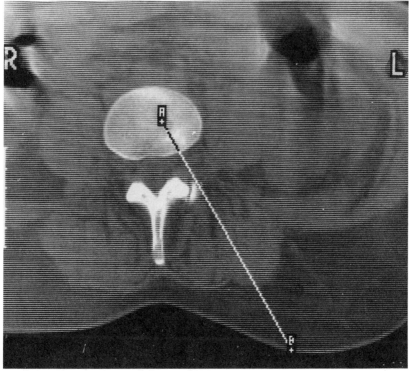

Figure 4–113 The trajectory of the needle is visible on this CT scan.

point of discussion. Obviously, in the operating room, because of the ruling discipline, sterility is more nearly guaranteed. On the other hand, there is a greater chance that the obtained X-rays will not be optimal. For the latter reason, we prefer operating in a room optimally equipped for angiography. This gives perfect radiological documentation, resulting in increased quality of the treatment and thus less chance for complications.

In our opinion, discography further improves the quality of the treatment. Injection of the enzyme into the annulus (whereby the enzyme does not come into contact with the nucleus) gives rise to a poorer outcome. On the other hand, a high correlation has been reported between the observation of the contrast medium in the area of the bulging disc and a good result of the treatment.[98] In addition, the availability of a discogram enhances documentation of the surgical procedure. At the same time there are rare cases in which the clinical findings indicate a herniated disc, but a CT scan and caudography do not sub-

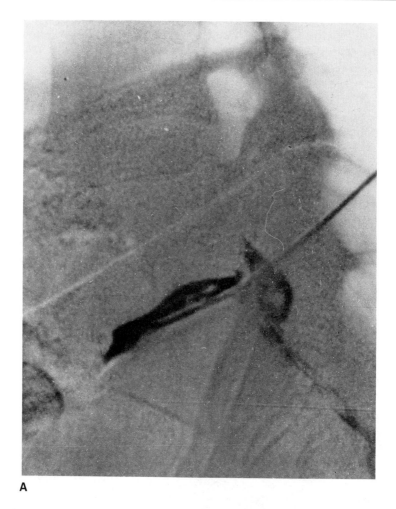

A

Figure 4–114 Subtraction view of a discogram of L5-S1 in a patient with a proven L5-S1 HNP at the right side. **A**, Lateral view. The contrast medium is clearly visible within and around the protruding disc. There is also some leakage of contrast medium along the posterior longitudinal ligament.

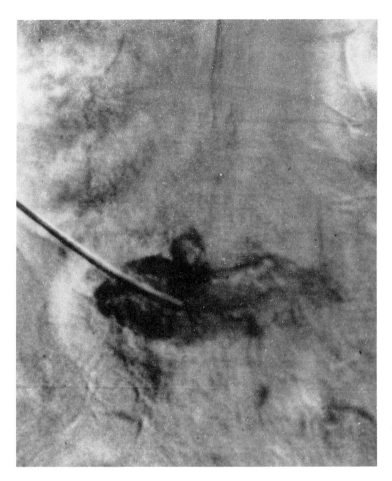

Figure 4–114 *B*, AP view. The needle comes from the right. On this somewhat oblique view, it is clearly evident that the contrast medium is projected paramedian at the right side, around and within the protruded nucleus.

stantiate this finding. A discogram can then provide the final confirmation of the diagnosis.

Relative to chemonucleolysis, discography alone does not have any proven negative influence on a normal intervertebral disc. Injection of contrast medium in rabbits did not cause any observable changes within the intervertebral disc. Follow-up studies in humans, through radiography and more recently through MRI, have also revealed that discography alone does not have any proven adverse effect on the intervertebral disc.[99]

Since some cases of severe neurological complications were observed in the United States, the manufacturers advised performing the procedure under local anesthesia, and the use of discography was discouraged. This was based on the fact that almost all of the complications occurred when the treatment was performed under general anesthesia whereby a discogram was also made. However, careful study of these complications revealed that often demonstrable technical mistakes were committed, causing contact of the enzyme and contrast medium with the subarachnoid space, which resulted in subarachnoidal bleeding.

We still prefer performing the procedure under general anesthesia, while the patient is constantly monitored. In a very large European study[100] even fewer complications were encountered in patients treated under general anesthesia.

There are indications that there is a negative influence of the contrast medium on the enzyme. If no changes are detectable on the discogram, there is no reason to inject the concerned disc.

One day after the treatment, the patient is able to start activities under the guidance of a physical therapist. An elastic orthopaedic corset is often beneficial in the first weeks. As a routine, the patient is administered diazepam (5 mg three times daily) and ibuprofen (200 mg three times daily). With this regimen the activation of the patient progresses very smoothly. The patient has to be reminded that he or she is not cured at that point, but on the way to recovery.

The patient can leave the hospital as soon as she or he prefers. Normally, this is the second day after the treatment. The average hospitalization time of patients undergoing chemonucleolysis in our facility in 1986 was 5.2 days (from day of admission to day of discharge).

Two to three weeks after the procedure, the patient should begin biking and swimming (backstroke). These activities enhance the recovery of the patient's physical condition during the period in which the vulnerable back is healing. After 6 weeks the patient further increases activities: emphasis is placed on physical conditioning and controlled flexibility exercises.

During the first weeks, it is impossible to predict the speed of the recovery. Later, when the patient looks back, he or she is often able to indicate a point when the recovery suddenly became apparent. This moment can vary from 1 week to several weeks.

When guiding the patient through the initial stage of recovery, it is important to emphasize the improvements and de-emphasize the residual complaints. Once improvement occurs, it is almost always followed by further improvement.

Complications

Chemonucleolysis may be called a safe procedure in our hands. After more than 1000 procedures performed in our region, severe complications have never been observed. There have been no instances of an anaphylactic reaction, the mortality rate is zero, and a temporary erythematosis occurred in only a small number of patients.

From the 780 patients treated in the orthopaedic department of the Roman Catholic Hospital in Groningen, from the period April 1980 to October 1, 1987, a bacterial discitis was encountered as a complication just once. In two patients there was an increase in the paresis of the extensor hallucis longus, which in one case was permanent and in the other reversible. A third patient, after 4 weeks, developed a total footdrop with severe dermatitis; fortunately this was only temporary. Some patients (usually female) reported temporary symptoms such as transient exanthema, urticaria, or itching several weeks after the treatment.

Thus, the chance for complications after chemonucleolysis is small. However, the rarely occurring more severe complications drew a significant amount of attention. After a very enthusiastic initial welcome, particularly in the United States, this led to a strong reduction in the application of chemonucleolysis. Perhaps this was due to the use of incorrect indications, which led to disappointing results, or it may be the consequence of the social climate that has risen from malpractice claims. Moreover, complications related to surgery of the lumbar HNP are generally not judged as strongly, even though they are usually more severe and occur more often. Of course it is important that complications be reported and analyzed. This has certainly led to further increases in the safety of chemonucleolysis.

Results

Assessing responses to treatment of a lumbar HNP is difficult. The indication for treatment almost always correlates with the amount of pain the patient is experiencing, while at the same time objective findings have to exist to support the diagnosis. In judging the final outcome, the patient's pain is the deciding factor; thus the result is not based solely on objective findings that may have resolved.

All the contemporary forms of treatment aim to relieve the irritation and/or compression of a nerve root. This does not necessarily mean that the treated disc and the whole motion segment will become normal again. On the contrary, one has to assume that there will be a degenerated motion segment as a residual situation. In a conservatively treated disc-related problem, this will also be the final status. Furthermore, comparison with the natural course of the disorder also has to be made. Actually, consensus is that a lumbar HNP is a self-limiting disease. In other words, after 10 years the average outcome of a treated patient versus an untreated patient shows no significant difference.

In every follow-up study one should note the time frame in which the follow-up is done, because further information can be obtained about the course of recovery. Some authors still have the opinion that the effect of the chemonucleolysis is nothing more than what would have occurred during the natural course of the disc disease. However, many authors agree with us that chemonucleolysis considerably accelerates the natural course. Furthermore, almost everyone is in agreement about the effect of chymopapain on the nucleus.

In a prospective CT study done by Konings et al,[101] it was demonstrated that the compression caused by the hernia had decreased in 20 of the 30 patients after 3 months, and that after 12 months the compression had disappeared in almost everyone (Figure 4–115) In relation to the narrowing of the intervertebral disc, a diffuse bulging of the annulus also occurred. None of the patients developed an epidural fibrosis, which is a well-known complication of surgical treatment. Experience

showed that the clinical recovery is often ahead of the radiological recovery.

In the past 7 years we performed several follow-up studies. Some of the studies were performed by independent examiners and included an extensive questionnaire. We used a classification system similar to those found in medical literature. The patient could choose to describe his or her recovery from the following categories:

- excellent (more than 85% improvement)
- good (50% to 85% improvement)
- fair (25% to 50% improvement)
- bad (no improvement).

In total, 384 patients (76.8%) scored excellent or good and 116 (23.2%) fair or bad. This questionnaire concerned 230 treatments with Discase and 270 with Chymodiactin.

From the first 300 patients treated with Chymodiactin with a follow-up of at least 6 months, 80% were considered successful (171 excellent, 68 good) and 20% were considered not successful (40 fair, 21 bad). The average age at time of treatment was 39 years (ranging from 14 to 73 years of age); in the patient group, 106 were female and 194 were male.

Assuming that there was in fact an indication for surgery in every patient, the success of the treatment can also be measured in the number of patients who required additional surgery after the chemonucleolysis. From the first 500 patients with a follow-up period of 0.5 to 5.5 years, 16 patients had undergone surgery once or twice (3.2%). Three patients (0.6%) underwent a repeated chemonucleolysis because of a recurrent radicular syndrome. This total of 19 patients is included in the category "unsuccessful."

Independent of the amount of success, some of the patients indicated that they experienced occasional pain in the back and/or leg. This pain mainly occurred during fatigue, which again emphasizes the necessity for good physical condition. In particular, the results in athletes generally were excellent. Among the treated patients were several soccer players from the highest division in the Netherlands. Other top athletes included professional golfers, basketball players, and Olympic handball players. It is widely known that one of the recent winners of the Wimbledon tennis tournament underwent a chemonucleolysis.

From the first 500 patients, 85% were no longer receiving medical or physical therapy treatment at the time of the follow-up study. Only 6% reported regular use of pain medication. Follow-up studies were also performed by independent examiners comparing the results in young patients, in patients 60 years and older, and in patients suspected of a having a sequestered disc. At an average of 24 months' follow-up of 18 patients with an average age of 14 to 19 years, the treatment result was rated good or excellent in 17 of the 18. In the meantime, none of the patients underwent further surgery. Other studies have also demonstrated the beneficial effect of chemonucleolysis in the juvenile lumbar HNP.

In contrast, it is assumed that chemonucleolysis is not an appropriate procedure in the treatment of older patients with lumbar HNP. For that reason, in 1978 we performed a follow-up study among patients older than 60 years. From the first 700 patients, 21 were older than 60 (average age 63 years and 11 months). Of the 21 patients only 1 had to undergo a facetectomy several months after the chemonucleolysis because of persisting complaints. There were no complications. After

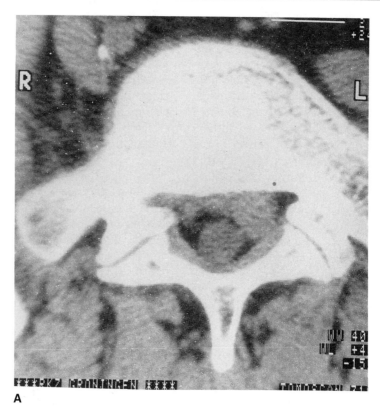

A

Figure 4–115 *A* and *B*, CT scan of a 60-year-old man, bedridden for several months due to a lumbar HNP of L5-S1, left.

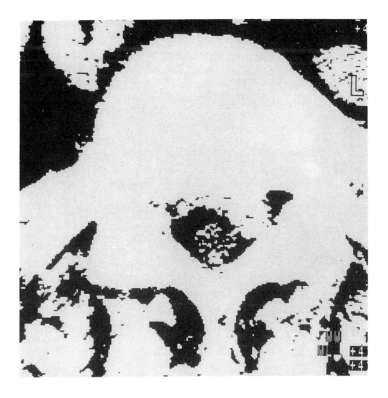

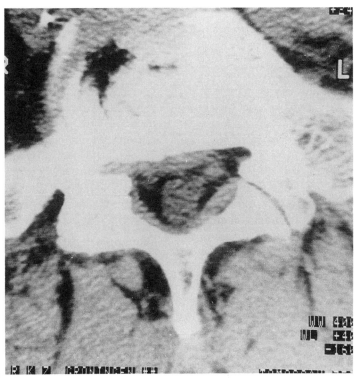

C

Figure 4–115 *C* and *D*, CT scan 4 years after chemonucleolysis. The patient is totally free of complaints, and the CT scan no longer indicates a herniation or epidural fibrosis. However, there are indications of disc degeneration, identifiable through the so-called vacuum phenomenon.

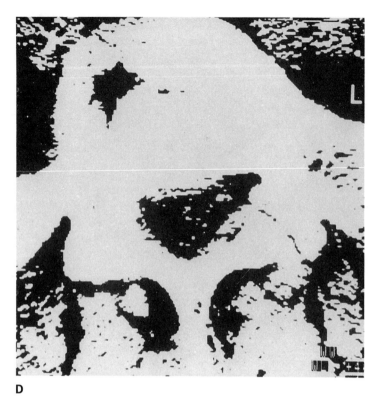

D

Figure 4–115 *C* and *D*, CT scan 4 years after chemonucleolysis. The patient is totally free of complaints, and the CT scan no longer indicates a herniation or epidural fibrosis. However, there are indications of disc degeneration, identifiable through the so-called vacuum phenomenon.

an average of 44 months (range 9 to 76 months), these patients were examined by an independent examiner. Two patients, in whom the results of the treatment were excellent, were deceased. In 15 of the remaining 18 patients, the results were excellent. There were no reported limitations during activities of daily living and there were no abnormal findings during the physical examination. In one patient the result was good (some residual back pain), and in two patients the result was classified as unsuccessful; however, they did not require further surgical treatment.

In 1986, we performed a retrospective radiological study in which localization of the herniation in relation to the intervertebral disc was determined. In the literature, some authors generalize that if the herniation is vis-

ible above or below the level of the disc, it is a contraindication for chemonucleolysis. From our study it can be concluded that there is no reason to exclude patients if the hernia is not visible at the level of the disc (Figure 4–116). Furthermore, if one interprets such a CT finding as a sequester, then a sequester is not a contraindication for chemonucleolysis.

Chemonucleolysis versus Surgery

Chemonucleolysis is still a heavily debated subject among its advocates and opponents. In comparing the results of chemonucleolysis and surgery, it is difficult to draw conclusions because many factors are involved that cannot be compared with each other.

Two regularly cited studies[102,103] demonstrate that chemonucleolysis is considerably less effective than surgery. The results of the chemonucleolysis in both of these series were so bad that the enzyme used in these studies (Discase) was examined afterward and was shown to be inactive.[98]

In a recently published study by Lavignolle et al[104] comparing the results of chemonucleolysis and microscopic surgery, no statistical significance was found. Postacchini et al[105] compared the results depending on the amount of nerve compression as determined by CT scan and/or caudography. Based on their study, they concluded that chemonucleolysis is the procedure of choice in small herniations and a good alternative procedure in average herniations, but that surgery offers better results in large herniations. However, the size of the latter group was very small.

Until now we have not found any reason not to perform chemonucleolysis in patients with a large herniation. In some patients the myelogram showed an almost complete block, but these patients enjoyed excellent treatment results after chemonucleolysis.

Publications written by skeptics will continue to appear in which it will be concluded that chemonucleolysis is not effective.[76] Several studies comparing surgical discectomy with chemonucleolysis have actually shown superior clinical results with surgery.[79,103,106–109] However, if a certain study shows that after chemonucleolysis, 20% of the patients still require surgery, this might reveal more about the treating physician than about the method. The physician has to learn to master the techniques of both discography and chemonucleolysis.

Because there are actual indications, based on many recent publications, for the effectiveness of chemonucleolysis, it is fair to state

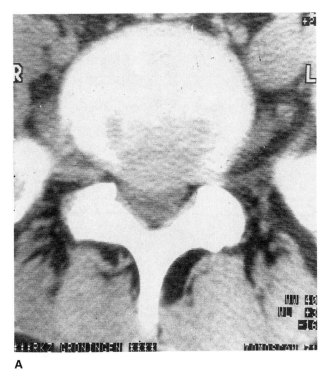

A

Figure 4–116 CT scan of a 24-year-old man. **A**, at the level of the L5-S1 disc no abnormalities are visible.

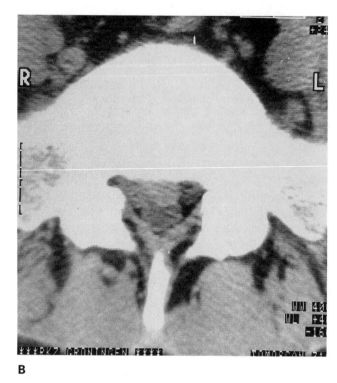

B

Figure 4–116 *B,* A large prolapse projected under the level of the disc and behind the sacrum. This is an excellent result after chemonucleolysis (follow-up period of over 1 year).

that after failure of conservative therapy in radicular irritation syndrome, two possibilities exist for treatment: chemonucleolysis and surgery. Each method has its advantages and disadvantages. The complications after chemonucleolysis are less in both quantity and severity; the spinal canal does not have to be opened, thus the proposition that chemonucleolysis is the last step in conservative treatment can be defended. Besides learning surgical techniques, surgeons should also learn chemonucleolysis in order to offer their patients a chance for optimal recovery. In surgery the spinal canal is opened, with all its advantages but also with disadvantages. Epidural fibrosis (arachnoiditis) is a well-known postoperative complication for which there still exists no effective treatment. The occurrence of such a fibrosis has yet to be observed after chemonucleolysis.

Conclusion

In summary, we can state that chemonucleolysis is an effective and safe treatment in meticulously selected patients with a lumbar HNP. Correctly preparing and guiding the patient is as important as the technical treatment itself. Moreover, it must be clear for everyone involved that a complete return to a normal situation can no longer be achieved; the motion segment remains degenerated. Finally, not only do these mechanical factors remain, but the subjective experience of the patient also plays a role in the outcome of the treatment.

PERCUTANEOUS DISCECTOMY

Percutaneous discectomy is a relatively new decompression method for lumbar disc prolapse. Under local anesthesia an aspirating/cutting cannula, the so-called nucleotome, is inserted into the disc whereby the nucleus is aspirated. Until now, the results achieved with this method appear to be promising. However, especially in the United States, accounts of a fair number of negative experiences have been published.[110] Not enough data, however, have been gathered to make a definitive judgment concerning this technique.

On the other hand, surgical treatment for lumbar disc prolapse has proved to be a rather risky procedure. Many complications can occur, such as damage to the ligaments, capsules of the zygapophyseal joints, nerve roots, and dura mater. Often adhesions and scar tissue develop due to a hematoma or to postoperative infections. Since the introduction of microsurgical techniques in 1975, these complications have been significantly reduced.

Besides chemonucleolysis, percutaneous discectomy should also be considered in the treatment of disc prolapse. Percutaneous discectomy was developed in 1974 by the Japanese surgeon Hijikata and his colleagues.[111] The method was further perfected in 1986 by the interventional radiologist Onik and co-workers.[112] In experienced hands, both of these methods have fewer complications than microsurgical treatment.

Indications

In percutaneous discectomy, the indications are the same as for chemonucleolysis, including the following:

- The absolute requirement is that the patient's radicular pain is more severe than the back pain.
- Neurological symptoms are present, such as an obviously positive Lasègue sign, possibly in combination with motor or sensory deficits.
- Conservative treatment has been administered for at least 6 weeks without re-

sult. In instances of an acute exacerbation, such as the occurrence of severe motor deficits, immediate application of the procedure may be required.

From the scarce statistics available, it is shown that the best results are obtained in young patients. In patients older than 45 years of age the results are mostly disappointing.

Contraindications

- In patients for whom back pain is the prevalent symptom
- In instances of a sequestered disc prolapse (indicated on CT scan or MRI)
- In patients older than 45 years of age with significant degenerative changes (precaution)
- In patients with spinal stenosis (detectable by CT scan)
- In patients who have undergone previous surgical treatment
- In patients who have undergone previous chemonucleolysis.

Procedure

As in the surgical microdiscectomy, percutaneous discectomy also consists of removing the prolapsed nucleus. However, the method of performance is completely different.

With the patient in the prone position under local anesthesia, a mandrin is inserted 8 cm from the midline. With the help of an image intensifier, and under radiological control, a trocar then glides over this mandrin, which is pushed in the direction of the prolapsed disc. In the annulus, an incision is made with the help of a trephine, after which the nucleotome is brought into the center of the disc. The nucleotome is a thin probe with a diameter of 2.8 mm and an opening at the end. By means of the subatmospheric pressure created within the probe, the disc material is suctioned up through the opening. In the opening a kind of "guillotine" is built in, cutting the aspirated material. Percutaneous discectomy can be applied at the levels L3-4, L4-5, and L5-S1.

One day before surgery, the patient should be admitted to the hospital for a full preoperative examination (blood tests, electrocardiogram, lung X-rays). At that time a relaxant premedication is also administered.

The procedure is not painful; the patient perceives only an uncomfortable feeling when the nucleotome penetrates into the disc. After this, the patient receives a sedative that allows him or her to remain relaxed during the entire procedure. Sedation is very important because the treatment can last 1½ to 1¾ hours, and even minimal movement of the patient can disturb the radiological orientation points.

The morning after the operation, the patient is allowed to go home, where he or she must remain flat in bed for 8 days. After that the patient may progress gradually to an upright sitting position whereby the low back is well supported by pillows. After 1 month, activities can be increased slowly up to maximal.

Complications

If the diagnosis is correct, there are minimal to no complications. In some cases a discitis can arise. Due to edema or a small hematoma, a very small number of patients may complain of transient paresthesia. However, if the patient does not comply with the imposed rest, there is a real chance for the development of edema or a large hematoma. In such instances, severe leg pain can arise.

If the procedure fails, operative microdiscectomy remains a viable option.

Results

In most cases, patients experience immediate relief. However, the pain disappears completely only after 2 to 6 weeks. The older the patient, the slower the recovery.

Results are considered to be excellent when the patient is completely asymptomatic. Results are considered good when the patient complains about some lumbar pain at the end of the day or after activity. When patients have constant back and/or leg pain, the results are considered to be poor.

According to international statistics,[113] an excellent result is achieved in 70% of all treated cases, a good result in 15%, and a poor result in 15%. The age-related observation of the results shows an 80% success rate in patients younger than 45 years and a success rate of only 37.5% in patients older than 45 years. For a quick overview of treatment in lumbar spine pathology, refer to Appendix A, Algorithms for the Diagnosis and Treatment of the Lumbar Spine Pathology.

REFERENCES

1. Mixter WJ, Barr JS. Rupture of the intervertebral disc with involvement of the spinal cord. *N Engl J Med.* 1934;211:210–215.

2. Coventry MB, Ghormley RK, Kernohan JW. The intervertebral disc: its microscopic anatomy and pathology, I: anatomy, development and pathology. *J Bone Joint Surg.* 1945;27:105–112.

3. Hirsch C, Nachemson A. A new observation on the mechanical behavior of lumbar discs. *Acta Orthop Scand.* 1954;23:254.

4. Hirsch C. The reaction of intervertebral discs to compression forces. *J Bone Joint Surg [Am].* 1955; 37:1188.

5. Virgin W. Experimental investigations into physical properties of intervertebral disc. *J Bone Joint Surg [Br].* 1951;33:607.

6. Junghans H. Cited by Schmorl G, Junghans H, eds. *The Human Spine in Health and Disease.* 2nd English ed. Stuttgart: Georg Thieme Verlag; 1968.

7. Nachemson A. Lumbar interdiscal pressure. *Acta Orthop Scand Suppl.* 1960;43.

8. Kulak RF, Belytschko TB, Schultz AB, Galante JO. Non-linear behavior of the human intervertebral disc under axial load. *J Biomech.* 1976;9:377.

9. White AA, Panjabi MM. *Clinical Biomechanics of the Spine.* Philadelphia: JB Lippincott Co; 1978.

10. Shirazi-Adl A, Shrivastava SC, Ahmed AM. Stress analysis of the lumbar disc-body unit in compression: a three-dimensional nonlinear finite element study. *Spine.* 1984;9:120.

11. Farfan HF, Huberdeau RM, Dubow HI. Lumbar intervertebral disc degeneration. The influence of geometrical features on the pattern of disc degeneration: a post mortem study. *J Bone Joint Surg [Am].* 1972;54:492–510.

12. Gracovetsky S, Farfan HF, Helleur C. The abdominal mechanism. *Spine.* 1985;10:317–324.

13. Farfan HF, Cossett JW, Robertson GH, Wells RV, Kraus H. The effects of torsion on the lumbar intervertebral joints: the role of torsion in the production of disc degeneration. *J Bone Joint Surg [Am].* 1970;52:468.

14. Merriam WF. The effects of postural changes in the inferred pressures within the nucleus pulposus during lumbar discography. *Spine.* 1984;9:405.

15. Rolander SD. *Motion of the Lumbar Spine with Special Reference to the Stabilizing Effect of Posterior Fusion.* Gothenburg, Sweden: Department of Orthopaedic Surgery, University of Gothenburg; 1966. Thesis.

16. Miles M, Sullivan WE. Lateral bending at the lumbar and lumbosacral joints. *Anat Rec.* 1961;139:387.

17. Cosetta JW, Farfan HF, Robertson GH, Wells RV. The instantaneous center of rotation of the third lumbar intervertebral joint. *J Biomech.* 1971;4:149–153.

18. Stokes IA, Bigalow LC, Moreland MS. Measurement of axial rotation of vertebrae in scoliosis. *Spine.* 1986;11:213.

19. Adams MA, Hutton WC. The effect of fatigue on the lumbar intervertebral disc. *J Bone Joint Surg [Br].* 1983;65:199–203.

20. Yang KH. King AI. Mechanism of facet load transmission as a hypothesis for low back pain. *Spine.* 1984;9:557–565.

21. Panjabi MM, Takata K, Goel VK. Kinematics of lumbar intervertebral foramen. *Spine.* 1983;8,4:348.

22. Waddell G. Psychological evaluation. Presented at the Lumbar Spine Instructional Course, organized by the International Society for the Study of the Lumbar Spine. May 11, 1991; Zürich, Switzerland.

23. Lasègue C. Considérations sur la sciaticque. *Arch Gen Med.* 1864;2:558.

24. Cyriax J. Dural pain. *Lancet.* 1978;4:919–921.

25. Krämer J. *Bandscheibenbedingte Erkrankungen.* Stuttgart: Georg Thieme Verlag; 1978.

26. Porter RW. *Management of Back Pain.* Edinburgh: Churchill Livingstone; 1986.

27. Waddell G, Reilly S, Torsney B, et al. Assessment of the outcome of low back surgery. *J Bone Joint Surg [Br].* 1988;70:723–727.

28. Macnab I, McCulloch J. *Backache.* 2nd ed. Baltimore: Williams & Wilkins; 1990.

29. Porter RW, Miller C. Gravity induced list. Presented to the International Society for the Study of the Lumbar Spine. *Dtsch Med Wochenschr.* 1984:257.

30. Krämer J. Zur Terminologie degenerativer Erkrankungen im Bereich der Wirbelsäule. *Man Med.* 1987;25:48–51.

31. Nachemson A. Low-back pain. Are orthopedic surgeons missing the boat? *Acta Orthop Scand. Suppl.* 1993 64(1):1–2. Editorial.

32. Weber H. Lumbar disc herniation: a controlled prospective study with ten years of observation. 1992 Volvo Award in clinical science. *Spine.* 1983;8:131–140.

33. Grantham VA. Backache in boys—a new problem? *Practitioner.* 1977;218:226–229.

34. Penning L. Functionele radio-anatomie van lumbale stenose. *Ned Tijdschr Man Ther.* 1990;9:36–48.

35. Verbiest H. Further experiences on the pathological influence of a developmental narrowness of the bone vertebral canal. *J Bone Joint Surg [Br].* 1955;37:576–583.

36. Rosenberg NJ. Degenerative spondylolisthesis. *J Bone Joint Surg [Am].* 1975;57:4.

37. Porter RW, Hibbert C. Calcitonin treatment for neurogenic claudication. *Spine.* 1983; 8:585–592.

38. Simkin PA. Simian stance: a sign of spinal stenosis. *Lancet.* 1982;1:652–653.

39. Johnsson K, Rosén J, Udén A. The natural course of lumbar spinal stenosis. *Acta Orthop Scand Suppl.* 1993;2511:67–68.

40. Charcot JMC. Sur la claudication intermittente observee dans un cas d'obliteration complete de l'une des arteres iliaques primitives. *Comptes Rend Soc Biol.* 1858;10:225–238.

41. Dyck P, Doyle JB. "Bicycle test" of van Gelderen in diagnosis of intermittent cauda equina compression syndrome. *J Neurosurg.* 1977;46:667–670.

42. Lamberton AJ, Bannister R, Worthington R, Seifert MH, Eastcott HHG. Claudication of the sciatic nerve. *Br Med J.* 1983;286:1785–1786.

43. Venner RM, Crock HV. Clinical studies of isolated disc resorption in the lumbar spine. *J Bone Joint Surg [Br].* 1981;63:491–494.

44. Wiltse LL, Newman PH, Macnab I. Classification of spondylolysis and spondylolisthesis. *Clin Orthop.* 1976;117:23–29.

45. Bird AH, Eastmond CJ, Hudson A, Wright B. Is generalised joint laxity a factor in spondylolisthesis? *Scand J Rheumatol.* 1980;9:203–205.

46. Hitoshi H. Spondylolysis in athletes. *Phys Sports Med.* 1980;8:75–79.

47. Young MH. Long term consequences of stable fractures of the thoracic and lumbar vertebral bodies. *J Bone Joint Surg [Br].* 1973;55:295–300.

48. Nordin BEC, Peacock M, Aaeon J, et al. *Clin Endocrinol Metab.* 1980;9:177–205.

49. Nordin BEC, Wright V, eds. *Osteoporosis: Bone and Joint Disease in the Elderly.* Edinburgh: Churchill Livingstone; 1983:167–180.

50. Stevenson JC, Whitehead ME. Postmenopausal osteoporosis. *Br Med J.* 1982;285:585–588.

51. Abel MS. Jogger's fracture and other stress fractures of the lumbosacral spine. *Skeletal Radiol.* 1985;13:221–227.

52. Cyriax J, Russel G. *Textbook of Orthopaedic Medicine.* 10th ed. *Treatment by Manipulation, Massage and Injection.* London: Baillière Tindall; 1980;2.

53. McKenzie RA. Prophylaxis in recurrent low back pain. *N Z Med J.* 1979;89:22–23.

54. McGavin JC. The McKenzie approach to spinal pain. *Phys Ther Forum.* 1988;7(27):1–4.

55. Nachemson A. Rational work-up for differential diagnosis. Presented at the Lumbar Spine Instructional Course, organized by the International Society for the Study of the Lumbar Spine; May 11, 1991; Zürich, Switzerland.

56. Matthews JA. De waarde van epidurografie bij de beoordeling van de weding van manipulatie en traktie bij lumbale discusproblemen. *Tijdschr Ned Vereninging Orthop Geneeskd.* 1981;1:23–43.

57. Hoorlinger XX. 1973.

58. Nordin M. Back schools. Presented at the Lumbar Spine Instructional Coure, organized by the International Society for the Study of the Lumbar Spine; May 11, 1991; Zürich, Switzerland.

59. Muller JWT. Klinische lessen: rugpijn. *Ned Tijdschr Geneeskd.* 1980;124:1857–1860.

60. Noordenbos W. *Pain.* Amsterdam: Elsevier; 1959. Dissertation.

61. Melzack R, Wall PD. Pain mechanisms, a new theory. *Science.* 1965;150:971–979.

62. Melzack R. *The Puzzle of Pain.* London: Penguin Science of Behavior; 1973.

63. Rexed B. The cytoarchitecture organization in the spinal cord in the cat. *J Comp Neurol.* 1952;96:415.

64. Dirksen R. Organisatie van het pijnsysteem. In: Booij H et al, eds. *Anesthesiologie.* Utrecht, Netherlands: Wetenschappelijke Uitgeverij Bunge; 1989:359–372.

65. Sanders M. Zenuwblokkade door RF-laesie. In: Booij H et al, eds. *Anesthesiologie.* Utrecht: Wetenschappelijke Uitgeverij Bunge; 1989:409–414.

66. Travel JG, Simons DG. *Myofascial Pain and Dysfunction: The Trigger Point Manual.* Baltimore: Williams & Wilkins; 1983.

67. Loeser JD, Fordyce WE. *Concepts of Pain: Chronic Low Back Pain.* New York: Raven Press; 1982.

68. Lloyd JW, Barnard JDW, Glynn CJ. Cryoanalgesia: a new approach to pain relief. *Lancet.* 1976;2:932.

69. Reese WES. Multiple bilateral subcutaneous rhizolysis of segmental nerves in the treatment of the intervertebral disc syndrome. *Ann Gen Pract.* 1971;26:126–127.

70. Sehgal AD, Gardner WJ. Place of intrathecal methylprednisolone acetate in neurological disorders. *Trans Am Neurol Assoc.* 1963;88:275–276.

71. Kepes ER, Duncalf D. Treatment of backache with spinal injections of local anesthetics, spinal and systemic steroids: a review. *Pain.* 1985;22:33–47.

72. Shealy CN. Percutaneous radiofrequency denervation of spinal facets: treatment for chronic back pain and sciatica. *J Neurosurg.* 1975;43:448–451.

73. Sluijter ME, Mehta M. Treatment of chronic back and neck pain by percutaneous thermal lesions. In: *Persistent Pain: Modern Methods of Treatment.* London: Academic Press; 1981;3:141–179.

74. Uematsu S. Percutaneous radiofrequency rhizotomy. *Surg Neurol.* 1974;2:319–324.

75. Moore DC. *Regional Block.* Springfield, Ill: Charles C Thomas, Publisher; 1968:123–137.

76. Nachemson A, Rydevik B. Chemonucleolysis for sciatica: a critical review. *Acta Orthop Scand.* 1988;59:56–62.

77. Deyo RA, Cherkin DC, Loeser JD, Bigos SJ, Ciol MA. Morbidity and mortality in association with operations on the lumbar spine: the influence of age, diagnosis and procedure. *J Bone Joint Surg [Am].* 1992;74:536–543.

78. North RB, Campbell JN, James CS et al. Failed back surgery syndrome: 5-year follow-up in 102 patients undergoing repeated operation. *Neurosurgery.* 1991;28:685–691.

79. Tullberg T, Isacson J, Weidenhielm L. Does microscopic removal of lumbar disc herniation lead to better results than the standard procedure? Results of a one-year randomized study. *Spine.* 1993;18(1):24–27.

80. Verbiest H. A radicular syndrome from developmental narrowing of the lumbar vertebral canal. *J Bone Joint Surg [Br].* 1954;36:230–237.

81. Bowen V, Shannon R, Kirkaldy-Willis WH. Lumbar spinal stenosis. *Childs Brain.* 1978;4:257–277.

82. Briggs H, Krause J. The intervertebral foraminotomy for relief of sciatic pain. *J Bone Joint Surg.* 1945;27:475–478.

83. Putti V. New conceptions in the pathogenesis of sciatica pain. *Lancet.* 1927:53–60.

84. Scaglietti O, Fontino G, Bartolozzi P. Technique of anatomical reduction of lumbar spondylolisthesis and its surgical stabilisation. *Clin Orthop.* 1976;117:164–175.

85. Shenkin HA, Hasj CJ. A new approach to the surgical treatment of lumbar spondylosis. *J Neurosurg.* 1976;44:148–155.

86. Getty CJM, Johnson JR, Kirwan EOG, Sullivan MF. Partial undercutting facetectomy for bony entrapment of the lumbar nerve root. *J Bone Joint Surg [Br].* 1981;63:330–335.

87. de Palma A, Rothman R. The nature of pseudarthrosis. *Clin Orthop.* 1968;49:113–118.

88. Turner JA, Ersek M, Herron L, Deyo R. Surgery for lumbar spinal stenosis: attempted meta-analysis of the literature. *Spine.* 1992;17:1–8.

89. Harrington PR, Dickson JH. Spinal instrumentation in the treatment of severe progressive spondylolisthesis. *Clin Orthop.* 1976;117:157–163.

90. Smith L. Enzyme dissolution of the nucleus pulposis in humans. *JAMA.* 1964;187:137–140.

91. Jeffery RM, Block JA, Schnitzer TJ, et al. Proteoglycan degradation after chemonucleolysis. Presented at the meeting of the International Society for the Study of the Lumbar Spine; May 24–28, 1987; Rome, Italy.

92. Gibson MJ, Buckley J, Mulholland RC, Worthington BS. The changes in the intervertebral disc after chemonucleolysis demonstrated by magnetic resonance imaging. *J Bone Joint Surg [Br].* 1986;68:719–723.

93. Dolan P, Adams MA, Hutton WC. The short-term effects of chymopapain on intervertebral discs. *J Bone Joint Surg [Br].* 1987;69:422–429.

94. Deutman R. Chemonucleolysis bij patiënten met hernia nuclei pulposi lumbalis. *Ned Tijdschr Geneeskd.* 1983;127:1385–1390.

95. Bradford DS, Cooper KM, Oegema TR. Chymopapain, chemonucleolysis, and nucleus pulposus regeneration. *J Bone Joint Surg [Am].* 1983;65:1220–1231.

96. Spencer DL, Miller JAA, Schults AB. The effects of chemonucleolysis on the mechanical properties of the canine lumbar disc. *Spine.* 1985;10:555–561.

97. Agre K, Wilson RR, Brim M, Medernott DJ. Chymodiactin postmarketing surveillance: demographic and adverse experience data in 29,075 patients. *Spine.* 1984;9:479–485.

98. Mulawka SM, Weslowski DP, Herkowitz HN. Chemonucleolysis, the relationship of the physical findings, discography and myelography to the clinical result. *Spine.* 1986;11:391–396.

99. Kahanovitz N, Arnoczky SP, Sissons HA, Steiner GC, Schwarz P. The effect of discography on the canine intervertebral disc. *Spine.* 1986;11,1:26–27.

100. Bouillet R. Complications de la nucleolyse discale par la chymopapaine. *Acta Orthop Belg.* 1987;53:250–260.

101. Konings JG, Williams FJB, Eutman R. The effects of chemonucleolysis as demonstrated by computerised tomography. *J Bone Joint Surg [Br].* 1984;66:417–421.

102. Crawshaw C, Frazer AM, Merriam WF, Mulholland RC, Webb JK. A comparison of surgery and chemonucleolysis in the treatment of sciatica: a prospective randomized trial. *Spine.* 1984;9:195–198.

103. Ejeskär A, Nachemson A, Herberts P, et al. Surgery versus chemonucleolysis for herniated lumbar discs: a prospective study with random assignment. *Clin Orthop.* 1983;174:236–242.

104. Lavignolle B, Vital JM, Baulny D, Grenier F, Castagnera L. Etudes comparées de la chirurgie et de la chimionucléolyse dans le traitement de la sciatique par hernie discale. *Acta Orthop Belg.* 1987;53,2:244–249.

105. Postacchini F, Lami R, Massobrio M. Chemonucleolysis versus surgery in lumbar disc herniations: correlation of the results to preoperative clinical pattern and size of the herniation. *Spine.* 1987;12:87–97.

106. van Alphen HAM, Braakman R, Berfelo M, Broere G, Bezemer PD, Kostanse PJ. Chemonucleolysis or discectomy? Results of a randomized multicentre trial in patients with a herniated intervertebral disc. *Acta Neurochir Suppl.* 1988;43:35–38.

107. Nordby EJ. Current concepts review chymopapain in intradiscal therapy. *J Bone Joint Surg.* 1983;65A,9:1350–1354.

108. Oppel U, Beyer HK, Fett H, Hedtmann A. Kernspintomographische Untersuchungen mit Kontrastmitteln beim Postdiskotomie-syndrom. *Orthopadie.* 1989;18:41–52.

109. Tregonning GD, Transfeldt EE, McCulloch JA, Macnab I, Nachemson A. Chymopapain versus conventional surgery for lumbar disc herniation: 10-year results of treatment. *J Bone Joint Surg.* 1991;73:481–486.

110. McCulloch JA. Surgical approach to herniated disc (microsurgery, chemonucleolysis, percutaneous nucleotomy). Presented at the Lumbar Spine Instructional Course, organized by the International Society for the Study of the Lumbar Spine; May 11, 1991; Zürich, Switzerland.

111. Hijikata S, Yamagishi M, Nakayama T, et al. Percutaneous discectomy: a new treatment method for lumbar disc herniation. *J Toden Hosp.* 1975;5:39.

112. Onik G, Helms CA, Ginsberg L, et al. Percutaneous lumbar discectomy using a new aspiration probe: porcine and cadaver models. *Radiology.* 1985;15:251–252.

113. Hellebuyck B. In alle zachtheid. *Jong Practicus.* 1989;33:28–31.

SUGGESTED READING

van Akkerveeken PF. *Lateral Stenosis of the Lumbar Spine.* Utrecht, Netherlands: Rijks University, Libertas Drukwerkservice BV; 1989. Thesis.

Allen DB, Waddell G. An historical perspective on low back pain and disability. *Acta Orthop Scand Suppl.* 1989;234:60.

Andrew T, Piggott H. Growth arrest for progressive scoliosis: combined anterior and posterior fusion of the convexity. *J Bone Joint Surg [Br].* 1985;67:193–197.

Archer IA, Diskson RA. Stature and idiopathic scoliosis: a prospective study. *J Bone Joint Surg [Br].* 1985;67:185–188.

Balderston RA, et al. The treatment of lumbar disc herniation: simple fragment excision versus disc space curettage. *J Spinal Disord.* 1991;4:22–25.

Barnes N, Thomas N. "Claudication" of the sciatic nerve. *Br Med J.* 1983;286:1785.

Barrett J. Mini-epidural injections for sciatica. *Man Med.* 1982;20:73–74.

Binns M. Joint laxity in idiopathic adolescent scoliosis. *J Bone Joint Surg [Br].* 1988;70:420–422.

Blaauw B, Schaafsma J, Blaauw-van Dischoeck B. Prolaps van de lumbale tussenwervelschijf bij kinderen en adolescenten. *Ned Tijdschr Geneeskd.* 1981;125:1404–1407.

Bogduk N, Long DM. Percutaneous lumbar medial branch neurotomy: a modification of facet denervation. *Spine.* 1980;5:193–200.

Bogduk N, Wilson AS, Tynan W. The human lumbar dorsal rami. *J Anat.* 1982;134:383–397.

Boger DC, Chandler RW, Pearce JG, Balciunas A. Unilateral facet dislocation at the lumbosacral junction. *J Bone Joint Surg [Am].* 1983;65:1174–1178.

Bolender NF, Schönström NSR, Spengler DM. Role of computed tomography and myelography in the diagnosis of central spinal stenosis. *J Bone Joint Surg [Am].* 1985;67:240–246.

Bough B, Thakore J, Davies M, Dowling F. Degeneration of the lumbar facet joints. *J Bone Joint Surg [Br].* 1990;72:275–276.

Bourque PR, et al. Selective calf weakness suggests intraspinal pathology, not peripheral neuropathy. *Arch Neurol.* 1990;47:79–80.

Bowman C, Dieppe P, Settas L. Remission of pseudo-spondylitis with treatment of Whipple's disease. *Br J Rheumatol.* 1983;22:181–182.

Brocher JEW. *Die Wirbelsäulenleiden und ihre Differentialdiagnose.* Stuttgart: Georg Thieme Verlag; 1962.

Brodon H. Inhibition-facilitation technique for lumbar pain treatment. *Man Med.* 1982;20:95–98.

Brokmeier AA. Manuelle therapie—Wirbelsäule—Bewegung und Funktionseinschränkung. *Krankengymnastik.* 1984;36:578–583.

Buchanan JR, Myers CA, Greer RB. A comparison of the risk of vertebral fracture in menopausal osteopenia and other metabolic disturbances. *J Bone Joint Surg [Am].* 1988;70:704–710.

Bunch WH, Chapman RG. Patient preferences in surgery for scoliosis. *J Bone Joint Surg [Am].* 1985;67:794–799.

Carmella G, Stanley VP, Utner M. Reliability in evaluating passive intervertebral motion. *Phys Ther.* 1982;62:436–444.

Cats A. De aandoeningen van de rug, I: juvenile kyfose (Morbus Scheuermann). *Reuma Wereldwijd.* 1984;8(2):1–4.

Cats A. De aandoeningen van de rug, II: osteoporose. *Reuma Wereldwijd.* 1984;8(3):1–4.

Cats A. De aandoeningen van de rug, III: spondylosis hyperostotica. *Reuma Wereldwijd.* 1984;8(4):1–4.

Choudhur AR, Taylor JC. Occult lumbar spinal stenosis. *J Neurol Neurosurg Psychiatry.* 1977;40:506–510.

Christodoulides AN. Ipsilateral sciatica of femoral nerve stretch test is pathognomonic of a L4-L5 disc protrusion. *J Bone Joint Surg [Br].* 1989;71:88–89.

Cicala RS, Thoni K, Angel JJ. Long term results of cervical epidural steroid injections of local anesthetics, spinal and systemic steroids: a review. *Clin J Pain.* 1989;5:143–145.

Citron N, Edgar MA, Sheehy J, Thomas DGT. Intramedullary spinal cord tumours presenting a scoliosis. *J Bone Joint Surg [Br]*. 1984;66:513–517.

Cohn ML, Huntington CT, Byrd S, Wooten DJ, Kochman C, Cohn M. Computed tomographic and electromyographic evaluation of epidural treatment for chronic low back pain. *Anesthesiology*. 1983;59:194. Abstract.

Colhoun E, McCall IW, Williams L, Cassar Pullicino VN. Provocation discography as a guide to planning operations on the spine. *J Bone Joint Surg [Br]*. 1988;70: 267–271.

Connolly RC. Chemonucleolysis. *J Bone Joint Surg [Br]*. 1977;59:1.

Cookson JC. Orthopedic manual therapy—an overview, II: the spine. *Phys Ther*. 1979;59:259–267.

Corrigan B, Maitlan GD. *Practical Orthopaedic Medicine*. London: Butterworth; 1983.

Crawshaw C, Kean DM, Mulholland RC, et al. The use of nuclear magnetic resonance in the diagnosis of lateral canal entrapment. *J Bone Joint Surg [Br]*. 1984;66:711–715.

Cuckler JM, Bernini PA, Wiesel SW, Booth RE, Rothman RH, Pickens GT. The use of epidural steroids in the treatment of lumbar radicular pain: a prospective, randomized, double-blind study. *J Bone Joint Surg [Am]*. 1985;67:63–66.

Cyriax J. *Textbook of Orthopaedic Medicine*. 7th ed. *Diagnosis of Soft Tissue Lesions*. London: Baillière Tindall; 1979;1.

Daruwalla JS, Balasubramaniam P. Moiré topography in scoliosis: its accuracy in detecting the site and size of the curve. *J Bone Joint Surg [Br]*. 1985;67:211–213.

Daruwalla JS, Balasubramaniam P, Chay SO, Rajan U, Lee HP. Idiopathic scoliosis: prevalence and ethnic distribution in Singapore schoolchildren. *J Bone Joint Surg [Br]*. 1985;67:182–184.

Deacon P, Berkin CR, Dickson RA. Combined idiopathic kyphosis and scoliosis: an analysis of the lateral spinal curvatures associated with Scheuermann's disease. *J Bone Joint Surg [Br]*. 1985;67:189–192.

Deacon P, Flood BN, Dickson RA. Idiopathic scoliosis in three dimensions: a radiographic and morphometric analysis. *J Bone Joint Surg [Br]*. 1984;66:509–512.

Defesche HFHG, Broere G. Het spinale hematom. *Ned Tijdschr Geneeskd*. 1980;124:157–160.

Dejung B. Die Verspannung des M. iliacus als Ursache lumbosacraler Schmerzen. *Man Med*. 1987;25:73–81.

Dekker M. Groningen, Netherlands: Rijks University; 1987. Dissertation.

Delisle B. Der Kreuzschmerz aus der Sicht des gynäkologen. *Physikalische Ther*. 1984;5:419–422.

Deyo RA. Conservative therapy for low back pain: distinguishing useful from useless therapy. *JAMA*. 1983;250:1057–1062.

Dickson RA. Conservative treatment for idiopathic scoliosis. *J Bone Joint Surg [Br]*. 1985;67:176–181.

Dimaggio A, Mooney V. Conservative care for low back pain: what works? Comparing rest, traction, bracing, manipulation and exercise. *J Muskuloskel Med*. 1987;4:27–34.

Dimaggio A, Mooney V. The McKenzie program: exercise effective against back pain. *J Musculoskel Med*. 1987;4:63–74.

Dorian L. Krankengymnastik oder Orthese zur Stabilisation der LWS? *Krankengymnastik*. 1981;33: 619–625.

van Duinen MTA. Radiculaire of pseudoradiculaire pijn? *Pijn*. 1983;7:1–7.

Duncan JAT. Chemical lumbar sympathectomy. *J Bone Joint Surg [Br]*. 1985;67:174–175.

Dunlop RB, Adams MA, Hutton WC. Disc space narrowing and the lumbar facet joints. *J Bone Joint Surg [Br]*. 1984;66:706–710.

Dyer CH. Should we be manipulating prolapsed intervertebral discs? *Br Osteopath J*. 1982;14:149–150.

Edgar MA. To brace or not to brace? *J Bone Joint Surg [Br]*. 1985;67:173–174.

Ekholm J, Arborelius UP, Németh G. The load on the lumbosacral joint and trunk muscle activity during lifting. *Ergonomics*. 1982;25:145–161.

Epstein JA, Epstein BS, Rosenthal AD, Carras R, Lavine LS. Sciatica caused by nerve root entrapment in the lateral recess; the superior facet syndrome. *J Neurosurg*. 1972;36:584–589.

Farfan HF. *Mechanical Disorders of the Low Back*. Philadelphia: Lea & Febiger; 1973.

Farfan HF. The scientific basis of manipulative procedures. *Clin Rheum Dis*. 1980;6:159–178.

Farwell SE. Complications following lumbar laminectomy. *Br Osteop J*. 1983;15:98–102.

Felsenthal G, Reischer MA. Asymmetric hamstring reflexes indicative of L5 radicular lesions. *Arch Phys Med Rehabil*. 1982;63:377–378.

Fidler MW, Plasmans CMT. The effect of four types of support on the segmental mobility of the lumbosacral spine. *J Bone Joint Surg [Am]*. 1983;65:943–947.

Fisk JR, DiMonte P, McKay S. Back schools: past, present and future. *Clin Orthop*. 1983;179:18–23.

Fisk JW, Baigent ML, HIll PD. The incidence of Scheuermann's disease: preliminary report. *Am J Phys Med*. 1982;61:32–35.

Fitzgerald RT. Sacroiliac strain. *Br Med J*. 1979;1,6173: 1285–1286.

Flatley TJ, Anderson MH, Anast GT. Spinal instability due to malignant disease: treatment by segmental spinal stabilization. *J Bone Joint Surg [Am]*. 1984;66: 47–52.

Floman Y. *Disorders of the Lumbar Spine*. Gaithersburg, Md: Aspen Publishers, Inc.; 1990.

Fredrickson BE, Baker D, McHolick WJ, Yuan HA, Lubicky JP. The natural history of spondylolysis and spondylolisthesis. *J Bone Joint Surg [Br]*. 1984;66: 699–707.

Frymoyer JW, Donaghy RMP. The ruptured intervertebral disc: follow-up report on the first case fifty years after recognition of the syndrome and its surgical significance. *J Bone Joint Surg [Am]*. 1985;67:113–116.

Frymoyer JW, Newberg A, Pope MH, Wilder DG, Clements J, MacPherson B. Spine radiographs in patients with low back pain: an epidemiological study in men. *J Bone Joint Surg [Am]*. 1984;66:1048–1055.

Füzesi L. Was liegt der Arthrosekrankheit zugrunde? *Rheuma Aktuell*. 1985;8:8.

Gabriel KR, Crawford AH. Magnetic resonance imaging in a child who had clinical signs of discitis: report of a case. *J Bone Joint Surg [Am]*. 1988;70:938–941.

Gaenslen FJ. Sacroiliac arthrodesis; indications, author's technique and end results. *J Am Med*. 89,24: 2031–2035.

Gallacchi G. Die synoviothese. *Rheuma Aktuell*. 1985; 8:7.

Graff KH, Prager G. Der "Kreuzschmerz" des Leichtathleten. Aspekte zur Sportpraxis. *Leichtathletik*. 1985;47:1687–1694.

Graff KH, Prager G. Der "Kreuzschmerz" des Leichtathleten (Fortsetzung aus LdLa Nr. 33-34/ 1985), II: Übungsauswahl. *Leichtathletik*. 1985; 48:1719–1726.

Graves JE, Pollock MI, et al. Quantitative assessment of full range of motion isometric lumbar extension strength. *Spine*. 1990;15:290–294.

Greenough CG, Dimmock S, Edwards D, Ransford AO, Bentley G. The role of computerized tomography in intervertebral disc prolapse. *J Bone Joint Surg [Br]*. 1986;68:729–733.

Grieve GP. *Common Vertebral Joint Problems*. Edinburgh: Churchill Livingstone; 1981.

Grieve GP. Lumbar instability. *Physiotherapy*. 1982;68: 2–9.

Grieve GP, ed. *Modern Manual Therapy of the Vertebral Column*. Edinburgh: Churchill Livingstone; 1986.

Guo-Xiang J, Wei-Dong X. Meralgia paraesthetica of spinal origin: brief report. *J Bone Joint Surg [Br]*. 1988;70:843.

Guo-Xiang J, Wei-Dong X, Ai-Hao W. Spinal stenosis with meralgia paraesthetica. *J Bone Joint Surg [Br]*. 1988;70:272–273.

Hagen R. Pelvic girdle relaxation from an orthopaedic point of view. *Acta Orthop Scand*. 1974;45:550–563.

Haldeman S. Spinal manipulative therapy: a status report. *Clin Orthop*. 1983;179:62–70.

Hall BB, McCulloch JA. Anaphylactic reactions following the intradiscal injection of chymopapain under local anesthesia. *J Bone Joint Surg [Am]*. 1983;65: 1215–1219.

Hall H, Iceton JA. Back school: an overview with specific reference to the Canadian back education units. *Clin Orthop*. 1983;179:10–17.

Halpin DS, Gibson RD. Septic arthritis of a lumbar facet joint. *J Bone Joint Surg [Br]*. 1987;69:457–459.

Hanley EN, Shapiro DE. The development of low back pain after excision of a lumbar disc. *J Bone Joint Surg [Am]*. 1989;71:719–720.

Hazel WA, Jones RA, Morrey BF, Stauffer RN. Vertebral fractures without neurological deficit: a long-term follow-up study. *J Bone Joint Surg [Am]*. 1988;70: 1319–1321.

Horm FC. Dynamische Wirbelsäulen—Therapie. *Physikalische Ther*. 1984;5:252–261.

Howie DW, Chatterton BE, Honw MR. Failure of ultrasound in the investigation of sciatica. *J Bone Joint Surg [Br]*. 1983;65:144–147.

Hsu LCS, Lee PC, Leong JCY. Dystrophic spinal deformities in neurofibromatosis: treatment by anterior and posterior fusion. *J Bone Joint Surg [Br]*. 1984; 66:495–499.

Ireland ML, Nicheli LJ. Bilateral stress fracture of the lumbar pedicles in a ballet dancer: a case report. *J Bone Joint Surg [Am]*. 1987;69:140–142.

Jackson CP, Brown MD. Is there a role for exercise in the treatment of patients with low back pain? *Clin Orthop*. 1983;179:39–45.

Jackson CP, Brown MD. Analysis of current approaches and practical guide to prescription of exercise. *Clin Orthop*. 1983;179:46–54.

Jensen GM. Biomechanics of the lumbar intervertebral disc: a review. *Phys Ther*. 1980;60:765–773.

Johansson JE, Barrington TW, Ameli M. Combined vascular and neurogenic claudication. *Spine*. 1982;7: 150–158.

Kadish LJ, Simmons EH. Anomalies of the lumbosacral nerve roots: an anatomical investigation and myelographic study. *J Bone Joint Surg [Br]*. 1984; 66:411–416.

Kambin P, Gellman H. Percutaneous lateral discectomy of the lumbar spine: a preliminary report. *Clin Orthop*. 1983;174:127–132.

Kempf HD, Lutz W. Das Karlsruher Rückenforum—eine "Rückenschule." *Krankengymnastik.* 1988;40: 373–376.

Ker NB, Jones CB. Tumors of the cauda equina: the problem of differential diagnosis. *J Bone Joint Surg [Br].* 1985;67:358–362.

Kirkaldy-Willis NH. Five common back disorders: how to diagnose and treat them. *Geriatrics.* 1978;33:12.

van Kleef JW. Lokale anaesthetica, fundamentele werkingsmechanismen en klinisch gebruik. *Ned Tijdschr Geneeskd.* 1982;126:1916–1921.

Knibbe JJ. Epidemiologie van lage rugklachten: een verkenning naar de oorzaak tot secundaire preventie. *Ned Tijdschr Fysiother.* 1987;97(7/8):169–174.

Kruls HJA. Over kinderen met scoliose. *Patient Care.* 1982;30:33.

Lackner K, von Schroeder S. Computertomographie der Lendenwirbelsäule. *ROFO.* 1980;2:124–131.

Lang SM, Moyle DD, Berg EW, et al. Correlation of mechanical properties of vertebral trabecular bone with equivalent mineral density as measured by computed tomography. *J Bone Joint Surg [Am].* 1988;70: 1531–1537.

von Lasch V, Treumann F, Holzgraefe M. Das LWS-Syndrom als Sportschaden beim Volleyball. *Dtsch Z Sportmedizin.* 1984;11:396–399.

Leu Hj. Die perkutane Nukleotomie: Technik, Indikationen und Erfahrungen seit 1979. In: *Jahrbuch der Orthopädie.* Zülpich: Biermann Verlag; 1989:13–25.

Lewith GT, Turner GM. Retrospective analysis of the management of acute low back pain. *Practitioner.* 1982;226:1614–1618.

Lilius G, Laasonen EM, Myllinen P, Harilainen A, Grönlund G. Lumbar facet joint syndrome: randomised clinical trial. *J Bone Joint Surg [Br].* 1989;71:681–684.

Lowe J, Libson E, Ziv I, Nyska M, Floman Y, Bloom RA, Robin GC. Spondylolysis in the upper lumbar spine: a study of 32 patients. *J Bone Joint Surg [Br].* 1978;59:582–586.

Maigne R. Low back pain of thoracolumbar origin. *Arch Phys Med Rehabil.* 1980;61:389–394.

Maitland GD. The slump test: examination and treatment. *Aust J Physiol.* 1985;31:215–219.

Mayer HM, Wolff R, Mellerowicz H, Brock M. Neurinom der Spinalwurzel L3 als Ursache belastungsabhängiger Lumboischialgien. *Sportverletzung Sportschaden.* 1988;2:35–38.

McCulloch JA. Chemonucleolysis. *J Bone Joint Surg [Br].* 1977;58:45–52.

McCulloch JA. Chemonucleolysis: experience with 2000 cases. *Clin Orthop.* 1980;146:128–143.

McDonald RS, Bell CMJ. An open controlled assessment of osteopathic manipulation in non specific low back pain. *Spine.* 1990;15:364–370.

Miller A, Stedman GH, Beisaw NE, Gross PT. Sciatica caused by an avulsion fracture of the ischial tuberosity: a case report. *J Bone Joint Surg [Am].* 1987;69: 143–144.

Muirhead A, Conner AN. The assessment of lung function in children with scoliosis. *J Bone Joint Surg [Br].* 1985;67:699–702.

Murtagh FR, Paulsen RD, Rechtine GR. The role and incidence of facet tropism in lumbar spine degenerative disc disease. *J Spinal Disord.* 1991;4:86–89.

Nachemson A. Work for all: for those with low back pain as well. *Clin Orthop.* 1983;179:77–85.

Niethard FU, Rompe G. Das lumbale Facettensyndrom. *Man Med.* 1981;19:49–53.

Panjabi MM, Greenstein G, Duranceau J, Nolte LP. Three-dimensional quantitative morphology of lumbar spinal ligaments. *J Spinal Disord.* 1991;4:54–62.

Papaioannou T. Scoliosis associated with limb-length inequality. *J Bone Joint Surg [Am].* 1982;64:59–62.

Paris SV. Spinal manipulative therapy. *Clin Orthop.* 1983;179:55–61.

Pearcy MJ, Tibrewal SB. Axial rotation and lateral bending in the normal lumbar spine measured by three-dimensional radiography. *Spine.* 1984;9:270–275.

Peltier LF. The classic: the "back school" of Delpech Montpellier. *Clin Orthop.* 1983;179:4–9.

Pincott JR, Davies JS, Taffs LF. Scoliosis caused by section of dorsal spinal nerve roots. *J Bone Joint Surg [Br].* 1984;66:27–29.

Pon A, Schlegel KF, Haasters J. Nukleolyse: Injektionstherapie des Bandscheibenleidens. *Dtsch Artzteblatt.* 1983;44:27–32.

Postacchini F. *Lumbar Spinal Stenosis.* Vienna: Springer Verlag; 1988.

Pott HG. "Reiter"—Infektionsfolge bei Prädisponierten. *Rheuma Aktuell.* 1985;8:4.

Putz R. Biomechanik der Wirbelsäule. *Krankengymnastik.* 1989;41:21–24.

Rabischong P, Louis R, Vignaud J, Massare C. The intervertebral disc. *Anat Clin.* 1978;1:55–64.

Raj PP. *Practical Management of Pain.* Chicago: Year Book Medical Publishers, Inc; 1986:683.

Reiter W. Der Kreuzschmerz aus der Sicht des Internisten. *Physikalische Ther.* 1985;6:21–25.

Roggendorf W, Brock M, Görge HH, Curio G. Morphological alterations of the degenerated lumbar disc following chemonucleolysis with chymopapain. *J Neurosurg.* 1984;60:518–522.

Rosomoff HL. Do herniated discs produce pain? *Clin J Pain.* 1985;1:91.

Santiesteban AJ. The role of physical agents in the treatment of spine pain. *Clin Orthop.* 1983;179:24–30.

Saunders HD. Use of spinal traction in the treatment of neck and back conditions. *Clin Orthop.* 1983;179:31–38.

Savini R, Gherlinzone F, Morandi M, Neff JR, Picci P. Surgical treatment of giant-cell tumor of the spine: the experience at the Instituto Ortopedico Rizolli. *J Bone Joint Surg [Am].* 1983;65:1283–1330.

Schatzker J, Pennal GF. Spinal stenosis, a cause of cauda equina compression. *J Bone Joint Surg [Br].* 1968;50:606–618.

Schönstrom NSR, Lindahl S, Willen J, Hansson T. Dynamic changes in the dimensions of the lumbar spinal canal: an in vitro experimental study. In: Schönstrom NSR. *The Narrow Lumbar Spinal Canal and the Size of the Cauda Equina in Man: A Clinical and Experimental Study.* Göteborg, Sweden: Sahlgren Hospital; 1988:64–75. Thesis.

Schroeder S, Rössler H. Orthesenversorgung der Lendenwirbelsäule bei chronischen Kreuzschmerzen. *Krankengymnastik.* 1981;33:625–634.

Scott JHS, Macleod J, eds. *Clinical Examination.* 6th ed. Edinburgh: Churchill Livingstone; 1983.

Shiqing X, Quanzhi Z, Dehao F. Significance of the straight-leg-raising test in the diagnosis and clinical evaluation of lower lumbar intervertebral-disc protrusion. *J Bone Joint Surg [Am].* 1987;69:517–522.

Siegal T, Tiqva P, Siegal T. Vertebral body resection for epidural compression by malignant tumors: results of forty-seven consecutive operative procedures. *J Bone Joint Surg [Am].* 1985;67:375–382.

Sluijter ME, Racz GN, eds. *Radiofrequency Lesions of the Communicating Techniques of Neurolysis.* Boston: Academic Press, Inc; 1989.

Snaith ML, Galvin SJ, Short MD. The value of quantitative radioisotope scanning in the differential diagnosis of low back pain and sacroiliac disease. *J Rheumatol.* 1982;9:435–440.

Snijders CJ, Snijder JGN. Biomechanische modellen in het bestek van rugklachten tijdens de zwangerschap. *Tijdeschr Soc Gezondheidszorg.* 1984;62:141–147.

Spengler DM. Chronic low back pain: the team approach. *Clin Orthop.* 1983;179:71–76.

Spengler DM. Current concepts review: degnerative stenosis of the lumbar spine. *J Bone Joint Surg [Am].* 1987:69:305–308.

de St Jon M, Bischof C. MRI kann Discographie ersetzen. *Man Med Aktuell.* 1987.

Stambough JL, Booth RE, Rothman RH. Transient hypercorticism after epidural steroid injection: a case report. *J Bone Joint Surg [Am].* 1984;66:1115–1116.

Steinrücken H. Diskussionsbeitrag: Zur Terminologie degenerativer Erkrankungen im Bereich der Wirbelsäule von J. Krämer. *Man Med.* 1987;25:56–59.

Stokes I, Greenapple DM. Measurement of surface deformation of soft tissue. *J Biomech.* 1985;18:1.

Sutton JR. In: *Current Concepts in Chemonucleolysis.* London: The Royal Society of Medicine;1984:72. International Congress and Symposium Series.

Svensson HO. Low back pain in forty to forty-seven year old men. *Scand J Rehabil Med.* 1982;14:55–60.

Svensson HO, Andersson GBJ. Low back pain in forty to forty-seven year old men: frequency of occurrence and impact on medical services. *Scand J Rehabil Med.* 1982;14:47–53.

Szappanos L, Szepesi K, Thomázy B. Spondylolysis in osteoporosis. *J Bone Joint Surg [Br].* 1988;70:428–430.

Szypryt DP, Twining P, Wilde GP, Mulholland RC, Worthington BS. Diagnosis of lumbar disc protrusion: a comprison between magnetic resonance imaging and radiculography. *J Bone Joint Surg [Br].* 1988;70:717–722.

Takata K, Inoue SI, Takahashi K, Ohtsuka Y. Swelling of the cauda equina in patients who have herniation of lumbar disc: a possible pathogenesis of sciatica. *J Bone Joint Surg [Am].* 1988;70:361–368.

Thomas LK, Hislop HJ, Waters RL. Physiological work performance in chronic low back disability: effects of a progressive activity program. *Phys Ther.* 1980;60:407–411.

Tollison CD, Kriegel ML. *Interdisciplinary Rehabilitation of Low Back Pain.* Baltimore: Williams & Wilkins; 1989.

Trettin H. Die Schonhaltung aus neurologischer Sicht. *Physikalische Ther.* 1986;7:198–206.

Troup JDG. Biomechanis of the vertebral column: its application to prevention of back pain in the population and to the assessment of working capacity in patients with lumbar spinal disability. *Physiotherapy.* 1979;65:238–244.

Vandeweerdt E. Lage rugpijn bij sportlui: manueel-diagnostische en therapeutische aspekten. Presented at a VVSS congress; November 5, 1983; Deipenbeek, Belgium.

Veldhuizen AG, Baas P, Webb PJ. Observations on the growth of the adolescent spine. *J Bone Joint Surg [Br].* 1986;68:724–728.

Verbiest H. *Neurogenic Intermittent Claudication: With Special Reference to Stenosis of the Lumbar Vertebral Canal.* Amsterdam: Elsevier Science Publishers; 1976:26–29.

Voorhoeve P, Admiraal, eds. *Pijn en Pijnbehandeling.* Lochem: De Tijdstroom; 1979.

de Vries J. Lage rugklachten en korsetten. *Ned Tijdschr Fysiother.* 1984;94:168–172.

de Vries J. Het Rainey flexion jacket, een korset bij lage rugpijn. *Ned Tijdschr Geneeskd.* 1987;131: 1813–1816.

Wantz GE. Ambulatory hernia surgery. *Br J Surg.* 1989;76:1228–1229.

Weitz EM. Paraplegia following chymopapain injection: a case report. *J Bone Joint Surg [Am].* 1984;66: 1131–1135.

White AA, Panjabi MM. *Clinical Biomechanics of the Spine.* Philadelphia: JB Lippincott Co; 1990.

White AJ, Derby R, Wynne G. Epidural injections for the diagnosis and treatment of low back pain. *Spine.* 1980;78–86.

Wiltse LL. Spondylolisthesis: classificaiton and etiology: symposium of the spine. *Am Acad Orthop Surg.* 1969:143.

Wiltse LL, Rocchio PD. Preoperative psychological tests as predictors of success of chemonucleolysis in the treatment of the low back syndrome. *J Bone Joint Surg [Am].* 1975;57:478–483.

Wirbser R. Therapiekonzept in der Krankengymnastik bei Morbus Bechterew. *Krankengymnastik.* 1989; 41:5–11.

Wood PM. Applied anatomy and physiology of the vertebral column. *Physiotherapy.* 1979;65:248–249.

Wright B. Hypermobile status. *Man Med.* 1981;19:78–80.

Wyke B. Neurological aspects of low back pain. In: Jayson M, ed. *The Lumbar Spine and Back Pain.* New York: Grune & Stratton; 1976;189–255.

Wynne AT, Nelson MA, Nordin BEC. Costo-iliac impingement syndrome. *J Bone Joint Surg [Br].* 1985;67: 124–125.

Yashon D. *Spinal Injury.* New York: Appleton-Century-Crofts; 1978.

Yasuma T, Ohno R, Yamauchi Y. False-negative lumbar discograms; correlation of discographic and histological findings in post-mortem and surgical specimens. *J Bone Joint Surg [Am].* 1988;70:1279–1289.

Yates O, Jenner J. Lage rugpijn—Welke oorzaak? Lage rugpijn is een van de meest voorkomende oorzaken van arbeidsverzuim en vormt een moeilijk diagnostisch probleem. *Mod Med.* 1980:42–45.

LUMBAR SPINE REVIEW QUESTIONS

1. Describe the capsular pattern of the lumbar spine.
2. What is the difference between a disc protrusion and a disc prolapse?
3. Which motion is usually the most limited in a disc protrusion? Which motion is usually the most limited in a disc prolapse?
4. In which age group is the nerve root compression syndrome usually seen?
5. Where is the pain usually located in a nerve root compression syndrome?
6. Which activity provokes the most pain/symptoms in a patient with neurogenic claudication?
7. Which provocation test often gives the first indication of a segmental lumbar instability? Describe the way in which the patient typically performs this test.
8. At which level does one most often see a degenerative spondylolisthesis?
9. In terms of physical therapy, what is the treatment of choice for a degenerative spondylolisthesis?
10. In which disorder is a spontaneous compression fracture most commonly seen?
11. Which lumbar vertebrae are most often affected in a traumatic compression fracture?
12. Which tests are indicative of a traumatic sprain of the superior iliolumbar ligament?
13. Which test is indicative of a traumatic sprain of the supraspinous ligament?
14. Which test is indicative of a traumatic strain of the erector spinae?
15. What is the treatment of choice for a traumatic sprain of the interspinous ligament?
16. What is the most common cause of Baastrup's disease?
17. What is the mechanism of injury in a traumatic kissing spine?
18. Describe the localization of pain in a lumbar zygapophyseal joint syndrome.
19. Which movements usually provoke the most pain in a lumbar zygapophyseal joint syndrome?
20. The spinal nerve of which neurological segment emerges between L4 and L5?
21. At which level is the L5 nerve root usually compressed by a disc?
22. What is an absolute indication for surgery in a lumbar disc prolapse?
23. What are the most positive tests during the functional examination of a patient with a primary posterolateral disc protrusion/prolapse?
24. When a patient with a lumbar disc protrusion has pain on the right side and is deviated to the left, on which aspect of the root is the compression occurring?
25. Give two absolute indications for a sacral epidural local anesthesia.
26. At which level does a spondylitic spondylolisthesis most often occur?
27. Which movement is most limited and painful in a lumbar retrolisthesis?
28. What is the ratio of men to women in a spondylitic spondylolisthesis?
29. What is the benefit of performing isometric abdominal muscle-strengthening exercises with the lumbar spine positioned in a slight lordosis?
30. Treatment with continuous lumbar traction is most indicated for which lumbar disorder?

LUMBAR SPINE REVIEW ANSWERS

1. Symmetrical limitation of lateral flexion and extension is more limited than flexion.

2. Disc protrusion: the outer annulus fibers are still intact and there are no neurological deficits.

   Disc prolapse: the nucleus pulposus breaks through the annulus and there are usually neurological deficits.

3. Disc protrusion: flexion.

   Disc prolapse: extension.

4. In people over 50 years of age.

5. In the leg, usually in the fifth lumbar dermatome.

6. Walking, especially downhill and descending stairs.

7. Active forward flexion.

   On returning from the flexed position, the patient places hands on the upper legs and "climbs" back up to the erect position.

8. L4-5.

9. Exercise therapy aimed at stabilization of the lumbar spine and decreasing intradiscal pressure.

10. Osteoporosis.

11. L1 and/or L2.

12. Forward flexion of the lumbar spine.

14. Resisted extension and ipsilateral lateral flexion.

15. Friction massage, and the patient must avoid pain-provoking movements during the recovery period.

16. Osteoporosis.

17. Hyperextension trauma.

18. Deeply localized vague pain in the back, sometimes radiating to the gluteal region and the thigh.

19. Combined movements of the lumbar spine (opposite movements of the coupling patterns).

20. L4.

21. L4-5.

22. S4 root compression (micturition problems).

23. Limited forward flexion; positive straight leg raise test in combination with neck flexion and extension of the foot.

24. The "shoulder" of the nerve root.

25. Primary posterolateral disc protrusion after approximately 3 months and a nerve root compression syndrome.

26. L5–S1.

27. Lumbar extension.

28. 3:1.

29. Decrease of the intradiscal pressure.

30. Lumbar syndrome, which occurs as a result of a slowly developing disc protrusion in which ipsilateral sidebending is more painful than contralateral sidebending.

IMPORTANT INFORMATION FOR PATIENTS WITH BACK PAIN

This handbook is based on the text of a booklet that was written especially for patients with back pain, due either to poor posture or to disc lesions. During the first visit, the patient is instructed to read the booklet at home. At the next appointment, the contents of the booklet are discussed, as the program described must be individually fitted to the patient.

Introduction

At least once during a lifetime, almost everyone experiences back pain, either temporarily or over an extended period. Usually, although the symptoms may be uncomfortable, the condition is not severe. If you are reading this text, then you already have been thoroughly examined by your physician and/or physical therapist. Although it is certain that your problem is painful, from a medical point of view it is considered harmless.

This handbook discusses the anatomy of the back, how back problems occur, and treatment and exercise programs for you to follow. Also included in the scope of this discussion of low back pain is pain that can be felt in the buttocks and legs. You have received this handbook from your doctor or physical therapist. Through attentive reading, you will realize that you are responsible for the most important part of your treatment. During your recovery, your therapist plays the role of the manager. To find out the details of your treatment plan, read on.

ANATOMY

In order to better understand the function of the back, a short anatomical overview is necessary.

The back consists of the *vertebral column* and its attached ribs. The main muscles of the back and abdomen are attached to the *ribs* and to the vertebral column. The vertebral column consists of 24 bones called *vertebrae*. The vertebrae are connected to each other in various ways:

- One connection between vertebrae is called a *disc*. Discs are found between the vertebrae and function as a kind of shock absorber. There is no disc between the first vertebra and the skull nor between the first two vertebrae.

- Another connection between vertebrae is called the *zygapophyseal joints*. Every vertebra has bony prominences called *articular processes*. All articular processes have contact with the articular process from the vertebra either directly above or directly below. These processes form the zygapophyseal joints (sometimes called the facet joints) (Figure 4–A–1). As in all joints (for instance, the knee, shoulder, or hip), the zygapophyseal joints are also surrounded and supported by a joint capsule.

- In addition, vertebrae are joined together in several different places by *ligaments*.

Vertebrae and Muscles

The vertebral column is divided into three sections. The first section contains the seven *cervical vertebrae*. These form the *cervical spine*. The highest cervical vertebra constitutes the connection of the spinal column to the head. The lowest cervical vertebra rests on the highest thoracic vertebra.

There are 12 vertebrae that form the second section, or *thoracic spine*. Twelve ribs are attached to the *thoracic vertebrae*, the upper 10 of which have either a direct or an

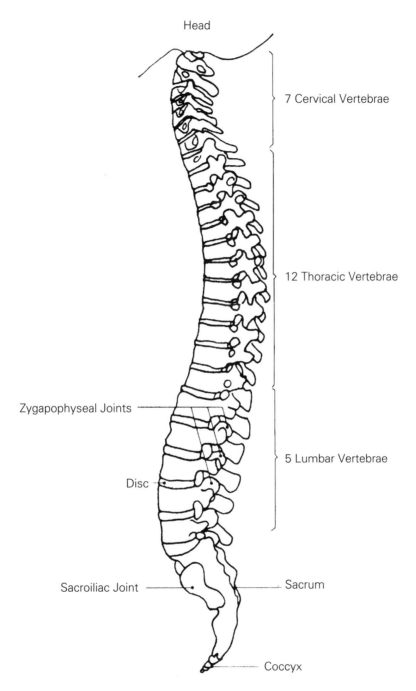

Figure 4–A–1 View of the vertebral column from the side.

indirect connection with the sternum at the front of the trunk. The lowest thoracic vertebra rests on the highest lumber vertebra.

The third section contains the five *lumbar vertebrae*, which form the *lumbar spine*. The lowest lumbar vertebra rests on the *sacrum*, which consists of five vertebrae that have grown together. At the lower end of the sacrum lies the *coccyx*, commonly called the tail bone (Figure 4–A–2).

The sacrum is connected to the pelvis through two *sacroiliac joints* (Figure 4–A–3). Therefore, these sacroiliac joints can also cause back pain. Simply stated, the verte-

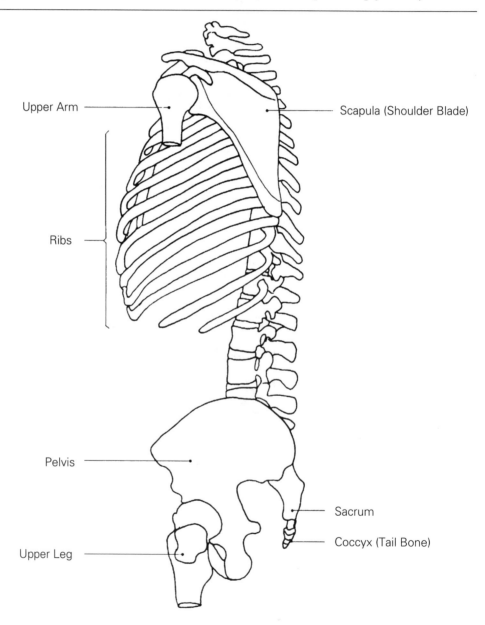

Figure 4–A–2 Side view of the vertebral column with ribs, scapula (shoulder blade), and pelvis.

bral column is the connection between the head and the pelvis.

The center of the vertebra contains a large opening through which the *spinal cord* runs. The spinal cord, part of the *nervous system*, directs a large amount of information to and from the brain. *Nerves* take this flow of information further to the arms and legs. These nerves arise from the spinal cord and leave the spinal column at approximately the level of the disc. Thus, when a disc is damaged, the *nerve root* found in that area can also become damaged and irritated. At the level of the cervical spine, this can lead to pain radiating down the arm into the fingers. With irritation of a nerve root in the lumbar area, pain can occur down the leg or even into the foot (Figure 4–A–4). A more detailed description of these symptoms is given later.

Usually, the abdominal, buttocks, and thigh muscles play the most significant role in the occurrence and treatment of back pain. Surprisingly, the back muscles are of the least

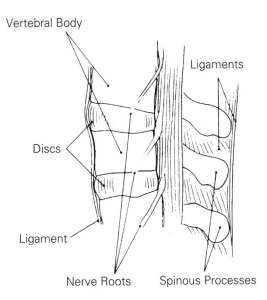

Figure 4–A–4 Longitudinal section through the spinal column.

importance. Later, this is discussed in more detail.

Quiz

Write down the correct label for each corresponding number on Figures 4–A–5 and 4–A–6, then compare with Figures 4–A–1 and 4–A–2.

Intervertebral Disc

Each intervertebral disc is at the center of a spinal segment. With the disc, a *spinal segment* consists of both adjacent vertebral bodies, the zygapophyseal joints with their capsules, the ligaments that connect both vertebrae to each other, and the exiting nerve roots (Figures 4–A–1 and 4–A–4).

To a large degree, the disc absorbs shock that occurs in the back during walking, running, and especially jumping. Of course, other parts of the body also have shock-absorbing functions. For example, let's say you jump down from a step. First, your feet take the shock, next the lower legs and knees, and so

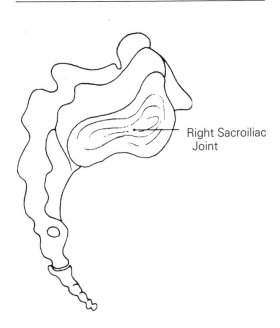

Figure 4–A–3 Side view of the sacrum.

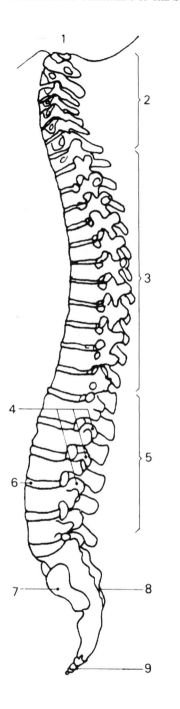

Figure 4–A–5 Side view of the vertebral column.

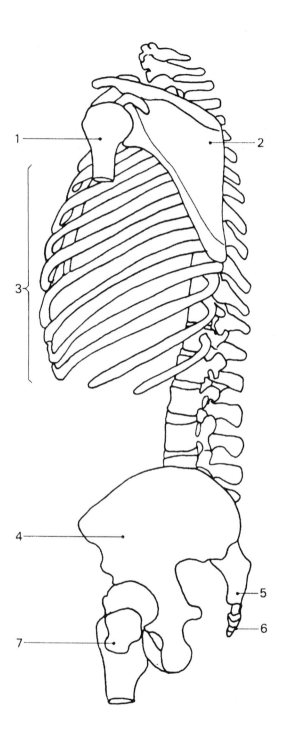

Figure 4–A–6 Side view of the vertebral column with ribs, scapula (shoulder blade), and pelvis.

on. The more the legs absorb the shock, the less load is placed on the discs.

Because the fibers in the outer layers of the disc run in different directions, not only is the shock that is applied from below absorbed, but so also are various other forces from different directions. This is why the disc is considered an unusually versatile and strong structure.

In the center of the disc, the "main shock absorber" is found, a gel-like core (*nucleus pulposus*), which constantly deforms during movements of the back (Figure 4–A–7).

Surprisingly, along with cartilage and connective tissue, the disc consists mostly of water. As people get older, the elasticity of the connective tissue decreases whereby the disc is less able to contain water and becomes thinner. This narrowing can be seen on X-ray films. The first discs to narrow are the ones on which most of the demand or stress has been placed over the years. In the low back this is the disc between the 4th and 5th lumbar vertebrae, but particularly the disc between the 5th lumbar vertebra and the sacrum. In shortened form, this is referred to as L4-5 and L5-S1 (Figure 4–A–8).

Narrowing of the disc is a natural part of the aging process. Therefore, do not get anxious when you hear, "Your back is significantly worn out in one area," or, "We find severe degeneration in your back." Because of the narrowing of the disc, more pressure is placed

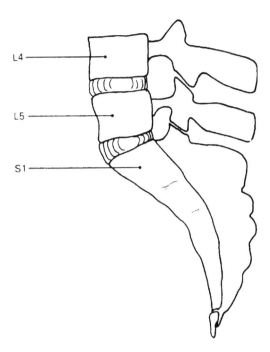

Figure 4–A–8 Sketch of the 4th and 5th lumbar vertebrae and the sacrum.

on the zygapophyseal joints (sometimes called facet joints), which then undergo "degenerative" changes. This so-called osteoarthrosis can be seen on X-ray films. Osteoarthrosis of the spine is termed *spondyloarthrosis*. Most of the time, as in narrowing of the disc, spondyloarthrosis does not cause any problem.

Organs with a good blood supply, such as the skin, heal quickly after an injury. Normally, scrapes or cuts on the skin heal within a few days. The less blood supply that an organ has, the slower the healing process will be. Because the disc has minimal to no blood supply, the healing is very slow, and along with it there is a loss of elasticity. As a result, the mobility of the back becomes limited.

Disc Lesions

Lesions of the disc are almost always due to poor technique in bending or lifting. Poor pos-

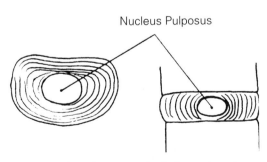

Nucleus Pulposus

Figure 4–A–7 Intervertebral disc, view from above and in a longitudinal cross-section core (nucleus pulposus).

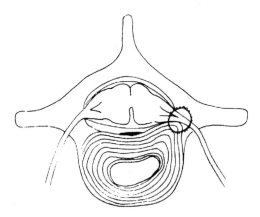

Figure 4–A–9 Lesion of the disc, stage 1.

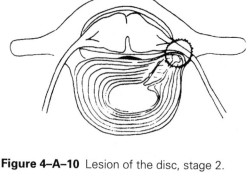

Figure 4–A–10 Lesion of the disc, stage 2.

ture or trauma, such as an accident, can also lead to disc lesions. Generally, these disc lesions can be divided into three stages.

Stage 1

The disc bulges slightly backward or backward and more to one side, which decreases the space available for the nerve root (Figure 4–A–9). One feels pain locally in the back. If the disc presses against the ligament (*posterior longitudinal ligament*) running in that area, the pain will be in the middle. If the pain is felt more to the right or more to the left, the disc is bulging more to that side.

Stage 2

In stage 2, one or more small tears have occurred in the disc. As a result the inner material (nucleus) can move to the outside of the disc. A complete escape of the material is restricted only by the outer layers of the disc (annulus fibers). This is called a *protrusion* (Figure 4–A–10). Pain occurring from this can be the same as in stage 1, or it can also be felt in the buttock region, or it can even radiate into the leg.

Stage 3

In stage 3, all of the outer layers of the disc are torn, through which the nucleus material

escapes. This is called a disc *prolapse* (Figure 4–A–11). Pain radiates into one leg and can be even more severe than the back pain. It is possible that pain is no longer felt in the back but now only in the leg.

Physicians and physical therapists can determine from which particular disc the problem is coming based on the type and location of the radiating pain. Pain at the back of the leg (sometimes called *sciatica*) usually indicates a lesion of the lowest disc (between L5 and S1). Generally, the larger the disc prolapse is, the easier it is to determine the correct diagnosis.

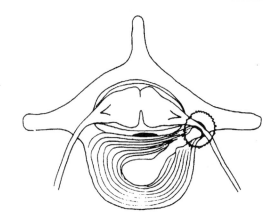

Figure 4–A–11 Lesion of the disc, stage 3.

Pressure on the nerve root can be so great that the normal electrical conduction is impossible. Sometimes this leads to a loss of strength in one or more muscles. Tingling or a general decrease in the sense of feeling in the leg or foot indicates a disturbance in sensation. Because pressure on the nerve root can also lead to a disturbance in the reflexes, during the clinical examination the knee and the heel cord reflexes are always tested.

HOW DOES BACK PAIN OCCUR?

The answer to this question is not easy. Back pain can actually be the manifestation of a wide variety of disorders. As already mentioned above, we are assuming that your back pain has no serious (malignant) cause. Unfortunately, there is much debate about what is the exact cause (and best treatment) of back pain. For instance, some people say that the zygapophyseal (or facet) joints are always responsible for causing back pain.

However, the disc and the ligaments or muscles must also be considered as the villains. In any case, science still cannot provide a definite or conclusive explanation for the phenomenon of low back pain. How the actual discussion stands can best be summarized as follows: At the center of the spinal segment is the disc. Many researchers are convinced that the first damage occurs in the disc. Every disc lesion results in a reaction of the entire spinal segment. Load on the zygapophyseal joints changes, which leads to abnormal tension on its capsule and ligaments. In some instances, the nerve root can even be irritated. Because all of the mentioned structures contain a lot of nerve fibers, pain can be caused by only one of the structures or by all of the structures combined.

Thus, we leave it open as to which structure is most responsible for your pain. Whether your pain comes from the disc or the zygapophyseal joints, it usually has no consequences regarding your treatment. Most back pain occurs as a result of poor posture or by improper lifting. Accidents, congenital defects, or even stress can also play a role in causing pain.

Good physical condition, particularly of the muscles, is an important requirement of maintaining correct posture. Muscles of the abdomen, buttocks, and particularly of the upper back area guarantee the correct position of the spine. Weakness of these muscles leads to an abnormally high load on the discs, the joint capsules, and ligaments, which in turn leads to pain.

Trauma can also be a cause of back problems. The trauma does not necessarily have to entail a violent injury to the body, such as falling down the stairs. Instead, something as apparently insignificant as spraining the ankle while stepping off a curb can lead to a severe back injury. Of course, severe accidents can cause severe injuries. Tears in ligaments and discs often accompany a vertebral fracture. However, back pain is often "only" a small muscle strain such as those seen in sports injuries.

SITTING, LIFTING, BENDING, LYING, STANDING, WALKING

Nachemson, a Swedish back expert, measured pressure in the discs of volunteers while they performed various positions and motions. He used the third lumbar disc to measure disc pressure. The resulting measurements of his tests are represented in Figure 4–A–12. For instance, it is obvious that the pressure during slouched sitting is always higher than it is in upright sitting. Kelsey, another researcher, found that work that involves a lot of sitting or a lot of driving is one of the most significant risk factors leading to a disc prolapse.

Below we have summarized the most significant results of the countless research studies that have been done in regard to back pain. The best protection for your back, besides good posture and strengthening the appropriate musculature, is to make sure that

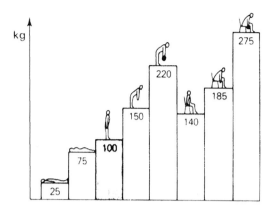

Figure 4–A–12 Pressure in the third lumbar disc during the following positions (from left to right): lying supine, sidelying, standing, standing and bending 20° forward, standing and bending 20° forward with a 20-kg weight, sitting without back support, sitting and bending 20° forward, sitting and bending 20° forward with a 20-kg weight.

you change your position and/or activity often throughout your day.

Sitting

In current times, sitting plays an important role in most jobs and in daily life. *Whenever possible, avoid sitting for long periods of time.* If prolonged sitting is unavoidable, support the low back with a posture pillow and tilt the back of the chair slightly backward. Every few minutes, simultaneously tense the abdominal and back muscles, holding for 6 seconds, during which you make yourself as tall as possible.

Make sure that there is adequate support for the legs. In chairs without an adjustable back or when sitting on a stool, it is important to sit actively. *Active sitting* means sitting up as straight as possible while tensing the abdominal and back muscles. It has been proven that by tensing the abdominal muscles the intra-abdominal pressure increases, leading to a decreased pressure in the disc (Figures 4–A–13A and 4–A–13B).

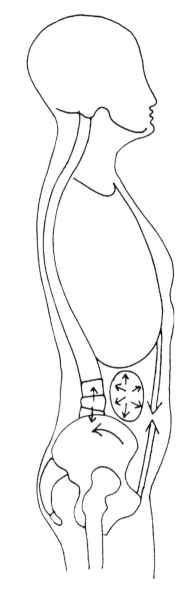

A

Figure 4–A–13A Increased pressure in the intra-abdominal space leads to decreased pressure in the disc.

When there is minimal pressure in the disc, the tension in the other spinal structures normalizes. Thus, one might see the disc as the middle point around which everything else revolves. Therefore, strengthening the abdominal muscles is very important. However,

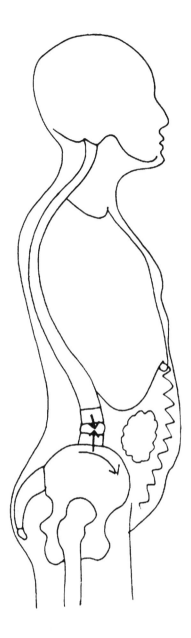

B

Figure 4–A–13B Less pressure in the intra-abdominal space leads to more pressure in the disc.

you may not bend the back during the exercises. Later we discuss some important abdominal exercises.

If you have an injured disc, every time you bend your back the center of the disc shifts backward. In this way, the nerve root or its

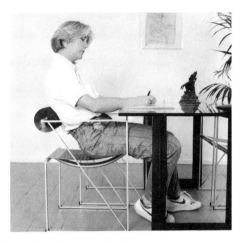

Figure 4–A–14 Poor sitting posture.

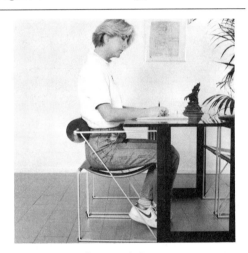

Figure 4–A–15 Correct sitting posture.

BY THE WAY, DO YOU HAVE GOOD POSTURE RIGHT NOW?
(Figures 4–A–14 to 4–A–18)

Bending and Lifting (Figures 4–A–19 to 4–A–24)

If you have ever had severe back pain, then you know that bending and lifting with a "hunched" back is impossible. Instead, keep your back straight and bend at the knees.

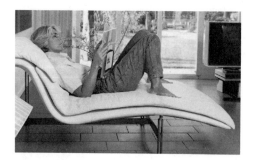

Figure 4–A–16 Poor sitting posture.

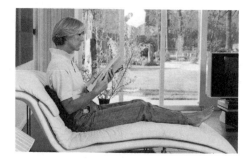

Figure 4–A–17 Correct sitting posture with the support of a posture pillow.

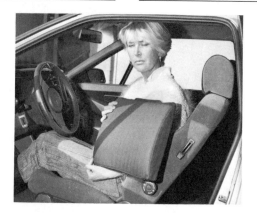

Figure 4–A–18 A posture pillow can also be used in the car.

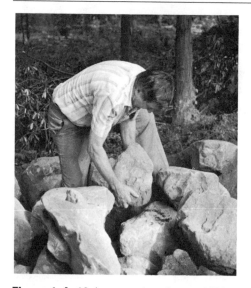

Figure 4–A–19 Incorrect bending and lifting.

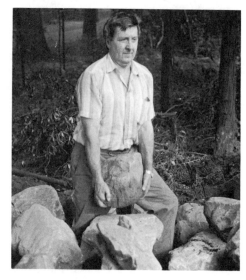

Figure 4–A–20 Correct bending and lifting.

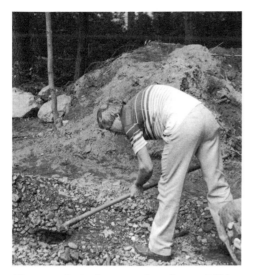

Figure 4–A–21 Incorrect bending and lifting.

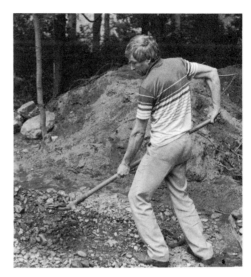

Figure 4–A–22 Correct bending and lifting.

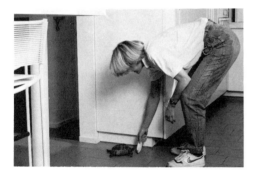

Figure 4–A–23 Incorrect bending.

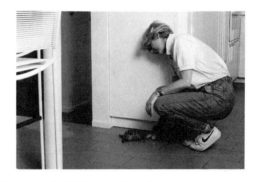

Figure 4–A–24 Correct bending.

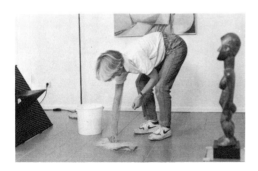

Figure 4–A–25 Incorrect bending.

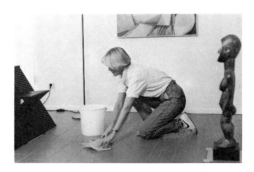

Figure 4–A–26 Correct bending.

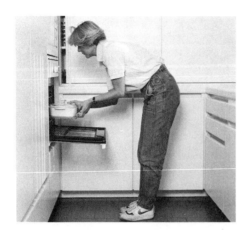

Figure 4–A–27 Incorrect bending.

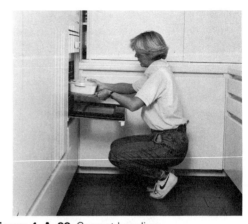

Figure 4–A–28 Correct bending.

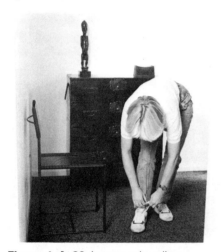

Figure 4–A–29 Incorrect bending.

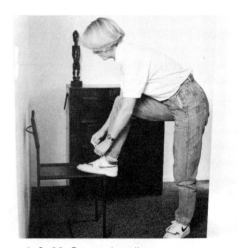

Figure 4–A–30 Correct bending.

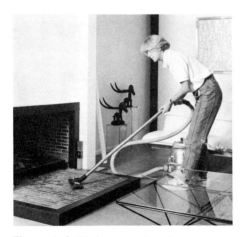

Figure 4–A–31 Incorrect bending.

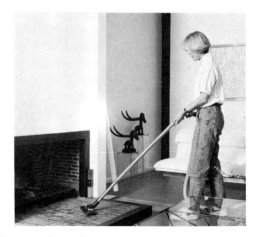

Figure 4–A–32 Correct bending.

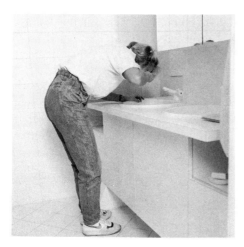

Figure 4–A–33 Incorrect bending.

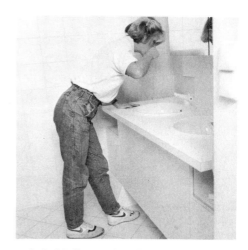

Figure 4–A–34 Correct bending.

sheath (*dura mater*) can become irritated, whereby pain can be felt in the back along with radiating pain in the leg. In order to prevent this, *you must keep the back erect but not too hollow.* Too much of a hollow in the back can jeopardize other areas of the spine.

Always bend at the knees when you have to bend and lift. This is assuming that your leg muscles are strong enough. If your legs need strengthening, pay particular attention to the leg exercises described later in this handbook. When you bend at the knees, simultaneously tighten your abdominal muscles.

Hold the object you are lifting as close as possible to your body.

Tightening your abdominal muscles also applies to such activities as vacuuming, brushing your teeth, working in the garden, and so on. Even though you might forget these tips at first, with time they will become a new habit and a valuable part of your everyday routine.

Lying (Figures 4–A–35 to 4–A–37)

You may think that when you lie down there is not much that can go wrong. How-

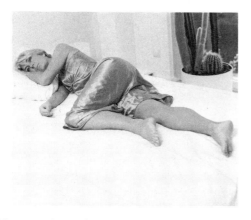

Figure 4–A–35 Correct posture in lying. Painful side up!

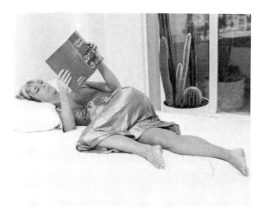

Figure 4–A–36 Correct posture for lying and reading. Painful side up!

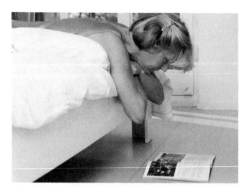

Figure 4–A–37 Alternative position for lying or reading.

ever, considering the fact that an individual spends at least one third of his or her life lying down, correct posture is very important. In addition, your mattress should be firm, with springs that are not too soft. If your bed is too soft, your back will rest in a position that is abnormally curved, and you may be occasionally awakened by pain. At home you can make sure that you have the proper bed, but what can you do when you are on the road or on vacation and the bed is too soft? Simply place the mattress on the floor and you will get through the night without pain. Of course, watch your posture when you lift the mattress down to the floor.

With some people it can be difficult to get accustomed to a firm mattress. In that case, choose one that is slightly less firm. You can determine the degree of firmness best for you by placing a board under your mattress or by sleeping with the mattress on the floor.

Do you like to sleep on your back, but have pain now when you do? Place a rolled-up hand towel or small pillow in the hollow of your back. Do you prefer to sleep on your side but hesitate to do so because of pain? Take care of the problem side of your back by lying on the side without pain and pulling up the top leg. Do you enjoy reading in bed? Try reading while lying on your stomach with the book on the floor. Even in lying, never spend prolonged periods in the same position. Change positions often.

No position or exercise should be painful. Many people erroneously think that they have to bear pain because "it must be good for my back." This is never true.

Have you ever had a real *lumbago* (acute and severe low back pain)? Then you know what pain is. As soon as you feel the threat of the lumbago coming on, lie down (to get rid of gravity). Place a pillow under your head, place one under your buttocks, and put your legs up on a stool or on several pillows. Some people find that they are most comfortable in a fetal position, which is sidelying with the legs pulled up. In any case, remain lying down until the pain goes away. This can take from minutes to hours.

Be careful when you do get up; make sure that you give your back maximal support. With hips and knees bent, turn on your side. As you bring both lower legs over the edge of the bed (in the clinic, over the edge of the treatment table), *tighten your abdominal muscles* and push yourself up with both hands. As soon as you are sitting, hold yourself maximally upright for 6 seconds. In so doing, you will again tighten your stomach, buttocks, and upper back musculature.

If you want to move from sitting to lying, do the same procedure but only in reverse.

Standing and Walking (Figures 4–A–38 and 4–A–39)

Prolonged standing is often miserable even for people without back problems; for people with back pain it can be pure torture. Hair stylists, waiters and waitresses, homemakers, factory workers, and surgeons, for instance, are people who have to stand frequently and often over long periods of time, placing an abnormal load on their backs. Assuming that the human back, as in four-legged animals, was originally created for horizontal posture, it is easy to understand that the erect position, particularly in standing, can lead to significant problems. Actually, certain existing ana-

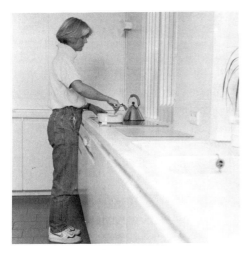

Figure 4–A–38 Proper standing posture, if the abdominal muscles are tightened.

tomical factors indicate that early in evolution the back was loaded quite differently than it is today.

What can we do to take some of the stress off the back when prolonged standing is unavoidable? First of all, constantly maintain tight stomach muscles. To achieve this, one needs a lot of exercise and training. Wearing proper shoes is also very important. A good

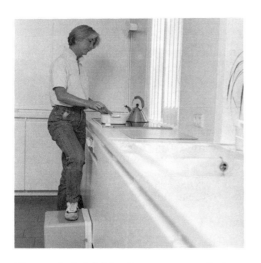

Figure 4–A–39 The best posture during prolonged standing: the feet are alternately placed on an 8- to 12-in high object.

shock-absorbing sole takes stress off the spine not only in standing (which is more or less walking in place) but also in walking.

During prolonged standing, load on the back can also be significantly decreased by alternately placing one foot on an elevated object that is about 12 in high. You will notice that tensing the abdominal muscles while alternating the weight-bearing leg makes standing much more comfortable.

Activities that involve partial standing and partial walking (such as a day of shopping or visiting a museum) can become much more enjoyable when one wears shoes with good shock absorption. Performing a 6-second isometric contraction of the abdominal muscles at regular intervals is also beneficial.

Proper jogging shoes offer the best shock absorption. If you are unable to wear this type of shoe due to work regulations, then choose a shoe with a rubber sole and heel instead of hard leather. Also place inlays or heel cups of a good shock-absorbing material in the shoes. Likewise, we recommend the same type of inlays for people with hip, knee, or ankle problems. Shock absorption can also be overdone. For example, you do not need shock-absorbing inlays in jogging shoes.

Patients with back problems often report that they prefer to stay moving rather than sit or stand for a long time. This makes sense, since during movement the abdominal muscles are more active, whereby the spine is more protected and under less stress.

When moving a heavy object, if you have the choice between pushing or pulling, always choose to push. Here the abdominal muscles will be tightened and thus protect the back. A heavy object can also be pulled by facing away from the object and pulling it with a rope (correct method). An incorrect method involves facing the object and pulling it backward. In this instance, the back muscles are tightened maximally, which brings the back into too much of a hollow.

WHILE YOU ARE READING NOW, DO YOU STILL HAVE GOOD POSTURE?

Assignment

Before you read further, please perform the following exercise: Sit up straight, tighten the abdominal and buttocks muscles (squeezing the buttocks together), make yourself as tall as possible, and hold for 6 seconds. Make sure that you keep breathing in a relaxed manner during the entire exercise. Then rest for 6 seconds, but remain sitting up straight. Repeat the exercise 10 times. This should take you about 2 minutes.

TEN COMMANDMENTS FOR A HEALTHY BACK

In addition to sitting, bending, lifting, lying, standing, and walking, there are numerous other situations that you will encounter on a daily basis that will need your attention. Below are our Ten Commandments for the Back. Make these a part of your daily routine.

1. Absolutely avoid sitting too long in the same position.
2. Bend and lift only with a straight back, tightened abdominal muscles, and bent knees.
3. Make sure that your abdominal, buttock, and thigh muscles are in optimal condition.
4. Sleep on a firm bed.
5. During prolonged standing, place one foot on a surface at a height of approximately 12 in.
6. Avoid exercises that bring the back into too much hollow or into an excessively hunched position.
7. Avoid wearing high-heeled shoes.
8. Wear shoes with good shock absorption.
9. Watch your nutrition and avoid too much stress. Being overweight is bad for the back.
10. Exercise daily, and if possible participate in a sport that protects your back.

DIAGNOSTICS

How can your doctor best determine what is wrong with your back? First of all, he or she will ask you several questions:

- What is your main complaint?
- Do you have pain? If so, where?
- Do you have a pins-and-needles sensation? If so, where?
- Do you have a feeling of muscle weakness? If so, where?
- Does your back feel stiff?
- When did the problems begin?
- When do you experience your problems?
  1. at rest
  2. during activities
  3. at night
  4. during the day

These questions are a part of a medical *history*. Additional questions are related to your profession, sport, hobby, general health, and family health. The last topic is of importance because certain back problems have a hereditary component. This means that your father, mother, or grandparents could have had similar problems.

Based on your answers to these questions, your doctor can identify the possible cause of your complaints. After taking your *history,* the doctor performs a *functional examination*. Tests are performed in both standing and in lying. Sometimes, in order for the doctor to get a complete picture, an X-ray will be taken (possibly with a contrast medium or a CT scan). Occasionally blood and urine laboratory tests are necessary. Once the *diagnosis* is determined, the doctor will recommend a treatment. Often this includes physical therapy.

In describing the following patient cases, we illustrate various types of back problems.

Example 1

A 40-year-old man describes a sudden, severe pain in his lower back that occurred while he was getting out of bed in the morning. It is impossible for him to stand upright and he finds that he is leaning slightly to the left. Because of the pain, he can do nothing more than lie back down and pull his knees up. This significantly decreases the pain but does not completely relieve it. His family physician makes a diagnosis of *acute lumbago* and prescribes several days of bed rest. One week later, he arrives at our clinic, already feeling much better, but bending is still difficult.

The treatment of this patient is left almost entirely to the principles of this handbook. If he follows the 10 commandments for a healthy back and exercises daily, he can be almost certain that he will never experience back pain again.

Example 2

A 32-year-old woman complains of irregularly occurring back pain, which she has had for the past 2 years. She usually experiences it during and after housecleaning activities. Vacuuming, for instance, is a "catastrophe."

During the functional examination, it was noted that the woman had very poor posture, as well as pronounced weakness in her abdominal, buttocks, and back muscles. She was given the appropriate information, which is also found in this handbook, with the recommendation that she exercise daily. The patient gradually improved. She occasionally experiences periods of discomfort; however, this does not interfere with her daily activities.

Example 3

A 50-year-old woman complains of 20 years of back pain. Sometimes the pain is so severe that she has to lie in bed for a few days. In the last 2 years, the pain has also radiated into her left leg, running from the back of her thigh to her heel.

During the functional examination, the patient could hardly bend forward. A straight leg raise of the left leg was only possible to about 50°, after which the patient felt her back pain, whereas the right leg was lifted to 90° without pain. This is called a *Lasègue sign*, and one says in this case, "Lasègue is positive at 50°," which means that the *sciatic nerve* is pinched. Usually this is caused by a protruding disc. Further examination showed no neurological deficits; in other words, muscle strength, sensation in the leg, and reflexes were normal.

A thorough explanation was given to the patient about her back problem, and she started physical therapy treatment consisting of traction. After her leg symptoms subsided, the patient was encouraged to perform daily exercises.

Example 4

A 34-year-old woman complains of acute back pain after a sneezing attack. Within a few hours, the pain is so severe in her back and both legs that she can hardly walk. Since the age of 14, she has had chronic back problems with occasional bouts of lumbago (severe back pain). Until this particular day, the patient's pain has never been so severe. The functional examination shows weakness in both calves, the Achilles (heel cord) reflex is absent on both sides, and the right heel feels numb. She is embarrassed to say that she has lost continence. This is an extremely important symptom and at the same time the only indication for surgery. (If surgery is not done for this type of disc prolapse, the incontinence can be permanent.)

The patient was referred immediately to a neurosurgeon and underwent surgery that same day. By the next morning, she could stand again and had almost no pain.

Example 5

A 15-year-old gymnast complains of back pain during all activities in which her back is bent significantly backward. When asked to demonstrate the most painful exercise for her, the gymnast bends over backward, placing her hands on the floor.

The functional examination did not bring about any more information other than that bending backward was painful. The spinous processes (these are small bony prominences of the spine, which you can feel [palpate] on yourself when rounding your back) in the low back were tender to palpation.

An X-ray, made while the gymnast stood in a backward-bent position, showed that the two painful spinous processes were touching each other. Of course, the rules in this handbook are not really appropriate for this young gymnast. Despite that, she was given information about the cause of her back pain, she was told to avoid the painful exercises for 2 months, and at the same time she received physical therapy. The patient had complete relief of pain after her treatment.

Example 6

An athletic 27-year-old man complains of almost 4 years of pain that alternates between his back and his buttock. Usually the pain is only on one side, but after several months the pain changes sides for no obvious reason. He has the most pain and stiffness in the morning. After several hours, the stiffness is gone. Actually, during and after sports activities, the patient has the least discomfort.

The patient felt that he was generally quite healthy, but after specific questioning, he admitted that some time earlier he had heel cord pain but had attributed that to jogging. Several months before, he also had intestinal problems, as well as a burning sensation in his eyes.

This history is very typical of a condition known as *ankylosing spondylitis*. It concerns an inflammatory process of the spine that usually begins in the sacroiliac joints (the two joints between the sacrum and the pelvis).

Sometimes it takes years to determine the final diagnosis, because the condition can be confirmed only after X-rays and blood tests.

Treatment consists of medication, along with advice as to appropriate posture and mobility exercises. The exercises specific for this problem are not addressed in this handbook.

Example 7

In our last example, a 29-year-old very active squash competitor complains of back pain regularly after each game. The pain radiates into both legs, but is relatively mild in nature. Also, the patient complains that his muscles are "too short."

No clear findings were obtained from the functional examination; certain movements were slightly painful, and a shortening was noted in the muscle that connects the spine with the upper leg (iliopsoas muscle). The patient's complaints pointed to a disruption of a lumbar vertebral arch, confirmed by X-ray. This type of fracture is called an *isthmic spondylolisthesis*.

Usually, treatment consists of careful stretching exercises for the shortened muscles (including the iliopsoas muscle mentioned above), along with intensive abdominal muscle-strengthening exercises (described in this handbook). Further explanation about the cause of the problem is also necessary, and the patient should follow nearly all of the recommendations and exercises in this handbook. Only in severe cases should surgery be considered.

Most back problems caused by poor posture, incorrect bending, or incorrect lifting are relatively harmless and occur between the ages of 35 and 45. With increasing age, fewer back problems are seen, even though changes on X-rays more frequently occur. This means that radiologically visible changes, in most instances, are not the cause of the back pain. Actually, the opposite is usually the case. Patients with severe complaints are often radiologically "healthy," whereas people with obvious "pathological" X-ray findings (e.g., severe osteoarthrosis, spondyloarthrosis) often have no pain at all (Figure

4–A–40). References frequently made to "congenital defects" are usually irrelevant. For example, the very often-diagnosed "scoliosis" (a sideways curve in the spine) can be found in practically everyone, although hardly anyone complains of pain. These so-called "congenital defects" are mostly just variations in nature and not real pathology.

Weekly, we hear at least one patient say that his or her lowest disc is "completely worn out" (or "degenerated" or "osteoarthrotic") and that the doctor said that he or she would have to learn to live with it. However, we are convinced that it is usually not the degenerated disc but rather the neighboring segment that is causing the problem. Patients frequently ask whether they will become more stiff because of the decreased mobility in the degenerated segment. Yes, but in such cases this is exactly what we want to happen, because not much more can happen to the degenerated segment and the spine still has a lot of other flexible segments. Have you ever noticed what happens on a bicycle when two links of the chain have rusted together? The chain continues to function well in spite of it.

In summary, we have established that there can be a variety of causes for your back pain. Therefore, make sure you have a thorough examination before you follow the advice and exercises in this handout.

TREATMENT

Many articles and books have been written regarding the treatment of low back pain. Most doctors and physical therapists have their own opinions about proper treatment. Unfortunately, even after many investigations, it is still not known which treatment is the best. In spite of the variety of treatment possibilities, ultimately you are the one who can relieve and even overcome your own back pain.

The most important conclusion that researchers agree on is that treatment (whether through medication, physical therapy, massage, electrical stimulation, ultrasound, hot packs, or cold packs) is always *symptomatic*. Therefore, in the first instance, one tries to relieve the symptoms. *Such treatment never reaches the root of the problem and therefore will never be healing in the actual sense.*

Manual therapy and traction are different in that they can affect the root of the problem. Many patients with back pain have excellent results with these types of treatments, *although this should never be seen as the only type of treatment to consider.* The patient should always receive thorough information about his or her back problem and should follow the principles of this handbook.

CONTINUE YOUR EXERCISE PROGRAM EVEN AFTER YOUR PAIN IS GONE!

The faster your condition improves, the more important it is to be aware of your posture and also to continue with your daily exercises. As in brushing your teeth, these exercises serve to prevent future problems.

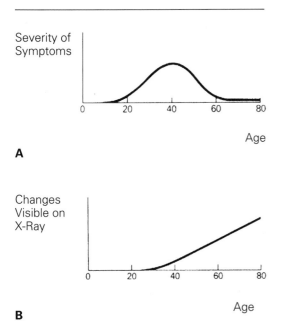

Figure 4–A–40 Discrepancy between severity of symptoms (***A***) and radiological (X-ray) findings (***B***).

Especially in cases of acute back pain, physical therapy and medications can offer a certain amount of pain relief in the first 10 to 14 days. To an even greater extent, this applies to manual therapy whereby the patient is able to begin the exercise program sooner. It has been shown that 3 months after the onset of back problems almost all patients, regardless of the type of treatment, are back to enjoying life again.

THE EXERCISE PROGRAM

There are numerous exercises for strengthening the abdominal muscles. Most have the disadvantage of forcing one to hunch the back, such as when one performs a sit-up from the lying position (sometimes with the feet fixed). Through the rounding of the back, the pressure in the disc increases, which either causes back pain or increases the already existing back pain. Actually, this is one of the most damaging exercises for the back. In the following section, exercises are described that strengthen the abdominal muscles and at the same time support the back.

Exercise 1

Starting position: Lie on your back on the floor with legs straight (a bed is generally too soft). Place a small towel roll (about 1½ to 2 in thick) in the hollow of your back. This exercise is performed in five phases.

Phase 1 (Figure 4–A–41)

Keeping your knees straight, push the backs of your heels (or the backs of your thighs) into the floor.

Phase 2 (Figure 4–A–42)

By contracting your abdominal muscles, tilt the pelvis backward. *The stomach is pulled in.*

Phase 3 (Figure 4–A–43)

While continuing to push your heels (or your thighs) into the floor, lift your head,

shoulders, and outstretched arms. *Maintain constant pressure between the heels or thighs and the floor.*

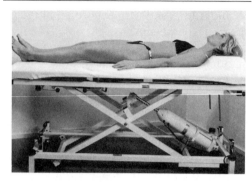

Figure 4–A–41 Exercise 1, Phase 1.

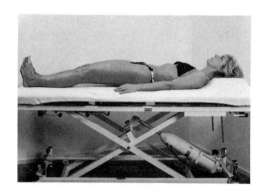

Figure 4–A–42 Exercise 1, Phase 2.

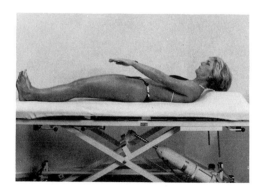

Figure 4–A–43 Exercise 1, Phases 3 and 4.

Phase 4 (Figure 4–A–43)

Keep breathing in a relaxed manner and try to come up as far as possible (normally you should not get farther than to lift your shoulder blades from the floor).

Phase 5

After 6 seconds, lower your upper body back down to the floor and rest for 2 to 3 seconds.

This exercise strengthens the straight abdominal muscle in particular. Repeat this exercise 10 times, twice daily. After resting for about 1 minute, go on to Exercise 2.

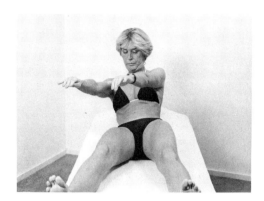

Figure 4–A–44A Exercise 2A.

Exercise 2 (Figures 4–A–44A and 4–A–44B)

This exercise is the same as Exercise 1, except that now the oblique abdominal muscles are trained. Instead of lifting the upper body straight up, this time as you come up bring your right shoulder more in the direction of your left knee. Then, the next time bring your left shoulder in the direction of your right knee. The same rules for the last exercise apply to this one. (See Exercise 1, phases 1, 2, 4, and 5.) Both of these exercises are ideal for strengthening the abdominal muscles. You will see that the strength and condition of your abdominal muscles will return quickly.

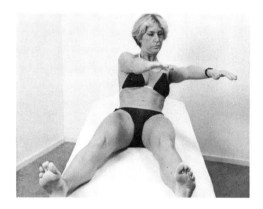

Figure 4–A–44B Exercise 2B.

Exercise 3 (Figure 4–A–45)

This exercise is similar to the first two exercises. Now the knees are bent and the back of the heels are hooked against a fixed point. While lifting the upper body, push your heels against the fixed edge, as if pulling the heels toward the body. Both the oblique and diagonal abdominal muscles are strengthened here.

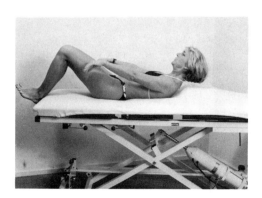

Figure 4–A–45 Exercise 3.

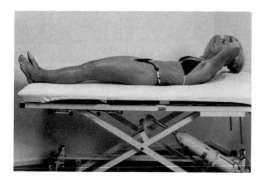

Figure 4–A–46 Exercise 4.

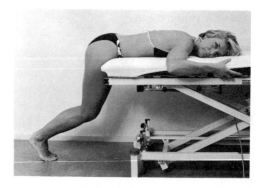

Figure 4–A–47 Exercise 5, Phase 1.

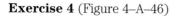

Exercise 4 (Figure 4–A–46)

The starting position is the same as with the first two exercises. Now place your hands, with fingers intertwined, behind your neck and repeat the first three exercises. To protect the cervical spine, as you are raising your upper body, push the back of your neck slightly into your hands. If you experience discomfort in your neck while performing Exercises 1, 2, or 3, then it is best that you perform them only as described here.

Exercise 5

The buttock and back muscles are strengthened with this exercise.

Starting position: Lie on your stomach on a single bed or some other elevated surface. With your hands at about the level of your head, grasp each side of the bed firmly. Both legs hang over the foot of the bed with the toes resting on the floor.

Phase 1 *(Figure 4–A–47)*

Straighten your knees, keeping your toes on the floor.

Phase 2 *(Figure 4–A–48)*

Slowly lift your legs, keeping your knees straight and staying below the horizontal. *Simultaneously tighten your abdominal muscles.* Hold this position for 6 seconds and

continue to breathe in a relaxed manner. Make sure that your upper body stays flat against the bed.

Phase 3

Slowly lower your legs back down until your toes touch the floor again. Relax for 2 to 3 seconds and then repeat the exercise.

Exercise 6 (Figure 4–A–49)

The musculature in the thoracic area of your back has the most influence on your posture.

Phase 1

Lie on your back with your knees bent. Rest both arms against the floor with your shoulders and elbows bent at 90° angles.

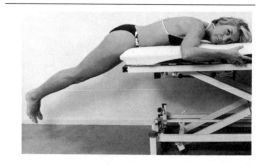

Figure 4–A–48 Exercise 5, Phase 2.

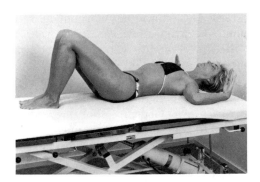

Figure 4–A–49 Exercise 6.

Phase 2

Maintain contact between your wrists and the floor, and point your fingers to the ceiling.

Phase 3

Tighten the abdominal muscles (this tilts the pelvis backward).

Phase 4

Push your wrists and elbows firmly into the floor and hold for 6 seconds. Continue to breathe in a relaxed manner. Rest for a few seconds, and repeat the exercise for a total of 10 times.

Exercise 7 (Figure 4–A–50)

We call this exercise the "ski exercise" because it strengthens the muscles at the front of the thighs. Strong thigh muscles are important for lifting.

Phase 1

Stand with your back against the wall. A chair or stool is placed between your lower legs and the wall.

Phase 2

Let your back slowly slide down the wall by bending your hips and knees. Stop just before reaching the stool. Do not sit down! Your thighs are now in a horizontal position.

Phase 3

Stay in this position as long as possible. By looking at the second hand on a clock or watch, count how long you are able to keep this position.

Phase 4

When you cannot hold the position any longer, slowly slide down farther until you are sitting on the stool.

Phase 5

Straighten and bend your knees several times before getting up.

Although it would be ideal, not everyone is able to perform all of the exercises two or three times daily. Therefore, we have established two programs, each of which takes only a minimum of 10 minutes. You may divide these 10 minutes throughout the day if necessary.

Program 1

Morning Exercises 1 and 2; 2 minutes
Exercise 5; 1 minute
Exercise 6; 1 minute
Exercise 7; as long as possible

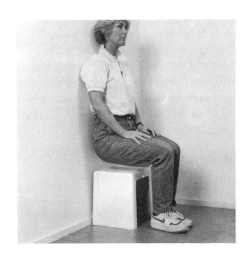

Figure 4–A–50 Exercise 7.

Evening   Exercise 3 (as Exercises 1 and 2); 2 minutes
Exercises 5, 6, and 7; as in morning

Program 2

Morning   Exercises 1 and 2; 1 minute
Exercise 4; 1 minute
Exercise 5; 1 minute
Exercise 6; 2 minutes
Evening   Exercise 4; 2 minutes
Exercise 5; 1 minute
Exercise 7; as long as possible

Of course, when you have time, you can always increase your program. Also, outside of these exercises, continually keep in mind your abdominal, buttock, and back muscles and your posture. Exercise regularly even when your pain is gone.

CONCLUSION

In summary, we want to emphasize again that it is not your doctor or your physical therapist who will alleviate your pain, but rather you yourself. Injections, electrical stimulation, medications, acupuncture, and so on are not the magic answers to back pain.

Sometimes there are patients for whom treatment has no effect at all. These patients often have severe back pain with pain in either one leg or both legs. Occasionally 2 or 3 days of bed rest may be helpful. Usually an MRI or CT scan is performed. Sometimes surgery for a prolapsed disc is necessary. After such operations, the advice in this handbook should again be followed.

SPORTS

As soon as you have significant improvement in your back pain you should return (in degrees) to some sports activities. Try swimming, not longer than half an hour, for instance, regularly changing the style or stroke. When you are completely pain free, you may increase your duration of swimming by 15 minutes each time. However, do not overdo it. In the first 3 months you should not swim more than three times per week.

In spite of the many negative reports, jogging is an excellent way to improve your physical fitness. Of course, there are a couple of rules to keep in mind: Run only in shoes with adequate shock absorption, and increase the amount of running very slowly. Although you may have been an avid runner before the onset of your back pain, begin jogging for only 2 minutes, at a relaxed pace. Make sure you land and push off correctly with your foot; land on the heel and roll off the forefoot.

Try the following training sequence:

Day 1   5 minutes
Day 2   —
Day 3   5 minutes, at a slightly faster pace
Day 4   —
Day 5   7 minutes
Day 6   7 minutes, at a slightly faster pace
Day 7   —
Day 8   10 minutes
and so on . . .

Slowly build up to jogging three times a week for half an hour. Sometimes people become real fanatics and have such fun jogging that eventually they even experience a "runner's high." We know former patients who have gone on to run marathons!

Biking is not considered a suitable sport for people who have had back problems, although one can try it as long as the back is kept straight. It is not advisable to return to such sports as hockey, rowing, racquetball, or baseball. Tennis and badminton are allowed but with the requirement that you have strong abdominal, buttock, back, and leg muscles.

In any case, we recommend that you consult your physician or physical therapist before beginning or returning to sports activities.

WE WISH YOU A SUCCESSFUL RECOVERY.

5

Thoracic Spine

5.1 FUNCTIONAL ANATOMY

An important function of the thoracic spine is protection of the organs located within the thorax. Therefore, mobility of the thoracic spine is not its primary purpose. Because of the cagelike construction of the ribs and spinal column, a considerable amount of mobility cannot be expected. However, the available mobility is very significant. Thus, besides describing anatomy and function of the thoracic spine and the ribs, attention is also given to the biomechanics of respiration.

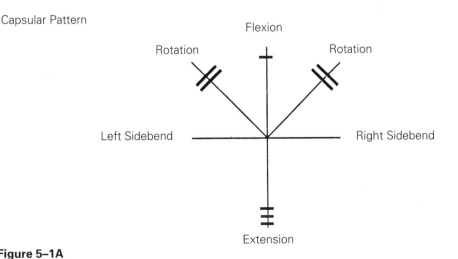

Figure 5–1A

Cross Line = LOM

SB not valid for test — seldom ⊕ c̄ disc, +
  combines c̄ rot. (except rib f.)   see p. 406

- Coupled Movements: Illustrated
- Combined Movements: A movement is combined when one of the motions in the coupled movement pattern is changed.

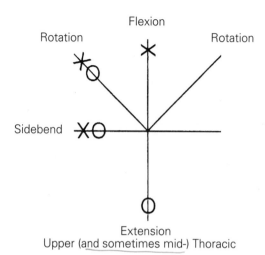

A *goes w/ cervical*

X = Flexion, ipsilateral
O = Extension, ipsilateral (cervical)

B *goes w/ lumbar*

X = Flexion, ipsilateral
O = Extension, contralateral (lumbar)

Figure 5–1B

The second to eighth thoracic vertebrae strongly resemble each other and contain the typical thoracic characteristics (Figure 5–2). The anterior-posterior (AP) diameter is almost equal to the transverse diameter (compared with the cervical vertebrae, which have a larger transverse diameter than AP diameter). The superior and inferior articular processes are located on the junction between body and pedicle. On each of these articular processes, an articular facet of the zygapophyseal joint is located. The superior articular facets are somewhat larger than the inferior facets. The intervertebral foramen, formed by two adjacent vertebrae, is rather small and round in comparison with the cervical and lumbar foramina. The spinous process is relatively large and points obliquely backward and downward. The transverse processes have two articular surfaces for the costal tubercles.

The first, ninth, tenth, eleventh, and twelfth thoracic vertebrae do not have the typical thoracic characteristics (Figure 5–3).

The upper costal articular facet at the lateral aspects of the first thoracic vertebral body has a peculiar form. These surfaces are almost round and articulate with the heads of only the first ribs. Otherwise, the form of this vertebra strongly resembles that of a cervical vertebra.

The ninth thoracic vertebra does not have the inferior costocapitular facets that one

$AP \geq T$

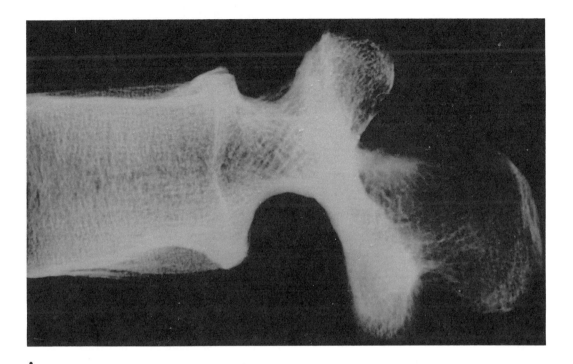

Figure 5–2 Typical thoracic vertebra (T2 to T8). **A**, X-ray; **B**, two thoracic vertebra, side view; **C**, thoracic vertebra, side view; **1**, body; **2a**, superior costocapitular demifacet (facet for articulation with the lower half of head of the rib); **2b**, inferior costocapitular demifacet (facet for articulation with the upper half of head of the rib); **3**, costotubercular facet; **4a**, superior articular (zygapophyseal) facet; **4b**, inferior articular (zygapophyseal) facet; **5**, transverse process; **6**, spinous process.

wedge 3.8

(N) Root far from disc, at foramina.
CVJ has disc as part of post med-aspect.

† Para-artic. spur in post. foramine, canal unknown
May press on N-T↑ kyphosis

3.8° × 12 = ave. 45°
total kyph. of Th-Spine

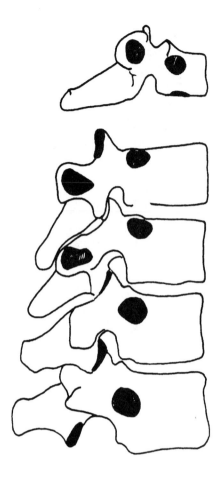

Figure 5–3 The first and the ninth to the twelfth thoracic vertebrae, side view.

would expect for the connections with the tenth ribs.

The tenth thoracic vertebra articulates with only the tenth ribs. The joint surfaces for the lower aspect of the heads of the ribs are located at the upper aspect of the vertebral body. Sometimes the articular surface on the transverse process for the costotransverse articulation is missing.

The eleventh thoracic vertebra articulates with the heads of only the eleventh ribs, and this only via a costovertebral connection. There are no costotransverse joints at the level of T11. The transverse processes here are small.

The twelfth thoracic vertebra articulates with only the twelfth ribs. The costal articular facets are located rather far posteriorly. The form of the vertebral body resembles that of a lumbar vertebral body.

Besides the absence of the joint surfaces for the ribs, the transition from the thoracic into the lumbar vertebral body type is also noticeable in the positions of the joint facets of the articular processes. This transition takes place rather abruptly. In one of the lower three thoracic vertebrae, the positions of the joint surfaces of the superior articular processes are characteristic of the thoracic vertebral body type, while at the same time the joint surfaces on the inferior articular processes have the typical lumbar position. (The lumbar facets are located in an almost sagittal plane). The vertebra where this most often occurs is usually the eleventh thoracic vertebra, but sometimes the tenth or the twelfth.

JOINTS

As previously mentioned, the mobility of the thoracic spine is limited due to the presence of the ribs and sternum. In addition, motion in the thoracic spine is dependent on the movements in the costovertebral and sternocostal connections, as well.

Intervertebral Discs

Thoracic discs, in comparison with lumbar and cervical discs, are relatively thin. This is understandable considering the limited mobility of the thoracic spine.   *Thin end plates*

Zygapophyseal Joints

The joint facets of the thoracic zygapophyseal joints lie almost in the frontal plane. There is a varying inclination in the transverse plane of 15° to 20° in relation to the frontal plane, running from ventrolateral to dorsomedial. In the parasagittal plane, there is an inclination in relation to the transverse plane of 60°, running from cranioventral to caudodorsal. The capsule is less lax, in comparison with the lumbar and cervical zygapophyseal joints.   *No meniscoid inclusions or folds in T4-8,*

Costovertebral Joints (Articulatio Capitis Costae)

The typical costovertebral joint is the connection between the head of the rib and two adjacent vertebral bodies (with the intervertebral disc) (Figure 5–4). In the capsule, the anterior costocentral (or radiate) ligament is located. This ligament runs from the ventral aspect of the rib, in three parts, as follows:

1. the cranial vertebra (pars superior)
2. the disc (pars intermedius)
3. the caudal vertebra (pars inferior)

The first, tenth, eleventh, and twelfth ribs each articulate with only one vertebra: the vertebra from the corresponding thoracic level. However, in these cases, the anterior

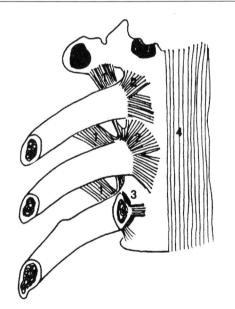

Figure 5–4 Typical costovertebral joints. *1*, the superior costotransverse ligament; *2*, the anterior costocentral (radiate) ligament; *3*, the intra-articular costocentral ligament; *4*, the anterior longitudinal ligament.

costocentral ligament is also connected to the cranial vertebra.

In the second to the ninth costovertebral joints, the intra-articular costocentral ligament is located. This ligament connects the head of the rib with the disc between the two adjacent vertebrae. It divides the articular cavity into two chambers. At the first, tenth, eleventh, and twelfth ribs, this ligament is absent; thus these joints have only a single chamber.

Costotransverse Joints (Articulatio Costotransversaria)

The costotransverse joint is the connection between the tubercle (facies articularis tuberculi costae) of a rib and the transverse process (fovea costalis processus transversus) of the corresponding vertebra (Figure 5–5). This joint is absent at the eleventh and twelfth ribs.

The capsule is relatively thin, but is reinforced by the costotransverse ligaments. The costotransverse ligament is located in the costotransverse foramen and connects the rib and the transverse process of the same level. The superior costotransverse ligament (which can be distinguished from the lateral costotransverse ligament and the costotransverse ligament itself) connects the neck of the rib and the transverse process of the vertebra located cranially. This ligament is penetrated by the intercostal nerves and by blood vessels. The stringlike lateral costotransverse ligament connects the rib with the tip of the transverse process of the corresponding vertebra.

Sternocostal Joints (Articulationes Sternocostales)

The first, sixth, and seventh rib cartilages are each linked to the sternum by a synchondrosis. The second to fifth ribs are each connected to the sternum through a synovial joint, whereby the cartilage of the corresponding rib articulates with a socketlike cav-

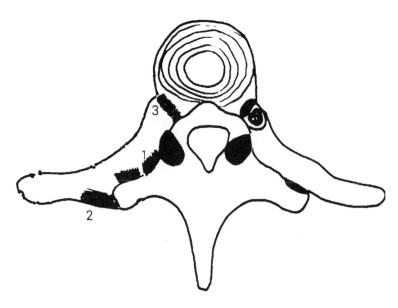

Figure 5–5 A typical costotransverse joint. *1*, Costotransverse ligament; *2*, lateral costotransverse ligament; *3*, intra-articular costocentral ligament.

ity in the sternum. The entire connection is surrounded by a capsule that is continuous with the perichondrium and the periosteum. The capsule is reinforced by ligaments. The radiate sternocostal ligament is a strong wide band running from the rib cartilage toward the sternum. At the level of the sternum, this ligament is interwoven with the sternocostal ligaments of the adjacent cranial and caudal joints. Fibers from these ligaments also intermingle with those of the opposite side, as well as with the insertion of the pectoralis major. At the second sternocostal junction (at the transition between the manubrium and the body of the sternum), there is always an intra-articular ligament. This is not always the case in the other sternocostal connections.

Very prominent. [handwritten annotation in margin]

Interchondral Joints (Articulationes Interchondrales)

Interchondral joints are found in the rib cartilage between the sixth and seventh, seventh and eighth, and eighth and ninth ribs. These synovial joints are located at the ventral aspect of the thorax, a few centimeters lateral of the mid-line. The joint capsule is reinforced by the interchondral ligament.

VASCULARIZATION

Vascularization of the thoracic part of the spinal cord and the meninges is mainly organized through the dorsal branches of the posterior intercostal arteries, with highly variable longitudinal anastomoses. From here, the vertebral bodies, joints, and nerve roots are also supplied. The part of the spinal cord between T4 and T9 is the most poorly vascularized region.[1]

see Ch [handwritten annotation in margin]

The venous drainage of the area runs through the anterior and posterior venous plexuses. They join the intervertebral vein, then the posterior intercostal vein, and later the azygos vein.

INNERVATION

The joints of the thoracic spine are innervated from the dorsal rami and the intercostal nerves. The mixed nerves of the paravertebral plexus also participate in the innervation.[2]

BIOMECHANICS

In relation to the mechanics of the thorax, two main aspects are distinguished: the movement of the thoracic spine and the movement of the ribs during respiration.

Kinematics of the Thoracic Spine

The mobility of the thoracic spine is limited in all directions. The movements in the sagittal plane (flexion-extension) are mainly limited by the position of the zygapophyseal joints and other bony structures such as the neural arch and the spinous processes. At the same time, the rib cage represents a ventral restraining factor. One can expect a total sagittal movement excursion of 2° to 6° per segment. More range of motion is possible in flexion than in extension.

The removal of the neural arches in anatomical specimens significantly increases the range of motion in the sagittal and transverse planes. This is in contrast to the situation in the lumbar spine, where such an increase in the amplitude of motion does not occur after the arches have been removed.

According to White,[3] the instant axis of rotation in flexion is located caudal to the disc of the specific segment, and in extension it is cranial to the disc. In sidebending, the instant axis of rotation is located within the disc at the convex side. In axial rotation, the axis moves from ventral to dorsal through the middle of the vertebral body.

During sidebending of a thoracic motion segment, the two facets on the inferior articular processes of the cranial vertebra move in opposite directions. The facet at the concave side (in left sidebending, the left facet) moves caudally. The facet on the convex side moves cranially.

Axial rotation in a thoracic motion segment leads to a torque within the disc which is greater than in the lumbar segments.

In relation to the question whether a coupling between axial rotation and sidebending exists in the thoracic spine, White[3] comes to an affirmative conclusion. In the upper part of the thoracic spine, this phenomenon is pronounced; in the middle and lower part of the thoracic spine, it is less apparent and also less consistent. During sidebending in the upper thoracic spine, the coupled axial rotation of the vertebral body is toward the concavity of the curve. Sidebending and rotation are ipsilateral. This coupling is the same in the midthoracic region. However, in many cases a contralateral axial rotation is observed in extension. In the lower thoracic spine, the coupling is ipsilateral during flexion and contralateral during extension (the same as in the lumbar spine).

Biomechanics of the Ribs

Costovertebral Connections

Movements in the costovertebral connections can be characterized as gliding motions with a small amplitude. The movements in the costovertebral and the costotransverse joints are functionally coupled with each other. A line connecting the centers of both joints represents the axis around which the movement of the rib takes place (Figure 5–6).

The axis of the lower ribs runs almost in the sagittal plane; for the upper ribs it runs practically in the frontal plane. The articular surfaces of the upper costotransverse joints are oriented roughly in the frontal plane; they are convex in a dorsal direction. The lower costotransverse joints are oriented more in a transverse plane and are flat (Figure 5–7). Because of these joint characteristics, movement of the upper ribs (the vertebrosternal ribs) increases the anterior-posterior diameter of the thorax, while movement of the lower ribs (the vertebrochondral ribs) increases the transverse diameter. *see p. 400*

Costocartilage and Sternum

During elevation of the ribs, the sternum rises and the costocartilage takes a more horizontal position. With further elevation, it rotates around its own longitudinal axis, a

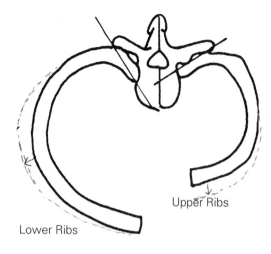

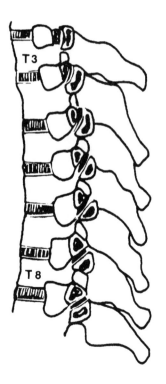

Figure 5–6 Axis of movement of the costovertebral connections.

Figure 5–7 Costotransverse joint surfaces.

forced rotation caused by the attachment of the ribs to the vertebral bodies. Meanwhile, the lower ribs move laterally and caudally in relation to the sternum.

Ribs and the Stability of the Spinal Column

Research has been done by Andriachi et al[4] in relation to the significance of the ribs for the stability of the spinal column. Guided by a mathematical model and computer simulations, the authors determined the stability of a normal spinal column with axial compression and the effect of the ribs on the stiffness of the spinal column during flexion. The properties of the costovertebral joints play an important role in this model.

The ribs and the sternum have a significant effect on the bending stiffness of the spinal column. There are indications that in extension the bending stiffness of the thoracic spine increases by a factor of 2. In flexion, the stiffness of the thoracic spine, with ribs and sternum, amounts to approximately 30% more, compared with a thoracic spine without ribs and sternum. In sidebending, the stiffness with ribs and sternum is approximately 45% more than that in the isolated spinal column, and during axial rotation approximately 30%. At the same time, Andriachi et al found that the spinal column with ribs and sternum can resist three times the compression force compared with an isolated spinal column.[4] *(prevents ventral translation)*

Aided by computer simulations, Andriachi et al also compared a normal spine with a scoliotic spine. In relation to the sidebending, only a small difference between the normal spine and the scoliotic spine was found. However, when traction was applied, the presence of ribs in the scoliotic spine caused a much smaller increase in the bending stiffness, compared with a normal spine. Based on these observations, it was calculated that the bending stiffness of a scoliotic spinal column amounted to only one-third that of a normal spinal column. In these calculations and simulations, the bending moments and the traction were applied at the level of T1.

Mechanics of Respiration

The deformability of the thorax as a whole is determined by the mobility and deformability of the composing thoracic parts. The costotransverse and costovertebral joints are important factors in this. During inspiration, the ribs are lifted around an axis that runs in a different direction in the upper (vertebrosternal) ribs than in the lower (vertebrochondral) ribs. As a result, the thorax is enlarged in a dorsal-ventral direction at its cranial aspect and in a more transverse direction at its caudal aspect.

The elasticity of the rib cartilage also has an influence. As the ribs elevate, the sternocostal angle changes, causing a torsion in the rib cartilage. This torsion is a dorsally directed rotation occurring around the longitudinal axis of the rib cartilage of the upper 10 ribs. The elasticity of the rib cartilage stores energy that is released again at the moment of "detorsion." The energy stored during inspiration is released again during expiration.

In general, the mechanism of the normal (not forced) respiration is as follows: because of the activity of the inspiratory muscles, energy (particularly elastic energy) is stored within the system, which is released when the inspiratory muscles relax. The available energy is the main factor responsible for normal expiration. Active muscle contraction takes place during forced expiration.

During inspiration a negative pressure develops within the pleural cavity. As a result, the lungs expand, causing a stretch and thus also storage of elastic energy. Because of the expansion of the lungs, air flow is directed inside (as long as the respiratory canals are not obstructed). Normally, the expiration occurs as a result of the "springing back" mechanism of the thorax and the lungs; a retraction of the lungs occurs and the air is pushed outward. By the way, even after maximal expiration, residual air is always left within the lungs.

5.2   EXAMINATION

For several reasons, discogenic lesions are seen much less frequently in the thoracic spine than in the cervical and lumbar spines. First, because of the presence of the ribs and the sternum, the flexibility of the thoracic spine is limited. Second, the posterior longitudinal ligament is much wider and stronger in the thoracic region than in the lumbar spine, making it difficult for disc material to bulge. At the same time, the intervertebral foramina lie cranial to the disc, leading to less rapid compression of the spinal nerve in the occurrence of a disc lesion. However, this does not mean that dural irritation cannot occur.

Approximately 60% of the thoracic disc prolapses are seen in the lower thoracic region, particularly T9 and T12, which is where the most flexion and extension take place.

Pain in the upper thoracic area (T1-4) is almost always caused by pathology of the cervical spine. Thus, examination and pathology of T1-4 are discussed in Chapter 6, Cervical Spine.

During the segmental functional examination of the thoracic spine, it is striking that the combined movements (in contrast to the normal "coupling patterns") are more often painful than the same movements in the lumbar or cervical spine. This can indicate pathology of the zygapophyseal joints or of the rib joints.

It is important to keep in mind that many internal organs can cause pain in the thorax, thus leading one to believe that there is a problem in the thoracic spine. Whenever the functional examination of the thoracic spine is negative, pathology of an internal organ should always be considered. Several internal organs can cause pain in the thorax:

- heart   C8-T8
- lungs   T3-10
- stomach   T5-9
- liver and gallbladder   T6-10
- spleen   T7-10
- caecum and duodenum   T6-10
- pancreas   T7-9
- appendix   T9-11
- kidneys   T9-L2

Pain located primarily on the right side may indicate a lesion of the liver, gallbladder, duodenum, ileum, or ascending colon. Pain located primarily on the left side may indicate a possible lesion of the heart, stomach, pancreas, spleen, jejunum, descending colon, or sigmoid colon. Of course, exceptions also occur; for example, in approximately 5% of all patients with angina pectoris, pain is referred to the right side.

OVERVIEW OF THE CLINICAL EXAMINATION

See Appx C.

General Inspection

- How does the patient enter the room? Observe
  1. Posture (flexed, deviated)
  2. Use of assistive devices (cane/crutch, wheelchair, corset, stretcher)
- How does the patient sit down, or does the patient prefer to remain standing?
  1. Is it painful to sit?
  2. What is the patient's sitting posture (kyphosis, straight back, lordosis, or deviated)?
- Note the patient's facial expression (fatigued or suffering).

History

If the patient clearly indicates that the complaints appear only during certain posi-

tions or movements, the history is primarily focused on a lesion of the musculoskeletal system. This may concern the thoracic vertebral column, the costovertebral connections, the costosternal connections, the sternum itself, or the thoracic musculature.

If the symptoms are not dependent on positions or movements, pathology of the internal organs should be suspected (among other things, note whether certain foods have an influence on the complaints).

Age

Age is of great importance in deciding the seriousness of specific lesions. A child with a severe kyphosis or scoliosis generally has minimal to no complaints. However, if the child has significant complaints, this may be an indication of an inflammation or a tumor.

Occupation, Hobby (Sport)

Working or participating in sports that encourage a kyphosis can lead to complaints or can increase already existing symptoms. Thus, a sport such as hockey would be contraindicated for an individual with Scheuermann's disease, at least in its active stage.

Chief Complaints

Does the patient complain of pain, a rash (herpes zoster), or an abnormal position of the spine, such as an abnormal kyphosis or scoliosis?

Herpes mostly in 60⁺ y.o. pts.

Onset

Did the symptoms have an acute onset, for instance during lifting a heavy object (this may indicate disc pathology), or a gradual onset, such as in the typical postural hyperkyphosis? In instances of trauma, the examiner should always rule out a thoracic fracture. Muscle lesions can occur during sports activities—much more often in the thoracic spine than in the cervical or lumbar spine.

Duration

When symptoms have been present for a long time, consider particularly postural problems, chronic disc pathology, or poor recovery in a self-limiting disorder such as Scheuermann's disease. However, it is also possible for all of these forms of pathology to be present in patients with acute complaints. *Also, Sx > 6 mo., get Symp. segmental reorganization.*

Localization of Complaints

In a prolapsed disc, pain due to irritation of the dura can have an extrasegmental radiation. Pain arising from the zygapophyseal joints is generally experienced locally. Segmental radiation (intercostal neuralgia) occurs as a result of irritation of the nerve or the presence of herpes zoster.

Sternal pain can be the result of a thoracic disc protrusion. However, in these instances the examiner first should rule out cardiac pathology. Arthritis in the manubriosternal joint can also cause pain in this area.

Factors That Influence Symptoms

Constant pain, independent of position or movement, can indicate pathology of the internal organs. Pain experienced only at night usually indicates either an inflammation or a tumor.

Pain during coughing, sneezing, or straining can indicate discogenic pathology or lesions of the costovertebral joints, the ribs (fracture), or the intercostal muscles.

Prior History

In many instances, recurring complaints indicate discogenic pathology. *or Sympath. As.*

Medication

For instance, it is important to note whether the patient is taking anticoagulants. In such cases, manipulations are contraindicated. Is the patient taking any medicine for internal problems?

Patient's Reaction to Symptoms

Does the patient try to function as normally as possible, or does the discomfort cause the patient to call in sick immediately, lie in bed, and/or take medications?

Specific Inspection

With the patient in standing position, inspect the patient from dorsal and ventral aspects and from both sides. What is the position of the pelvis? Is there an obvious leg length difference?

Note the patient's posture. Is there an abnormal kyphosis? If so, is it curved or angular? In instances of an abnormal kyphosis, the shoulders are often protracted and the distance between the medial borders of the scapulae and the vertebral column is increased. An abnormal kyphosis can result in a flat back, a round back, or a round-hollow back.

In a scoliosis, the asymmetry is particularly noticeable: the waist triangles are unequal; sometimes on one side they are completely gone. Often there is a noticeable gibbus (hump). *ribs,*

From the front, the sternal region is especially noted. An arthritis of the manubriosternal joint is usually conspicuous because of local swelling and occasionally also local redness of the skin. In such instances, always check the patient's eyes (to see whether an iritis is also present); ankylosing spondylitis can *begin* with an arthritis of the manubriosternal joint; however this arthritis can also occur *during* the disease process.

Swelling of the second rib especially can indicate Tietze syndrome.

Palpation

If there is visible swelling, it should be palpated for its consistency. Lipomas are frequently seen in the upper thoracic region; in these instances, the swelling is freely movable over the underlying musculature. An arthritis of the manubriosternal joint causes a firm swelling; the same is true for swelling occurring in Tietze syndrome. (rib 2/manubrium)

Palpation of the painful region is *never* performed before the functional examination.

Functional Examination

If the patient complains of pain in the upper thoracic area, the cervical spine functional examination should be performed first. Functionally, the first three to four thoracic vertebrae belong to the cervical spine. Also, problems in the cervical spine often project pain into the upper thoracic region. + v/u versa

Before the functional examination, determine whether the patient is experiencing symptoms at that specific moment. Note whether the symptoms change per test during the functional examination. Furthermore, it is imperative always to compare the affected with the nonaffected side. This means that both sides are tested, first the nonaffected side (to have an idea of what is "normal") and then the affected side.

During the functional examination, attention is given to the following:

- *articular signs* (which motions are painful and/or limited?)
- *dural and root signs* (stretch tests for the dura mater and the nerve roots; in adhesions and/or impingement of these structures, severe pain is provoked by these tests)
- *muscle signs* (which muscles are painful during the resisted tests?)
- *central neurological signs* (for instance, the Babinski foot sole reflex in a spastic gait pattern) Hyper-reflex. ז Sp. Col. injury
- *other causes for the symptoms* (for instance, pathology of the internal organs)
- *pain behavior of the patient*

The examination is performed with the patient in standing, lying supine, and prone, and it consists of a basic functional examination and a segmental functional examination. The segmental functional examination is performed only when the basic functional examination provides insufficient information or when the appropriate treatment techniques provide minimal to no relief of symptoms. This happens more often in the thoracic spine than in the lumbar or cervical spine.

TESTS FOR BASIC FUNCTIONAL EXAMINATION

In Sitting

Cerv. Exam if T4+up? upper th. only

Tests for Upper Thoracic Pathology

5.1 Scapular retraction (T1, T2)
5.2 Ulnar nerve stretch test (C8-T1)

Active Tests

5.3 Flexion
5.4 Flexion with neck flexion (dural stretch) (+ hk extension)
5.5 Extension
5.6 Left sidebend
5.7 Right sidebend
5.8 Left rotation   ז lumbar left, ipsi. SB.
5.9 Right rotation

Passive Tests

5.10. Left rotation   + O.P.
5.11. Right rotation   " "
5.12. Left rotation with neck flexion (dural stretch)
5.13. Right rotation with neck flexion (dural stretch) - ↑rot. ז Flexion. Retest Dura. - Slump

Resisted Tests

5.14. Left rotation
5.15. Right rotation
5.16. Flexion
5.17. Left sidebend
5.18. Right sidebend

Neurological Examination

5.19/20 Patellar tendon reflex (left/right)

5.21/22 Achilles tendon reflex (left/right)

5.23/24 Foot sole reflex (left/right)

In Prone

5.25. Active extension

5.26. Passive extension

5.27. Resisted extension

In Supine

5.28. Resisted flexion

5.29. Resisted flexion with left rotation

5.30. Resisted flexion with right rotation

TESTS FOR SEGMENTAL FUNCTIONAL EXAMINATION

In Sitting

Active General Tests

5.31. Flexion with left sidebend and left rotation

5.32. Flexion with right sidebend and left rotation

5.33. Flexion with right sidebend and right rotation

5.34. Flexion with left sidebend and right rotation

5.35. Extension with right sidebend and left rotation

5.36. Extension with left sidebend and left rotation

5.37. Extension with left sidebend and right rotation

5.38. Extension with right sidebend and right rotation

Passive General Tests

5.39. Extension with left sidebend and left rotation

5.40. Extension with right sidebend and left rotation

5.41. Extension with left sidebend and right rotation

5.42. Extension with right sidebend and right rotation

Passive Local Tests

5.43. Dorsal translation, in weight bearing

5.44. Extension in weight bearing

5.45. Extension with left sidebend and right rotation in weight bearing

5.46. Extension with right sidebend and left rotation in weight bearing

In Prone

5.47. Ventral translation

5.48. Axial rotation test

In Sidelying

5.49. Dorsal translation

5.50. Extension in non–weight bearing

5.51. Extension with left sidebend and right rotation in non–weight bearing

5.52. Extension with right sidebend and left rotation in non–weight bearing

If both the basic and the segmental examinations of the thoracic spine are negative, an examination of the ribs is performed. Should this examination also be negative, it is very likely that there is not a problem with the musculoskeletal system.

TESTS FOR EXAMINATION OF THE RIBS

Test for the First Rib, Costovertebral Joint

5.53/54. Test for mobility and end-feel

Tests for the Second to the Twelfth Ribs

5.55/56. Position test (left/right)

5.57/58. Springing test (left/right)

5.59/60. Testing active mobility of the ribs (left/right)

5.61/62. Testing costotransverse joints for mobility, end-feel, and pain provocation (left/right)

5.63/64. Testing costovertebral and costotransverse mobility (left/right)

5.65/66. Testing passive mobility of the ribs (left/right)

PALPATION

After the functional examination, the suspected affected structure can be palpated for local tenderness. This particularly applies to the muscle lesions that are found more often in the thoracic region than in the lumbar or cervical region. In the thoracic region, lesions of the following muscles are found:

- pectoralis major
- latissimus dorsi
- intercostal muscles
- serratus anterior
- inferior serratus posterior
- rectus abdominis
- internal oblique abdominal muscle
- external oblique abdominal muscle

SUPPLEMENTARY EXAMINATION

If necessary, the following supplementary examinations can be performed:

- radiological examination (functional views, myelography, computed tomography [CT] scan)
- magnetic resonance imaging (MRI)
- bone scan
- spinal tap
- laboratory tests

DESCRIPTION OF TESTS FOR BASIC FUNCTIONAL EXAMINATION

See Tests for Basic Functional Examination for specific types of tests according to matching number.

As with the lumbar and the cervical spines, during the various tests a distinction is made between coupled movements (mostly ligamentous restriction) and combined movements (restricted mostly by the facets).

The direction of the coupling (and thus also of the combined motions) in the lower thoracic segments (T8-9 and below) is the same as in the lumbar spine. In the upper thoracic segments (T3-4 and above), the direction of the coupling is the same as in the cervical spine.

The "silent zone" of the thoracic spine, which is from T4 to T8, has an inconsistent coupling pattern in extension. Therefore, some thoracic three-dimensional movements in extension can be either coupled or combined, depending on the amount of extension possible in these thoracic segments.

The upper thoracic segments (T1 to T4) are tested in the cervical spine functional examination. The thoracic functional examination mainly involves the segments T4-5 to T9-10, whereas the T10 to T12 segments are included in the lumbar spine functional examination.

Upper thoracic complaints are best examined by performing the functional examination for the cervical spine (see Chapter 6). In addition, the following two tests should also be performed. (Keep in mind that neck flexion causes a stretch on the dura at all levels.)

Tests for Upper Thoracic Pathology: In Sitting

5.1 Scapular Retraction (T1, T2)

Position of the Patient

The patient sits on the treatment table with the arms relaxed and the hands resting in the lap.

Position of the Examiner

The examiner stands either in front of or behind the patient.

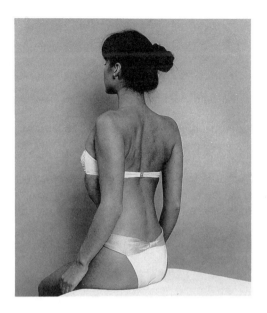

Test 5.1

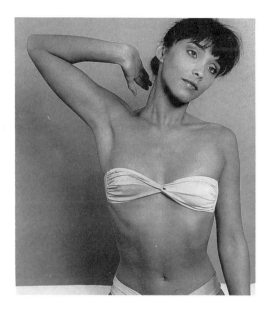

Test 5.2

Performance

The patient brings both shoulders as far backward as possible, whereby the thoracic spine is in extension. Hence, the nerve roots of T1 and T2 are brought under a stretch. The test is very seldom positive, only in the instance of an upper thoracic disc protrusion or when there is a tumor in this area.

5.2 Ulnar Nerve Stretch Test (C8, T1)

Position of the Patient

The patient sits on the treatment table with arms relaxed at the sides.

Position of the Examiner

The examiner stands behind the patient.

Performance

Under guidance and instruction from the examiner, the patient starts from a position of shoulder girdle depression and retraction, and then abducts the shoulder 90°, position-ing it in maximal external rotation and extension, with the elbow in maximal flexion and pronation. Wrist extension and radial deviation are then added. Finally, the head is brought into contralateral sidebend. In this way, the mobility of particularly the C8 and T1 roots and that of their peripheral extensions (ulnar nerve) are tested. If the patient's local pain is provoked, it may be the result of a stretch on the root due to a disc lesion and/or a tumorous process at the level of T1-2 (disc lesions are rarely found at this level).

Active Tests

Examination of the active motions described below is performed to determine the range of motion and the pattern of the movement. In instances when a limitation of motion is found, the examiner must determine whether it is in the form of a capsular pattern or a noncapsular pattern. If pain is provoked, the precise location should be noted.

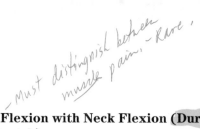

— Must distinguish between muscle pain. — Rare.

Active Tests: In Sitting

5.3 Flexion

Position of the Patient

The patient sits on the treatment table, at the short end. The thighs, which are slightly abducted, rest fully on the table and the feet are placed flat on the floor. The hands are placed on the thighs, with the arms in a relaxed position. The lumbar spine should be in its normal lordosis.

Position of the Examiner

The examiner stands or sits next to the patient.

Performance

1st Press LB flat (flex it)

The patient is instructed to bring the shoulders in the direction of the hips. By palpating the thoracolumbar junction with one hand, the examiner controls the moment when the movement progresses into the lumbar spine.

In thoracic disc pathology, flexion is usually very painful and severely limited.

5.4 Flexion with Neck Flexion (Dural Stretch)

Position of the Patient

Same as for test 5.3.

Position of the Examiner

Same as for test 5.3.

Performance

The patient is instructed to bring the shoulders in the direction of the hips, subsequently maximally flexing the trunk (also in the lumbar spine). At the end of the flexion, the patient then brings the chin as far as possible to the chest.

When dural irritation is suspected (usually as the result of a disc protrusion), this test is usually positive. In other words, the symptoms increase when the patient brings the cervical spine into flexion and diminish again upon lifting the head. If the test is negative, the examiner can straighten one or both of the patient's knees, as well as bring the ankles

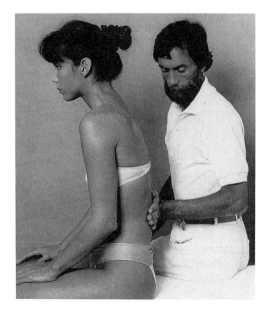

Test 5.3

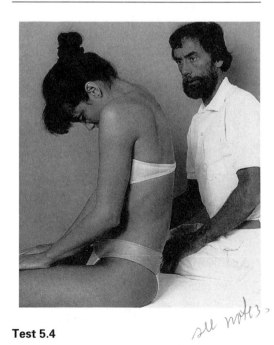

Test 5.4

see notes.

into dorsiflexion (extension). In this way, the dura is brought under even more stretch via the sciatic nerve. *+ Then n/e extension should ↓ pain ⎯ dural release tension,*

5.5. Extension

Position of the Patient

Same as for test 5.3.

Position of the Examiner

The examiner stands or sits next to the patient. One hand palpates the spinous processes of T12 and L1 (the thoracolumbar junction) in order to monitor the moment when the movement progresses into the lumbar spine.

Performance

Try arms over chest, lift arms up

The patient brings the sternum forward until the examiner notes movement in the thoracolumbar junction (this brings the patient's center of gravity forward). From this slightly forward position of the trunk, the patient is instructed to extend the thoracic spine without moving the cervical spine.

Significant limitations of extension are generally seen in patients with Scheuermann's disease, ankylosing spondylitis, osteoporosis, and disc pathology. In the last instance, the limitation of motion is also very painful.

5.6. Left Sidebend *— 🚩 Rib fx?*

5.7. Right Sidebend *Not much Th. spine stress*

Position of the Patient

Same as for test 5.3. Now the patient crosses the arms in front of the chest, resting the hands on the shoulders.

Position of the Examiner

The examiner stands behind the patient.

Performance

The patient is instructed to bend the trunk sideways, whereby the imaginary axis of rotation lies at the crossing point of the arms. The shoulders should remain in the frontal plane.

In disc pathology, the sidebend is usually the easiest motion to perform. Generally,

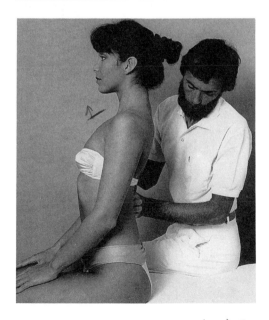

Test 5.5 *Arms crossed on chest. Lift arms upward.*

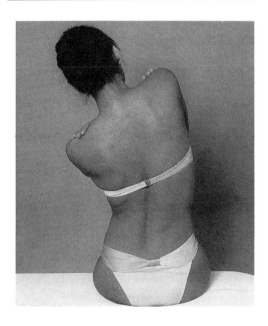

Test 5.6

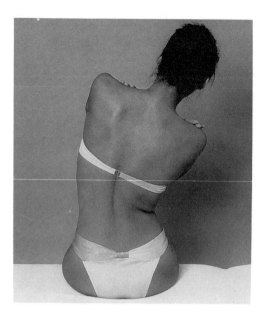

Test 5.7

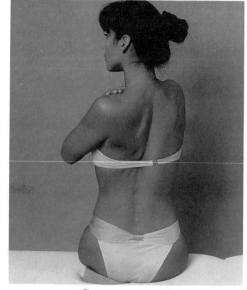

Test 5.8   *wedge or pillow.*

flexion, extension, and the rotations are the most limited and painful motions in instances of disc lesions.

5.8.   Left Rotation

5.9.   Right Rotation

Position of the Patient

Same as for tests 5.6 and 5.7.

Position of the Examiner

The examiner stands or sits behind the patient.

Performance

To prevent lumbar rotation as much as possible, a small sandbag or wedge is placed first under the patient's left buttock and then under the right buttock. When the wedge lies under the left buttock, a left sidebending and right rotation occurs in the lumbar spine. The patient is now instructed to rotate as far as possible to the left, without rotating the cervi-

5.8

Keep lumbar neutral, not flexed,

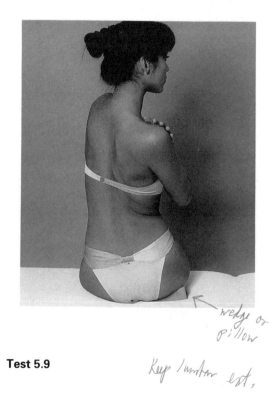

Test 5.9   *wedge or pillow*

Keep lumbar ext,

cal spine. In this way, the lumbar spine is locked, combined, in left sidebend with ipsilateral rotation. Thus the left rotation occurs mostly in the thoracic spine. In the same way, right rotation is tested (wedge under right buttock).

Pain at the end range of the rotation is often the first sign of disc pathology.

Passive Tests

In examining the passive motions described in the following tests, the range of motion is compared with the active movements. Often, it is possible to move farther in the passive motions than in the active motions. Determining the end-feel is of great importance here. As with the active motions, the provocation of pain is also noted.

Passive movements with flexion components are not performed, because by so doing a possible disc protrusion can be aggravated. In the thoracic spine, this is especially significant given the small diameter of the vertebral canal. The danger of spinal cord compression is much greater than in the other areas of the spinal column.

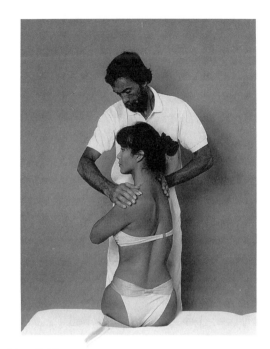

Test 5.10

Passive Tests: In Sitting

5.10   Left Rotation

5.11   Right Rotation

Position of the Patient

The patient sits on the treatment table. The slightly abducted thighs rest fully on the table and the feet are placed flat on the floor. The patient crosses the arms in front of the chest, resting the hands on the shoulders.

If left rotation is to be performed, a small sandbag or wedge is placed under the patient's left buttock. For right rotation, a small sandbag or wedge is placed under the right buttock. The lumbar spine should be in its normal lordosis.

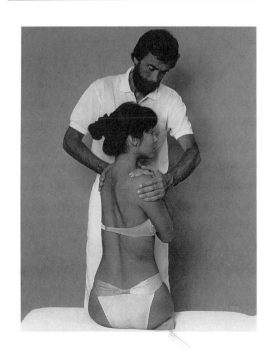

Test 5.11

Position of the Examiner

The examiner stands in front of the patient, and in order to stabilize the patient's legs, places the patient's knees between the examiner's knees.

For the left rotation, the examiner's right hand is placed on the patient's right hand, which is resting on the left shoulder. The examiner's left hand is placed just behind the patient's right shoulder.

Performance

The examiner rotates the patient to the left. At the end of the motion, the patient is asked to exhale audibly. Then, in order to determine the end-feel, at the end of the exhalation slight overpressure is exerted into the direction of the rotation. The same procedure is repeated for right rotation.

5.12.   Left Rotation with Neck Flexion (Dural Stretch)

5.13.   Right Rotation with Neck Flexion (Dural Stretch)

Position of the Patient

Same as for tests 5.10 and 5.11.

Position of the Examiner

Same as for tests 5.10 and 5.11.

Performance

The performance of this test is similar to that for tests 5.10 and 5.11, except that now at the end of the rotation motion, the patient is instructed first to bring the chin as far as possible to the chest, and then to flex the entire spinal column by bringing the shoulders toward the hips. At the end of the motion, the patient can again exhale, so that the maximal amount of rotation and flexion can be reached.

This is not a test to gain an impression about thoracic rotation; instead, it is a stretch test of the dura. If the patient's symptoms are

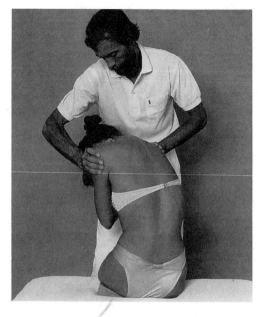

Test 5.12

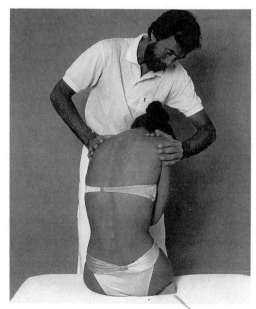

Test 5.13

Combine
A, ® rot,
P, over P,
Neck flex ext,
↑ LB flex
↑ P, rot, - no over P,
nk flex, ext,
If all is ⊖, Add knee extension

now provoked in the end position, the patient is asked to raise the head. If the symptoms diminish, the test is considered positive for a dura irritation.

If the test is negative, the examiner can straighten one or both of the patient's knees, as well as bring the ankles into dorsiflexion (extension). In this way the dura is brought under even more stretch via the sciatic nerve.

Resisted Tests: In Sitting

In the thoracic region, pathology of the muscles is seen much more often than in the lumbar and cervical regions. These disorders usually involve overuse injuries or traumatic lesions of the abdominal muscles, the intercostal musculature, the pectoralis major, or the latissimus dorsi. During the resisted tests described below, patients complain primarily of pain; weakness is seldom found.

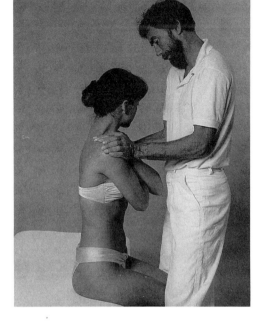

Test 5.14

5.14. Left Rotation

5.15. Right Rotation

Position of the Patient

Same as for tests 5.6 and 5.7.

Position of the Examiner

Same as for tests 5.10 and 5.11.

Performance

When testing resisted left rotation, the examiner's left hand is placed on the patient's left hand, which is resting on the right shoulder. The right hand is placed against the posterior aspect of the patient's left shoulder, just medial to the scapula. The patient is now instructed to rotate the trunk to the left while the examiner applies isometric resistance. The opposite is performed when testing resisted right rotation.

This test is usually positive only in traumatic lesions of the intercostal muscles.

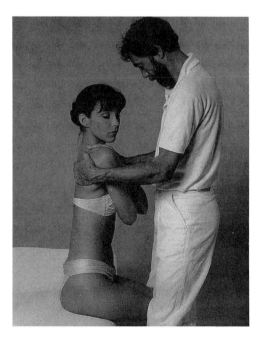

Test 5.15

Slump test:
sit @ nedge, Flex trnk too
® SB
® rot
Extend RLE
then Ext. neck,

5.16. Flexion

Position of the Patient

Same as for test 5.3.

Position of the Examiner

While standing next to the patient, the examiner places one hand against the patient's sternal manubrium and the other hand at the patient's thoracolumbar junction.

Performance

The patient is instructed to bring the sternum in the direction of the hips while the examiner applies isometric resistance. In this test, the abdominal muscles in particular are tested for strength and pain provocation. If a lesion of the abdominal muscles is suspected, then further tests can be performed to distinguish between the various abdominal muscles. (See tests 5.28 to 5.30.)

5.17. Left Sidebend

5.18. Right Sidebend

Position of the Patient

Same as for test 5.3.

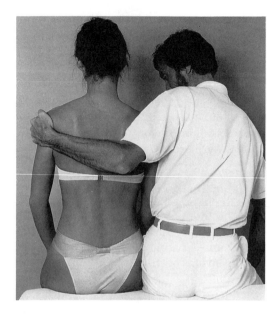

Test 5.17

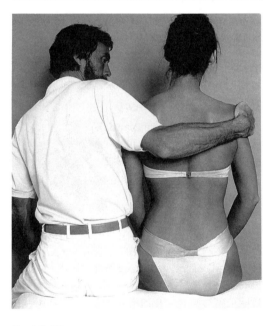

Test 5.18

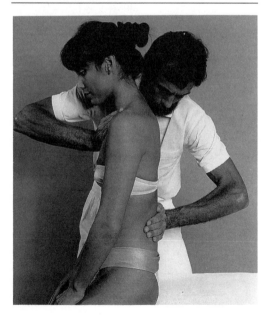

Test 5.16

Position of the Examiner

While sitting next to the patient, the examiner places the hand closest to the patient on the patient's farthest shoulder. In order to fix the patient's trunk, the examiner sits with the lateral aspect of his or her pelvis against the lateral aspect of the patient's pelvis.

Performance

The patient is instructed to sidebend away from the examiner (pushing into the hand on the shoulder). The examiner applies isometric resistance. The test is repeated on the other side.

In this test, mainly the ipsilateral back extensors are tested, and to a lesser degree also the oblique abdominal muscles and the intercostal muscles. Generally, a lesion of the intercostal muscle will cause pain during this test.

Neurological Tests: In Sitting

The neurological examination is performed with the specific goal of ruling out central neurological pathology according to the tests described below.

5.19/20. Patellar Tendon Reflex (Left/ Right)

Position of the Patient

The patient sits with the lower legs hanging over the treatment table. (The feet should not touch the floor.)

Position of the Examiner

The examiner stands or sits in front of the patient.

Performance

The patellar tendon is tested via the patellar ligament between the tibial tuberosity and the apex of the patella.

This test is significant in patients with thoracic spinal cord pathology.

5.21/22. Achilles Tendon Reflex (Left/ Right)

Position of the Patient

Same as for test 5.19/20.

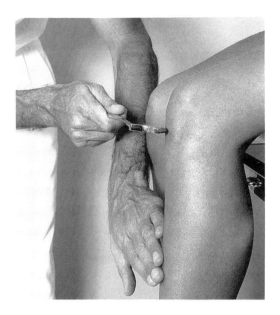

Test 5.19/20

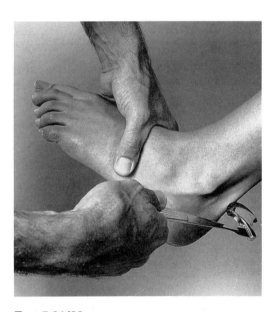

Test 5.21/22

Position of the Examiner

The examiner squats or sits in front of the patient.

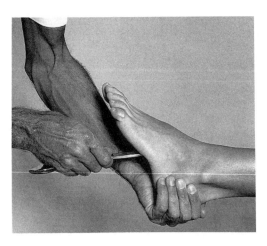

Test 5.23/24

Performance

With one hand, the examiner holds the patient's foot in extension (dorsiflexion). The other hand tests the Achilles tendon reflex.

As with the patellar tendon reflex, this test is also significant in patients with thoracic spinal cord pathology.

5.23/24.   Foot Sole Reflex (Left/Right)

Position of the Patient

Same as test for test 5.19/20.

Position of the Examiner

The examiner squats or sits in front of the patient.

Performance

With moderate pressure against the sole of the patient's foot, the examiner moves the pointed end of the reflex hammer from the lateral side of the heel over the lateral side of the sole, to the base of the fifth metatarsal, and then from there, medial to the base of the first metatarsal.

Normally, the patient pulls the foot away and flexes the toes. However, other reactions from the patient are also possible. The pathological Babinski reflex includes extension of the great toe, spreading of the other toes, and flexion of the knee and hip. The presence of a Babinski reflex indicates a serious central disorder.

Active General Tests: In Prone

The interpretation of tests in prone, described below, is similar to that for the corresponding tests in sitting except that now the effect of gravity is eliminated. In cases of minor disc pathology, one frequently notes that pain that occurs in sitting is often absent during the same tests in lying.

5.25.   Active Extension

Position of the Patient

The patient lies prone, with the legs slightly spread and the hands folded under either the chin or the forehead.

Position of the Examiner

The examiner stands next to the patient.

Performance

The patient is instructed to lift the trunk as high as possible (extension). Range of motion and pain provocation are noted.

5.26   Passive Extension

Position of the Patient

The patient lies prone.

Position of the Examiner

The examiner stands next to the patient.

Performance

Various methods exist by which to perform this test. In instances when the patient is larger than the examiner, the patient is instructed to take the prone-on-elbows position, whereby the trunk hangs in extension (Test 5.26A). The patient is then asked to make a deep exhalation to allow the thoracic

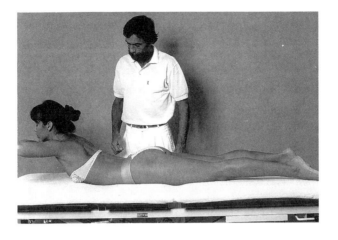

Test 5.25

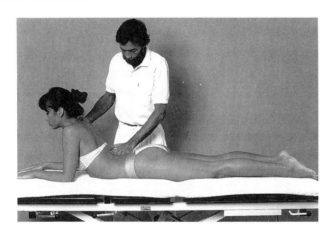

Test 5.26A

Press: start
distal, then up
level by level.

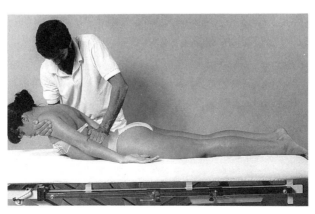

Test 5.26B

L/R Hands,
palms down clasped under
forehead.

Lift pt. to
neutral ext.
Tx
over press

spine to hang even more in extension. If pain is not yet provoked, the examiner exerts overpressure through the spinous processes of the extended thoracic spine.

Alternative Performance. The alternative method is applicable only when the patient is not too heavy (Test 5.26B). With his or her cranial arm and hand, the examiner grasps across the ventral upper aspect of the patient's thorax at the level of the shoulders. The caudal hand is placed at the level of the L1 and L2 spinous processes. The examiner then extends the patient's trunk, monitoring with the caudal hand that the movement does not go into the lumbar spine. At that point, the upper lumbar spine is fixed and slight overpressure is exerted by the cranial arm. Range of motion and pain provocation are noted.

5.27. Resisted Extension

Position of the Patient

The patient lies prone with the arms resting alongside the trunk.

Position of the Examiner

The examiner stands next to the patient. The cranial hand is placed between the patient's scapulae; the caudal arm fixes the thighs just proximal to the knees.

Performance

The patient is instructed to lift the shoulders and trunk as far as possible. The examiner then exerts isometric resistance. This tests the back extensors for strength and pain provocation.

If the examiner suspects a lesion of the abdominal muscles, the following additional tests can be performed in supine.

Active Tests: In Supine

5.28. Resisted Flexion

Position of the Patient

The patient lies supine with the hips and knees flexed 90°; the feet rest against the raised end of the treatment table.

Position of the Examiner

The examiner stands next to the patient. One hand is placed at the patient's sternal manubrium and the other hand is placed on the patient's knees.

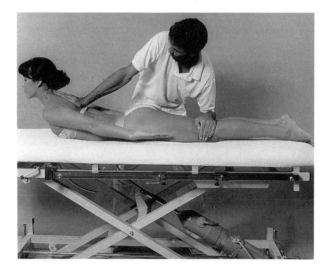

Test 5.27

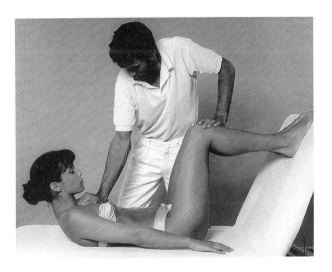

Test 5.28

Performance

The patient is instructed to bring the sternum in the direction of the hips. The therapist then applies isometric resistance. This tests chiefly the straight abdominal muscles for strength and pain provocation.

5.29. Resisted Flexion with Left Rotation

5.30. Resisted Flexion with Right Rotation

In the same manner as for test 5.28, the oblique abdominal muscles are tested. The examiner now places the cranial hand against the anterior aspect of the patient's shoulder, and the patient is instructed to bring that shoulder in the direction of the contralateral hip. The test is then repeated with resistance applied against the opposite shoulder.

DESCRIPTION OF TESTS FOR SEGMENTAL FUNCTIONAL EXAMINATION

See Tests for Segmental Functional Examination for specific types of tests according to matching number.

If the basic functional examination of the thoracic spine provides insufficient information, the segmental functional examination of the thoracic spine is performed. The segmental functional examination is also indicated when the basic functional examination was positive but the appropriate treatment resulted in minimal to no improvement or when improvement with the appropriate treatment plateaus and the patient is left with residual symptoms.

The following tests serve to examine the segmental mobility of the thoracic spine. The segmental functional examination of the thoracic spine focuses on segments T4-5 to T9-10 and is performed from cranial to caudal.

Hypomobility without neurological deficits can be an indication for treatment with manual mobilization. In instances of hypermobility or instability, depending on severity, stabilization exercises, a corset, or even surgery may be indicated. In order to be able to perform the segmental examination precisely—and especially to be able to interpret the findings—much experience is necessary.

Active General Tests: In Sitting

During the active general tests, the examiner observes the curvature of the thoracic

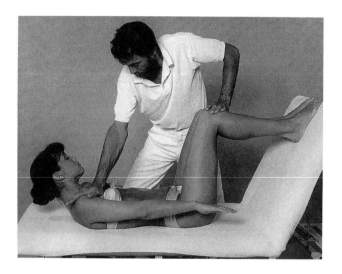

Test 5.29

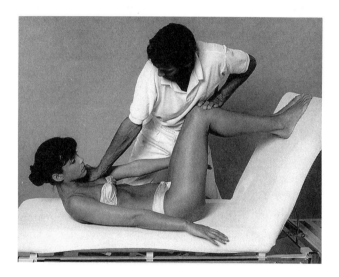

Test 5.30

spinal column and notes any provocation of the patient's symptoms.

5.31. Flexion with Left Sidebend and Left Rotation

Position of the Patient

The patient sits on the treatment table. The slightly abducted thighs rest fully on the table and the feet are placed flat on the floor. The patient crosses the arms in front of the chest, resting the hands on the shoulders.

The lumbar spine should be in its normal lordosis.

Position of the Examiner

The examiner stands or sits behind the patient. One hand palpates the spinous proc-

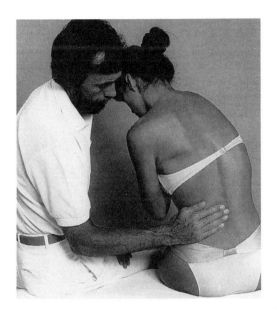

Test 5.31

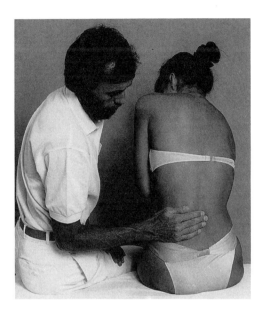

Test 5.32

esses of T12-L1 (the thoracolumbar junction) to monitor the moment that the movement progresses into the lumbar spine.

Performance

The patient is asked to perform *simultaneously* the following motions: flexion (see test 5.3), left sidebend (see test 5.6), and left rotation (see test 5.8). The lumbar spine should remain in its normal lordosis. *(? wedge)*

5.32. Flexion with Right Sidebend and Left Rotation

In the same manner as described for test 5.31, the patient is asked to perform flexion, right sidebend, and left rotation.

5.33. Flexion with Right Sidebend and Right Rotation

In the same manner as described under test 5.31, the patient is asked to perform flexion, right sidebend, and right rotation.

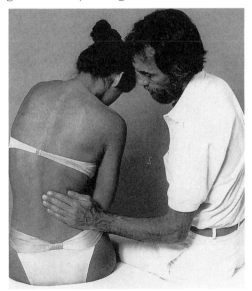

Test 5.33

5.34. Flexion with Left Sidebend and Right Rotation

In the same manner as described under test 5.31, the patient is asked to perform flexion, left sidebend, and right rotation.

5.35. Extension with Right Sidebend and Left Rotation

Position of the Patient

Same as for test 5.31.

Position of the Examiner

Same as for test 5.31.

Performance

The patient is asked to perform *simultaneously* the following motions: extension (see test 5.5), right sidebend (see test 5.7), and left rotation (see test 5.8).

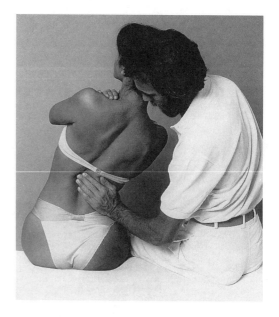

Test 5.35

5.36. Extension with Left Sidebend and Left Rotation

In the same manner as described under test 5.35, the patient is asked to perform extension, left sidebend, and left rotation.

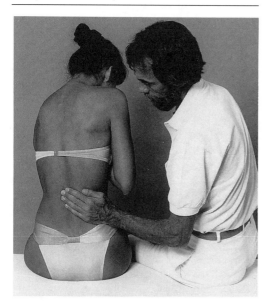

Test 5.34

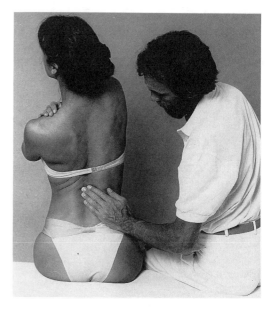

Test 5.36

5.37. Extension with Left Sidebend and Right Rotation

In the same manner as described under test 5.35, the patient is asked to perform extension, left sidebend, and right rotation.

5.38. Extension with Right Sidebend and Right Rotation

In the same manner as described under test 5.35, the patient is asked to perform extension, right sidebend, and right rotation.

Passive General Tests: In Sitting

The following passive tests are performed to determine the range of motion, end-feel, and pain provocation. As previously mentioned in the basic functional examination, passive movements with flexion components are not performed, because in so doing a possible disc protrusion can be aggravated.

Only when the entire segmental functional examination does not provide sufficient infor-

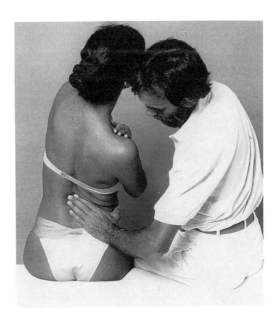

Test 5.38

mation should the passive tests (with overpressure) be performed in flexion.

5.39. Extension with Left Sidebend and Left Rotation

Position of the Patient

Same as for test 5.31.

Position of the Examiner

The examiner stands at the right side of the patient.

Performance

The examiner places the left hand at the level of the L1 and L2 spinous processes, with the fingers resting directly caudal from the right 12th rib. The forearm is positioned perpendicular to the patient's back.

The examiner's right arm is crossed over the patient's crossed arms and the right hand is placed on the patient's right hand, which is resting on the left shoulder (as pictured). Another method for the examiner consists of

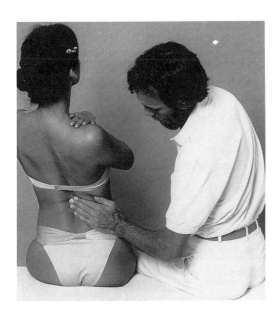

Test 5.37

sit ē hip at 70° flex , easier to extend.

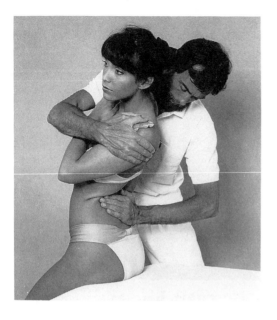

Test 5.39

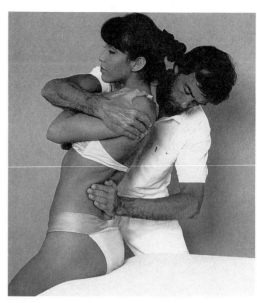

Test 5.40

reaching up between the patient's crossed arms with the right arm, placing the right hand on the patient's left shoulder.

The examiner's sternum or the anterior aspect of the right shoulder rests against the lateral aspect of the patient's right shoulder, and in so doing holds the patient's shoulder girdle between the right hand and trunk.

The motion that follows is induced by movement of the examiner's trunk: the examiner now sidebends to the left, rotates to the left, and flexes, which results in extension, left rotation, and left sidebend (respectively) of the patient's trunk. The patient is brought into the end range of this movement, and the examiner then exerts slight overpressure in order to determine the end-feel.

5.40. Extension with Right Sidebend and Left Rotation

In the same manner as described for test 5.39, the examiner brings the patient into extension, left rotation, and right sidebend. The

examiner now has to make trunk extension (with slightly flexed knees) in order to bring the patient's trunk into a right sidebend. End-feel is determined by exerting slight overpressure.

5.41. Extension with Left Sidebend and Right Rotation

Position of the Patient

Same as for test 5.39.

Position of the Examiner

The examiner stands at the patient's left side.

Performance

In the same manner as described for test 5.39, the examiner now brings the patient into extension with right rotation and left sidebend. In order to do this, the examiner performs, respectively, a right sidebend, right rotation, and extension of his or her trunk. At

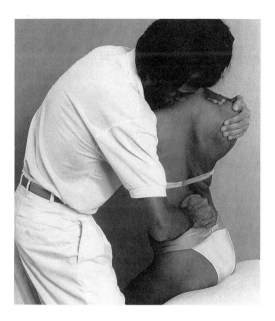

Test 5.41

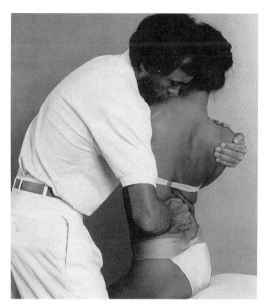

Test 5.42

the end of the patient's range of motion, the examiner exerts overpressure in order to determine the end-feel.

5.42. Extension with Right Sidebend and Right Rotation

In the same manner as described in tests 5.40 and 5.41, the examiner brings the patient into extension, right sidebend, and right rotation. End-feel is determined by exerting slight overpressure.

Passive Local Tests: In Sitting

5.43. Dorsal Translation, in Weight Bearing *(NWB = 5.49)*

Position of the Patient

The patient sits on the short side of the treatment table, legs slightly abducted, and feet resting flat on the floor. The lumbar spine is in its normal lordosis. The arms are crossed in front of the trunk with the hands resting on the shoulders.

Position of the Examiner

The examiner stands next to the patient.

Performance

The examiner places one hand on the spinous processes below the segment to be tested with the fingers pointing in a cranial direction. The tip of the middle finger rests in the interspinous space of the segment to be tested and has contact with the tip of the cranial spinous process. The other hand rests against the patient's arms at the point where they cross.

The examiner exerts pressure in a dorsal direction, perpendicular to the local curvature of the thoracic spine. In so doing, the dorsoventral diameter of the thorax decreases. Initially, the examiner experiences little resistance: pre-tension is taken up from the soft tissue structures and the ribs. At the point when the resistance increases, generally a small amount of dorsal movement is still possible. The examiner exerts dorsal pres-

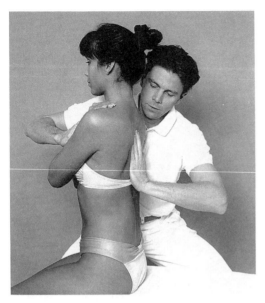

Test 5.43A T4–5 Level

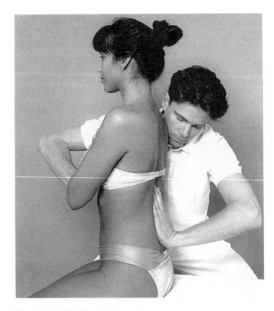

Test 5.43C T9–10 Level

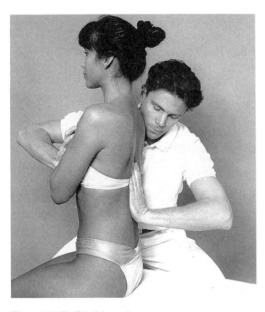

Test 5.43B T6–7 Level

the amount of movement and the end-feel.

As the more caudal segments are tested, the crossed point of the patient's forearms is also shifted more caudally (Test 5.43B and Test 5.43C). Visual control is possible through the examiner's arm, which is placed in a perpendicular position on the local curvature of the thoracic kyphosis.

5.44. Extension in Weight Bearing

Position of the Patient

Same as for test 5.43.

Position of the Examiner

While standing next to the patient, the examiner grasps the patient's farthest shoulder, placing the arm either on top of or underneath the patient's crossed arms. The tips of the index and middle fingers of the other hand are placed in the interspinous spaces of two adjacent segments, whereby the ring finger stabilizes the caudal spinous process of the caudal segment (Test 5.44A).

sure until the end of the translation motion has been reached, and then performs a slight overpressure (Test 5.43A). The tip of the middle finger placed in the interspinous space of the segment being tested registers

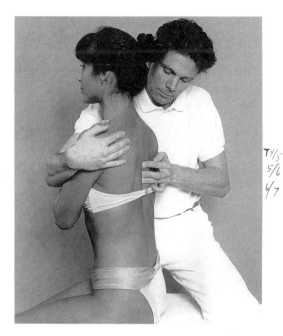

Test 5.44A

Feel for Closure

Test 5.44B

Performance

The examiner fixes the patient's shoulder girdle between hand and thorax (placing either sternum or anterior shoulder against the lateral aspect of the patient's closest shoulder). The examiner brings the patient's thoracic spine into extension by performing a sidebend of his or her trunk (Test 5.44B).

T4/5
5/6
6/7

The imaginary axis of rotation runs through the segment being tested, thus the farther caudal the segments being tested, the greater the amount of extension required to reach these segments.

The fingers palpate the amount of movement, whereby the index finger should feel a "closing" (extension) of the cranial segment before the middle finger registers motion in the caudal segment.

⊕ test = poor closure.

5.45. Extension with Left Sidebend and Right Rotation in Weight Bearing

Position of the Patient

Same as for test 5.43.

Position of the Examiner

Same as for test 5.44. The examiner stands on the patient's left side.

Performance

The examiner places one hand on the patient's back in such a way that the extended thumb lies parallel to the vertebral column. The thumb rests against the lateral aspect (closest to the examiner) of the caudal spinous process of the segment to be tested, and the rest of the hand fixes the caudally lying segments. The end of the thumb is in the interspinous space of the segment to be tested, and the tip has contact with the caudal aspect of the cranial spinous process.

By placing the fingers of the fixing hand well below the ribs corresponding to the segment being tested, the examiner ensures that the rotation motion is not restricted (Test 5.45A).

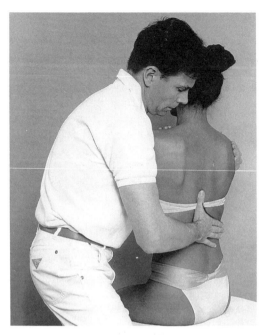

Test 5.45A Beginning position.

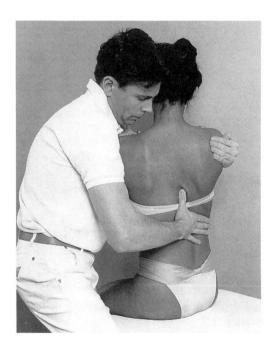

Test 5.45B End position.

The examiner brings the patient's trunk into a simultaneous extension, left sidebend, and right rotation. The thumb palpates the amount of motion and compares it with the adjacent segments (Test 5.45B).

5.46.   Extension with Right Sidebend and Left Rotation in Weight Bearing

In the same manner as described for test 5.45, the examiner tests extension with right sidebend and left rotation. The examiner now stands on the patient's right side (Test 5.46A) and brings the patient into simultaneous extension, right sidebend, and left rotation (Test 5.46B).

Passive Local Tests: In Prone

5.47.   Ventral Translation *for Scheuermann's pt. c̄ excessive ROM ax, irritating lev to hyper mobil d*

Position of the Patient

The patient lies prone on the treatment table. The table is positioned at the examiner's midthigh level. The patient's head should be in a neutral position with arms resting alongside the body.

If the patient has a pronounced kyphosis, the head of the table can be adjusted slightly downward or a small firm pillow can be placed under the thorax.

Position of the Examiner

The examiner stands next to the patient at the level of the thoracic spine.

Performance

The examiner places the ulnar side of the hand (the midpoint of the fifth metacarpal) against the spinous process. The other hand reinforces the first hand, whereby the fingers are placed in the palm, the bases of both the hypothenar and thenar eminences rest on the radial aspect of the second metacarpal, and the thumb lies against the dorsum of the hand. Both arms are extended (Test 5.47A).

Get vert, Extension

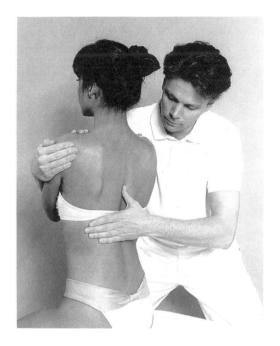

Test 5.46A Beginning position.

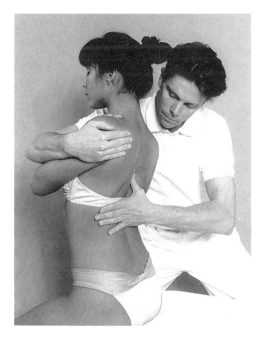

Test 5.46B End position.

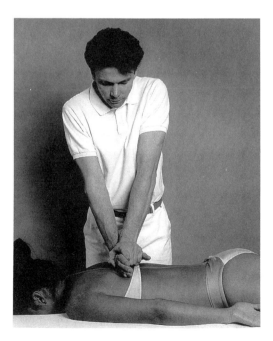

Test 5.47A   *Sp. process.*
more extension of ZAJ

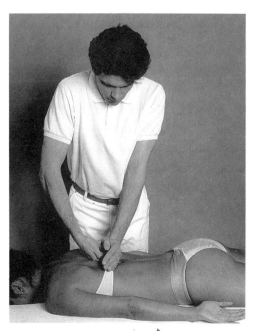

Test 5.47B   *Transverse process*
+ little flex   ZAJ

stabilize caudal, press ī cephalic th

The bisector of the angle formed by both arms should be vertical to the local curvature of the patient's kyphosis. To ensure this position, it may be necessary for the examiner to shift slightly more caudal or cranial.

The examiner now exerts pressure ventrally, until all of the pre-tension has been taken up from the thorax, after which the segment is brought into its maximal ventral translation. Per segment, this is performed several times in order to determine the local movement. At the end of the last test movement, slight overpressure is exerted to determine the end-feel.

Alternative Performance

Another method of testing the ventral translation is performed by exerting ventral pressure against the transverse processes.

The dorsal aspect of the index and ring fingers (at the level of the distal interphalangeal joints) is placed against the transverse process of the vertebra to be tested. The middle finger rests in flexion. The examiner reinforces the first hand by placing the ulnar aspect of the other hand against the palmar aspect of the distal interphalangeal joints of the ring and index fingers. The reinforcing hand is positioned vertical to the local curvature of the kyphosis, and the arm remains extended (Test 5.47B).

The rest of the test is performed as described above. With this alternative performance, a purer translatory movement in the traction direction occurs in the zygapophyseal joint.

Besides testing the amount of translation and the end-feel for each segment, provocation of pain is also clinically significant.

5.48   Axial Rotation Test

Position of the Patient

Same as for test 5.47.

Position of the Examiner

The examiner stands at the head of the treatment table.

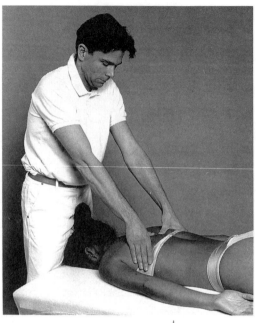

Test 5.48

Performance

The examiner places the end phalanx of each thumb opposite to each other on the lateral aspect of two adjacent spinous processes. The caudal thumb fixes and the cranial thumb moves the segment's cranial vertebra.

The rotation is tested first in one direction from cranial to caudal. Then the opposite rotation is tested, again from cranial to caudal.

Besides testing the amount of translation and the end-feel for each segment, the provocation of pain is also clinically significant.

Passive Local Tests: In Sidelying

5.49.   Dorsal Translation   (NWB)

Position of the Patient

The patient lies in a stable sidelying position, close to the ventral edge of the treatment table. The head and the waist are supported by small pillows to allow the spine to

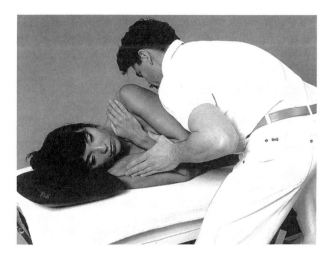

Test 5.49A

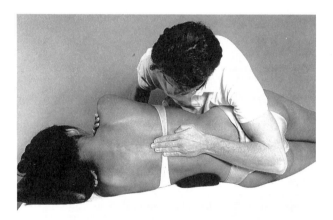

Test 5.49B

rest in a neutral position in the frontal plane. In the sagittal plane, the normal physiological curves of the spine are present. The patient's arms are held crossed in front of the body with the hands resting on the shoulders (Test 5.49A).

Position of the Examiner

The examiner stands in front of the patient at the level of the patient's abdomen.

Performance

The examiner places the caudal hand on the spinous processes below the segment to be tested with the fingers pointing in a cranial direction. The tip of the middle finger rests in the interspinous space of the segment to be tested and has contact with the tip of the cranial spinous process (Test 5.49B).

The other hand is placed against the patient's arms at the point where they cross.

The examiner exerts pressure in a dorsal direction, perpendicular to the local curvature of the thoracic spine. In so doing, the dorsoventral diameter of the thorax decreases. Initially, the examiner experiences little resistance: the pre-tension is taken up from the soft tissue structures and the ribs.

At the point when the resistance increases, generally a small amount of dorsal movement is still possible. The examiner exerts dorsal pressure until the end of the translation motion has been reached, and then performs a slight overpressure. The tip of the middle finger placed in the interspinous space of the segment being tested registers the amount of movement and the end-feel.

As the more caudal segments are tested, the crossed point of the patient's forearms are also shifted more caudally. Visual control is possible through the examiner's arm, which is placed perpendicularly on the local curvature of the thoracic kyphosis.

The advantage of this test in sidelying versus in sitting is that it is generally easier to test the amount of dorsal translation without the influence of gravity.

5.50. Extension in Non–Weight Bearing

Position of the Patient

The same as for test 5.49, except that a pillow is not placed under the patient's head.

Position of the Examiner

The examiner stands in front of the patient at the level of the patient's thorax.

Performance

The examiner's cranial hand is placed on the upper thoracic vertebrae; the patient's head rests in a neutral position on the examiner's forearm whereby the mandible and mastoid process are supported and the ear is not covered.

The examiner's trunk is positioned against the upper aspect of the patient's trunk. In this way, the patient's shoulder girdle and the examiner's hand and trunk form one unit.

The tips of the index and middle fingers of the other hand are placed in the interspinous spaces of two adjacent segments, whereby the ring finger stabilizes the caudal spinous process of the caudal segment.

The examiner rotates his or her trunk, which brings the patient's thoracic spine into extension. At the same time, to create a fulcrum at the segment being tested, the fingertips of the cranial hand exert ventral pressure against the spinous process of the segment's cranial vertebra. For the segments that can-

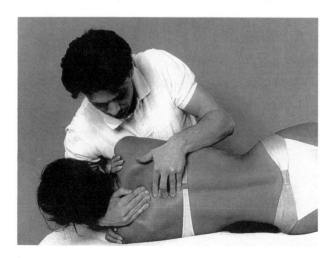

Test 5.50

$T_4 \rightarrow T_{10}$ Ventral PA $\overline{P}$ on caudal Sp. Process not be reached by the cranial hand, the examiner exerts general ventral pressure with the fingertips while bringing the patient's thorax into extension.

The imaginary axis of rotation runs through the segment being tested, thus the farther caudal the segments being tested lie, the greater the amount of extension required to reach these segments. The fingers palpate the amount of movement, whereby the index finger should feel a "closing" (extension) of the cranial segment before the middle finger registers motion in the caudal segment.

5.51. Extension with Left Sidebend and Right Rotation in Non–Weight Bearing

Position of the Patient

Same as for test 5.49. The patient lies on the left side. If the patient is particularly mobile, a slight left sidebend can be prepositioned by shifting the small pillow at the waist more cranially under the midthoracic ribs.

Position of the Examiner

Same as for test 5.49.

Performance

The examiner's caudal forearm is placed flat against the patient's back, whereby the middle finger, reinforced by the index finger, rests against the lateral aspect (closest to the table) of the caudal spinous process of the segment being tested. The tip of the middle finger has contact with the caudolateral aspect of the tip of the segment's cranial spinous process. The examiner's cranial hand is placed against the patient's left hand, which is resting on the right shoulder.

By pushing the patient's right shoulder in a dorsal direction, the patient's trunk is now moved simultaneously into extension, left sidebend, and right rotation. The trunk is then returned to its neutral position, and the examiner repeats this motion several times.

While the examiner's caudal hand and forearm fix the rest of the patient's spine, the middle finger palpates the amount of motion and compares it with that in the adjacent segments.

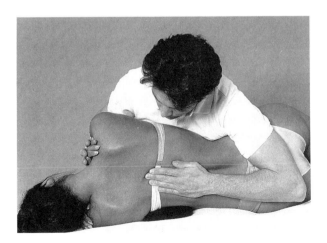

Test 5.51

5.52.   Extension with Right Sidebend and Left Rotation in Non–Weight Bearing

In the same manner as described in test 5.51, the non–weight-bearing extension, right sidebend, and left rotation are tested. Here the patient lies on the right side. By pushing the patient's left shoulder in a dorsal direction, the patient's trunk is now moved simultaneously into extension, right sidebend, and left rotation. Again, the examiner's middle finger palpates the amount of motion in the segment and compares it with that in the adjacent segments.

If both the basic and segmental examinations of the thoracic spine are negative, an examination of the ribs is performed. Should this examination also be negative, it is very likely that there is not a problem with the musculoskeletal system.

DESCRIPTION OF TESTS FOR EXAMINATION OF THE RIBS

See Tests for Examination of the Ribs for specific types of tests according to matching number.

Pathologies of the costovertebral connections, as well as the costosternal and costochondrosternal connections, are seldom seen. Arthritides can occur in every joint, and thus also in the rib joints. However, this rarely occurs. Limitations of motion can be seen in some patients with chronic obstructive pulmonary disease (COPD) as a result of inflammatory disorders such as ankylosing spondylitis, and occasionally after a trauma (for instance, after a rib fracture). Occasionally a limitation of motion can occur after a chronic lung inflammatory disorder.

During examination and treatment of the ribs, it is important that the patient knows how to perform stomach breathing versus chest breathing. If necessary, the patient may have to be instructed in the different forms of breathing beforehand.

Test for the First Rib, Costovertebral Joint

5.53/54.   Test for Mobility and End-Feel

Position of the Patient

In the literature, various positions for testing the first rib are described. Each position

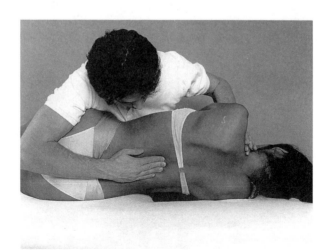

Test 5.52

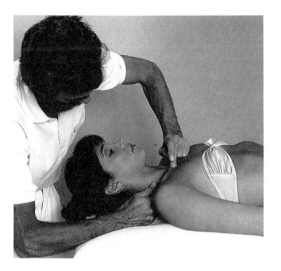

Test 5.53/54A Localization of first rib.

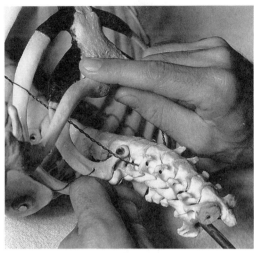

Test 5.53/54B Skeletal model.

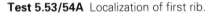

has different advantages and disadvantages; for instance, when the head is positioned in an ipsilateral rotation, the rib is easier to palpate, but the tension from the trapezius is greater.

Here the patient is examined with the head in a neutral position, supported by a small pillow if necessary (depending on the patient's thoracic kyphosis). The arms rest alongside the body.

Position of the Examiner

The examiner stands or sits at the head of the treatment table. The spinous process of T1 and the superior angle of the scapula are localized. If the right side is to be tested, the examiner places the radial aspect of the right index finger's proximal phalanx on the cranial aspect of the first rib at the level of the C7-T1 interspinous space and cranial to the superior angle of the scapula. The first rib is palpated through the trapezius.

The index finger of the other hand can palpate the rib cartilage of the first rib just caudal to the sternal end of the clavicle. However, this is not a testing finger; palpation of this area offers only a confirmation that the first rib is moving.

Performance

The amount of movement is determined during relaxed breathing of the patient. With the cranial hand, the examiner moves the rib in a caudal, ventral, and contralateral direction. The optimal direction of movement varies significantly; the examiner may have to change the direction of motion slightly in order to find the optimal direction.

The end-feel is determined by slight overpressure, performed at the end of a deep exhalation. The amount of movement and end-feel are always compared with those of the other side.

Tests for Second to Twelfth Ribs

5.55/56. Position Test (Left/Right)

Position of the Patient

The patient sits at the foot of the examination table with the feet resting flat on the floor.

Position of the Examiner

The examiner stands next to the patient, opposite the side to be tested.

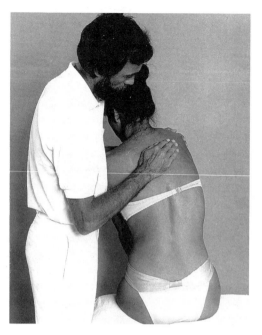

Test 5.55/56A

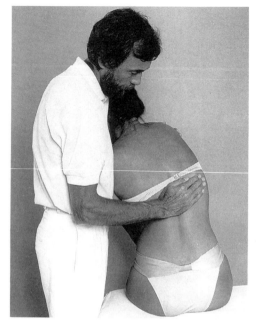

Test 5.55/56B

Performance

If the right side of the patient is to be tested, the examiner's left hand grasps the patient's right shoulder, bringing the trunk into a simultaneous flexion, left sidebend, and left rotation. With the right hand, the examiner palpates the posterior angle of the ribs from cranial (Test 5.55/56A) to caudal (Test 5.55/56B) in one smooth motion. The same is then repeated from caudal to cranial (not shown). The test is performed on both sides. When testing the left side, the patient is positioned in flexion, right sidebend, and right rotation.

Normally during this test, a regular wave-like course of alternating rib and intercostal space is palpated. If a rib is in a position of inspiration, this can generally be detected in the form of a sharp upper edge when palpating in the cranial-to-caudal direction. During the caudal-to-cranial palpation, if the sharp lower edge of a rib is detected, that rib is likely in a position of expiration.

Examples of pathological positions include the position of inspiration seen particularly in patients with COPD and positions of expiration occurring traumatically or in patients with ankylosing spondylitis.

5.57/58. Springing Test (Left/Right)

Position of the Patient

The patient sits at the foot of the treatment table with the feet resting flat on the floor.

Position of the Examiner

The examiner stands at the patient's side, opposite the side to be tested.

Performance

If the right side of the patient is to be tested, the examiner's left hand grasps the patient's right shoulder, bringing the trunk into a simultaneous flexion, left sidebend, and right rotation. The examiner places the the-

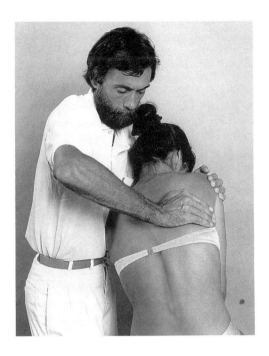

Test 5.57/58

---

nar eminence of the right hand on the posterior angle of the second rib of the patient's right side. Maintaining moderate pressure, the examiner slides the thenar eminence over the posterior angle of all the ribs, starting cranially and ending caudally. When testing the left side, the patient is positioned in flexion, right sidebend, and left rotation.

Alternative Performance
(not pictured)

In the above-described test and position of the patient, the pressure from the testing hand pushes in a direction opposite to the rotated position of the patient. This can result in a ventral movement of the rib, as well as a rotation of the segment. In order to obtain movement *only* from the rib, an alternative testing position can be used; when testing the right side, the examiner brings the patient into a simultaneous flexion, right sidebend, and left rotation. When testing the left side,

the patient is positioned in flexion, left sidebend, and right rotation.

As described above, the examiner places the thenar eminence of the right hand on the posterior angle of the second rib of the patient's right side. Maintaining moderate pressure, the examiner slides the thenar eminence, starting cranially and ending caudally, over the posterior angle of all the ribs.

Normally, the somewhat springy, elastic movement of the rib is palpated. The ribs are pushed ventrally and then spring back in a dorsal direction. If the motion is limited in one rib's costovertebral and/or costotransverse joints, a hard end-feel is palpated at that rib instead of the normal ventral yielding and springing back.

In some disorders, motion in the ribs' costovertebral and costotransverse joints is limited, resulting in an absence of the springing-back feeling. The most obvious example of this is in ankylosing spondylitis.

5.59/60. Testing Active Mobility (Left/ Right)

Position of the Patient

The patient sits at the foot of the treatment table.

Position of the Examiner

The examiner can stand either in front of or behind the patient.

Performance

The examiner places the fingertips of both hands in the intercostal spaces on the right and left sides of the patient.

In examining the ribs 2 through 4, the fingertips are placed at the ventral aspect of the intercostal spaces, and the patient is asked to bring both arms from 90° flexion into elevation (Test 5.59/60A).

In examining the ribs caudal to the fourth, the fingertips are placed at the lateral aspect of the intercostal spaces, and the patient is

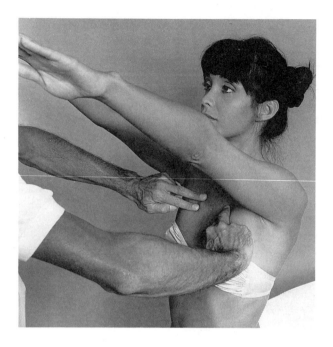

Test 5.59/60A

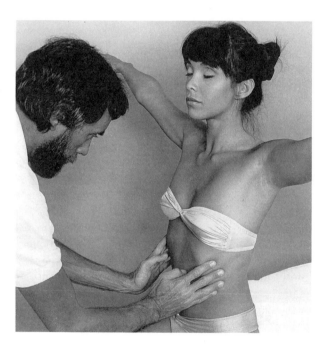

Test 5.59/60B

asked to bring both arms from 90° abduction into elevation (Test 5.59/60B).

The examiner compares the cranial movement of the ribs on both sides.

5.61/62. Testing Costotransverse Joints for Mobility, End-Feel, and Pain Provocation (Left/Right)

Position of the Patient

The patient lies prone with the arms resting alongside the body and the head in a neutral position. If the posterior angle of a rib is covered by the medial position of the scapula, the patient hangs the arm of the side being tested over the edge of the table. In so doing, the scapula is brought into protraction, allowing the posterior angle to be palpated.

Position of the Examiner

The examiner stands next to the patient, opposite the side to be tested. After localizing

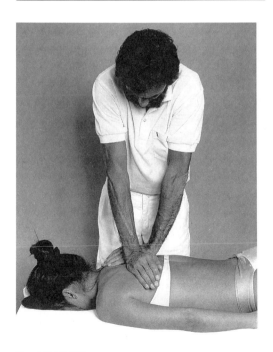

Test 5.61/62

the posterior angle of the rib, the examiner places the proximal part of the hypothenar eminence on that part of the rib. To fix the movement segment, the hypothenar eminence of the other hand is placed on the transverse processes of the corresponding vertebrae closest to the examiner.

Performance

With the arm extended, the examiner moves the posterior angle of the rib in a ventral direction. This motion is repeated several times, each time reaching the end of the range of motion. At the end of the last motion, the patient is instructed to exhale deeply; at the end of the exhalation, slight overpressure is given to determine the end-feel.

This test is performed on the first through the tenth ribs. For the first through the sixth ribs, the direction of motion is ventral and lateral, perpendicular to the local curvature of the kyphosis. From the seventh to the tenth ribs, the direction of motion is ventral, lateral, and cranial. The eleventh and twelfth ribs do not have costotransverse joints.

The examiner registers the amount of motion, end-feel, and pain provocation.

5.63/64. Testing Costovertebral and Costotransverse Mobility (Left/Right)

Position of the Patient

The patient lies supine with the arms resting alongside the body. This test can also be performed in sitting.

Position of the Examiner

The examiner stands at the head of the treatment table.

Performance

The costovertebral and costotransverse mobility of the ribs is determined during maximal inhalation and exhalation. The second rib is localized directly lateral from the

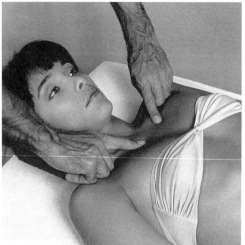

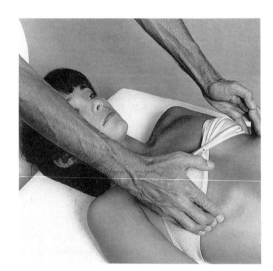

Test 5.63/64A   **Test 5.63/64B**

angle of the sternum. To determine mobility, the tips of the palpating fingers are placed bilaterally in the space between the first and second ribs (Test 5.63/64A).

Because the upper ribs rotate more in the frontal plane and the lower ribs rotate more in the sagittal plane, as the examiner tests more caudally the fingers are placed more laterally between the ribs (Test 5.63/64B).

In examining the eleventh and twelfth ribs, information is registered only in regard to the costovertebral mobility.

5.65/66.   Testing Passive Mobility (Left/Right)

Position of the Patient

The patient lies in supine for testing the mobility of the cranial ribs, and in sidelying for testing the mobility of the caudal ribs (5 to 12). This test can also be performed in sitting.

Position of the Examiner

The examiner stands at the head of the treatment table.

Performance

The examiner grasps the patient's upper arm just proximal to the elbow and elevates the arm through flexion in order to test the cranial ribs (Test 5.65/66A), or through abduction when testing the caudal ribs (Test 5.65/66B). At the same time, the fingers of the other hand palpate several intercostal spaces. The cranial ribs are palpated from the ventral aspect and the caudal ribs are palpated from the lateral aspect.

As the examiner brings the patient's arm into elevation, the palpating fingers should register that the ribs move in a cranial direction and that the intercostal spaces widen.

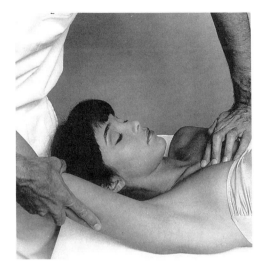

Test 5.65/66A

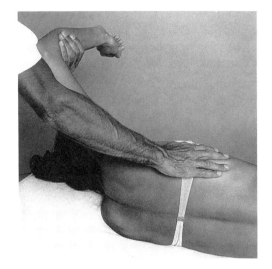

Test 5.65/66B

5.3   PATHOLOGY

all Appx C.

PRIMARY DISC-RELATED DISORDERS

In this book, disorders are considered to be primary disc-related disorders when the initial impressions indicate that the patient's signs and symptoms are caused by a lesion of the disc. In some cases, the causal role of the disc is not yet scientifically proved. However, in our view the evidence is convincing enough to consider these primary disc-related disorders nonetheless.

In the thoracic region, pathology of the intervertebral disc is seldom seen. Only 2% of all demonstrable disc lesions are localized in the thoracic spine. However, many people have symptoms in the thoracic area that are probably discogenic in nature but the cause cannot yet be confirmed. This particularly concerns symptoms that occur during certain work positions, especially the kyphosed posture and/or positions.

Thoracic Posture Syndrome

In people who perform work that involves a lot of sitting, meaning prolonged periods of kyphosed posturing, low back pain as well as neck and/or thoracic pain can arise. It is assumed that a dorsal shift of the thoracic disc occurs, whereby pressure is gradually increased on the posterior longitudinal ligament and the dura mater. In addition, overloading occurs on the other dorsal ligaments and the paravertebral musculature. Which of these structures is the primary cause of the complaints is still unknown.

Clinical Findings

- The patient complains of central thoracic pain during sitting, which increases as the day goes on. During the night and in the morning, the patient has no complaints. Lifting and carrying heavy objects increase the pain. If the patient corrects this posture or lies down, the symptoms disappear immediately—at least in the beginning stage. In later stages, it can take hours before the symptoms eventually decrease and disappear.
- In the functional examination, some of the passive tests can be "felt" at end-

range. Real pain cannot be provoked in the functional examination.

- If the patient is experiencing these symptoms *at the moment* the examination takes place, then one of the dura tests is usually positive. Usually this involves flexion of the entire spine, including the cervical spine.

Treatment

Treatment focuses primarily on the cause of the problem. In other words, along with information as to the cause of the symptoms, the patient must also change his or her posture. If necessary, the working environment must be adjusted. At the same time, it is advisable for the patient to perform daily specific muscle-strengthening exercises for the thoracic back extensors and the scapula adductors. (See Appendix 4–A, Patient Handbook.)

If the patient has considerable pain, continuous mechanical traction can be applied. This treatment should be given daily for at least 2 weeks. The duration of the traction should be increased gradually from 15 minutes to 30 minutes.

Posterolateral Disc Protrusion

Except in the thoracic posture syndrome, thoracic disc pathology is almost always the result of a trauma. Usually the injury involves axial compression, such as occurs in a fall on the buttocks or when carrying a heavy object with the thoracic spine in flexion. The trauma could be recent or could have taken place years previously.

In the differential diagnosis, a disorder of the internal organs should be considered.

Clinical Findings

- The patient complains of localized paravertebral pain. The symptoms usually come on during prolonged sitting or as a result of a movement in which the thoracic spine was flexed. In lying, the patient has no complaints. The pain sel-

dom radiates; if it does, it is usually extrasegmental and due to dural irritation.

- Coughing, sneezing, and straining can increase the pain.
- In the functional examination, one of the rotation motions is usually painful and limited, both actively and passively. Sometimes active flexion is also painful.
- Stretch on the dura is almost always positive (neck flexion with flexion of the entire spine, or neck flexion with one of the thoracic rotations).
- CT scan or MRI can confirm the diagnosis.

Treatment

Without treatment, a chronic recurring problem can develop, often including periods without pain lasting for months. Usually mobilization of the thoracic spine with axial separation is very effective. After this treatment, the patient should perform regular mobility (rotation) exercises as well as muscle-strengthening exercises (for the back extensors and the scapula adductors). In addition, the patient must receive extensive information regarding the problem, along with instruction in proper posture and body mechanics.

Posterolateral Disc Prolapse

As in posterolateral disc protrusion, posterolateral disc prolapse (Figure 5–8) usually concerns a post-traumatic syndrome. The most significant difference between the two is that in a disc prolapse intercostal neuralgia arises.

In the differential diagnosis, malignant tumors have to be considered. This usually involves a bronchial carcinoma or Pancoast's tumor. Breast carcinomas and mediastinal and paravertebral tumors initially can resemble an innocent intercostal neuralgia. However, the most frequent cause of an intercostal neuralgia is herpes zoster.

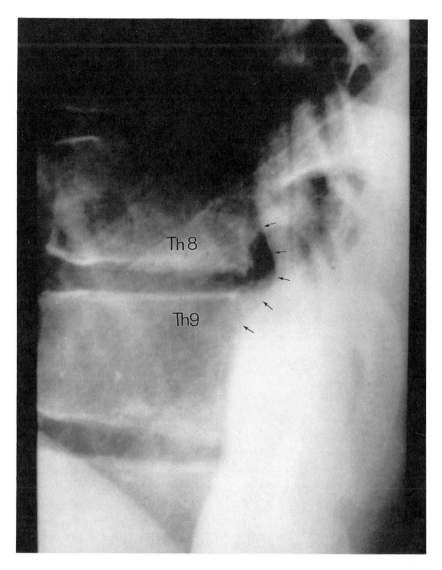

Figure 5–8 A massive thoracic disc prolapse is seen on a conventional lateral X-ray with myelography at the level of T7 to T10 in a 35-year-old patient with a disc prolapse at T8-9. The dural sac, filled with contrast medium, is pushed away by the disc prolapse (**arrows**).

Clinical Findings

- The most significant symptom is the intercostal neuralgia. In some patients, pain is experienced only at the sternum, without local thoracic pain. Often, taking a deep breath is painful. In considering the differential diagnosis, ruling out a myocardial infarct is important—in these cases, taking a deep breath usually is not painful.

- Coughing, sneezing, and straining increase the symptoms.

- In the functional examination various motions can be painful. Flexion, as well as extension, and either one or both rotations are painful and limited, both actively and passively.

- The dural stretch tests are usually positive.
- Myelo-CT scan and/or MRI confirm the diagnosis.

Treatment

Information regarding the lesion and ergonomic advice are of great importance. In many instances, mobilization with axial separation is very effective. As with a thoracic disc protrusion, muscle strengthening of the back extensors and the scapula adductors is indicated.

The prognosis is varied. Some patients have complete relief of their pain after one manipulation, whereas other patients improve very gradually and take 1 month to recover.

Posterocentral Disc Prolapse

The posterocentral disc prolapse (Figure 5–9) concerns a rare but dangerous lesion. Carson et al[5] estimate the frequency of this lesion to be in 1 per 1 million per year. Because the spinal canal is narrower in the thoracic region than in the lumbar and cervical regions, spinal cord compression and neurological deficits can occur rapidly.

A study done by Fidler and Goedhart[6] shows evidence that of the 215 described cases of thoracic disc prolapse, by far most occurred in the lower thoracic region. In this study, the most frequently affected intervertebral discs were T11-12, T10-11, and T9-10, while not one prolapse was found in the C7 to T4 region.

Clinical Findings

- The patient usually complains of severe local pain in the back with radiating symptoms in the corresponding dermatome. In instances of a lower thoracic prolapse, pain can also be experienced in the abdomen on that side. Motor defi-

cits are seldom seen; however, disturbances in sensation in the form of hyperesthesia are frequently seen.
- Coughing, sneezing, straining, and sometimes taking a deep breath are very painful.
- Findings in the functional examination vary, depending on the location of the prolapse. In a central disc prolapse, in particular, the long tracts of the spinal cord can become compromised, with a resulting complete transverse lesion or possibly a Brown-Séquard syndrome in which one-half of the spinal cord is compressed. This lesion can be either partial or total. The possible spastic paresis of the leg is on the same side as the disc prolapse, while below this level on the opposite side the sensations of pain and temperature are disturbed.
- In some patients, it is impossible to perform almost every motion, and in other patients there is only a limitation of flexion and/or a rotation of the thoracic spine.
- To confirm the diagnosis, myelography, a CT scan, and particularly an MRI are utilized.

Treatment

In some mild cases, conservative treatment, bed rest, or cautious continuous traction (refer to Chapter 4, section 4.4, Treatment) can alleviate the symptoms. However, as soon as there are signs or symptoms of spinal cord compression, surgery is indicated.

Spondylodiscitis

Spondylodiscitis is an inflammation of the intervertebral disc that usually has a hematogenic cause. It is seen primarily in children between 4 and 5 years of age and in adults over 50. The distribution between gender is the same for each age span.

The lumbar spine is the most frequently affected region; in adults, the disorder is also

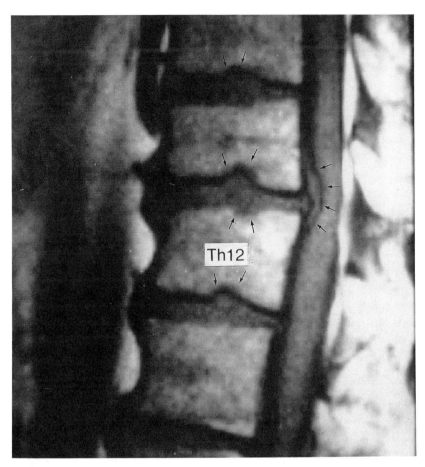

Figure 5–9 A massive thoracic disc prolapse is shown on an MRI of the lower thoracic spine in a 49-year-old patient with a disc prolapse (***right arrows***) at the T11-12 level. Compression of the spinal cord is obvious. The Schmorl's nodules in the vertebral bodies of T10, T11, and T12 (***middle arrows***) indicate Scheuermann's disease.

seen in the midthoracic area of the spinal column. However, occasionally in adults the inflammation can be found in the cervical column; in children localization in the cervical spine is seen sporadically.

Because the disorder in the thoracic spine is seen only in adults, the discussion here is limited to spondylodiscitis in adults. This is generally considered to be a septic process. There is a subacute form as well as a chronic form.

It is important to differentiate between spondylodiscitis and tumors. One of the most frequently seen tumors manifesting itself in the thoracic spine is Kahler's disease (multiple myeloma) (Figures 5–10 to 5–12).

Clinical Findings

- The patient complains of either an acute or a gradual onset of pain in the back with radiating symptoms around the side and sometimes even into the legs. The symptoms increase during loaded activities of the spinal column.

- In the functional examination, there are active as well as passive thoracic spine

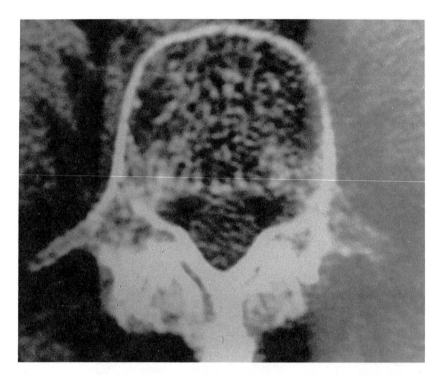

Figure 5–10 A CT scan at the level of T8 in a patient with severe midthoracic pain shows the presence of Kahler's disease (multiple myeloma). There is severe destruction of the vertebral body. The normal trabecular pattern of the bone has completely disappeared.

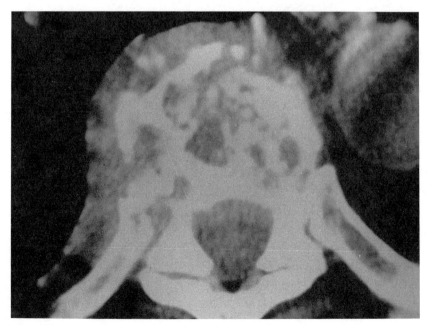

Figure 5–11 A CT scan at the level of T8 in a patient with severe thoracic pain radiating into both legs reveals spondylodiscitis, destruction stage.

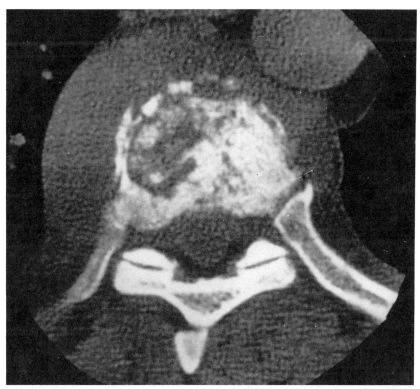

Figure 5–12 A CT scan at the level of T10 in a patient with severe thoracic pain reveals spondylodiscitis, destruction stage, caused by Pott's disease (tuberculosis of the spinal column).

limitations of motion in a capsular pattern (symmetrical limitations of motions of rotation).

- Radiologically, various stages can be differentiated: a destruction stage, a reparation stage, and an end-stage.[7]

Treatment

Treatment consists of bed rest and the appropriate antibiotics. Surgery is indicated only when the patient does not react well to the conservative treatment. An exception to this is a threatening transverse lesion; in this case, surgical intervention is absolutely indicated.

SECONDARY DISC-RELATED DISORDERS

In this book, secondary disc-related disorders are disorders in which a primary disc lesion was experienced earlier, the normally occurring physiological degeneration of the segment is accelerated, or, due to trauma, normal adaptation to the degeneration is made impossible. Thus, it always involves situations in which extreme disc degeneration is later coupled with changes in the zygapophyseal joints. This leads to narrowing of the spinal canal and the intervertebral foramen. In some cases, the causal role of an earlier primary disc-related problem is not yet confirmed. However, in our view the evidence is convincing enough to consider these as "secondary disc-related disorders" nonetheless.

Secondary disc-related disorders are seen mostly in the lumbar spine, to a lesser degree in the cervical spine, and very rarely in the thoracic spine. This may be explained by the fact that primary thoracic disc pathology is so seldom present.

TRAUMATIC DISORDERS

In this book, traumatic disorders include not only lesions of which the patient is aware of the traumatic onset, but also lesions such as "spontaneous" fractures in which a prolonged degenerative process has been present. Also included in this category are the non–disc-related) disorders that may or may not have a traumatic onset.

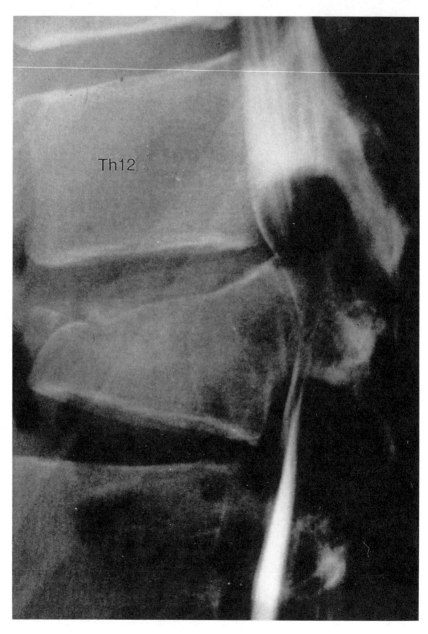

Figure 5–13 Conventional myelogram at the level of the thoracolumbar junction in a patient who sustained a compression trauma after falling from a great height. The vertebral body of L1 is significantly compressed at its ventral aspect (see also Figure 5–14).

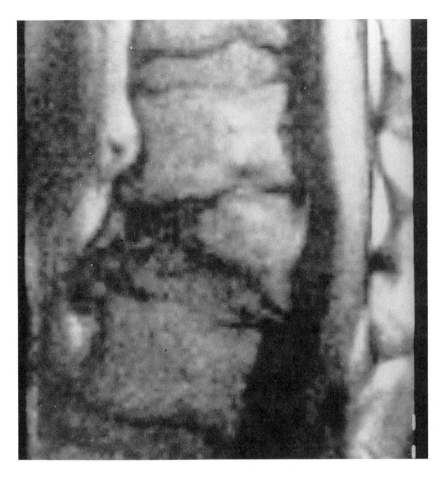

Figure 5–14 MRI of the thoracolumbar junction in a patient who sustained a significant fall. There is a wedge-shaped compression fracture of the T12 vertebral body. In both cases (this one and the one in Figure 5–13), a dorsal shifting of the posterior wall of the vertebrae occurred, resulting in a decreased anterior-posterior diameter of the spinal canal with compression of the medullary cone.

Traumatic Compression Fracture

A traumatic compression fracture can occur at any age and is the result of an axial force acting on the flexed thoracic spine. In the thoracic spine, the most frequently affected vertebral body is T12, and in the lumbar spine it is L1 and L2 (Figures 5–13 to 5–16).

Clinical Findings

- The patient experiences acute pain immediately after a traumatic event. Every movement is extremely difficult, due to pain. The patient should have X-ray films taken immediately.
- Conventional X-rays demonstrate the fracture, but the severity of the fracture is best indicated in a CT scan. Often there is also damage to one or more intervertebral discs. However, neurological lesions seldom occur.

Treatment

Treatment consists of bed rest until the pain has diminished enough to allow cautious

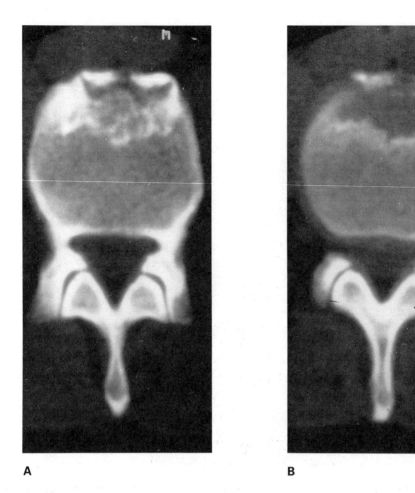

A   **B**

Figure 5–15 CT scan at the level of L2 in a patient who underwent an earlier hyperflexion trauma. A compression fracture is visible at the anterior ventral aspect of the vertebral body.

movement. This can take days to weeks. During the recovery, the patient should be encouraged to swim and walk as much as possible. The ultimate prognosis is good. Some patients continue to experience slight, intermittent symptoms.

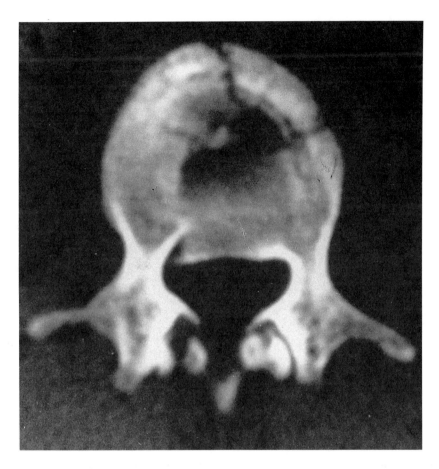

Figure 5–16 CT scan at the level of T12 in a patient who experienced a severe axial trauma. A "burst" fracture is seen with a dorsal shifting of the back wall of the vertebral body.

Spontaneous Compression Fracture

"Spontaneous" compression fractures are most often seen in women over 60 years of age and are almost always the result of osteoporosis (Figure 5–17). One or more vertebral bodies can either gradually or suddenly collapse. The acute fracture causes severe back pain, while the gradually occurring fracture causes chronic pain.

Clinical Findings

- A significant kyphosis is noted, which is usually curved but sometimes also can be angular. Because of the compensatory increase in the cervical and lumbar lordoses, many patients also complain of cervical and/or lumbar pain.

- In the functional examination, various findings can be expected. Flexion can cause pain; extension is usually impossible to perform and can cause pain due to "kissing spines" (approximation of the spinous processes). Sidebend can be painful as a result of compression of the twelfth rib against the ilium. In most cases, rotation is severely limited and can also be painful.

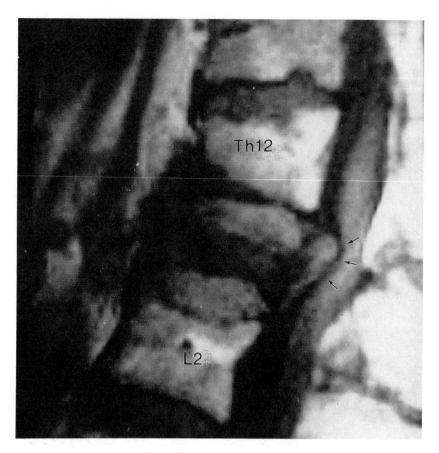

Figure 5–17 MRI of the thoracolumbar junction in a 73-year-old patient with osteoporosis. There is a compression fracture of the L1 vertebral body. The vertebral body has a flattened form, while the adjacent disc spaces appear to be relatively normal. The spinal cord is significantly compromised because of the fragmented vertebral body (**arrows**).

- X-rays demonstrate the decisive diagnostic findings and usually show the characteristic "codfish" vertebrae.

Treatment

In the acute fracture, several days of bed rest may be necessary. However, it is very important to keep these periods of bed rest as short as possible, because inactivity promotes osteoporosis. Initial activity such as walking, biking, or swimming should be encouraged. Movement is the most important way of stopping the demineralization process. Specific conservative treatment, such as extension exercises or prescribing a corset, generally causes an increase rather than a decrease in the symptoms. (The costoiliac compression syndrome is discussed under Other Disorders.)

Slipped Rib Tip Syndrome (Costa Fluctuans)

When the nineth and/or tenth rib have not merged with the ventral rib cage or are loosened due to a trauma to the ventral rib cage, an impingement of the soft tissue in this area can occur during some movements. People with a kyphotic posture or a hyperkyphosis may be predisposed to this syndrome. The disorder can also have a traumatic onset, for instance, as a result of a car accident in which the driver is not wearing a seat belt and the lower ribs are pushed against the steering wheel. Also, a vigorous trunk rotation can cause the ninth or tenth rib to be torn loose. This can happen in such sports as discus throwing, shot put, javelin throwing, and golfing.

In the differential diagnosis, the examiner should consider lesions of the thoracic spine and/or the costovertebral joints, as well as lesions of the abdominal muscles.

Clinical Findings

- The patient complains of local pain that can be provoked by sidebend and rotation to the affected side. The so-called hooking maneuver is also positive: the patient sits in a kyphosis and the examiner hooks the fingers under the rib cage, then pulls in a ventrocranial direction.
- Palpation of the free rib ends causes sharp local pain.

Treatment

If the disorder is due to poor posture, the primary treatment consists of correcting the posture. In some cases, infiltrating the free rib end with a local anesthetic gives lasting pain relief. In severe cases, the corresponding intercostal nerve can be blocked or the affected rib(s) can be removed surgically.

Strain of the Intercostal Muscles

Strain of the intercostal muscles is almost always due to a traumatic event, and in most cases occurs as a result of a rib fracture. Usually the muscles between two or more ribs are affected.

Clinical Findings

- The pain is very local. Inhaling and exhaling deeply, particularly in acute cases, can be painful.

- In the functional examination, the resisted tests are usually negative.
- The exact location of the lesion can be determined by means of palpation. Because of the local tenderness, differentiation from an intercostal neuralgia is rather simple.

Treatment

Transverse friction, regardless of the duration of the lesion, is almost always curative within a few treatments. (Other relevant muscle lesions are discussed under Other Disorders.)

FORM ABERRATIONS OF THE SPINAL COLUMN

In discussing form aberrations of the spinal column, disorders characterized primarily by abnormal kyphosis/lordosis/scoliosis are considered, along with the chronic disorders that affect the morphology of the spinal column as a whole. More localized chronic disorders are discussed under Other Disorders.

Thoracic Kyphosis

A kyphosis is a curve in the spinal column in the sagittal plane, with its convexity dorsal. Differentiation is made between hyperkyphosis and hypokyphosis. Whether or not the kyphosis can be considered abnormal is determined by radiological measurements.

Almost every growth disturbance at the ventral aspect of the spinal column (vertebra or disc) can have a kyphosing effect because the height of the affected structure diminishes due to load. The subsequent result is that the adjacent parts of the vertebral column compensate by increasing their curvature. Thus, various form aberrations of the back occur (Figure 5–18), as follows.

- *Hollow-round back.* The hollow-round back is a thoracic hyperkyphosis with intensified (compensatory) lordotic

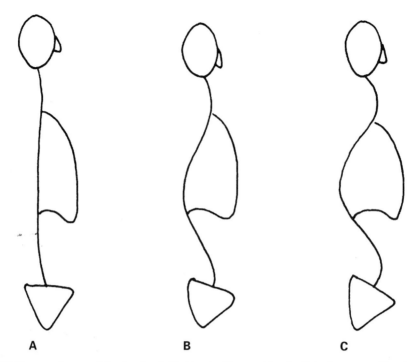

Figure 5–18 Various forms of the back. **A**, Flat back; **B**, round back; **C**, hollow-round back.

curves of the cervical and lumbar spines; thus, all of the curves in the sagittal plane are increased. The apex of the kyphosis is shifted from the normal localization, T6, caudally—usually to T8.

- *Round back*. If the thoracolumbar junction is affected, the thoracic kyphosis extends caudally. In this instance, the lumbar lordosis is shortened. The lumbar lordosis does not compensate by increasing. One speaks of a round back when the apex of the thoracic kyphosis has shifted toward the thoracolumbar junction.
- *Flat back*. If the lumbar spine is affected, causing a decrease in the lumbar lordosis, the thoracic kyphosis compensates by diminishing. The result is a flat back.

The result of these abnormal curvatures is a decreased ability to absorb the loads working on the spine. Therefore, the spine acts as a rigid rod. In a flat back; in a round back, as well as in a hollow-round back, the very mobile transition zones are overloaded. This mainly involves the lower cervical region and the lumbosacral region. Because the kyphotic region is usually more rigid, symptoms seldom occur. If they do occur, they are usually temporary.

Causes of Abnormal Thoracic Kyphosis

The abnormal thoracic kyphosis is divided into the following categories:

- congenital kyphosis
- acquired kyphosis, with the subcategory of kyphosis due to systemic disorders

Congenital Kyphosis

- *Dorsal Wedge Vertebra.* The dorsal wedge vertebra is seen mostly in the first lumbar and the first thoracic vertebrae. The angular kyphosis that results is usually severely progressive (Figure 5–19). In the upper thoracic spine, this ultimately can lead to paraplegia through spinal cord compression.
- *Block Vertebra.* The block vertebra is based on a disturbance in the embryological segmentation. The block vertebra is identified on X-ray by the smooth ventral concave border, which differentiates it from, for instance, traumatically occurring block vertebrae (synostosis after a fracture) (Figure 5–20).
- *Spina Bifida Manifesta (Meningomyelocele).* A meningomyelocele can cause a kyphosis, a lordosis, or a scoliosis. If a kyphosis is the result, it is short, curved, and rigid (Figures 5–21 and 5–22).

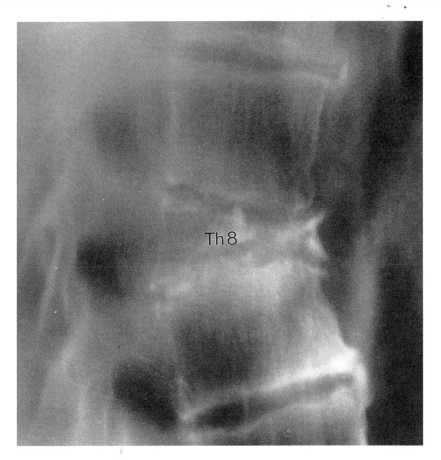

A

Figure 5–19 X-ray of the midthoracic spine in an adult man with a congenital angular kyphosis. **A**, Conventional lateral view. The vertebral body of T8 is wedge shaped.

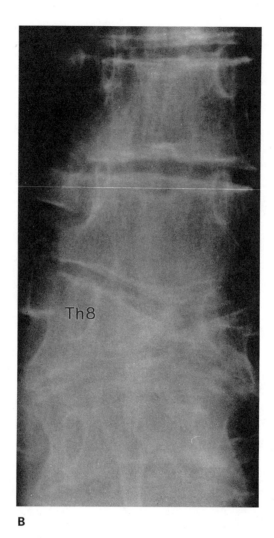

B

Figure 5–19 *B,* Conventional anterior-posterior view. The wedge shape appears here to be more a bow tie.

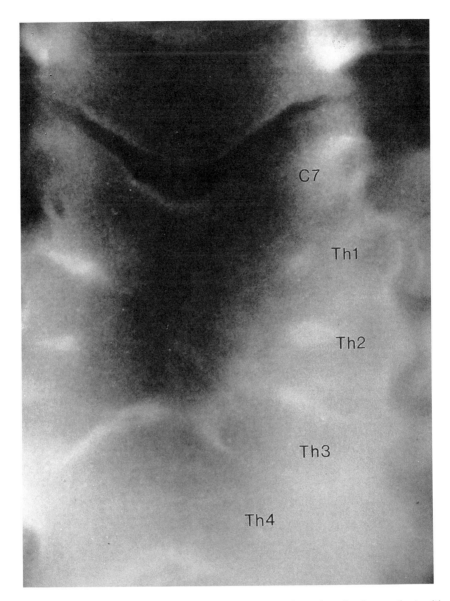

Figure 5–20 Conventional anterior-posterior X-ray of the upper thoracic spine in a patient with a con-genital upper thoracic angular kyphosis. There is a block vertebra (fusion) of C7 to T5; in this picture, T5 is difficult to distinguish.

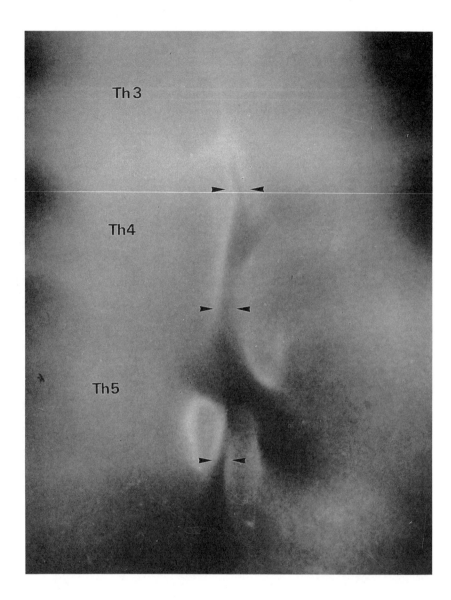

Figure 5–21 Anterior-posterior tomogram of the upper thoracic spine in a patient with an angular thoracic kyphosis. The vertebrae T3 to T5 have grown together completely. In the median plane, where the spinous processes should be (***arrowheads***), there is only an open space: this is a spina bifida.

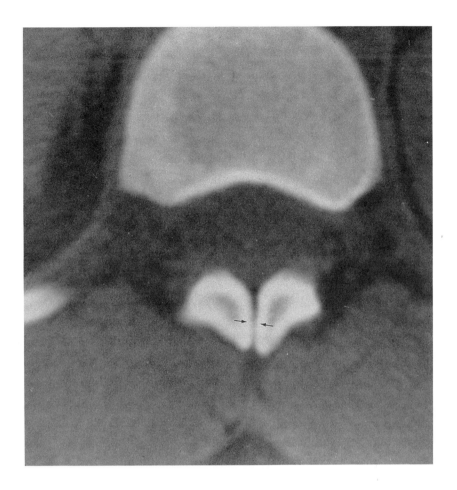

Figure 5–22 CT scan at the level of the T12 in a patient with a slight lower lumbar kyphosis. The patient has spina bifida occulta. The two parts of the spinous process have not fused.

Acquired Kyphosis

- *Poor Posture*. Poor posture is the most common cause of an abnormal kyphosis in children. For a large part, the sitting posture at school is responsible for this postural problem.

  Treatment consists simply of correcting the posture. If the appropriate exercises are initiated too late (after the age of 14), there is a possibility that the acquired posture can no longer be completely corrected.

- *Scheuermann's Disease*. By far the most frequent cause of an abnormal kyphosis is Scheuermann's disease, which is a growth disturbance. ✗

- *Rachitis*. A reversible kyphosis can sometimes be seen in young children with rachitis. Because of a softening of the bones and a weakening of the muscles, an increased thoracolumbar kyphosis occurs. Without treatment, this kyphosis will stiffen progressively. However, with the appropriate causal and local treatment, full recovery is possible.

✗ Osteo chondrosis weak end plates, onset age 11-14 y.o. commonest: see several irregular end plates, ↑ wedge form. May have cranial protrusions of disc (Schmorl's nodes)?

- *Leukemia in Children.* Leukemia in children leads to osteoporosis of the vertebral body. Usually a thoracolumbar lordosis occurs.
- *Vertebral Fracture.* Because of compression of the anterior part of the vertebral body, vertebral fractures can result in an angular kyphosis. In children, this is the case particularly when the growth plates of the vertebrae are affected. Usually T12, L1, or L2 is involved. Sometimes two or more vertebrae are fractured (Figure 5–23).
- *Osteoporosis.* In osteoporosis, predominantly seen in women after menopause, ventral compression fractures of the osteoporotic thoracic vertebrae can occur (Figure 5–24).

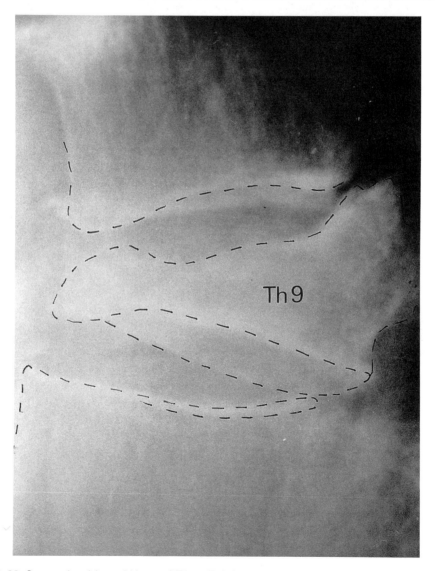

Figure 5–23 Conventional lateral X-ray of T8 to T10 in a patient who underwent a severe trauma. There is a severe compression fracture of T9 with wedge-shaped flattening.

- *Vertebra Plana and Platyspondylisis.*
Vertebra plana constitutes a rare disorder that occurs in the third year of life in the lower thoracic spine. It occurs as a result of an eosinophilic granuloma. Over the course of years, the radiologically visible flat vertebra develops into a normal vertebra again. Platyspondylisis

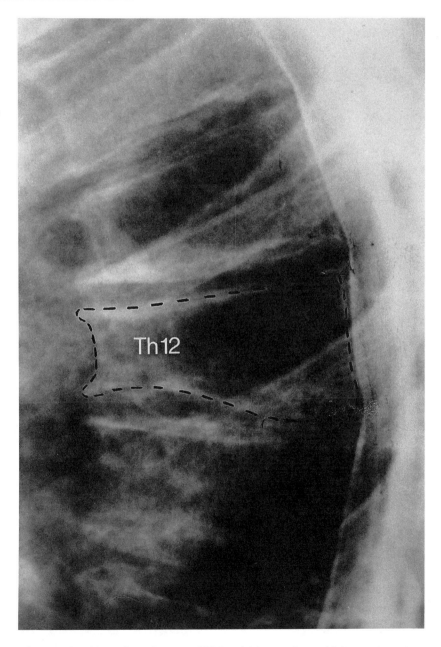

Figure 5–24 Conventional lateral myelogram of T10 to L1 in a patient with lower thoracic complaints. There is lower thoracic kyphosis due to osteoporosis in very wide and flat vertebrae (platyspondylisis). T12 has a clearly recognizable wedge form (indicated by the broken lines).

is an abnormal widening and flattening of the vertebrae (congenital), usually without clinical significance (Figure 5–25).

- *Iatrogenic Kyphosis.* As a result of a laminectomy in children who are still growing, in many cases a progressive kyphosis occurs. After such surgery, the patient should be very closely followed by the physician in order to control the possible development of a kyphosis.

- *Inflammations and Tumors.* In cases of tumors and inflammations of the spinal column, pain at rest, especially at

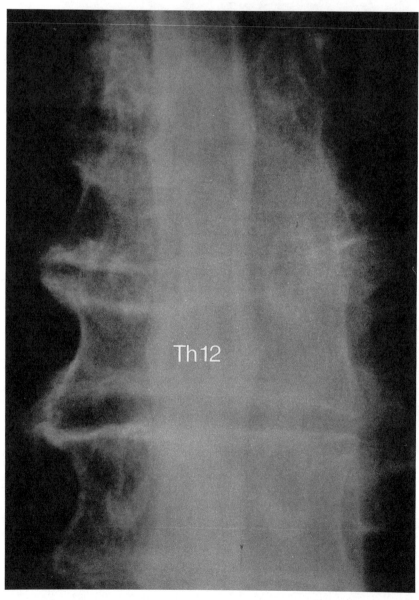

Figure 5–25 Conventional lateral myelogram of T10 to L1 in a patient with lower thoracic/upper lumbar symptoms. There is platyspondylisis of T12.

night, is the first symptom. The pain can increase during activity. The abnormal kyphosing of the affected part of the spinal column usually occurs long after the onset of the symptoms. In many instances, the functional examination indicates limitations of motion in the capsular pattern. At the same time, there is often local percussion pain or pain when falling back onto the heels from a tiptoe position (Figures 5–26 and 5–27).

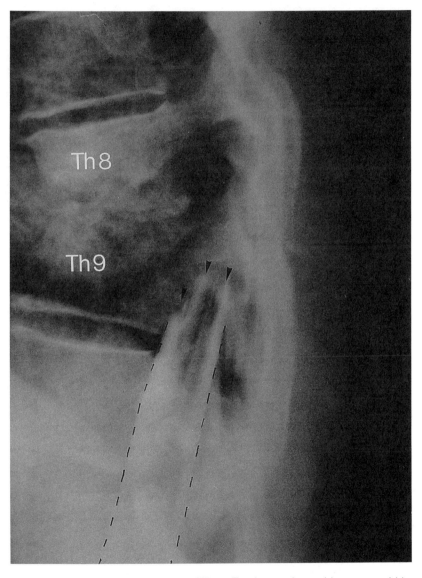

Figure 5–26 Conventional lateral myelogram of T7 to T11 in a patient with severe midthoracic symptoms and spinal cord symptoms. The vertebral bodies of T8 and T9 are flattened into a wedge shape and have completely fused together, caused by Pott's disease (tuberculosis of the spine). Due to compression of the spinal cord, there is a complete stop (***arrowheads***) of the column (***broken lines***) of contrast fluid, which was injected caudally.

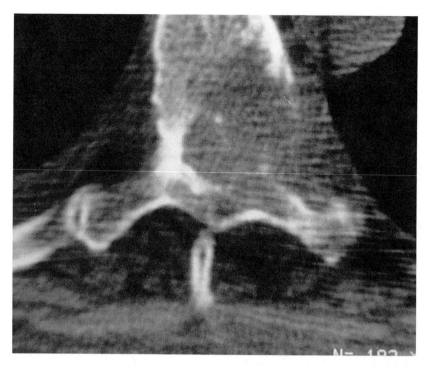

Figure 5–27 CT scan at the level of T8 in a patient with severe midthoracic complaints and significant symptoms of spinal cord compression. There is complete destruction of the bone and filling of the spinal canal due to a tumor.

Kyphosis in Systemic Disorders

- *Osteogenesis Imperfecta.* In this disease, spontaneous fractures occur frequently. The disorder involves not only the long bones of the body, but also the vertebrae. Radiologically, the typical picture of the biconcave "fish" vertebrae is demonstrated along with an abnormally high intervertebral space. The severity of the collapse of the vertebrae determines the severity of the kyphosis.

- *Hypothyroidism.* In hypothyroidism (insufficient function of the thyroid gland), a deformation of L1 and L2 can develop as an early sign, with a resultant thoracolumbar kyphosis. However, with hormonal treatment this kyphosis is completely reversible.

- *Chondrodystrophy.* Chondrodystrophy is a hereditary disturbance of the endochondral ossification. This results in underdevelopment of the longitudinal growth, with normal growth in width of the affected vertebrae. Thus a kyphosis of the thoracolumbar junction is seen as a result of the wedge-shaped vertebrae. The lumbar spine is markedly short, with a very strong lordotic lumbosacral kink. Because of this, many chondrodystrophic dwarfs have complaints of back pain.

- *Muscle Diseases.* During sitting, patients with progressive muscular dystrophy and patients with myotonia often have a flaccid total kyphosis as a result of their inability to sit erect. In standing, the pelvis tips forward, and a maximal lordosis occurs, often with a dorsally prominent cervicothoracic junction. Usually, the vertebral column remains mobile.

Clinical Findings

- The kyphosis is best judged from the side. A plumb line running along the most prominent part of the spinal column is used in order to define the depth of the lordoses (cervical and lumbar).

- If the thoracic kyphosis is increased, the scapulae and shoulders are generally in a protracted position. In most cases, this leads to a shortening of the pectoral muscles, which results in the inability to correct actively the forward-bent posture. In inspection from the dorsal aspect, the distance between the medial borders of the scapula and the spinous processes is greater than it is under normal circumstances.

- The spinous processes in the kyphosed part of the thoracic spine are usually more visible and sometimes the skin in this area is hyperpigmented because of pressure against chair backs. In many cases, the ribs are positioned more ventrally in the transverse plane and therefore the typical form of the thoracic spine (the so-called sarcophagus cover form) becomes apparent when the patient performs forward flexion (Figure 5–28). In some cases this form is not present, but one can observe an increased kyphosis in combination with a funnel-shaped chest.

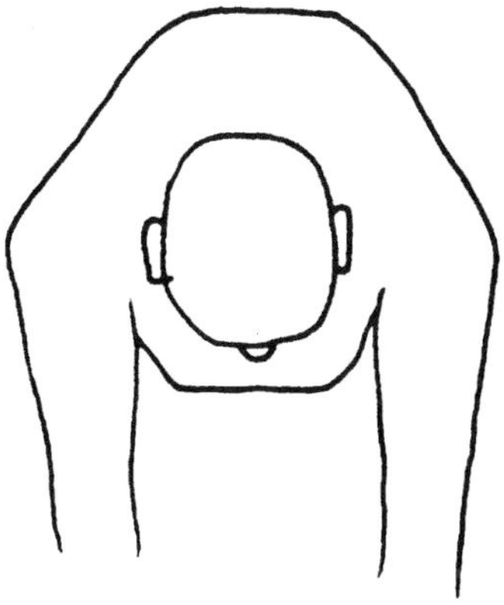

There are various methods of measuring the kyphosis. Determining the depth of the lordotic curves (cervical and lumbar) in relation to the plumb line hanging along the most prominent part of the kyphosis is a quick way of obtaining a general impression (Figure 5–29). However, the measurements obtained, to a certain extent, are dependent on the posture. Thus these measurements are not reliable.

A better method of measuring is through goniometry using the Debrunner kyphosometer[8] (Figure 5–30). The instrument measures an angle, the kyphosis angle. This is defined as the angle between the upper and lower measuring surfaces of the instrument. The margin of error amounts to approximately 3° to a maximum of 5°. The difference between the kyphosis angles in various positions gives a good impression of the mobility of the kyphotic spine.

Each end of the measuring instrument is gently pushed into place against two spinous processes: cranial on T2-3 and caudal on T11-12. (In determining the curve of the lum-

Figure 5–28 Sarcophagus cover form of the thoracic spine, according to Henke.[8]

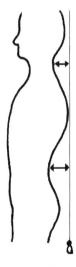

Figure 5–29 Measuring the lordosis of the cervical and lumbar regions by use of a plumb line, according to Henke.[8]

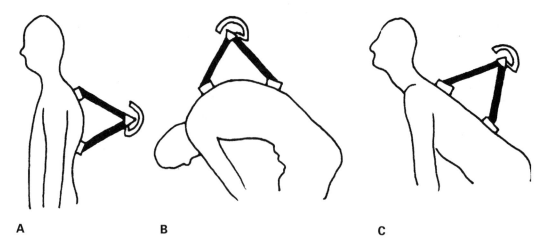

A   **B**   **C**

Figure 5–30 Angle measurement with the kyphosometer developed by Debrunner.[8] The angle of kyphosis is measured as the angle between the instrument's measuring surfaces (the small white rectangles). **A**, In standing; **B**, in maximal flexion, with flexed hips; **C**, in maximal extension, with flexed hips, according to Henke.[8]

bar spine the instrument is placed on T12-L1 and the sacrum.)

Measurements are made in three positions: in relaxed standing, in maximal flexion, and in extension with flexed hips. The normal values of the thoracic kyphosis amount to approximately 30° in standing, 50° in flexion, and 8° in maximal extension.

If such clinical examination indicates a fixed kyphosis, although it may be only to a small degree, X-ray films of the spine should be taken in standing and from two directions. It does not have to be a total view; however, the three curves should be visible in order to be measurable (Figure 5–31). Only when surgery is being considered should functional views be performed in order to determine the possibility of decreasing the curvature. On the X-ray films, the following variables are measured:

- the size of the kyphosis, especially the distance between the "end vertebrae"; this means the cranial and caudal vertebrae that make the greatest angle to the horizontal
- the most dorsally prominent point on the curve; this so-called "apex vertebra" is

generally the most wedge shaped and, in cases of scoliosis, is also the most rotated

- the kyphosis in degrees, the angle between a perpendicular line coming from the cranial aspect of the cranial end vertebra and a perpendicular line coming from the caudal aspect of the caudal end vertebra
- the vertebral rotation, if a scoliosis is present

Treatment

The treatment of an abnormal kyphosis is dependent on the cause. The goal of the treatment is prevention of an irreversible postural deformity. A hyperkyphosis is often progressive until growth stops and then continues to increase even after that. In many instances, after growing has stopped, a fixed abnormal posture causes neck and/or back complaints. During the growing period, an abnormal kyphosis rarely causes discomfort; if this is the case, the complaints are almost always temporary. Thus pain should never be the criterion for the necessity of treatment.

Until growing has stopped, every patient with a round back, a hollow-round back, or a

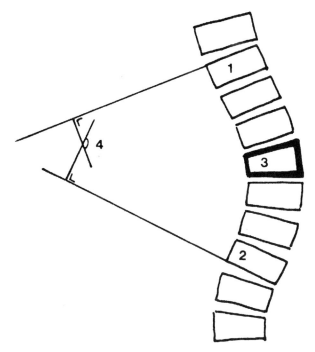

Figure 5–31 The measurement of kyphosis on a lateral X-ray film. *1*, Cranial end vertebra; *2*, caudal end vertebra; *3,* apex vertebra; *4,* kyphosis angle.

flat back should be followed on a regular basis. Before entry into puberty (the adolescent "growth spurt"), seeing the patient every 8 to 12 months is sufficient; afterward checking the patient every 6 months is necessary. Radiological control is performed only when the measurements indicate a reason for it.

Surgery. Indications for a surgical correction are usually determined by the angle of the kyphosis. In a normal spine, the thoracic kyphosis in standing measures approximately 30°, the lumbar lordosis to the upper border of the sacrum is approximately 40°, and the lumbosacral junction is almost straight. Deviations of 10° more or 10° less fall within the norm. In a round or hollow-round back, if the angle of kyphosis in standing is more than 50°, or if in a flat back the thoracic kyphosis amounts to less than 10°, operative treatment is indicated. In the flat back, the severity of the lumbar spine kyphosis is the decisive factor. In addition, the amount of progression,

the growth reserve (see Scoliosis), and the rigidity of the affected part of the spine are significant. In borderline cases, these can be the determining factors in selecting treatment: surgery versus bracing.

Congenital hyperkyphotic curves are the most frequent indication for surgical correction. In this instance, a posterior spondylosyndesis (fusion) is performed as early as possible. If the operation is performed too late, much more extensive surgery is required.

Also, in disorders that are coupled with paralysis, or in tumors, inflammations, and fractures, surgery is generally indicated. After growth is complete, if a severe kyphosis causes chronic back pain that does not respond to conservative treatment, surgery also should be considered.

Bracing. Treatment by means of bracing can be used only during the growth period. There has to be at least 1 year of growth reserve (see Scoliosis) still available. Treatment through bracing is utilized much more often than surgical correction.

The brace extends the spine, taking the load off the ventral aspect of the vertebral column. As a result, the vertebral bodies develop more quickly on their ventral sides and the spinal column continues to grow in the normal form (as long as this position is maintained for many months). Because the spinal column grows 24 hours per day, it is extremely important that the brace be worn both day and night.

In principle there are two kinds of braces: a passive brace and a passive-active brace. The passive brace (plaster brace) is rarely used because the vertebral column tends to stiffen while the thorax remains rather small. Another disadvantage is that the passive brace cannot be removed for daily hygiene.

In the passive-active brace, there are only a few contact points with the trunk, which allows for freedom of movement and development. Patients have the tendency to move away from the upholstered contact points of the brace and in so doing actively correct themselves. In addition, an intensive, but simple, exercise program is provided. For instance, the patient should participate in the customary school physical education program while wearing the brace. However, performing gymnastics on various apparatuses as well as jumping exercises should be avoided because of the great risk of accidents. The brace can be taken off for approximately 1 hour per day in conjunction with washing, bathing, or swimming. The brace is also taken off for part of the time during the daily exercise program.

Currently three different types of braces are being utilized: the Milwaukee brace, the Bähler brace, and the Boston brace. The type of brace worn is determined by the form of the back (and the orthopaedist's experience with the type of brace). Thus, the Bähler brace is usually used in mild cases of rounded back and in mild cases of flat back; the Milwaukee

brace is mainly suitable for the hollow-round back and is also applied in severe round and flat backs. The Boston brace is also employed for correction of hollow-round backs. Moreover, research is being conducted in several places to improve the quality of the types of braces now in use.

In treating with braces, the following phases are differentiated:

- a period of increasing the kyphosis correction, during which the brace is frequently adjusted
- a period in which the settings of the brace remain the same and in such a way that, if at all possible, the vertebral column is slightly overcorrected; this overcorrection is recommended because during the weaning-off phase, an average relapse of 6° occurs
- a period of weaning off the brace

Generally the brace has to be worn between 1½ and 2 years. Exactly when to begin weaning off the brace is determined by X-ray. The intervertebral spaces should no longer be wedge shaped, and radiologically there should be no difference in posture with or without the brace. The patient is weaned off the brace slowly in order to prevent relative overload of the back and loss of the correction. Usually the wearing time of the brace is reduced by 1 hour every 2 weeks. After about 6 months, the brace is only worn at night. For the next 3 months, the patient continues to wear the brace only at night.

Exercise. A nonfixed kyphosis (usually a postural anomaly or a beginning Scheuermann's disease) generally can be very well treated with an intensive exercise program. A partly fixed (hypomobile) kyphosis cannot be corrected only through exercises. Therefore, it is absolutely necessary that an orthopaedist evaluate a patient's abnormal kyphosis. The treatment should also be determined by the orthopaedist rather than the family physician or a physical therapist. In instances where the kyphosis is completely fixed, exercise therapy should not be prescribed.

Exercise therapy offers the best results when performed rigorously. The patient should perform the program daily at home and should be seen regularly by the physical therapist. Initially, the therapist should see the patient three times per week, later gradually decreasing to one time per week, and finally one time per month. Of course, this can vary significantly between individuals; it also depends on how quickly the patient learns the exercises and how dedicated the patient is.

The exercise program should consist of five different exercises at the most. The often-preached "multi-variational programs" tend to be confusing, and they lead to less efficient outcomes in comparison with a simple program consisting of a few exercises that have been scientifically proven to be effective.[8] The program includes stretching exercises for the pectoralis major and minor muscles, mobilizing exercises for the thoracic vertebral column (particularly to improve extension), and muscle-strengthening exercises for the thoracic spine extensors and the scapula adductors. In addition, special attention is given to correcting the posture in relation to all activities in the daily life of the patient.

Scheuermann's Disease

Next to the kyphotic postural abnormalities, Scheuermann's disease is the second most common cause of an abnormal thoracic kyphosis (hyperkyphosis). This disorder manifests itself during the pubescent years, generally at the age of 11. Scheuermann thought that the disease was based on an avascular necrosis of the "epiphyses" of the vertebral body. However, his supposition was not correct because the bony rings of the vertebral body do not contribute to the growth of the vertebral body. Therefore, Scheuermann's "epiphyses" could better be called the "apophyses."

The cartilage of the end-plates has, more or less, apparent openings into the collagenous fiber system. In Scheuermann's disease, the end-plates in these zones are pushed against the vertebral body due to pressure from the intervertebral discs. The end-plate can crack, thus making it possible for disc material to bulge into the vertebral body (Schmorl's nodules) (Figure 5–9). These bulges are pathognomonic for Scheuermann's disease.

In today's literature, there is still much discussion as to the exact cause of Scheuermann's disease. For instance, Bradford et al[9] consider the weak areas in the vertebral body to be due to a form of juvenile osteoporosis.

Clinical Findings

- Clinically, in many cases the thoracic kyphosis is conspicuous (Figure 5–32).
- In the local segmental functional examination, the movement in extension is limited. Often, especially in the early stages, the pectoralis major and minor muscles are found to be shortened.
- The diagnosis is determined on the basis of X-ray findings. The radiological examination demonstrates the following characteristic changes:
  1. Schmorl's nodules, possibly with sclerosis at the edges (bony reaction)
  2. irregular boundaries with indentations of the end-plates
  3. wedge-shaped deformation of the affected vertebrae and the end-plates
  4. increase of the anterior-posterior diameter of the affected vertebral body
  5. decrease of the corresponding intervertebral discs, as well as the intervertebral spaces
- Only a very small number of all the patients with radiologically confirmed Scheuermann's disease have notable symptoms. However, especially in young

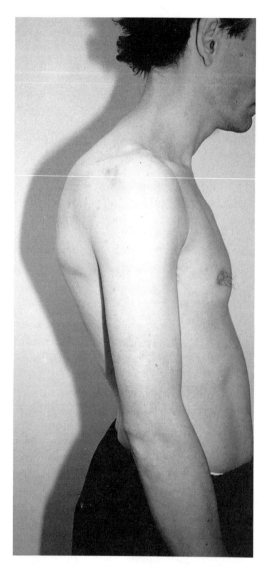

Figure 5–32 Patient with an increased kyphosis due to Scheuermann's disease.

athletes, Scheuermann's disease can lead to significant symptoms.[10]

Treatment

If the patient has no complaints, treatment is initiated only in the presence of an obvious hyperkyphosis. In this instance, it is extremely important to start the exercise program as quickly as possible. Chances are great that the thoracic kyphosis will stiffen if an exercise program is not prescribed in time.

Treatment consists of stretching the pectoralis major and minor muscles, cautious mobilization of the thoracic spine, and muscle-strengthening exercises for the thoracic spine extensors and the scapula adductors. In addition, instruction in proper posture, specifically related to various daily activities, is given.

Sports activities in which prolonged or frequent kyphosing is involved, such as hockey and rowing, as well as "fighting" sports such as judo and wresting, should be avoided. By contrast, swimming (breast stroke, crawl) should be encouraged; swimming requires constant "anti-kyphosing" activity, at least if it is performed in the correct manner.

In some cases, depending on the progression and severity of the kyphosis, treatment with a brace and sometimes even surgical treatment are indicated.

Scoliosis

A scoliosis is a curvature of the spinal column in the frontal plane. Almost everyone has a slight scoliosis of no clinical significance. Differentiation is made between *structural* and *functional* scoliosis.

Functional scoliosis is generally due to a postural deviation and is reversible. Structural scoliosis is irreversible. There are almost always changes in the forms of the vertebrae, along with deformation of the ribs in the thoracic region. (One should also keep in mind that some grotesquely scoliotic patients are often best treated by psychotherapy; they may have hysterical scoliosis.)

A functional scoliosis can arise from an antalgic lateral shift of the vertebral column, such as when a lumbar nerve root is compressed. Usually this occurs as the result of a disc protrusion or prolapse, and in rare cases it is due to a tumor or inflammation.

A structural scoliosis is always coupled with a rotation of the vertebrae. The vertebral bodies rotate toward the convexity. In most cases, a torsion of one part, or of several parts, of the vertebral column is noted without an accompanying pelvic obliquity. If a pelvic obliquity is observed, it is often due to a difference in the leg length. In addition, a flexion contracture of the hip or knee, as well as an adducted or abducted position of one or both hips, can also cause an obliquity of the pelvis. Nonetheless, in diagnosing a scoliosis, palpation to determine the presence of a pelvic obliquity or asymmetry remains important: the height of both anterior superior iliac spines and both posterior superior iliac spines is compared.

Because of the rotation in the thoracic spine, which always occurs in a structural scoliosis, the ribs are also "taken along" in this rotation and deformed. Thus, on the convex side of the scoliotic curve, a hump from the ribs occurs. Gravity continuously forces the scoliosis to be more lateral. The pressure constantly increases on the concave side and constantly decreases on the convex side. During growth the vertebrae take on an even more wedged shape. In general the trunk musculature has the same effect as gravity, further reinforcing the process. With the increasing curvature, the thorax becomes increasingly more deformed.

Respiration also intensifies the rotation. Because the ribs rotate along with the vertebrae, the ribs on the convex side are found more at the back and on the concave aspect they are found more at the side. During inhalation, the chest cavity pushes outward and forces the ribs on the concave side forward, while the ribs on the convex side are forced backward. In addition, the force of the intercostal musculature is transferred via the ribs onto the vertebrae as fixed points. Owing to the deformation already present, on the concave side this force goes beyond the transverse processes acting upon the vertebral body; on the convex side the force acts upon the transverse processes. This too results in a further rotation of the vertebrae.

During growth, the concave side of the scoliosis comes under more and more pressure, while the convex side experiences less pressure. Because of this, the concave side gradually has more bone growth, whereby minimal compensation of the curvature occurs. The actual compensation occurs through additional curves above and below the main curve. Through these secondary curves, the ultimate posture remains erect: the body still stands "in line."

The secondary curves are initially functional, but as the patient grows older, they become structurally fixed as well. Furthermore, in some cases of severe progression an originally secondary curve can become a second primary curve. Even a nonoptimally compensated curve will end up again with the spine in a vertical course. In this way the simplest form of scoliosis arises, the so-called C-scoliosis, consisting of one primary and two secondary curves. The more often occurring completely compensated scoliosis consists of two primary and two partial curves. (In most cases, this concerns one initial primary curve with three accessory curves.) In rare cases, a scoliosis consists of two equally strong primary curves, a so-called double curve.

The primary curve can be differentiated from the compensatory curves by the greater degree of curvature, the more pronounced vertebral deformation and rotation, and the greater rigidity. However, one has to take into account that the rigidity is determined by the localization; thus, for instance, a scoliosis in the thoracic spine is always much more rigid than in the lumbar spine.

With an eye on early diagnosis of scoliosis, extensive investigations have been performed in schools. In the literature, the percentages of children with scoliosis varies from 2% to 15% of all schoolchildren. This large difference in percentages can be explained in the fact that some examiners recorded even the slightest asymmetry as a scoliosis, while others included only the curves of 10° or more. Girls tend to have a scoliosis more often than boys. Of all the children with a scoliosis, only 2 to 4 per 1000 ultimately are treated.

As children get older, the chance of a scoliosis increases. The chance that a scoliosis will be progressive increases if it amounts to 20° before the age of 7 or amounts to 30° before puberty. Thoracolumbar and double scolioses are more often progressive than the localized thoracic or lumbar scolioses. In most cases, when growing stops, the progression of the scoliosis also stops. However, some scolioses continue to increase even after the cessation of growth. Pregnancy can also have an unfavorable influence.

The progression of a scoliosis in children also depends on the cause of the scoliosis.

Causes of Scoliosis

There are several causes for structural scoliosis.

- *Osteogenic Scoliosis.* Osteogenic scoliosis is the result of an intrathoracic process or of a specific bone disease. It can also be congenital, for instance, in the presence of a wedge vertebra.
- *Neurogenic Scoliosis.* Neurogenic scoliosis can be congenital, but it is usually the result of poliomyelitis or another acquired nerve disorder.
- *Myogenic Scoliosis.* Myogenic scoliosis can be congenital or the result of a muscular dystrophy or other muscle disease.
- *Idiopathic Scoliosis.* The largest group of the structural scolioses is "idiopathic." Generally in an idiopathic scoliosis, the higher the primary curve is localized, the more progressive it is. Of course, the earlier a scoliosis appears, the longer the remaining amount of growth. The age groups can be divided as follows:

- infantile scolioses (0 to 3 years)
- juvenile scolioses (4 to 9 years)
- adolescent scolioses (10 years until growing stops)

Adolescent scolioses have a better prognosis than the juvenile or infantile scolioses, despite the fact that the greatest period of growth occurs during puberty. In general, the idiopathic scolioses in the adolescent age group increase by 1° per month, while in the remaining groups the progression amounts to 5° per year. Ultimately an idiopathic scoliosis, if untreated, can cause severe deformity of the vertebral column.

Clinical Findings

- The functional examination usually gives little information.
- Through the inspection, the examiner establishes the presence of a lumbar, a thoracolumbar, a thoracic, or a C-scoliosis (Figure 5–35).
- The radiological examination is very important; by using the Cobb[8] method, the scoliosis can be accurately measured (Figures 5–33 and 5–34).

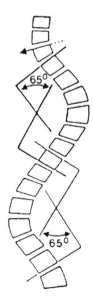

Figure 5–33 Measuring a scoliosis on an X-ray, according to Cobb.[8]

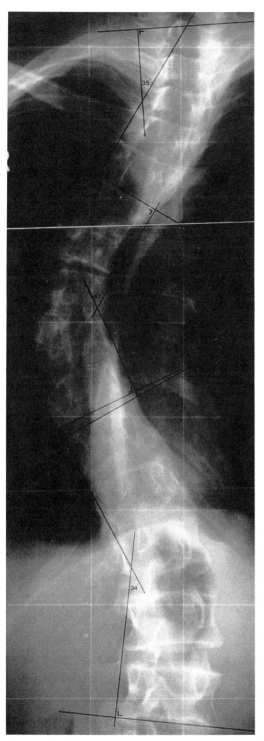

Figure 5–34 Anterior-posterior conventional X-ray of the entire spinal column with angles measured at various levels.[8]

Consequences of an Idiopathic Scoliosis

- *Back Pain.* Although back pain occurs in scoliotic patients, statistically it is not present more often than it is in patients without a scoliosis.
- *Diminished Lung Function.* In people with an idiopathic scoliosis, the vital capacity is significantly reduced. With severe curves, the diminished lung function itself can lead to severe heart problems and ultimately to death.

Treatment

Lately there has been much discussion about the appropriate treatment of an idiopathic scoliosis.[11] These debates mostly take place in the area of physical therapy. It is assumed that, in many instances, a scoliosis can be very favorably influenced through exercise treatment. It is certainly a fact that by visual inspection the scoliosis sometimes appears to have improved; however, radiological evidence shows that usually the torsion of the vertebral body actually increases. At present, this discussion has ceased, and there now remains only the choice of whether to treat by bracing or surgery. Exercise treatment is still considered very important, but only as supportive therapy.

In treatment with a brace, both the Boston and the Milwaukee braces are used. Generally, a brace should be worn until growth has stopped. Weaning off the brace takes place first during the day and must progress very gradually over a period of several months. The brace still has to be worn at night for at least 1 year. During the growth spurt in puberty, wearing the brace is crucial. In every case, during this period, the brace should be worn 23 hours per day.

An indication for treatment with a brace is a progressive scoliosis with a curve of at least 15°. If the scoliosis initially is diagnosed in children over 10 years of age and the curve amounts to 20°, treatment with a brace is indicated, even without the demonstration of progression.

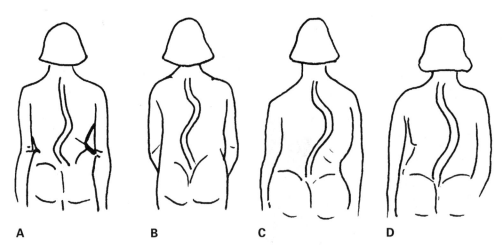

A   **B**   **C**   **D**

Figure 5–35 Various types of scolioses. **A**, Lumbar scoliosis; **B**, thoracolumbar scoliosis; **C**, thoracic scoliosis; **D**, C-scoliosis, according to Henke.[8]

It is extremely important that the treatment with bracing is very carefully applied. Parents and children should ensure that the cushioned contact points are always correctly located and that the brace always closes well. Curves of 40° or more are not suitable for treatment through bracing. In these cases, surgical treatment is indicated.

Another determining factor for the treatment is the expected growth reserve. This is determined by radiologically visible "Risser signs." The apophysis of the iliac crests ossify during the pubescent growth spurt from ventral to dorsal and ultimately merge with the pelvis from dorsal to ventral. This ossification is divided into five stages (Figure 5–36). Another, even more precise, method in predicting the end of the growth of the vertebral column is the radiological record of the fusion of the vertebral body apophyses with the vertebral body. The apophyses ossify between the ages of 7 and 12, and then begin to merge with the vertebral body at age 14 or 15.

OTHER DISORDERS

The fact that the pathology discussed under Other Disorders does not fall under the categories of primary disc-related disorders, secondary disc-related disorders, traumatic

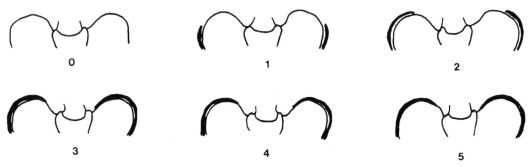

0   1   2

3   4   5

Figure 5–36 The Risser stages. The ossification stages are represented in increasing numbers: the higher the figure, the lower the remaining growth reserve, according to Henke.[8]

lesions, and postural deviations of the vertebral column does not imply that these disorders are less important. In a number of cases, there is a partial overlap with the earlier types of pathology.

Forestier's Disease

Forestier's disease is also known as "ankylosing hyperostosis" or "diffuse idiopathic skeletal hyperostosis (DISH)." (See also Chapter 11, Imaging Techniques, and Figure 11–14.) This disorder is characterized by a diffuse calcification or ossification of the anterior longitudinal ligament. Large osteophytes form at the anterior aspect of the vertebral bodies, which can fuse together. The disease progresses very slowly. The first symptoms can be manifested at the age of 40. However, at this age making a diagnosis is very difficult because the classic radiological findings usually are not clearly present until over the age of 60. The disease affects men twice as often as women.

The cause of this disorder is unknown. Some patients suffer from a manifest or latent form of diabetes mellitus (17% to 50%).[12]

Clinical Findings

- Often the patients are athletic and in the middle-aged group; they complain of stiffness and moderate pain, particularly in the morning and in the evening, as well as after prolonged sitting. The stiffness is localized especially in the thoracic spine, and to a lesser degree in the thoracolumbar junction or lumbar spine. There is no pain at night, and the pain does not radiate.
- The symptoms are also dependent on the weather. In wet and cold weather, the symptoms increase; they decrease during sports activities, in warm weather, and with the application of local heat modalities.
- Many patients regularly take aspirin to decrease their symptoms.

- In 10% to 20% of patients, dysphagia (swallowing disturbance) is the most significant complaint. The dysphagia is caused by cervical osteophytes (particularly from the vertebral bodies of C3 and C4) at the level of the cricoid.[12] On swallowing films of the esophagus, the indentations from the osteophytes are seen (Figure 5–37).
- Many patients also have complaints other than of a spinal origin. Mostly they concern the symptoms in tendons and joints, particularly in the elbow. Heel pain is also a frequent symptom, leading one to suspect an Achilles insertion tendopathy. However, the functional examination of the painful joints and tendons is negative.
- The lumbar lordosis is practically straight, whereas the thoracic kyphosis is slightly increased. In approximately half of the patients, the active and passive motions of the spinal column are not limited. The remainder of the patients experience a decreased sidebend first, then diminished rotation, and finally decreased flexion/extension.
- Radiologically, Forestier's disease is differentiated from spondylitis deformans (rheumatoid spondylitis), disc degeneration, and ankylosing spondylitis based not only on positive findings but also on negative findings. Findings characteristic of Forestier's disease include calcium deposits and abnormal bony formation along the ventrolateral side of at least four adjacent vertebral bodies, with or without button-shaped protrusions at the level of the intervertebral disc. In regard to the negative findings, there should be no significant narrowing of the intervertebral discs, phenomena of degenerative disc aberrations must be absent, and there must be no signs of ankylosing of the intervertebral joints, or of erosion, sclerosis, or fusion of the sacroiliac joints.

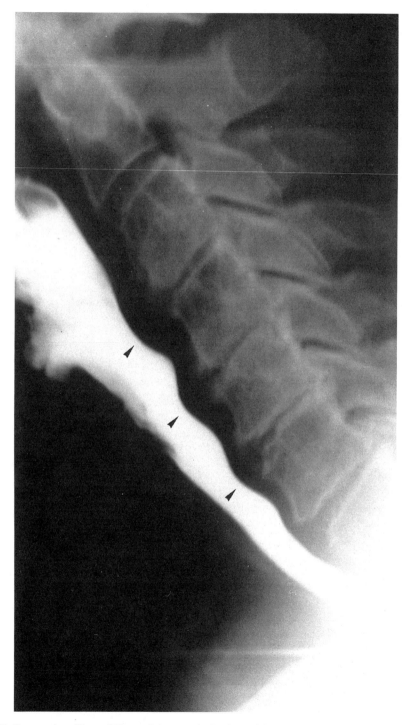

Figure 5–37 Conventional lateral X-ray of the cervical spine with contrast medium in the esophagus in a 73-year-old patient with difficulty swallowing and a severe form of Forestier's disease in the thoracic spine. At the level of the ventral osteophytes of the cervical vertebrae (*arrowheads*), there are obvious indentations in the esophagus.

Treatment

Because the etiology of this disorder is unknown, causal treatment is impossible. The disease does not lead to disability, and the prognosis is good. The treatment is aimed at decreasing the symptoms. If necessary, aspirin is prescribed. All kinds of modalities related to warmth and heat can be utilized; in general, a warm climate quickly diminishes the symptoms.

Costoiliac Compression Syndrome

The costoiliac compression syndrome is a complication in patients with osteoporosis or, in rare cases, in patients with generalized severe disc degeneration. The distance from the lowest rib and the iliac crest is decreased in such a way that a mechanical irritation between the two bony structures occurs. This disorder is seen most often in women.

Clinical Findings

- The patient complains of pain in the back and/or in the side, in the area of the twelfth rib. The pain can be either constant or intermittent. The pain increases during sitting, particularly on a low chair, during trunk rotation, and during walking.
- In the functional examination, sidebend to the affected side is the most painful motion. On palpation during this motion, compression between the twelfth rib and the iliac crest is noted.

Treatment

Conservative treatment, at its best, offers only temporary relief of the pain. The only effective measure is surgical resection of the twelfth rib.

Manubriosternal Joint Monoarthritis

The manubriosternal joint is an amphiarthrosis between the manubrium and the body of the sternum, with fibrocartilaginous tissue between the bony structures. A part of the fibrocartilaginous tissue develops a synovial joint space, making the joint a possible location for the occurrence of an arthritis. (A similar situation is present in the pubic symphysis.) In the joint, movement occurs during respiration, particularly during deep inhalation.

The manubriosternal joint is frequently affected in rheumatoid arthritis, spondylitis ankylopoietica, psoriatic arthritis, and Reiter's disease.

A monoarthritis can also occur without obvious etiology. This disorder is seen more frequently in women than in men. The patients are usually between 20 and 45 years of age.

In considering the differential diagnosis, angina pectoris should be ruled out.

Clinical Findings

- The patient complains of constant local pain, which increases with coughing, sneezing, straining, and exertion (sport). Sometimes this pain radiates intermittently to the shoulders or to the left shoulder and arm.
- There is local swelling and tenderness. The functional examination demonstrates an increase in pain with every movement and in taking a deep breath.
- Blood tests should be performed in order to differentiate from the earlier-mentioned systemic diseases.
- The radiological examination confirms the diagnosis. In particular, the lateral view indicates the pathological changes of the manubriosternal joint. In addition, radiologically this disorder can be differentiated from other arthritides, tumors, and Paget's disease.

Treatment

Most patients react very well to a local injection of 1 to 2 mL of a corticosteroid.

Tietze Syndrome

Tietze syndrome is characterized by a painful swelling of the costosternal cartilage of sometimes the first, usually the second, and less often the third rib. The disorder occurs more often on the left side than on the right side. The pathogenesis is unknown. Also, the pathology itself is unclear. Electron microscopic examination and radiological examination have not been able to demonstrate any specific changes.

Clinical Findings

- The patient complains of either an acute or a gradual onset of pain in the affected region, which increases with deep respiration, coughing, and sneezing. Sometimes the pain radiates to the shoulder.
- Local palpation is painful, and in most cases there is obvious swelling.

Treatment

This disorder is self-limiting, but it can last for a period that varies from weeks to years. In some cases, the pain is so severe that treatment is necessary. An injection of corticosteroid into the painful swelling may be helpful.

It is significant to note that the shortest ribs, which have a connection with the body of the sternum, are always involved. This gives rise to the possibility that Tietze syndrome might be caused by a dysfunction of the corresponding segments of the upper thoracic spine. Thus, the anterior localization of the pain is a manifestation of a dysfunction of the junction of the vertical and horizontal kinetic chains, vertical being the spinal column and horizontal being the ribs and their connections. With this in mind, patients may also benefit from mobilization of these thoracic segments and the vertebral-rib connections.

Lesion of the Pectoralis Major

Although the pectoralis major is important mainly for movement of the shoulder, the rare strain of the muscle belly and the even more rare partial tear or total rupture are discussed here because the pain is usually experienced in the thorax. This lesion is almost always the result of a sports injury, usually in gymnasts, pole vaulters, swimmers, and athletes participating in the various fighting sports.

Clinical Findings

- The pain is experienced in the craniolateral aspect of the ventral side of the thorax, just caudal to the clavicle, and can radiate to the medial aspect of the upper arm to the elbow.
- In the functional examination, passive elevation of the arm with overpressure in a dorsal direction is painful. This test is also positive in lesions of the latissimus dorsi and of the tendon of the long head of the biceps brachii. Differentiating from a lesion of the latissimus dorsi is accomplished through palpation; differentiating from a lesion of the biceps is determined by means of the functional examination of the shoulder (particularly the resisted tests and the biceps stretch test).
- Resisted adduction of the shoulder is painful, and resisted shoulder internal rotation is seldom positive. Resisting the combined movements of adduction and internal rotation is usually the most painful test. Another test that clearly provokes the symptoms is pushing the hands together with the arms positioned horizontally in front of the body.
- Lesions of this muscle generally are localized just caudal to the clavicle, or in the most caudolateral part of the muscle close to the ribs.
- A partial tear or total rupture generally occurs at the level of its insertion on the humerus. In this case, the patient has severe acute local pain and is almost unable to give resistance against adduction and internal rotation because of the pain.

Very often, shortening of the pectoralis major muscles is noted without symptoms being caused by the muscle itself. This shortening can be the result of a hyperkyphosis such as in Scheuermann's disease. It is also possible for this shortening to lead to symptoms from other structures, such as in a thoracic outlet compression syndrome.

Treatment

Treatment consists of transverse friction massage or, in very acute cases, an injection of a local anesthetic. After the transverse friction, the muscle also should be stretched cautiously.

Stretching exercises, performed several times throughout the day, are indicated in patients with muscle shortening due to a hyperkyphosis or thoracic outlet compression syndrome.

Insertion Tendopathy of the Pectoralis Minor

The insertion tendopathy of the pectoralis minor muscle is a rare lesion, which is almost exclusively seen in javelin throwers. However, shortening of the pectoralis muscles is frequently seen as the result of a hyperkyphosis. A similar shortening can be one of the causes of a thoracic outlet compression syndrome.

Clinical Findings

- The patient complains of local pain during throwing. The pain is never so severe that the patient has to stop the sports activity completely.
- The basic functional examination of the shoulder is almost always negative. In many instances, the so-called throwing test is positive. Protraction of the shoulder against resistance is sometimes positive only after provocation (performing the throwing activity several times before being examined).
- There is always local tenderness on the medial caudal aspect of the coracoid process.

Treatment

Treatment consists of transverse friction massage and stretching.

Strain of the Latissimus Dorsi

As in lesions of the pectoralis major and pectoralis minor, lesions of the latissimus dorsi are almost always the result of a sports injury, usually in gymnasts, ballet dancers, and participants in the fighting sports.

Clinical Findings

- The patient usually has local pain.
- Resisting the combined motion of adduction and internal rotation of the shoulder is especially painful. The examiner differentiates lesions of the pectoralis major from lesions of the teres major by palpation; however, the latter is almost never seen.
- The most frequent localization of the lesion is just ventrolateral to the scapula.

Treatment

Treatment with transverse friction massage and stretching exercises is very effective.

Lesions of the Abdominal Muscles

Patient history is very important in helping to differentiate among a problem with the internal organs, a lesion of the abdominal muscles, and a pathology in the sacroiliac joint and/or pubic symphysis. One expects to find lesions of these muscles only in athletes or after abdominal surgery—particularly after surgery for an inguinal hernia. Lesions of the rectus abdominis are seen more frequently than lesions of the oblique abdominal muscles.

Clinical Findings

- The patient complains of local pain.
- If the rectus abdominis is affected, raising both straight legs against resistance is particularly painful. If pain is experienced in the groin, the first consideration is a lesion of the iliopsoas. Differentiation can be made by performing the

basic functional examination of the hip; resisting the combined motion of flexion and external rotation of the hip is particularly painful in instances of an iliopsoas lesion.

- If one of the oblique abdominal muscles is affected, in most cases resisted trunk rotation is painful. The external oblique abdominal muscle allows contralateral trunk rotation, and the internal oblique muscle allows ipsilateral trunk rotation.

- In adolescents between the ages of 14 and 16, painful resisted trunk rotation usually indicates an avulsion fracture of the iliac crest.

- The rectus abdominis muscle is most often affected just above the navel, or just above the pubic symphysis. In the former instance, trunk extension performed simultaneously with arm elevation is very painful.

- Lesions of the oblique abdominal muscles are usually located close to the iliac crest. If the pain is located on the right side, the examiner should rule out the possibility of chronic appendicitis. One possibility for making this differentiation is to have the patient maximally contract the abdominal muscles on the right side and then palpate again for the most painful spot. If the patient still experiences obvious pain, a lesion of the abdominal muscle is indicated, because the internal organs are no longer palpable due to the contraction of the muscles. The patient then relaxes the muscles, and the palpation is repeated with the same pressure. If the pain was less during the previous palpation, but is now very obvious, the lesion probably lies within the abdomen.

Pain located below the navel almost always occurs in combination with a lesion of the hip adductors and the pubic symphysis (pubalgia).

Treatment

Transverse friction massage and, as soon as the functional examination is negative, muscle-strengthening exercises usually result in pain relief. In instances of an avulsion fracture of the iliac crest, the patient should rest for a few weeks. In other words, all activity of the oblique abdominal muscles should be avoided.

Herpes Zoster

Herpes zoster is a viral disorder of the dorsal ganglion of one or more nerve roots. As a result, pain and skin eruptions develop in one or more dermatomes. Especially in the acute phase, the pain can be very intense.

In most cases the disorder is self-limited and does not last longer than 2 to 3 weeks. However, especially in older patients, the pain can sometimes last much longer. This situation is called a postherpetic neuralgia.

Herpes zoster can occur at any level of the entire spinal column; however, it is most often localized in the thoracic region. The disorder is not dependent on age; however, it is seen less often in children than in adults, and is seen much more often in persons over 70 years of age.

According to deMorages and Kierland,[13] the incidence varies from 0.7 case per 1000 people per year in children younger than 10 years to 10.1 cases per 1000 per year in people older than 70 years. In the group over 70 years of age, the chance of a postherpetic neuralgia is 35% to 50%.

Clinical Findings

- The patient complains of often severe pain in one or more dermatomes.

- On inspection, the characteristic skin eruptions are present.

- The functional examination is negative.

Treatment

In almost all cases, an epidural administration of 1 mL of triamcinolone acetonide

(40 mg/mL) offers quick relief of pain. The epidural injection is given one segment cranial to the affected segment. The effect is probably based on the disappearance of the perineural edema, stopping the destruction of the nerve roots.

A modern concept of treatment is the administration of an oral virustatic (acyclovir). This relieves not only the pain, but the skin eruptions as well. In addition, the postherpetic pain decreases considerably.

Refer to Appendix C for condensed diagrams on Differential Diagnosis of Thoracic Spine Pathology.

5.4 TREATMENT

INTRODUCTION

Treatment (in terms of manual therapy) for symptoms in the thoracic region is initiated only on the condition that the complaints could be provoked during the functional examination of the thoracic spine or ribs. If it is not possible to reproduce the patient's symptoms during the functional examination, the patient is asked to provoke the symptoms, for instance, by performing the exercise or maneuver or by assuming the particular position that usually brings on the complaints. In instances when a similar provocation cannot be performed in the examining room, the functional examination is repeated during the patient's next visit. If it remains impossible to provoke the patient's symptoms, treatment should not be initiated until a clear diagnosis has been made. It may still be possible that there is pathology of the internal organs or that the patient has herpes zoster.

If the symptoms occur only during prolonged sitting in a kyphotic posture, the treatment is aimed primarily at improving the patient's posture and, if necessary, improving the patient's working environment.

If articular and/or dural signs are present, the lesion is very likely primary disc related. In this instance, the treatment should begin with soft tissue techniques in preparation for mobilization. The techniques appropriate for these lesions are *always* performed *in combination with axial separation*. This is very important because mobilization techniques without traction can increase a disc protrusion. In the thoracic spine, this can be extremely dangerous because of the relatively small diameter of the spinal canal whereby a disc protrusion or prolapse can quickly result in compression of the spinal cord.

In performing the rotation mobilization techniques, first the nonpainful or least painful rotation is mobilized before mobilizing in the more or most painful direction. If treatment is applied in the opposite order, the symptoms often increase. These are empirical findings for which there is currently no explanation.

Instruction in proper posture is almost always necessary, along with accompanying postural exercises. The patient should be thoroughly informed as to the rationale of the exercises. If necessary, ergonomic advice is also given.

In the functional examination, if the combined movements are painful (or in cases when they are more painful than the coupled motions), pathology of the zygapophyseal joints is suspected. In these instances, the mobilization techniques are also performed in combination with axial separation because these techniques also have a favorable influence on zygapophyseal joint dysfunction.

If the clinician is certain that the patient has a zygapophyseal joint problem and the general techniques with axial separation do not result in improvement, then, based on findings from the segmental functional examination, local segmental techniques can be performed.

In zygapophyseal joint dysfunction, treatment with the local segmental techniques usually progresses from techniques that emphasize traction, to techniques that emphasize rotation, and finally to techniques that emphasize extension. After the mobilization, it is very important to maintain mobility by means of simple exercises; this prevents recurrence.

Despite treatment with axial separation techniques and the local segmental techniques, if there still is no or insufficient improvement, and if there is reason from the history to believe that there may be a dysfunction of the ribs, a specific examination of the ribs is performed. If this examination is positive, the treatment is directed appropriately. After improvement, simple exercises are again given to maintain the increased mobility.

As already mentioned in the sections regarding examination and pathology, muscle lesions in the thoracic region can also be the cause of the symptoms. These lesions are found much more frequently in the thoracic region than in the cervical and lumbar spine regions. In these instances, transverse friction, stretching, and/or muscle-strengthening exercises are usually indicated. Refer to Appendix A for condensed diagrams on Treatment in Disorders of the Thoracic Spine.

SOFT TISSUE TECHNIQUES

Transverse Friction of the Rotatory Muscles (Figure 5–38)

In the thoracic region, local transverse friction of the vertebral and paravertebral musculature can be applied as a method of pain relief. Although the resisted motions rarely cause pain in the thoracic spine, in many cases transverse friction can relieve local pain temporarily, after which mobilizations can be performed. Generally, in the thoracic spine the rotatory muscles can cause local tenderness. They run in a direction from craniomedial to caudolateral.

Position of the Patient

The patient lies prone with the arms resting alongside the body and the head in a neutral position. Depending on the amount of the patient's thoracic kyphosis, the head of the table can be lowered slightly or a firm pillow can be placed underneath the trunk. (This ensures a neutral position of the thoracic spine and prevents too much lordosis in the cervical spine.)

Position of the Therapist

The therapist stands next to the patient at the level of the thoracic spine.

Performance

The friction is best performed with the thumbs. The direction of the transverse friction is transverse to the running of the muscle fibers, thus from caudomedial to craniolateral.

Transverse Stretching of the Erector Spinae (Figure 5–39)

Position of the Patient

The patient lies prone with the arms resting alongside the body and the head in a neutral position. Depending on the amount of the patient's thoracic kyphosis, the head of the table can be lowered slightly or a firm pillow can be placed underneath the trunk. (This

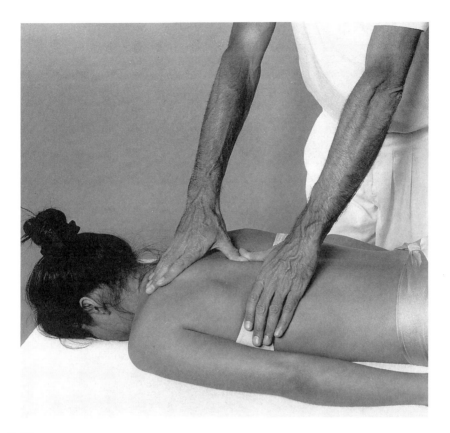

Figure 5–38

ensures a neutral position of the thoracic spine and prevents too much lordosis in the cervical spine.)

Position of the Therapist

The therapist stands next to the patient at the level of the thoracic spine.

Performance

The technique can be performed using the thumb, the heel of the hand, the thenar eminence, or the thumb reinforced by the thenar eminence of the other hand. As illustrated, the thumb (reinforced by the thenar emi-

nence of the other hand) hooks against the erector spinae at the segment of the thoracic spine being treated. A transverse stretch is performed by pushing either away from (after hooking against the medial aspect of the erector spinae) or toward (after hooking against the lateral aspect of the erector spinae) the spinal column, without rubbing over the muscle.

This technique can be performed in a general manner or per segment. The transverse stretching is performed slowly and held for about 1 second at the end of each movement. The hands of the therapist then return to the

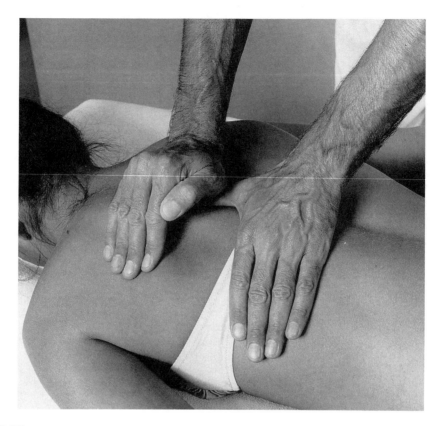

Figure 5–39

initial position, and the maneuver is repeated in a rhythmic manner for several minutes.

Besides having a pain-relieving effect, this technique is particularly useful in preparation for the following techniques, in which the erector spinae are treated with simultaneously performed movements.

Transverse Stretching of the Erector Spinae with Simultaneously Performed Sidebend of the Thoracic Spine (Figure 5–40)

Position of the Patient

The patient is positioned in sidelying close to the edge of the table, with the painful side up. A small pillow is placed under the patient's head, and the patient rests either with both hands placed between the pillow and the head or with both arms crossed in front of the body.

If the patient is very mobile and the therapist chooses to emphasize the stretch component of this technique, a small pillow can be placed under the patient's thorax, bringing the thoracic spine into slight sidebend.

When emphasizing movement, no pillow is placed under the thoracic spine. Instead, a small pillow or towel roll may be placed underneath the lumbar spine to ensure a neutral position of the spine.

Position of the Therapist

The therapist stands in front of the patient. The treatment table is positioned at the level of the therapist's greater trochanter.

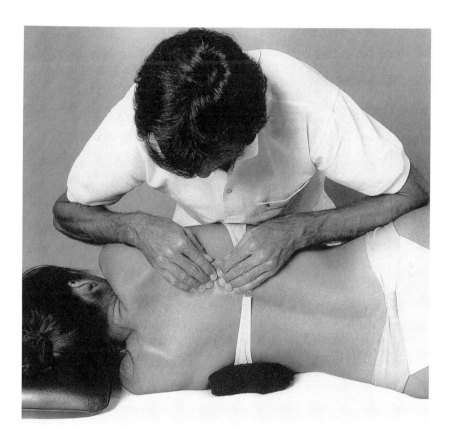

Figure 5–40

Performance

The therapist places the fingers of both hands at the medial side of the upper-lying erector spinae. The therapist's caudal arm rests on the lateral aspect of the patient's ribs and pelvis. The cranial arm lies against the lateral aspect of the cranial ribs and along the lateral border of the scapula. The prominence of the humeral head serves as a base of support. With the fingers, the therapist now pulls the erector spinae in a lateral direction. At the same time, the therapist's arms push the patient's pelvis caudal and the shoulder cranial.

This technique can be performed in a general manner or per segment. The transverse stretching is performed slowly and held for about 1 second at the end of each movement.

The patient is then returned to the initial position and the maneuver is repeated for several minutes in a rhythmic manner.

Both for pain relief and in preparation for mobilization, this technique can be performed on both sides. This technique is also beneficial in preparation for the following technique.

Transverse Stretching of the Erector Spinae with Simultaneously Performed Extension, Sidebend, and Coupled Rotation of the Thoracic Spine (Figure 5–41)

Position of the Patient

The patient is positioned in sidelying close to the edge of the table, with the painful side

[handwritten notes: pre position S.B ī Lt position] Flex pts arm to move scap, to get to mid-Th. higher Th. OR mid Th]

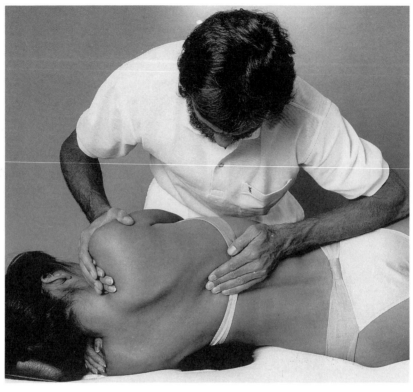

Rot.

Figure 5–41

up. A small pillow is placed under the patient's head and the patient rests either with both hands placed between the pillow and the head or with both arms crossed in front of the body.

If the patient is very mobile and the therapist chooses to emphasize the stretch component of this technique, a small pillow can be placed under the patient's thorax, bringing the thoracic spine into slight sidebend.

When emphasizing movement, no pillow is placed under the thoracic spine. Instead a small pillow or towel roll may be placed underneath the lumbar spine to ensure a neutral position of the spine.

Position of the Therapist

The therapist stands in front of the patient. The treatment table is positioned at the level of the therapist's greater trochanter.

Performance

With the fingers and with the entire ulnar side of the caudal hand, the therapist hooks the medial edge of the upper-lying erector spinae muscle. The other hand has contact with the ventrocranial aspect of the upper-lying side of the thorax. If the patient's arms are crossed in front of the trunk with the hands resting on the shoulders, the therapist can use the upper-lying hand as a point of support.

By pushing the upper-lying shoulder in a dorsal direction, the therapist brings the patient's thoracic spine into extension, sidebend, and coupled rotation. At the same time, the therapist's caudal hand attempts to bring the erector spinae in the opposite direction while the forearm stabilizes the rest of the patient's spine and pelvis.

This technique can be performed in a general manner or per segment, whereby the caudal hand moves segment by segment from cranial to caudal. The transverse stretching is performed slowly and held for about 1 second at the end of each movement. The patient is then returned to the initial position and the maneuver is repeated for several minutes in a rhythmic manner.

Transverse Stretching of the Erector Spinae with Simultaneously Performed Flexion, Sidebend, and Ipsilateral Rotation of the Thoracic Spine (Figure 5–42)

In the same manner as described for the previous technique, movement also can be performed in flexion in preparation for specific joint mobilization.

Position of the Patient

See previous technique.

Position of the Therapist

See previous technique.

Performance

With either the thumb or the thenar eminence of the caudal hand, the therapist pushes against the lateral edge of the upper-lying erector spinae. The other hand is placed on the craniodorsal aspect of the patient's upper-lying shoulder. The therapist's cranial hand moves the patient's trunk in a ventral direction, which results in flexion, sidebend,

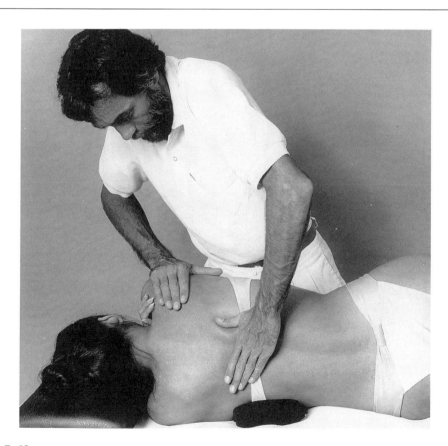

Figure 5–42

and ipsilateral rotation. At the same time, the other hand attempts to pull the erector spinae in the opposite direction.

This technique can be performed in a general manner or per segment, whereby the caudal hand moves segment by segment from cranial to caudal. The transverse stretching is performed slowly and held for about 1 second at the end of each movement. The patient is then returned to the initial position and the maneuver is repeated for several minutes in a rhythmic manner.

LOCAL SEGMENTAL PAIN-RELIEVING TECHNIQUES

Ventral Vibration and Oscillation
(Figure 5–43)

Position of the Patient

The patient lies prone with the arms resting alongside the body and the head in a neutral position. Depending on the amount of the patient's thoracic kyphosis, the head of the table can be lowered slightly or a firm pillow can be placed underneath the trunk. (This ensures a neutral position of the thoracic spine and prevents too much lordosis in the cervical spine.)

Position of the Therapist

The therapist stands next to the patient at the level of the thoracic spine.

Performance

The therapist places both thumbs, one on top of the other, on the spinous process of the

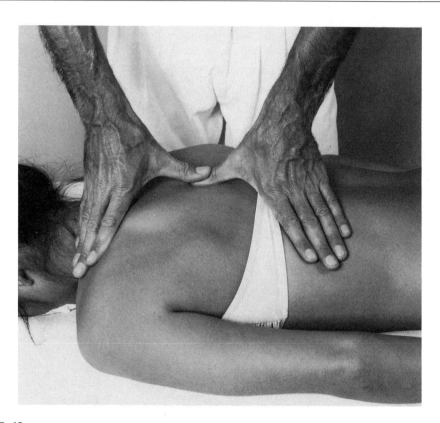

Figure 5–43

painful segment. By performing local manual vibration in a ventral direction, initially a diminishing of the local pain results. The therapist can then make a transition from local vibration to rhythmic movement (oscillation) so that, besides pain relief, very minimal mobilization also occurs. The vibration and oscillation can also be alternated.

In the same way, this technique can be applied to the transverse processes or to the ribs. In the latter case, dysfunction of the costotransverse joint is present.

Vibration and Rhythmic Movement in a Rotation Direction (Figure 5–44)

Position of the Patient

The patient lies prone with the arms resting alongside the body and the head in a neutral position. Depending on the amount of the patient's thoracic kyphosis, the head of the table can be lowered slightly or a firm pillow can be placed underneath the trunk. (This ensures a neutral position of the thoracic spine and prevents too much lordosis in the cervical spine.)

Position of the Therapist

The therapist stands at the head of the patient.

Performance

The therapist places one thumb against the lateral aspect of the caudal spinous process of the segment being treated. The other thumb rests against the opposite side of the cranial

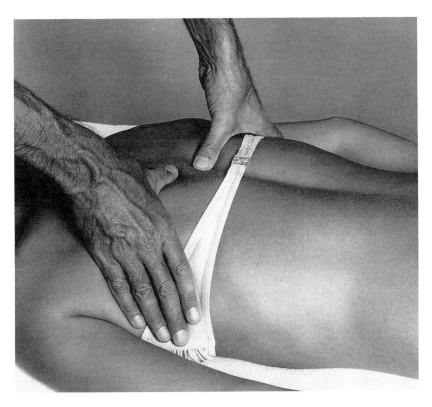

Figure 5–44

spinous process. When performing the technique, the caudal thumb fixes while the cranial thumb performs the rhythmic motion.

In contrast to the rotational mobilizations in which the first rotation is always *away* from the painful direction, in this technique the direction for treatment is *toward* the painful rotation. Also, here the therapist can begin with a manual vibration and then make a transition into rhythmic movements within the limits of pain. Afterward the vibration and oscillation can be alternated.

MOBILIZATION TECHNIQUES FOR THE THORACIC SPINE

The following techniques (both general and local) can be performed in various ways: They can be held for a period of time, from several seconds to several minutes (the patient continues to stomach-breathe). The techniques can also be performed as a manipulation: at the end of the patient's exhalation and immediately before the next inhalation, the therapist takes up the pre-tension and accentuates the movement in the appropriate direction. To emphasize pain relief, they can be performed in the form of vibrations and oscillations as well.

Segmental Separation in Sitting: General (Figures 5–45A–D)

Position of the Patient
(Figure 5–45A)

The patient sits as close to the edge of the table as possible, with the legs either straddling the width of the table (when sitting at the short end) or with the legs resting on the table (when sitting at the long end). The arms are crossed in front of the chest with the

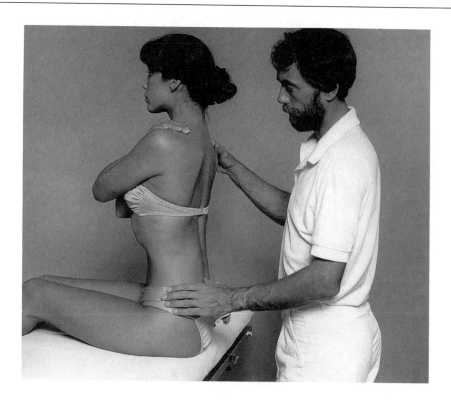

Figure 5–45A Position of the patient.

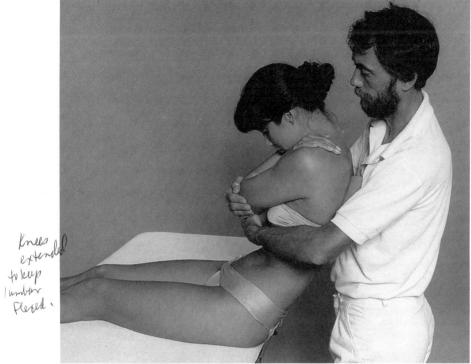

Knees
extended
to keep
lumbar
flexed.

Stand in stride
leaning fward
toward pt.

Figure 5–45B Step 1.

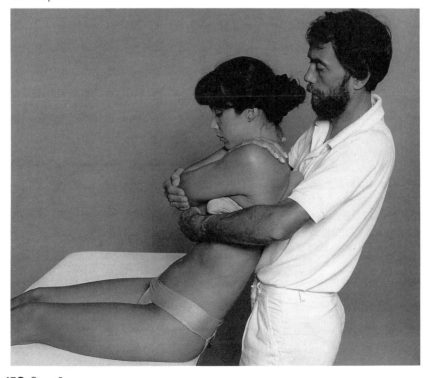

Figure 5–45C Step 3.

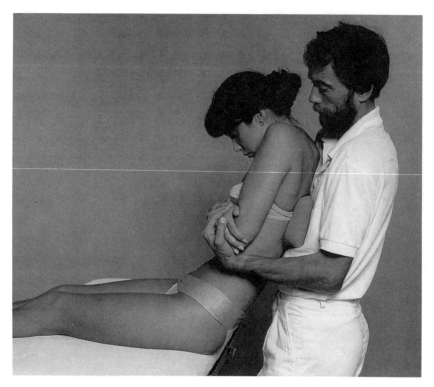

Figure 5–45D Segmental separation, lower thoracic spine.

hands resting on the shoulders. If the therapist is right-handed, the patient's right hand is placed on the left shoulder and the left hand is placed on the right shoulder (Figure 5–45A).

Position of the Therapist

The therapist stands behind the patient with the legs in stride, whereby the left leg is in front (if the therapist is right-handed). The treatment table is placed at a height so that the affected segment is at the level of the therapist's sternum. Placing a small, rolled-up towel between the patient and the sternum is recommended.

Performance

Step 1 (Figure 5–45B). The therapist grasps the patient's elbows: the right elbow with the left hand and the left elbow with the right hand. The patient leans backward and relaxes against the therapist, whereby the thoracic spine has contact (through the towel) with the therapist's sternum. The spinal column is now completely kyphosed.

Step 2. The therapist pulls the patient's elbows away from each other (bringing the patient's shoulders into more adduction) and pushes the patient's elbows into the thorax. The patient is instructed to take a deep breath. The moment the patient begins to breathe in, the therapist checks to see whether the patient is completely relaxed; this is best determined by bringing the patient's thorax in alternating right and left rotation. If the patient is not entirely relaxed, this procedure cannot be performed.

Step 3 (Figure 5–45C). During the exhalation, the therapist takes maximal pre-tension by pulling the patient's elbows farther away from each other and by pushing them into the patient's thorax. Simultaneously, the therapist straightens his or her knees slightly and brings the sternum in a cranial and ventral direction.

To emphasize the lower thoracic segments, the patient crosses the forearms and slightly grasps more distally either on the arms or at the elbows. The towel and the therapist's sternum are placed accordingly, at the lower thoracic region (Figure 5–45D).

Segmental Separation in Standing: General (Figures 5–46A–B)

Position of the Patient

The patient stands with the arms crossed in front of the chest and the hands resting on the shoulders. If the therapist is right-handed, the patient first places the right hand on the left shoulder and the left hand on the right shoulder (Figure 5–46A).

As mentioned in the previous technique, to emphasize the lower thoracic segments, the patient can cross the arms and rest the hands more caudally on the upper arms or slightly grasp the elbows.

Position of the Therapist

The therapist stands behind the patient with the legs in stride. If the therapist is right-handed, the left leg is placed in front.

Performance

Step 1 (Figure 5–46A). The therapist grasps the patient's elbows: the right elbow with the left hand and the left elbow with the right hand. The patient leans backward and relaxes against the therapist, whereby the thoracic spine has contact (through the towel) with the therapist's sternum. The spinal column is now completely kyphosed.

Step 2. The therapist pulls the patient's elbows away from each other (bringing the patient's shoulders into more adduction) and pushes the patient's elbows into the thorax.

The patient is instructed to take a deep breath. The moment the patient begins to breathe in, the therapist checks to see whether the patient is completely relaxed; this is best determined by bringing the patient's thorax in alternating right and left rotation. If the patient is not entirely relaxed, this procedure cannot be performed.

Step 3 (Figure 5–46B). During the exhalation, the therapist takes maximal pre-tension by pulling the patient's elbows farther away from each other and by pushing them into the patient's thorax. Simultaneously, the therapist straightens his or her knees slightly and brings the sternum in a cranial and ventral direction.

The advantage to this technique in standing is that the axial separation component is much greater. The disadvantage is that it cannot be performed when the therapist is significantly shorter than the patient.

Segmental Separation: Local (Figure 5–47)

Position of the Patient

See previously described separation techniques.

Position of the Therapist

See previously described separation techniques.

Performance

To emphasize the separation in one thoracic segment, a wedge can be used. It is placed on the transverse processes of the segment's cranial vertebra. In the same way, a segment can be emphasized by placing a sandbag or small towel roll on the spinous process of the segment's cranial vertebra. The technique is then performed in the same manner as described for the other segmental separation techniques. It is called the *mitnehmen* (take with) technique; the wedge takes the cranial vertebra with it in a cranial direction.

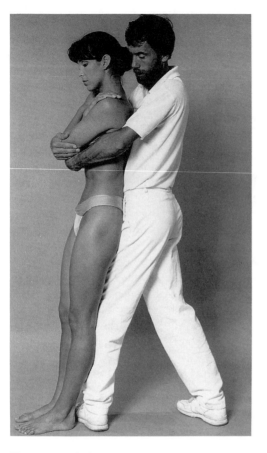 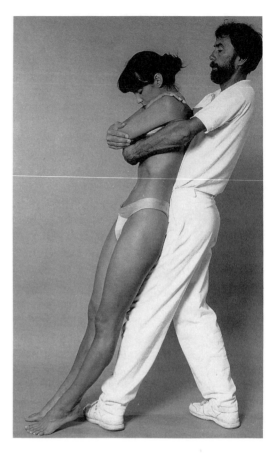

Figure 5–46A Step 1.

Figure 5–46B Step 3.

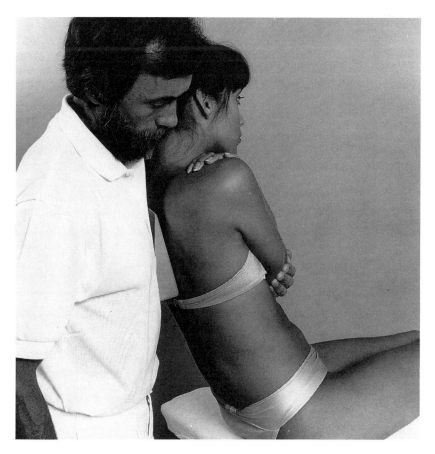

Figure 5–47

axial stretch, good c̄ facet
& disc.

Segmental Traction: Local (Figure 5–48)

Position of the Patient

See previously described separation techniques.

Position of the Therapist

See previously described separation techniques.

Performance

To emphasize the traction in one thoracic segment, a wedge can be used. It is placed on the transverse processes of the segment's caudal vertebra. In the same way, a sandbag or towel roll can be placed on the spinous process of the segment's caudal vertebra. As in all of the other separation techniques, it is important to ensure that the crossed point of the patient's arms lies at the level of the segment's cranial vertebra.

The therapist grasps the patient's elbows: the right elbow with the left hand and the left elbow with the right hand. The patient leans backward and relaxes against the therapist, whereby the thoracic spine has contact (through the towel) with the therapist's sternum. The spinal column is now completely kyphosed.

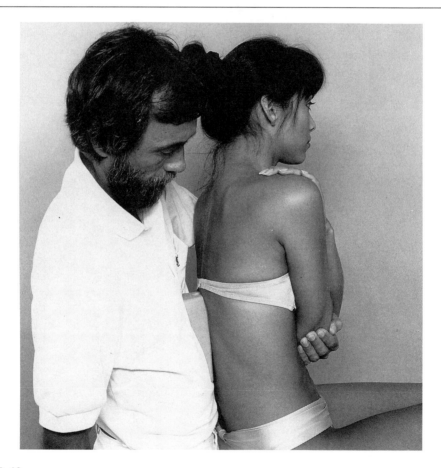

Figure 5–48

capsule stretch

The therapist applies pre-tension by pulling the patient's elbows away from each other (bringing the patient's shoulders into more adduction) and into the thorax. The patient is instructed to take a deep breath.

As the patient begins to breathe in, the therapist checks to see whether the patient is completely relaxed; this is best determined by bringing the patient's thorax in alternating right and left rotation. If the patient is not entirely relaxed, this procedure cannot be performed.

During the exhalation, the therapist takes maximal pre-tension by pulling the patient's elbows farther away from each other and by pushing them into the patient's thorax. The therapist's legs and sternum remain in the same position in order to fix the segment's caudal vertebra and all of the segments caudal to that. By retracting and elevating his or her shoulders, the therapist pulls through the patient's crossed arms, taking the segment's cranial vertebra in a dorsocranial direction. This technique is called the *gegenhalten* (hold against) technique because the caudal vertebra is held in relation to the cranial vertebra.

THREE-DIMENSIONAL MOBILIZATION TECHNIQUES

In treating the thoracic spine with three-dimensional techniques (both general and local), the rules of the "coupling patterns" are followed whenever possible.

In describing the following techniques, the rules applying to the lower thoracic spine are incorporated. The coupling for the lower thoracic spine is the same as for the lumbar spine: in flexion the coupling is ipsilateral, and in extension the coupling is contralateral. Upper thoracic problems (which rarely occur) are not addressed in the following descriptions.

In mobilizing the midthoracic spine (T4 to T8), the therapist first has to determine whether the coupling is in the same or in the opposite direction during extension. This is easy to test by positioning the patient in extension and sidebend, and then by bringing in first an ipsilateral rotation and then a contralateral rotation. The rotation that is easiest to perform is the coupled rotation. If it appears that the patient has an ipsilateral coupling in extension, a rotation opposite to that shown in the following techniques should be performed.

The following techniques (both general and local) can be performed in various ways: They can be held for a period of time, from several seconds to several minutes (the patient continues to stomach-breathe). The techniques can also be performed as a manipulation: at the end of the patient's exhalation and immediately before the next inhalation, the therapist takes up the pre-tension and accentuates the movement in the appropriate direction. To emphasize pain relief, they can be performed in the form of vibrations and oscillations as well.

Mobilization in Axial Separation by Means of Rotation, Extension, and Coupled Sidebend: General
(Figure 5–49)

Position of the Patient

The patient lies on the nonpainful side (with the painful side up). If the patient is very mobile, then a small pillow can be placed under the midthoracic region in order to bring the patient into a slight sidebend. In mobilizing the rotation, the rotation is performed first in the direction that is not (or is the least) painful.

Position of the Therapist

The therapist stands at the ventral aspect of the patient. The treatment table is positioned at the level of the therapist's patellas.

Position of the Assistants

One assistant sits on the floor at the head of the treatment table and grasps both of the

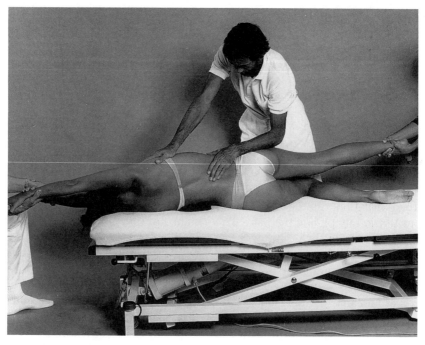

*OR put & pt's
hand on her
ribs & mob
there.*

Figure 5–49

Ext, ① SB, ℝ rot.

patient's wrists. Another assistant sits or stands at the foot of the table and uses both hands to grasp the patient's upper-lying leg, just above the malleoli.

The assistants are positioned directly opposite each other and make an angle of approximately 30° in respect to the long axis of the treatment table. In relation to the patient, the diagonal runs from dorsocranial to ventrocaudal.

Performance

The therapist positions the patient's bottom leg in approximately 45° hip flexion. The therapist places the cranial hand on the patient's upper-lying pectoral region. The caudal hand is placed at the level of the lumbar spine in such a way that the radial side of the middle finger hooks underneath the lateral aspect of the L1 spinous process. The lumbar spine and pelvis are stabilized by placing the caudal forearm against the lateral aspect of the lumbar spine and the elbow at the pelvis.

The therapist instructs both assistants to pull on the patient's arms and upper-lying leg. This axial separation should never be painful because the subsequent muscle splinting makes it almost impossible to perform the mobilization. The mobilization takes place by moving the patient's top shoulder and upper thoracic area in a dorsal and cranial direction.

After performing this technique, the patient is re-examined (one or two of the previously painful tests are repeated). If improvement is noted, the treatment should continue with the same technique. If the results indicated no improvement, the patient is mobilized in the other rotation direction.

When this technique is performed as a manipulation, the patient is asked to inhale deeply, and during the exhalation the axial separation and rotation are performed simultaneously. The rotational impulse is applied just after the end of the exhalation phase (and before the patient begins to inhale again).

Mobilization in Axial Separation by Means of Rotation, Flexion, and Coupled Sidebend: General

(Figure 5–50)

Position of the Patient

See previous technique.

Position of the Therapist

See previous technique.

Position of the Assistants

See previous technique.

Performance

The therapist positions the patient's top leg in extension and the bottom leg in approximately 45° of hip flexion. The therapist places the cranial hand just caudal to the patient's upper-lying scapula and on the dorsal aspect of the ribs. The other hand grasps the ventral aspect of the patient's pelvis (the anterior superior iliac spine).

The assistants grasp the patient's wrists and top leg. As with the previous technique, a diagonal of approximately 30° in relation to the long axis of the table is also made. However, here the diagonal runs from ventrocranial to dorsocaudal in relation to the patient.

The therapist instructs both assistants to pull on the patient's arms and upper-lying leg. This axial separation should never be painful. While the caudal hand stabilizes the pelvis, the therapist moves the patient's shoulder and upper thoracic region in a ventral direction.

After performing this technique, the patient is re-examined (one or two of the previously painful tests are repeated).

When this technique is performed as a manipulation, the patient is asked to inhale deeply, and during the exhalation the axial

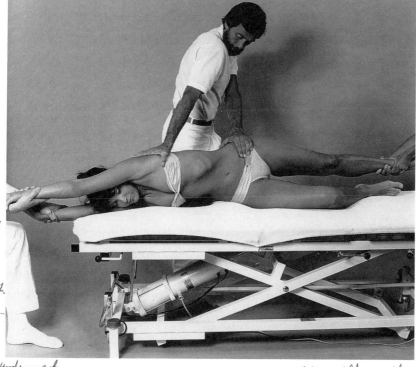

Figure 5–50

[handwritten annotations:] if raise head up get Th. ⓛ SB to ↑ rigidity of upper Th J Option, to focus on Low Th.

To ↑ Low Th rigid to mob upper Th, Try ↑ Lumbar ext.

OR: leg Falls off table to ↑SB

Hold shlds, then pull at pelvis

Flex Ⓡ SB Ⓡ rot

Direct. of glide of fault.

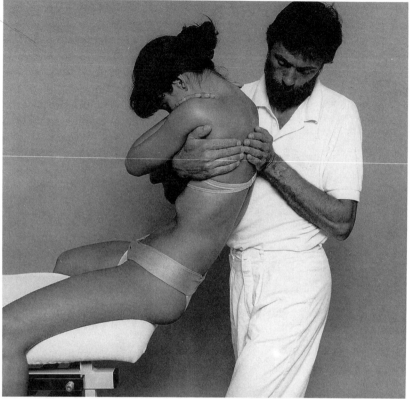

Figure 5–51A Step 1.

separation and rotation are performed simultaneously. The rotational impulse is applied just after the end of the exhalation phase (and before the patient begins to inhale again).

Axial Separation with Rotation in Sitting: General or Local
(Figures 5–51A–C)

Position of the Patient

The patient sits at the short end of the treatment table with the legs straddling each side. The patient sits on both ischial tuberosities as close to the edge of the table as possible. The arms are crossed in front of the chest with the hands resting on the shoulders.

Position of the Therapist

The therapist stands behind the patient closest to the side to which the patient will be rotating. The legs are in a stride position.

Performance

Step 1 (Figure 5–51A). From ventral, the therapist brings one forearm underneath the

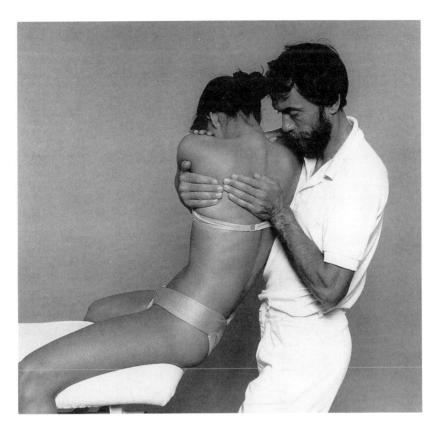

Figure 5–51B Step 2.

patient's crossed arms and grasps the dorsal aspect of the patient's thorax. The ulnar aspect of the hand rests on the rib corresponding to the cranial vertebra of the segment being treated. The base of the hypothenar eminence of the other hand (in particular, the pisiform) is placed against the lateral aspect (on the side of the therapist) of the spinous process of the segment's cranial vertebra. An alternative placement for the hypothenar eminence of that hand is on the cranial vertebra's transverse process (on the side far-

thest away from the therapist). This alternative hand placement is not shown. The therapist's forearm points in a cranial, ventral, and lateral direction.

Step 2 (Figure 5–51B). The patient now relaxes completely, leaning back against the therapist (the lumbar spine is in a kyphosis). The therapist rotates the patient's trunk toward the therapist. The patient is supported by the therapist's trunk.

To better localize the mobilization, the therapist brings the patient's trunk into a

Omer says put on Transverse Process
Push it into rot. (RP)
Pulling same rib around (RP).

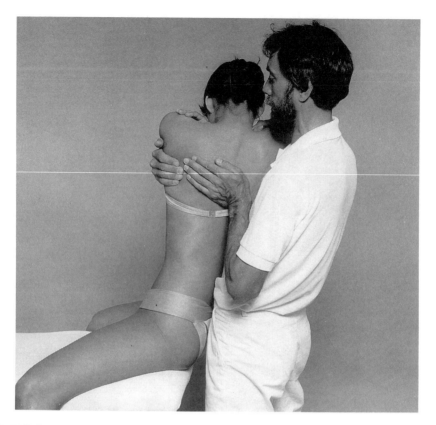

Figure 5–51C Step 3.

slight sidebend that is opposite to the mobilizing rotation, ensuring that this sidebend occurs only in the segments caudal to the one being mobilized. Now the thoracic and lumbar segments caudal to the segment being treated are locked. The segment being treated remains in its normal thoracic kyphosis.

SB by side shift, hips stay in same place.

Step 3 (Figure 5–51C). The mobilization occurs when the therapist personally performs a trunk rotation in the same direction as the mobilizing rotation. At the same time, the therapist's spine is extended.

To perform this technique as a manipulation, the patient is asked to inhale deeply, and during the exhalation maximal pre-tension is taken up. An extra rotational/axial-separation impulse is applied just after the end of the exhalation phase (and before the patient begins to inhale again).

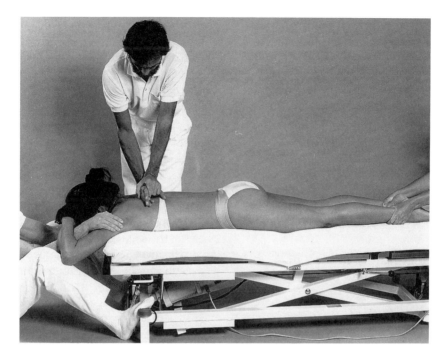

Figure 5–52

Dorsoventral Manipulation with Axial Separation (Figure 5–52)

Position of the Patient

The patient lies prone on the treatment table with the forehead resting on the hands.

Position of the Therapist

The therapist stands next to the patient at the level of the segment to be treated. The treatment table is placed at the level of the therapist's patellas.

Position of the Assistants

One assistant sits on the floor at the head of the table and, with both hands, reaches underneath the patient's forearms and over the patient's upper arms to grasp the patient's shoulders as proximally as possible. At this point, the patient is asked to slide both arms and head off the table, supported by the assistant. The other assistant grasps both of the patient's ankles just proximal to the malleoli (Figure 5–52).

Performance

The therapist's hands are placed at the level of the affected segment; the hypothenar eminence of the cranial hand rests against the spinous process while the other hand supports the cranial hand in such a way that the thumb lies on the dorsum of that hand and the fingers are placed between the fingers and the thumb of the cranial hand.

The patient is instructed to inhale deeply. During the exhalation, the assistants apply the axial separation by pulling on the patient's shoulders and legs while the therapist takes up maximal pre-tension. Just after the end of the exhalation phase, and before the patient begins to inhale again, the therapist quickly exerts overpressure by means of an abrupt nod of the head.

In general, this technique can be performed only when the patient does not have any complaints of low back pain. Because the segments cranial and caudal to the treated segment also move during the mobilization, this technique is not very local. However, it is often a very effective technique.

This technique can be performed without axial separation only when there are still minor residual symptoms after first utilizing the segmental separation techniques in sitting and/or in standing (see the section, Dorsoventral Manipulation without Axial Separation).

Traction Mobilization of the Zygapophyseal Joints in Supine
(Figures 5–53A–C)

Position of the Patient

The patient lies supine on the treatment table, with the arms crossed in front of the chest and the hands resting on the shoulders. The hips and knees are flexed.

Position of the Therapist

The therapist stands next to the table at the level of the patient's thorax.

Performance

The therapist places a mobilization wedge under the transverse processes of the segment's caudal vertebra (Figure 5–53A). The cranial hand supports the patient's head and neck and, if necessary, also the thoracic segments cranial to the zygapophyseal joints being mobilized. The index finger of the cranial hand palpates between both spinous processes of the segment being treated (depending on the level, the spinous processes lie 2 to 4 cm caudal to the zygapophyseal joints). This palpation is possible because of the groove in the mobilization wedge (Figure 5–53C).

The therapist's caudal hand makes contact with the crossing point of the patient's forearms. The patient's arms should cross at the level of the sternal attachment of the rib com-

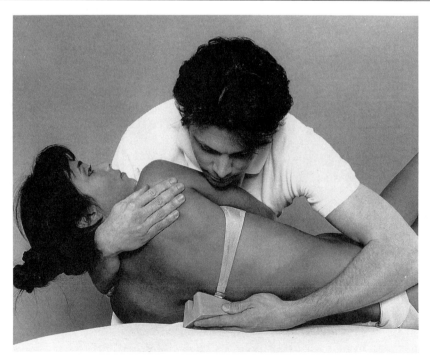

Figure 5–53A

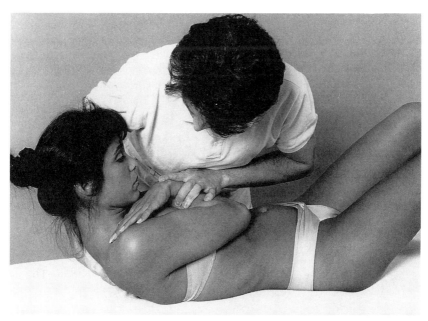

Figure 5–53B

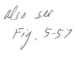

also see
Fig. 5-57

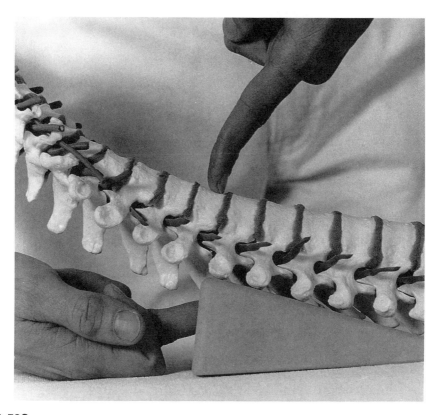

Figure 5–53C

ing from the segment's cranial vertebra. The therapist now brings the patient's thorax into flexion, only to the point where the segment just cranial to the segment being treated is flexed. The mobilization takes place by performing pressure via the patient's forearms in a dorsocranial direction (Figure 5–53B). Slack is first taken up from the thorax (particularly from the ribs), before an actual traction occurs in the zygapophyseal joints.

If necessary, the head of the table can be raised to support the patient's head, neck, and thoracic spine in flexion. The wedge and segment being treated should be positioned just below the hinge of the table, whereby the segment being mobilized remains in its normal thoracic kyphosis.

This traction technique also can be performed as a manipulation. Again, the pretension is taken up at the end of the patient's exhalation, after which the manipulative impulse is performed.

Traction Mobilization of the Zygapophyseal Joints in Sitting
(Figure 5–54)

Instead of using a wedge, in the same manner as described for the previous technique, the edge of the treatment table can be used to perform local segmental traction in the zygapophyseal joints. The cranial spinous process of the segment being treated is positioned above the edge of the table. The technique is

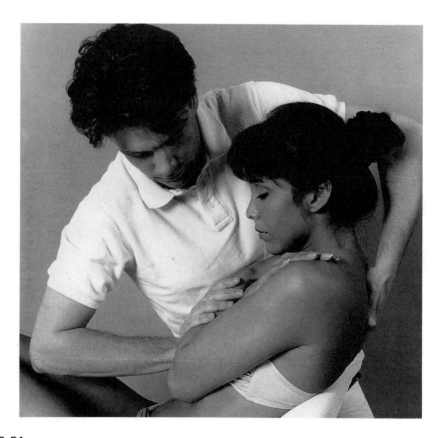

Figure 5–54

T4 & below.

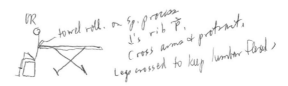

performed as described for the previous technique. A disadvantage here is that the amount of pressure on the caudal spinous process is rather great.

Dorsoventral Manipulation without Axial Separation (Figure 5–55)

The dorsoventral manipulation can be performed with or without axial separation: *with* axial separation in patients with articular or dural signs, and *without* axial separation in patients with zygapophyseal joint dysfunction.

Position of the Patient

The patient lies prone with the head in a neutral position. The arms rest alongside the body.

Position of the Therapist

The therapist stands next to the patient at the level of the segment being treated. The treatment table is positioned to a height allowing for the therapist to stand with the arms straight and shoulders vertically positioned over the hands.

Performance

The therapist's hands are placed at the level of the affected segment. The hypothenar eminence of the cranial hand rests against the spinous process while the other hand supports the cranial hand in such a way that the thumb lies on the dorsum of that hand and the fingers are placed between the fingers and the thumb of the cranial hand (Figure 5–55).

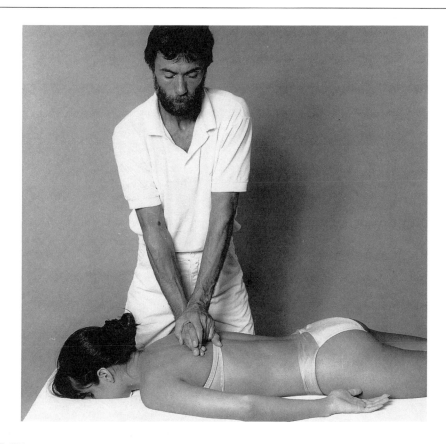

Figure 5–55

The patient is instructed to inhale deeply. Just after the end of the exhalation phase, and before the patient begins to inhale again, the therapist quickly exerts overpressure by means of an abrupt nod of the head.

SEGMENTAL ROTATION MOBILIZATION TECHNIQUES

The local traction and separation techniques generally are followed by the local rotation techniques. The direction of the rotation in each technique is initially determined by the painful rotation. The rotation techniques are always performed first in the nonpainful direction. The following rotation mobilization techniques are performed only in patients with a zygapophyseal joint dys-

function. *Rotation without axial separation can lead to dangerous consequences in patients with disc lesions.*

Segmental Rotation Mobilization in Prone (Figures 5–56A and 5–56B)

Position of the Patient

The patient lies prone with the head in a neutral position. The arms rest alongside the body.

Position of the Therapist

The therapist stands next to the patient at the level of the segment to be treated. The therapist stands on the side of the patient to which the mobilizing rotation will occur. (In other words, for a right rotation mobilization, the therapist stands at the right side of the

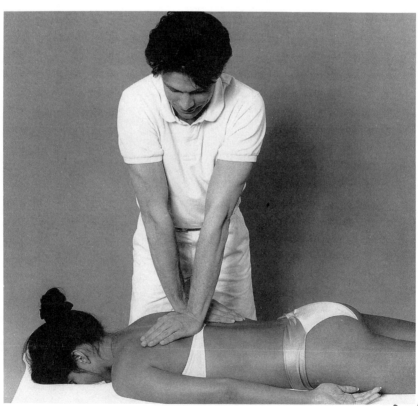

Figure 5–56A

For Facet only. Not if disc involve

T1-3 Too Rigid.   *T3-4, preposition head in same rotation.*   *∠ between arms is ⊥ to kyphosis.*

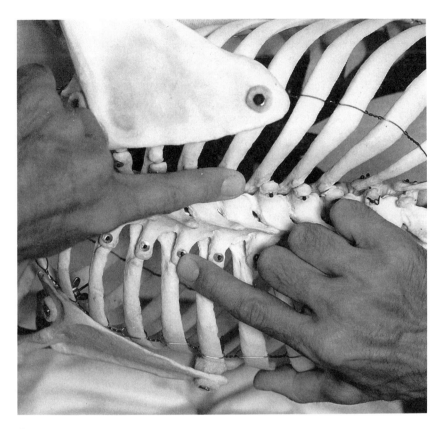

Figure 5–56B

---

patient.) The treatment table is positioned to a height allowing the therapist to stand with the arms straight and shoulders vertically positioned over the hands.

Performance

With the thenar eminence of the caudal hand, the therapist makes contact with the cranial vertebra's transverse process on the side farthest away. The therapist places the hypothenar eminence of the cranial hand on the caudal vertebra's transverse process on the side closest to the therapist.

The therapist's arms are extended and the shoulders are positioned vertically above the hands (Figure 5–56A). Pressure is now exerted against the cranial transverse process in a cranial and ventral direction while the caudal transverse process is stabilized by pressure exerted in a caudal and ventral direction (Figure 5–56B). This results in a segmental rotation of the segment's cranial vertebra in relation to the caudal vertebra. The rotation occurs in the direction of the therapist.

This technique also can be performed as a manipulation. The patient is asked to inhale deeply. During the exhalation, maximal pretension is taken up, and then just at the end of the exhalation and before the patient again takes a breath, the short, abrupt overpressure is applied.

Segmental Rotation Mobilization in Supine (Figures 5–57A–C)

This technique is an alternative mobilization for the Segmental Rotation Mobilization in Prone.

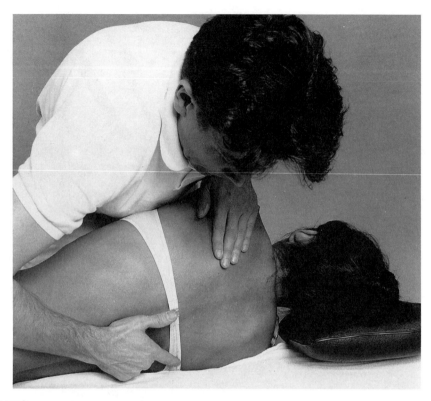

Figure 5–57A

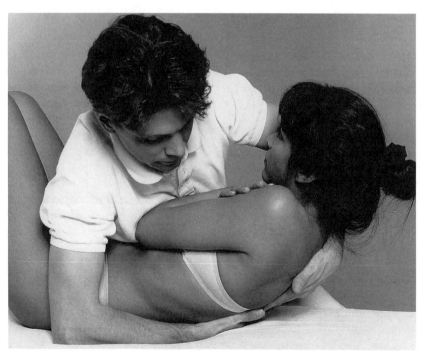

Figure 5–57B

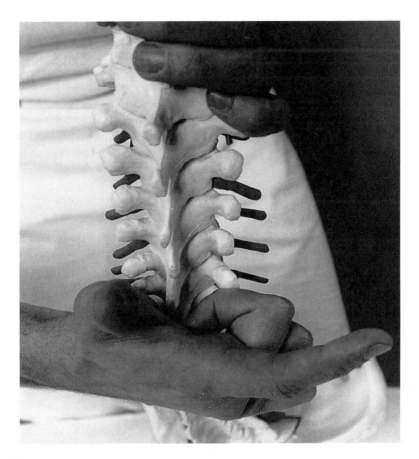

Figure 5–57C

Position of the Patient

The patient lies supine with the arms crossed in front of the chest and the hands resting on the shoulders. The patient's arms should cross at the level of the sternal attachment of the rib coming from the cranial vertebra of the segment to be treated. To prevent too much pressure directly on the ribs, the forearm farthest from the therapist is crossed on top of the other forearm. The patient's head initially is supported by a pillow.

Position of the Therapist

The therapist stands next to the patient opposite the side to which the rotation will occur. (In other words, if a left rotation mobi-

lization is performed, the therapist stands at the patient's right side.)

Performance

With the cranial hand, the therapist grasps the dorsal aspect of the patient's opposite shoulder and rolls the patient over toward him or her in such a way that the thoracic spine no longer lies against the treatment table (Figure 5–57A). The caudal hand makes contact with the segment to be treated: the thumb is in maximal retroposition, the index finger is in maximal extension, and the other fingers are in maximal flexion ("pistol grip"). The base of the thenar eminence (in particular, the tuberosity of the scaphoid) is placed on the caudal vertebra's transverse process.

At the same time, the dorsal aspect of the middle phalanx of the middle finger is placed against the cranial vertebra's transverse process (Figure 5–57C).

The patient is then "rolled back" into the supine position whereby the therapist's hand remains positioned exactly as just described. With the cranial arm, the therapist now supports the patient's head, neck, and thoracic spine (cranial to the segment being treated) and flexes the patient's thoracic spine only to the point where the segment just cranial to the segment being treated is flexed. The segment being treated remains in its normal thoracic kyphosis (resting position).

Next, the therapist's sternum is placed on the patient's arms, just at the point where they cross (Figure 5–57B). The mobilization is performed by the therapist's exerting pressure from the trunk, through the patient's trunk, in a craniodorsal direction. The resulting rotation in the segment is in the direction away from the therapist.

As described in the other techniques, this technique also can be performed as a manipulation.

Mobilization in the Gliding Direction through Extension, Rotation, and Coupled Sidebend: Local Technique for the Upper-Lying Zygapophyseal Joint (Figure 5–58)

Position of the Patient

The patient lies on the nonpainful side (with the painful side up). If the patient is very mobile, a small pillow can be placed under the midthoracic region, to pre-position in a slight sidebend. The head rests on the table, encouraging the sidebend component of the technique. The arms are crossed in front of the chest with the hands resting on the shoulders. The treatment table is adjusted to the level of the therapist's greater trochanter.

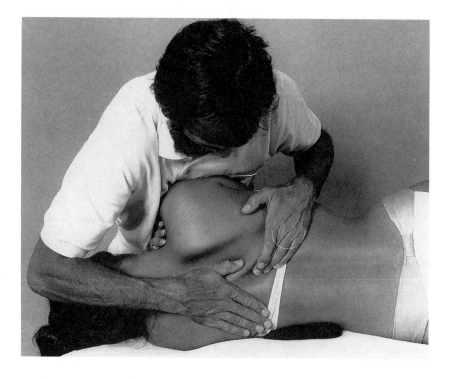

Figure 5–58

Position of the Therapist

The therapist stands facing the patient at the level of the segment to be treated.

Performance

With the caudal hand, the therapist fixes the caudal vertebra of the segment to be treated by placing the end phalanx of the middle finger against the lateral aspect of the spinous process (on the side lying closest to the table). The rest of the hand and forearm can rest along the patient's lumbar spine and pelvis (not shown) to stabilize the thoracic and lumbar segments lying caudal to the segment being treated.

The thumb of the cranial hand is placed against the lateral aspect of the spinous process (on the opposite side of the caudal hand's middle finger). At the same, time the therapist's trunk is placed against the patient's crossed arms and the therapist holds the patient's upper thoracic area and shoulder girdle between the upper body and the cranial hand (and forearm).

While fixing with the caudal hand, the therapist moves the patient's upper-lying shoulder in a dorsal, caudal, and medial direction. This diagonal results in an extension, sidebend, and coupled rotation. Because the patient's shoulder girdle (along with the segments cranial to the segment being treated) and the therapist's trunk move as one unit, the motion is performed by a rotation and slight forward flexion of the therapist's upper body.

Mobilization in the Gliding Direction through Flexion, Rotation, and Ipsilateral Sidebend: Local Technique for the Upper-Lying Zygapophyseal Joint (Figure 5–59)

Position of the Patient

The patient lies on the nonpainful side (with the painful side up). If the patient is very mobile, a small pillow can be placed under the midthoracic region in order to pre-

position in a slight sidebend. The head rests on the table, encouraging the sidebend component of the technique. The patient's arms are crossed in front of the chest with the hands resting on the shoulders. The treatment table is adjusted to the level of the therapist's greater trochanter.

Position of the Therapist

The therapist stands facing the patient at the level of the segment to be treated.

Performance

With the caudal hand, the therapist fixes the caudal vertebra of the segment to be treated by placing the end phalanx of the thumb against the lateral aspect of the spinous process (upper side). The rest of the hand and forearm rest along the patient's lateral lumbar spine and pelvis, to stabilize the thoracic and lumbar segments lying caudal to the segment being treated. The tips of the index and middle fingers of the cranial hand are placed against the lateral aspect of the spinous process (on the side lying closest to the table). At the same time, the therapist's trunk is placed against the patient's crossed arms and the therapist holds the patient's upper thoracic area and shoulder girdle between the upper body and the cranial hand (and forearm).

While fixing with the caudal hand and arm, the therapist moves the patient's upper-lying shoulder in a ventral, cranial, and lateral direction. This diagonal results in a flexion, sidebend, and ipsilateral rotation. Because the patient's shoulder girdle (along with the segments cranial to the segment being treated) and the therapist's trunk move as one unit, the motion is performed by a rotation and slight sidebend of the therapist's upper body.

Segmental Extension Mobilization in Supine (Figure 5–60)

Position of the Patient

The patient half-sits against the raised end of the treatment table with the thoracic seg-

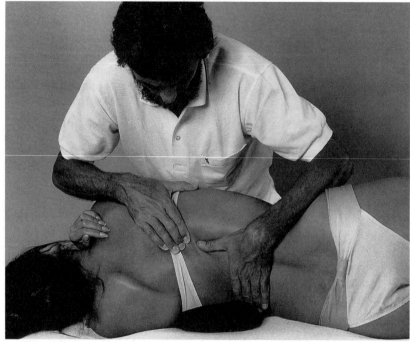

Hand on pt's head.

Figure 5–59

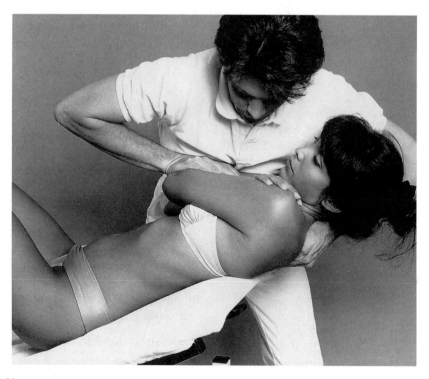

Figure 5–60

ments cranial to the segment being treated over the edge of the table. The cranial spinous process of the segment being treated is also positioned above the edge of the table. The patient's arms are crossed in front of the chest with the hands resting on the shoulders. The patient's arms should cross at the level of the sternal attachment of the rib coming from the cranial vertebra of the segment being treated.

Position of the Therapist

The therapist stands next to the patient at thorax level.

Performance

With the cranial arm, the therapist supports the patient's head, neck, and the part of the thoracic spine hanging over the edge of the table. The tip of the therapist's index finger has contact with the spinous process of the cranial vertebra of the segment being treated. The spinous process of the caudal vertebra (along with the thoracic and lumbar segments caudal to it) is fixed against the table. The other hand grasps the point where the patient's forearms cross. The therapist now exerts slight pressure via the patient's arms, through the thorax in a craniodorsal direction. In so doing, traction in the zygapophyseal joints occurs.

Next, the part of the patient's trunk lying over the table is brought into extension. This extension occurs in the following way: the hand lying against the patient's back exerts pressure in a ventrocaudal direction, while at the same time the ventrally positioned hand maintains the traction in a dorsocranial direction. The therapist's sternum comes into contact with the lateral aspect of the patient's shoulder and induces the extension motion in the patient's thoracic spine by personally performing a sidebend.

This technique generally is performed for several seconds or minutes in a slow rhythmic manner. The end position is held for approximately 1 second before returning to the initial position, and then the motion is repeated.

Unilateral Segmental Extension Mobilization in Supine (Figure 5–61)

This technique is often very effective in dysfunctions of the lower thoracic segments.

Position of the Patient

The patient half-sits against the raised end of the treatment table with the thoracic segments cranial to the segment being treated over the edge of the table. The cranial spinous process of the segment being treated is also positioned above the edge of the table. The patient's arms are crossed in front of the chest with the hands resting on the shoulders. The patient's arms should cross at the level of the sternal attachment of the rib coming from the cranial vertebra of the segment to be treated.

Position of the Therapist

The therapist stands next to the patient at thorax level, opposite the side to be treated. (In other words, if the left zygapophyseal joint of a segment is being treated, the therapist stands at the patient's right side.)

Performance

With the cranial arm, the therapist supports the patient's head, neck, and the part of the thoracic spine hanging over the edge of the table. The tip of the index finger has contact with the spinous process of the cranial vertebra of the segment being treated. The spinous process of the caudal vertebra (along with the thoracic and lumbar segments caudal to it) is fixed against the table. The other hand grasps the point where the patient's forearms cross. The therapist now exerts slight pressure via the patient's arms, through the thorax in a craniodorsal direction. In so doing, traction in the zygapophyseal joints occurs.

In the same way as described in the previous technique, the part of the patient's trunk lying over the edge of the table is brought into extension. At the same time, the patient is brought into a sidebend away from the thera-

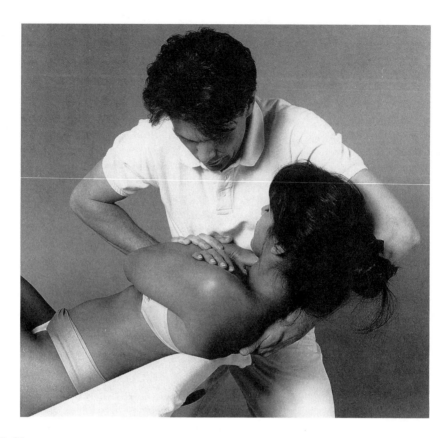

Figure 5–61

pist, along with a simultaneous coupled rotation. For example, in treatment of a segment's left zygapophyseal joint, the patient is brought into extension, left sidebend, and right rotation.

This technique generally is performed for several seconds or minutes in a slow, rhythmic manner. The end position is held for approximately 1 second before returning to the initial position, and then the motion is repeated.

Segmental Mobilization through Extension, Rotation, and Coupled Sidebend in Sitting (Figure 5–62)

Position of the Patient

The patient sits on both ischial tuberosities at the edge of the short end of the treatment table. The feet rest flat on the floor. The hips are flexed approximately 70° to maintain a neutral lordosis in the lumbar spine. The patient crosses the arms in front of the chest with hands resting on the shoulders.

To lock the segments below the segment being treated, a wedge or sandbag can be placed under the patient's ischial tuberosity at the side to which the therapist will be rotating the patient's thoracic spine. In so doing, the therapist must ensure that the subsequent sidebend occurs only in the segments caudal to the one being treated. For instance, if the technique includes a left rotation, the sandbag is placed under the patient's left ischial tuberosity. This induces a left sidebend and right rotation in the thoracic and lumbar segments caudal to the one being treated. The segment to be treated remains in its neutral kyphosis (resting position).

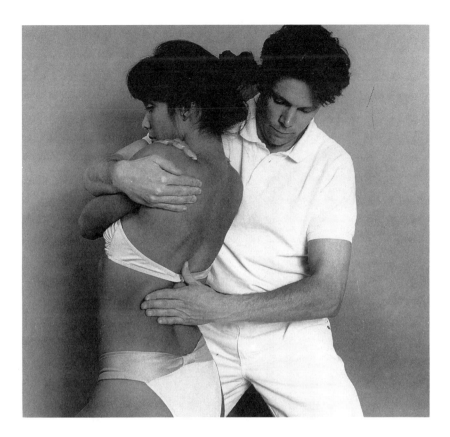

Figure 5–62

Position of the Therapist

The therapist stands next to the patient, opposite the side to which the patient will be rotated. (When making a left rotation, the therapist stands at the right side of the patient.)

Performance

From ventral, the therapist brings an arm over the patient's crossed arms and grasps the dorsal aspect of the patient's shoulder that is farthest away (as shown). Another way of holding the patient is for the therapist to reach up between the patient's crossed arms with an arm and then grasp the patient's shoulder that is farthest away. Either the therapist's sternum or anterior aspect of the shoulder is placed against the lateral aspect of

the patient's other shoulder. In so doing, the patient's shoulder girdle is now held between the therapist's hand and trunk.

To fix the segment's caudal vertebra, the therapist places a thumb against the lateral aspect of the spinous process, at the side closest to the therapist. The fingers of this hand are placed against the other side of the patient's back, ensuring that its contact with the lower segments and ribs does not interfere with the ensuing mobilization movement. Through a movement of the therapist's trunk, the patient's thoracic spine is brought into extension, sidebend, and coupled rotation.

This technique generally is performed for several seconds or minutes in a slow rhythmic manner. The end position is held for approximately 1 second before returning to the initial position, and then the motion is repeated.

The technique is very effective as a mobilization technique and also in proprioceptive training of the segment.

TREATMENT OF MUSCLE LESIONS

Transverse Friction of the Intercostal Muscles (Figure 5–63)

Lesions of the intercostal muscles usually occur as a result of a direct trauma, often involving a rib fracture.

Position of the Patient

The patient lies supine on the treatment table with the arms resting at the sides.

Position of the Therapist

The therapist sits or stands next to the patient at the level of the lesion.

Performance

The transverse friction is best performed with the tip of the middle finger reinforced by the index finger. The transverse friction consists of a movement parallel to the ribs. Often two or three muscle groups in adjacent intercostal spaces are affected. At least 10 minutes of transverse friction should be performed per localization. Despite the duration of the lesion, the problem is almost always cured in one to three sessions of transverse friction.

Transverse Friction of the Pectoralis Major (Figure 5–64)

In the functional examination, resisted adduction and internal rotation of the shoulder are painful.

Position of the Patient

The patient sits against the inclined head of the treatment table.

Position of the Therapist

The therapist sits next to the treatment table, facing the patient.

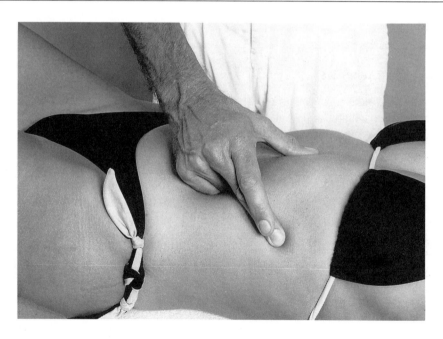

Figure 5–63

Performance

If the patient's left side is affected, the therapist grasps the area of the lesion between the thumb and index finger of the left hand. These fingers form a type of "O-grip." Pressure is applied between the thumb and the index finger, to the point where the patient experiences very slight pain. The therapist moves the hand in a ventral and caudal direction during the friction phase and in the opposite direction during the relaxation phase.

The treatment is generally very successful; within three to six treatments, the patient has complete relief of pain.

In addition to the transverse friction, stretching should be performed. In very acute instances, an injection of a local anesthetic can be very helpful. Partial tears or total ruptures require 3 to 6 weeks of local rest.

Stretching of the Pectoralis Major
(Figures 5–65A–C)

In general, the function of the pectoralis major is adduction and internal rotation of the humerus. With the arm fixed in abducted elevation, the muscle assists in elevation of the thorax (accessory breathing muscle). The muscle is also active during forced inhalation, such as in certain sports activities and in some cases of COPD.

The function of the various parts of the muscle are as follows:

- *pars abdominalis.* depression of the shoulder girdle and adduction of the hu-

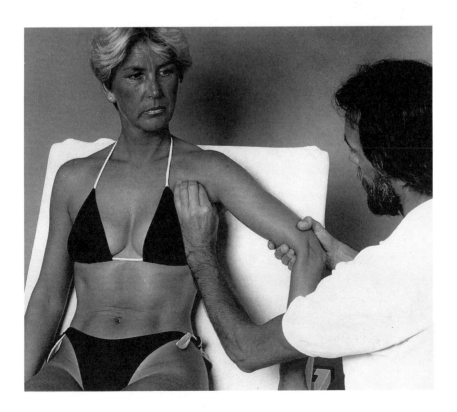

Figure 5–64

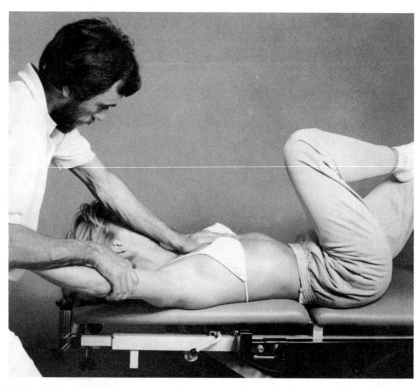

Figure 5–65A Initial position.

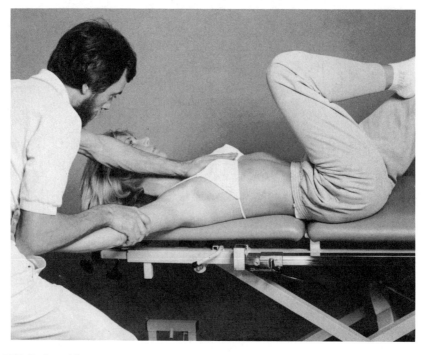

Figure 5–65B End position.

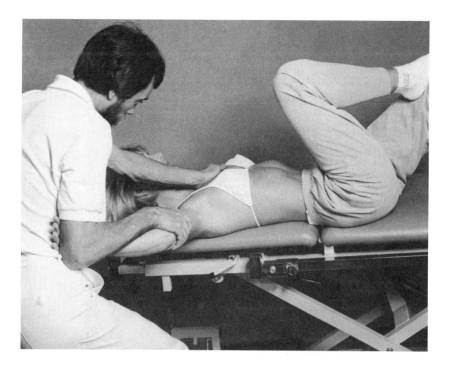

Figure 5–65C Stretching of the pars clavicularis.

merus in the direction of the opposite hip

- *pars sternocostalis.* adduction of the humerus in the direction of the opposite nipple
- *pars clavicularis.* horizontal adduction of the humerus

Position of the Patient

The patient lies supine with the side to be stretched as close to the edge of the treatment table as possible. One leg is positioned with the hip and knee slightly flexed and the foot resting on the table. The hip and knee of the other leg are brought into even more flexion, whereby the foot of that leg is placed just proximal to the knee of the leg resting on the table. This positioning prevents the lumbar spine from lordosing during the stretching. The patient's arm lies in abducted elevation and external rotation. The amount of abduc-

tion depends on which part of the pectoralis major is to be stretched.

Position of the Therapist

The therapist stands at the head of the table next to the patient's affected side. If the right side is to be stretched, the therapist uses the left hand to fix the right aspect of the patient's thorax (pars abdominalis) or the sternum (pars sternocostalis and pars clavicularis). The right hand grasps the patient's upper arm just proximal to the elbow, and the patient's forearm is held between the therapist's forearm and the trunk.

Performance

Very gradually, the patient's arm is now brought farther into elevation and external rotation, with respect for pain and muscle splinting:

- maximal elevation: pars abdominalis

- approximately 125° elevation: pars sternocostalis
- approximately 90° elevation: pars clavicularis.

During the stretching, some patients experience paresthesia in part of the hand and/or fingers. This is probably due to compression of part of the brachial plexus underneath and against the coracoid process.

Generally, it is beneficial to stretch the pectoralis major on both sides. The therapist can perform a bilateral stretch by fixing the patient's thorax to the treatment table with a mobilization belt. In this instance, the therapist stands behind the supine patient at the head of the table. The patient should also stretch several times per day at home.

Transverse Friction of the Pectoralis Minor (Figure 5–66)

In the rare insertion tendopathy of the pectoralis minor, the basic functional examination is negative. In some cases, resisted protraction of the shoulder is painful. The lesion almost always involves the insertion at the coracoid process.

Position of the Patient

The patient sits against the inclined head of the treatment table.

Position of the Therapist

The therapist sits on a chair, next to and slightly behind the patient.

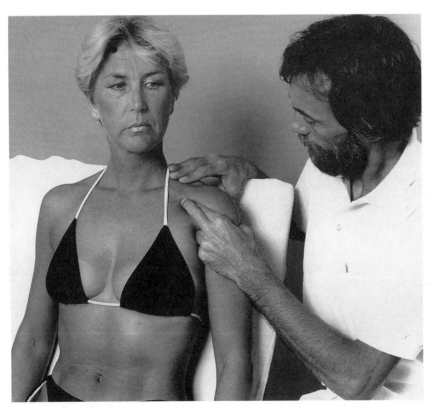

Figure 5–66

Performance

The transverse friction is performed with the index finger, reinforced by the middle finger. If the patient's left side is to be treated, the therapist uses the left hand to perform the technique. The tip of the index finger is placed at the medial aspect of the coracoid process. During the friction phase, the therapist's hand moves from medial to lateral in such a way that the finger maintains contact with the coracoid process.

In addition to the transverse friction, stretching exercises should also be performed. The patient generally experiences a full recovery in 2 to 3 weeks of treatment.

Stretching of the Pectoralis Minor
(Figure 5–67)

The function of the pectoralis minor with a fixed thorax is chiefly a tipping of the scapula. If the scapula is fixed, the muscle assists in lifting the thorax (accessory breathing muscle).

Position of the Patient

The patient lies in supine with the shoulder (scapula) over the edge of the table.

Position of the Therapist

The therapist stands next to the affected side of the patient. The therapist grasps the

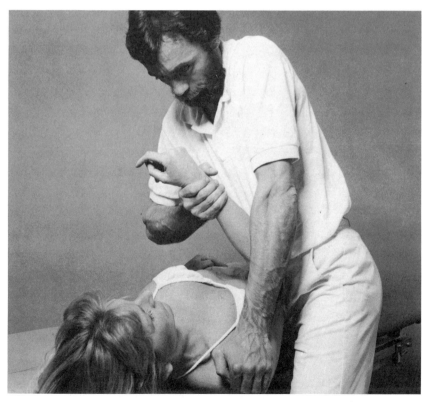

Figure 5–67

Stretch Pect. Minor

patient's forearm just proximal to the wrist. If the right side is to be stretched, with the right hand the therapist brings the patient's upper arm into internal rotation, slight adduction, and approximately 70° flexion. The left hand is placed on the anterior aspect of the patient's right shoulder.

Performance

The patient's shoulder is slowly brought into a craniodorsal direction. At the end of the range of motion, the stretch can be increased by instructing the patient to exhale deeply. Here too, it is recommended to stretch both the right and left sides. The patient should also stretch several times per day at home. When the patient stretches at home, both sides should be stretched simultaneously.

Transverse Friction of the Latissimus Dorsi (Figure 5–68)

Strain of the latissimus dorsi rarely occurs and is almost exclusively the result of a sports injury. The lesion is usually located just ventrolateral to the scapula. In the functional examination, resisted adduction and internal rotation of the shoulder are painful.

Position of the Patient

The patient sits on a chair or stool next to the short side of the treatment table. The arm is abducted approximately 45° and the forearm rests on the table.

Position of the Therapist

The therapist sits diagonally behind the patient, next to the end of the long side of the treatment table.

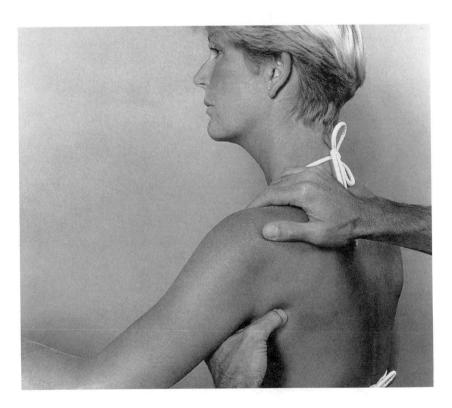

Figure 5–68

Performance

If the patient's left side is affected, the therapist uses the index finger and thumb of the left hand to grasp the affected area of the latissimus dorsi from ventral and dorsal, respectively. The transverse friction is performed by bringing the index finger and thumb together and then moving the whole hand in a ventrolateral direction. Generally, only a few treatments with transverse friction are needed for a full recovery.

In addition to the transverse friction, stretching exercises should also be performed. Muscle-strengthening exercises also should be included in the treatment program because of the significant chance for recurrence.

Transverse Friction of the Rectus Abdominis (Figure 5–69)

Strain of the rectus abdominis is seldom seen as a solitary lesion; most of the time the patients also have a pubalgia, with predominantly groin pain. In the functional examination, resisted trunk flexion is painful. Lifting both extended legs from a supine position is especially painful.

Position of the Patient

The patient lies on the treatment table with a pillow under the knees and the arms resting alongside the body.

Position of the Therapist

The therapist sits or stands next to the patient at the level of the lesion.

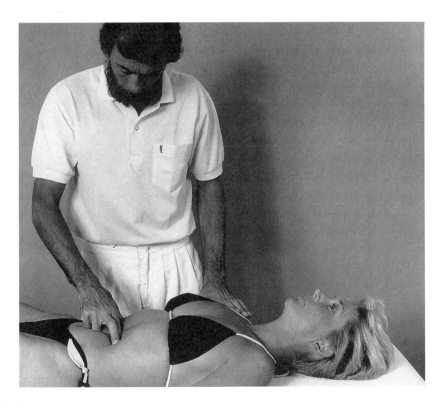

Figure 5–69

Performance

The precise area of the lesion is located; usually strain of the rectus abdominis occurs just cranial to the navel or just cranial to the pubic symphysis. The transverse friction is best performed with one or more fingertips, depending on the size of the lesion. The transverse friction is applied transverse to the running of the muscle fibers and from a medial to a lateral direction. Generally, complete recovery is achieved in 2 to 3 weeks of treatment.

Muscle-stretching (trunk extension) as well as muscle-strengthening exercises should be included in the treatment program. The muscle strengthening should be initiated only after the functional examination is negative.

MOBILIZATION OF THE COSTOVERTEBRAL CONNECTIONS

Mobilization of the First Rib: Costotransverse Joint (Figure 5–70)

Position of the Patient

The patient lies supine with the arms alongside the body. For the same reasons mentioned in describing the first rib mobility test, the first rib is mobilized with the patient's head in a neutral position. The head can be supported on a small pillow, depending on the amount of thoracic kyphosis.

Position of the Therapist

The therapist sits or stands at the head of the treatment table. If the patient's left side is

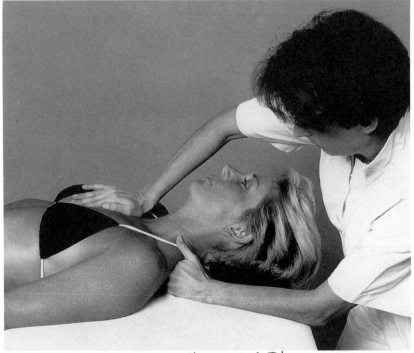

Figure 5–70

to be treated, the therapist uses the left hand to perform the mobilization. The therapist places the radial side of the index finger's middle phalanx on the dorsal aspect of the first rib's posterior angle. The wrist is held in slight extension. The ulnar side of the mobilizing hand rests on the treatment table, and the elbow is flexed approximately 45°. The heel of the other hand fixes the patient's sternum.

Performance

The mobilization is performed with the patient breathing normally. By a slight radial deviation of the wrist, the therapist moves the first rib in a ventrolateral direction. The mobilization is performed in a slow, rhythmic manner for several minutes.

Mobilization of the First Rib: Costovertebral Joint (Figure 5–71)

Position of the Patient

The patient lies supine with the arms alongside the body. For the same reasons mentioned in describing the first rib mobility test, the first rib is mobilized with the patient's head in a neutral position. The head can be supported on a small pillow, depending on the amount of thoracic kyphosis.

Position of the Therapist

The therapist sits or stands at the head of the treatment table. If the patient's left side is to be treated, the therapist uses the left hand to perform the mobilization. The therapist

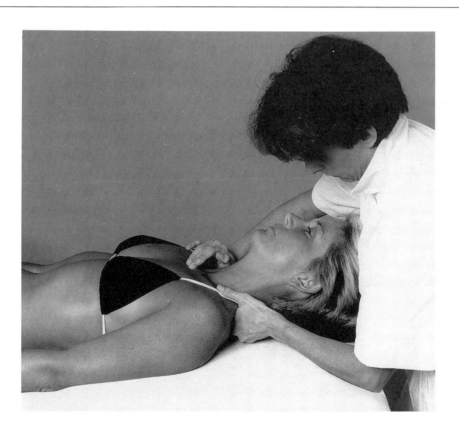

Figure 5–71

places the radial side of the index finger's middle phalanx on the cranial aspect of the first rib's posterior angle. The wrist is held in slight ulnar deviation, the forearm is held in slight supination, and the elbow is flexed approximately 90°.

Performance

While the patient exhales as deeply as possible, the first rib is brought into a caudal, ventral, and contralateral direction. The patient is then asked to stomach-breathe; in this way the first rib hardly moves, and the mobilization can be maintained for several seconds or minutes. The index finger of the opposite hand palpates the first rib between the sternal end of the clavicle and the second rib (which is found directly lateral to the sternal manubrium).

Mobilization of the First Rib: Costovertebral Joint with Simultaneous Stretching of the Scalene Muscles
(Figures 5–72A and 5–72B)

Position of the Patient

The patient lies supine, with the head over the end of the table. The arms rest alongside the body.

Position of the Therapist

The therapist sits or stands at the head of the treatment table. If the left side is to be treated, the therapist's right hand grasps the patient's occiput. The patient's head rests on the therapist's forearm and is held between the forearm and trunk. The upper cervical spine is stabilized by positioning it in flexion.

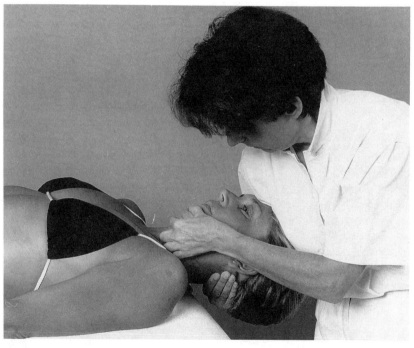

Figure 5–72A

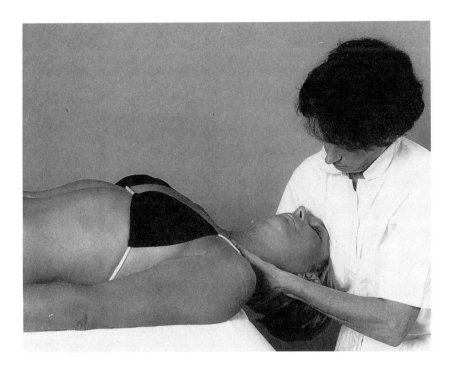

Figure 5–72B

This is done by pulling on the occiput and simultaneously pushing the forehead (with the anterior aspect of the right shoulder) and the chin (with the other hand) (Figure 5–72A). The radial side of the left index finger's proximal phalanx is then placed on the cranial aspect of the first rib's posterior angle.

Performance

Dorsal glide (flex C-1-2-3)
The head is very gradually (with respect for pain and muscle splinting) brought into extension, sidebend ~~toward~~ *away* the side being treated, and contralateral rotation.* The head is then held in this position while the first rib is mobilized in a caudal, ventral, and con-

tralateral direction (Figure 5–72B). During the mobilization, the cervical spine is held in slight (protective) traction.

Self-Stretch of the Scalene Muscles
(Figures 5–73A–E)

Position of the Patient

The patient sits on the treatment table or on a chair, with a large towel or bedsheet, folded, over the shoulder of the affected side. The patient sits on one end of the towel and holds the other end firmly with both hands. In so doing, the first rib is fixed in a caudal direction.

* toward painful side.

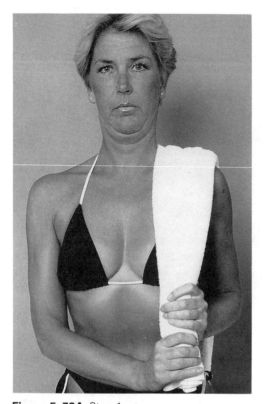

Figure 5–73A Step 1.

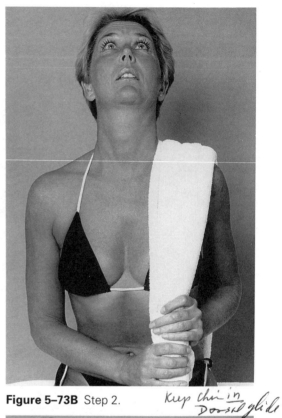

Figure 5–73B Step 2. *Keep chin in Dorsal glide*

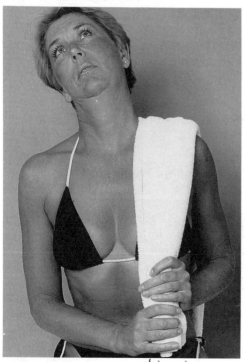

Figure 5–73C Step 3. *chin in D.G. Contra SB —*

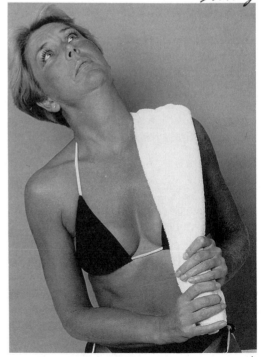

Figure 5–73D Step 4. *add rotation* *Keep chin down or look down.*

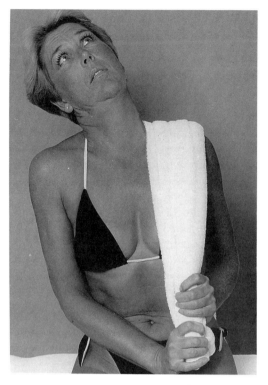

Figure 5–73E Step 5.   *Chin down,*

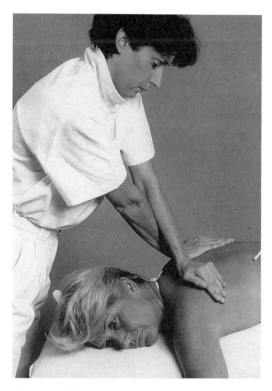

Figure 5–74

Performance

Step 1 (Figure 5–73A). The patient pulls the chin in as far as possible.

Step 2 (Figure 5–73B). Keeping the chin in, the patient brings the head as far as possible into extension.

Step 3 (Figure 5–73C). While maintaining this position (from steps 1 and 2), the patient now performs a sidebend away from the side to be stretched.

Step 4 (Figure 5–73D). From this position, the patient then rotates the head in the direction of the side being stretched.

Step 5 (Figure 5–73E). To stretch the scalene muscles, the patient is instructed to exhale deeply and at the same time to pull the towel downward, bringing the first rib into an even more caudal position.

Step 6. The patient should then stomach-breathe for 20 to 60 seconds to maintain the stretch. If paresthesia or more than a slight in-

40⁺.

crease in pain arises, then the exercise should be stopped.   *Several x/day.*

Mobilization of Ribs 1 through 6: Costotransverse Joints (Figure 5–74)

Position of the Patient

The patient lies prone with the arms resting alongside the body. Depending on the amount of the patient's thoracic kyphosis, the head of the table can be lowered, or a very firm pillow can be placed under the thorax. The patient's head is rotated toward the side to be treated.

Position of the Therapist

The therapist stands at the head of the treatment table.

Performance

The therapist positions the patient's trunk in side flexion toward the side to be treated.

To make the upper ribs more accessible to palpation, the arm on that side hangs over the edge of the table, bringing the scapula into protraction.

If the left side is to be treated, the therapist places the hypothenar eminence of the left hand on the posterior angle of the rib to be mobilized. The hypothenar eminence of the other hand fixes the transverse processes of the corresponding vertebrae on the opposite side. The direction of the mobilization is perpendicular to the local kyphosis and slightly lateral.

Mobilization into Inspiration of Ribs 2 through 6: Costovertebral Joints
(Figures 5–75A and 5–75B)

Position of the Patient

The patient lies supine, with the arms resting alongside the body and the head in a neutral position.

Position of the Therapist

The therapist stands at the head of the treatment table at the patient's affected side.

Performance

If the right side is to be treated, the radial side of the therapist's right metacarpophalangeal II joint and index finger (or the thenar eminence) hooks against the cranial aspect of the rib lying caudal to the affected rib. The placement of the hand on the rib is lateral to the rib cartilage and ventral on the thorax. While the therapist monitors and prevents any cranial movement of the rib, the patient brings the right arm as far as possible into elevation through flexion. The patient's arm is fixed between the therapist's upper arm and trunk.

Phase 1. While preventing the caudal rib from moving in a cranial direction, the therapist mobilizes the affected rib into inspiration

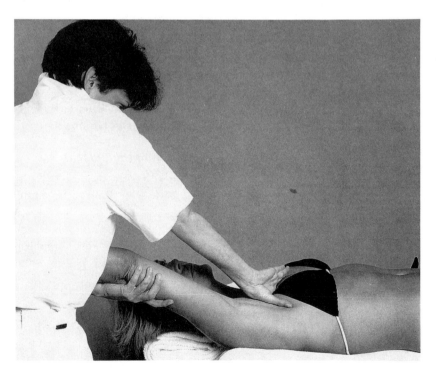

Figure 5–75A Initial position.

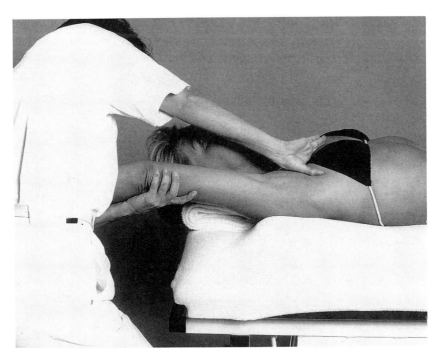

Figure 5–75B End position.

by passively bringing the patient's arm slowly and rhythmically farther into elevation (Figure 5–75A).

Phase 2. Now the patient is instructed to inhale deeply (emphasizing chest-breathing), while the therapist holds the caudal rib in its exhalation position. Simultaneously, elevation of the affected rib is promoted when the therapist brings the patient's arm even farther into elevation. During the mobilization, the patient should stomach-breathe in a relaxed manner.

Phase 3. While maintaining the maximal elevation of the arm, the therapist asks the patient to exhale maximally and accompanies the caudal movement of the rib, thereby increasing the intercostal space. After completely exhaling, the patient performs abdominal breathing while the therapist holds the rib in its new caudal position.

Note: In order to intensify the mobilization, a small pillow or towel can be placed underneath the scapula, allowing the patient's arm to be brought into even more elevation.

Mobilization into Expiration of Ribs 2 through 6: Costovertebral Joints
(Figure 5–76)

Position of the Patient

The patient lies supine with the arms resting alongside the body and the head in a neutral position.

Position of the Therapist

The therapist stands at the head of the treatment table at the patient's affected side.

Performance

If the right side is to be treated, the radial side of the therapist's right metacarpophalangeal II joint (or the thenar eminence) hooks against the cranial aspect of the af-

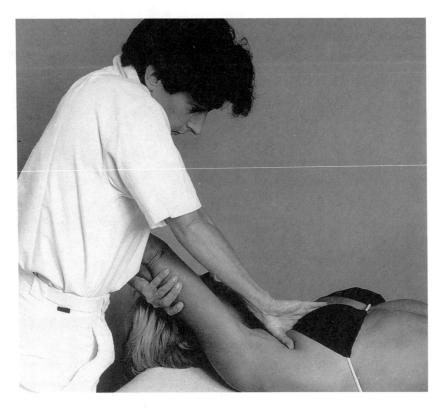

Figure 5–76

fected rib. The placement of the hand on the rib is lateral to the rib cartilage and ventral on the thorax. Without pulling the affected rib farther cranial into inspiration (monitored by the therapist's right hand), the patient brings the right arm as far as possible into elevation through flexion. The patient's arm is fixed between the therapist's upper arm and trunk.

Phase 1. While maintaining the position of the patient's arm, the therapist mobilizes the affected rib caudally, in a slow, rhythmic manner.

Phase 2. Still maintaining the elevated position of the arm, the therapist asks the patient to exhale as deeply as possible. The therapist accompanies the rib in the direction of the exhalation and holds the rib in this position while the patient continues with stomach-breathing.

Phase 3. While fixing the affected rib, the therapist instructs the patient to inhale deeply and at the same time tries to maintain the caudal position of the rib. During this inhalation, the therapist also increases the arm elevation, thereby stretching the intercostal structures.

Mobilization of Ribs 7 through 10: Costotransverse Joints
(Figure 5–77)

Position of the Patient

The patient lies prone, with the arms resting alongside the body. Depending on the amount of the patient's thoracic kyphosis, the head of the table can be lowered, or a very firm pillow can be placed under the thorax.

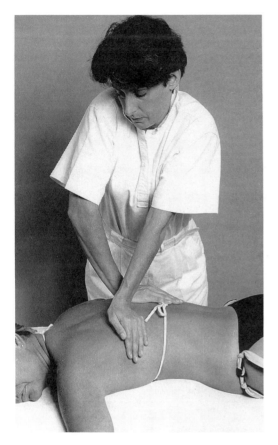

Figure 5–77

The patient's head is rotated toward the side to be treated.

Position of the Therapist

The therapist stands next to the patient, opposite the side to be treated.

Performance

The therapist positions the patient's trunk in sidebend toward the side to be treated. To make the upper ribs more accessible to palpation, the arm on that side hangs over the edge of the table, bringing the scapula into protraction. If the left side is to be treated, the therapist places the hypothenar eminence of the

left hand on the posterior angle of the rib to be mobilized. The hypothenar eminence of the other hand fixes the transverse processes of the corresponding vertebrae on the opposite side. The mobilization is performed in a ventral, lateral, and cranial direction.

Mobilization into Inspiration of Ribs 7 through 10: Costovertebral Joints
(Figure 5–78)

Position of the Patient

The patient lies on the nonaffected side, with the head in neutral (supported on a pillow).

Position of the Therapist

The therapist stands behind the patient at the head of the treatment table.

Performance

If the right side is to be treated, the radial side of the therapist's right metacarpophalangeal II joint and index finger (or the thenar eminence) hooks against the cranial aspect of the rib lying caudal to the affected rib. While the therapist monitors and prevents any cranial movement of the rib, the patient brings the right arm as far as possible in elevation through abduction. The patient's arm is fixed between the therapist's upper arm and trunk.

Phase 1. While preventing the caudal rib from moving in a cranial direction, the therapist mobilizes the affected rib into inspiration by passively bringing the patient's arm slowly and rhythmically farther into elevation.

Phase 2. Now the patient is instructed to inhale deeply (emphasizing chest breathing) while the therapist holds the caudal rib in its exhalation position. Simultaneously, elevation of the affected rib is promoted when the therapist brings the patient's arm even far-

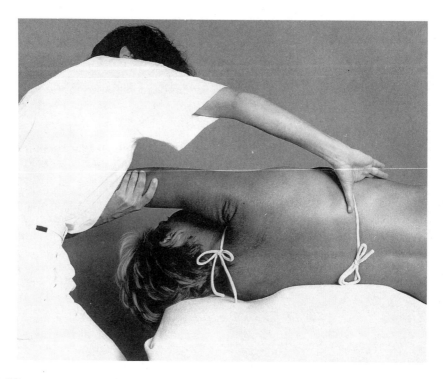

Figure 5–78

or hypo thenar,

ther into elevation. During the mobilization, the patient should stomach-breathe in a relaxed manner.

Phase 3. While maintaining the maximal elevation of the arm, the therapist asks the patient to exhale maximally and accompanies the caudal movement of the rib, thereby increasing the intercostal space. After completely exhaling, the patient performs abdominal breathing while the therapist holds the rib in its new caudal position.

Mobilization into Expiration of Ribs 7 through 10: Costovertebral Joints
(Figure 5–79)

Position of the Patient

The patient lies on the nonaffected side, with the head in a neutral position (supported on a pillow). The hip of the top leg is positioned in extension and slight adduction.

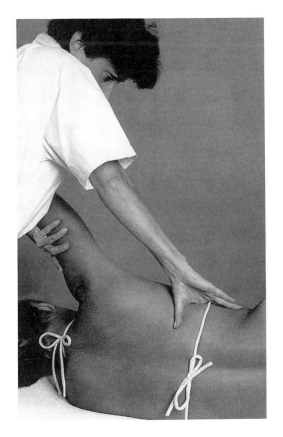

Figure 5–79

Position of the Therapist

The therapist stands behind the patient at the head of the treatment table.

Performance

If the right side is to be treated, the radial side of the therapist's right metacarpophalangeal II joint (or the thenar eminence) hooks against the cranial aspect of the affected rib. Without pulling the affected rib farther cranial into inspiration (monitored by the therapist's right hand), the patient brings the right arm as far as possible into elevation through abduction. The patient's arm is fixed between the therapist's upper arm and trunk.

Phase 1. While maintaining the position of the patient's arm, the therapist mobilizes the affected rib caudally in a slow, rhythmic manner.

Phase 2. Still maintaining the elevated position of the arm, the therapist asks the patient to exhale as deeply as possible. The therapist accompanies the rib in the direction of the exhalation and holds the rib in this position while the patient continues with stomach-breathing.

Phase 3. While fixing the affected rib, the therapist instructs the patient to inhale deeply and at the same time tries to maintain the caudal position of the rib. During this inhalation, the therapist also increases the arm elevation, thereby stretching the intercostal structures.

REFERENCES

1. Dommisse GF. The blood supply of the spinal cord. *J Bone Joint Surg [Br]*. 1974;56:225.

2. Vrettos XC, Wyke BD. Articular reflexogenic systems in the costovertebral joints. *J Bone Joint Surg [Br]*. 1974;56:382.

3. White AA. Analysis of the mechanics of the thoracic spine in man. *Acta Orthop Scand Suppl*. 1969;127.

4. Andriachi T, Schultz A, Belytschko T, Galante J. A model for studies of mechanical interactions between the human spine and rib cage. *J Biomech*. 1974;7:497–507.

5. Carson J, Gumpert J, Jefferson A. Diagnosis and treatment of thoracic intervertebral disc protrusions. *J Neurol Neurosurg Psychiatry*. 1971;34:68–77.

6. Fidler MW, Goedhart ZD. Excision of prolapse of thoracic intervertebral disc. *J Bone Joint Surg [Br]*. 1984;66:518–522.

7. Jansen BRH. Spondylodiscitis: een onderzoek naar de mogelijkheden van haematogene ontsteking van de tussenwervelschijf. Delft, Netherlands: WD Meinema; 1977. Thesis.

8. Henke G. *Rückenverkrümmungen bei Jugendlichen*. Bern, Switzerland: Verlag Hans Huber; 1982.

9. Bradford DS, Brown DM, Moe JH, Winter RB, Jowsey J. Scheuermann's kyphosis: a form of osteoporosis? *Clin Orthop*. 1976;118:10–15.

10. Swärd F, Hellstrom M, Jacobson B, Pëterson L. Back pain and radiologic changes in the thoraco-lumbar spine of athletes. *Spine.* 1990;15:124–128.

11. Aufdemkampe G. Opvattingen over skoliose in 100 jaar "Tijdschrift." *Ned Tijdschr Fysiother.* 1990;100:226–242.

12. van der Korst JK. *Gewrichtsziekten.* Utrecht: Bohn, Scheltema & Holkema; 1984.

13. deMorages JM, Kierland RR. The outcome of patients with herpes zoster. *Arch Dermatol Syphilol.* 1957;75:193.

SUGGESTED READING

Andrew T, Piggott H. Growth arrest for progressive scoliosis: combined anterior and posterior fusion of the convexity. *J Bone Joint Surg [Br].* 1985;67:193–197.

Archer IA, Dickson RA. Stature and idiopathic scoliosis: a prospective study. *J Bone Joint Surg [Br].* 1985;67:185–188.

Barker ME. Manipulation in general medical practice for thoracic pain syndromes. *Br Osteopathic J.* 1983;15:95–97.

Bergsmann O, Eder M. *Funktionelle Pathologie und Klinik der Wirbelsäule, Band 2: Funktionelle Pathologie und Klinik der Brustwirbelsäule.* Stuttgart: Gustav Fischer Verlag; 1982.

Bohlman HH, Zdeblick TA. Anterior excision of herniated thoracic discs. *J Bone Joint Surg [Am].* 1988;70:1038–1047.

Bolender NF, Schönström NSR, Spengler DM. Role of computed tomography and myelography in the diagnosis of central spinal stenosis. *J Bone Joint Surg [Am].* 1985;67:240–246.

Cats A. De aandoeningen van de rug (1): juveniele kyfose (morbus Scheuermann). *Reuma Wereldwijd.* 1984; 8(2):1–4.

Cats A. De aandoening van de rug (2): osteoporose. *Reuma Wereldwijd.* 1984;8(3):1–4.

Cats A. De aandoening van de rug (3): spondylosis hyperostotica. *Reuma Wereldwijd.* 1984;8(4):1–5.

Citron N, Edgar MA, Sheehy J, Thomas DGT. Intramedullary spinal cord tumours presenting as scoliosis. *J Bone Joint Surg [Br].* 1984;66:513–517.

Cyriax J. Diagnosis of somatic thoracic disorders. Presented at the British Association of Manipulative Medicine Symposium; March 12, 1967; Royal Army Medical College, Westminster, London.

Daruwalla JS, Balasubramaniam P. Moiré topography in scoliosis: its accuracy in detecting the site and size of the curve. *J Bone Joint Surg [Br].* 1985;67:211–214.

Daruwalla JS, Balasubramaniam P, Chay SO, Rajan U, Lee HP. Idiopathic scoliosis: prevalence and ethnic distribution in Singapore schoolchildren. *J Bone Joint Surg [Br].* 1985;67:182–184.

Deacon P, Berkin CR, Dickson RA. Combined idiopathic kyphosis and scoliosis: an analysis of the lateral spinal curvatures associated with Scheuermann's disease. *J Bone Joint Surg [Br].* 1985;67:189–192.

Deacon P, Flood BM, Dickson RA. Idiopathic scoliosis in three dimensions: a radiographic and morphometric analysis. *J Bone Joint Surg [Br].* 1984;66:509–512.

Defesche HFHG, Broere G. He spinale hematoom. *Ned Tijdschr Geneeskd.* 1980;124:157–160.

Dickson RA. Conservative treatment for idiopathic scoliosis. *J Bone Joint Surg [Br].* 1985;67:176–181.

Ditton JN. Intralesional triamcinolone-bupivacaine in the treatment of post-herpetic neuralgia. *Problems in Pain.* Toronto: Pergamon Press; 1980:262–266.

Edgar MA. To brace or not to brace? *J Bone Joint Surg [Br].* 1985;67:173–174.

Ernst WK. Angeborene und konstitutionelle Fehlformierungen im Thoraxbereich im Kindesalter. *Krankengymnastik.* 1988;40:379–382.

Fisk JW, Baigent ML, Hill PD. Incidence of Scheuermann's disease: preliminary report. *Am J Phys Med.* 1982;61:32–35.

Flatley TJ, Anderson MH, Anast GT. Spinal instability due to malignant disease: treatment by segmental spinal stabilization. *J Bone Joint Surg [Am].* 1984;66:47–52.

Fredrickson BE, Baker D, McHolick WJ, Yuan HA, Lubicky JP. The natural history of spondylolysis and spondylolisthesis. *J Bone Joint Surg [Am].* 1984;66:699–707.

Hsu LCS, Lee PC, Leong JCY. Dystrophic spinal deformities in neurofibromatosis: treatment by anterior and posterior fusion. *J Bone Joint Surg [Br].* 1984;66:495–499.

Ker NB, Jones CB. Tumors of the cauda equina: the problem of differential diagnosis. *J Bone Joint Surg [Br].* 1985;67:358–362.

Krämer J. *Bandscheibenbedingte Erkrankungen.* Stuttgart: Georg Thieme Verlag; 1978.

Lewith GT, Field J, Machin D. Acupuncture compared with placebo in post-herpetic pain. *Pain.* 1983;17:361–368.

Maigne R. Low back pain of thoracolumbar origin. *Arch Phys Med Rehabil.* 1980;61:389–394.

Muller JWT. Rugpijn. *Ned Tijdschr Geneeskd.* 1980;124: 1857–1860.

Nötges A. Differentialdiagnose und Therapie des Thoraxschmerzes aus kardiologischer Sicht. *Krankengymnastik.* 1988;40:377–378.

Panjabi MM, Brand RA, White AA. Mechanical properties of the human thoracic spine. *J Bone Joint Surg [Am].* 1976;58:642–652.

Papaioannou T. Scoliosis associated with limb-length inequality. *J Bone Joint Surg [Am].* 1982;64:59–62.

Pincott JR, Davies JS, Taffs LF. Scoliosis caused by section of dorsal spinal nerve roots. *J Bone Joint Surg [Br].* 1984;66:27–29.

Roberts AP, Connor AN, Tolmie JL, Connor JM. Spondylothoracic and spondylocostal dysostosis. *J Bone Joint Surg [Br].* 1988;70:123–126.

Sachs B, Bradford D, Winter R, Lonstein J, Moe J, Willson S. Scheuermann kyphosis: follow-up of Milwaukee-brace treatment. *J Bone Joint Surg [Am].* 1987;69: 50–57.

Savini R, Gherlinzoni F, Morandi M, Neff JR, Picci P. Surgical treatment of giant-cell tumor of the spine: the experience at the Istituto Ortopedico Rizzoli. *J Bone Joint Surg [Am].* 1983;65:1283–1330.

Siegal T, Tiqva P, Siegal T. Vertebral body resection for epidural compression by malignant tumors: results of forty-seven consecutive operative procedures. *J Bone Joint Surg [Am].* 1985;67:357–382.

Sobotta J, Becker H. *Atlas der Anatomie des Menschen.* Munich: Urban & Schwarzenberg; 1972.

Waddell G. Psychological Evaluation. Presented at the Lumbar Spine Instructional Course, organized by the International Society for the Study of the Lumbar Spine; May 11, 1991; Zürich, Switzerland.

Waddell G, Reilly S, Torsney B, et al. Assessment of the outcome of low back surgery. *J Bone Joint Surg [Br].* 1988;70:723–727.

Welter HF, Thetter O, Schweiberer L. Kompressionssyndrome der oberen Thoraxapertur. *Muench Med Wochenschr.* 1984;126:1122–1125.

Williams PL, Warrick R, Dyson M, Bannister LH, eds. *Gray's Anatomy.* New York: Churchill Livingstone; 1989.

Wyke B. Morphological and functional features of the innervation of the costovertebral joints. *Folia Morphol.* 1975;23:296–305.

Wyke B. The neurological basis of thoracic spinal pain. *Rheumatol Phys Med.* 1970;10:356–367.

Yates D, Jenner J. Lage rugpijn—welke oorzaak? *Mod Med.* January 1980:42–45.

THORACIC SPINE REVIEW QUESTIONS

1. What is the capsular pattern of the thoracic spine?
2. In the thoracic postural syndrome, when do patients have *relief* of their pain?
3. What is the most common cause of a thoracic posterolateral disc protrusion?
4. What is the most significant clinical difference between a posterolateral disc protrusion and a posterolateral disc prolapse?
5. What neurological findings are most often present in a posterolateral disc prolapse?
6. With which imaging technique can one best evaluate a posterolateral disc prolapse?
7. Why can a posterolateral disc prolapse be so dangerous?
8. In which age group is spondylodiscitis most frequently seen?
9. From which primary tumors are metastases in the thoracic spine most often seen?
10. Where is the characteristic radiation of pain that occurs in incidence of a thoracic spondylodiscitis?
11. Which pathology should be suspected with findings of pain on local percussion and pain when falling back onto the heels from a tiptoe position?
12. Which disorders in the thoracic spine manifest a limitation of motion in the capsular pattern?
13. What is the etiology of a spondylodiscitis?
14. Spontaneous compression fractures in the thoracic spine are seen most in which age group? Are they seen more often in males or females?
15. What is the usual cause of a traumatic compression fracture in the lower thoracic spine?
16. In osteoporosis, why is extension of the thoracic spine often painful and limited?
17. With which imaging technique can one best evaluate a traumatic compression fracture?
18. A manubriosternal joint arthritis is seen most frequently in which age group?
19. Which disorders are seen most often in the thoracic spine?
20. What is the treatment of choice for an arthritis of the manubriosternal joint?
21. List four disorders of the thoracic spine in which pain is provoked with coughing, sneezing, and straining.
22. With which imaging technique can one best visualize manubriosternal joint arthritis?
23. In Tietze's syndrome, where is the pain and swelling usually localized?
24. Which muscle lesions could lead one to think that there is a problem in the thoracic spine?
25. What is most often the cause of an intercostal neuralgia?
26. In thoracic spine pain, pathology from which structures should always be ruled out first?
27. At what age does Scheuermann's disease usually begin?
28. Posterocentral disc prolapses of the thoracic spine are seen most often at which level?
29. From where does upper thoracic pain usually originate?
30. What is the physiological coupling of motion in the midthoracic region?

THORACIC SPINE REVIEW ANSWERS

1. Symmetrical limitation of rotations.
2. Relief of pain is experienced during movement and while lying down. Often in the chronic stage, pain relief is achieved only after a few hours of lying down.
3. A traumatic axial loading of the thoracic spine.
4. In a posterolateral disc prolapse, an intercostal neuralgia is usually manifested.
5. None.
6. By means of a CT scan or MRI.
7. In the thoracic spine, the spinal cord has little room. Thus, prolapses of the disc relatively quickly result in compression of the spinal cord.
8. Over age 50 years.
9. Bronchial carcinoma and Pancoast tumor.
10. The pain radiates into the side and/or into the legs.
11. Inflammation and tumors.
12. Tumors, inflammations, and severe degenerative changes.
13. Caused by the hematogenic spreading of a microorganism to the disc.
14. In women over age 60 years.
15. As the result of a traumatic axial load on the flexed vertebral column.
16. Because of the collapse of the vertebrae, the spinous processes lie closer to each other. During extension, a painful compression can occur:" kissing spine" also called Baastrup syndrome.
17. By means of a CT scan.
18. Between ages 20 and 45 years.
19. The thoracic postural syndrome and Scheuermann's disease.
20. An injection with a corticosteroid.
21. Posterolateral disc prolapse, posterocentral disc prolapse, manubriosternal arthritis, and Tietze's syndrome.
22. By means of a technetium scan (bone scan).
23. At the level of the costosternal cartilage of the second rib, left more often than right.
24. Lesions of the intercostal muscles, the pectoralis major, and the latissimus dorsi.
25. Herpes zoster.
26. Internal organs.
27. At the age of 11 years.
28. In the lower thoracic region.
29. Of cervical origin.
30. For flexion, the coupling is ipsilateral. For extension, the coupling varies, depending on the flexibility of the midthoracic spine. In some people, it is an ipsilateral coupling; in others, the coupling is contralateral.

6

Cervical Spine

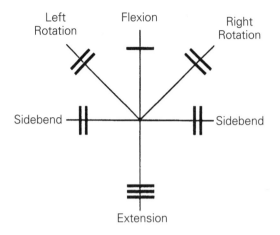

Figure 6–1A Capsular Pattern

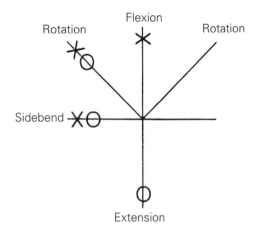

```
X = Flexion, ipsilateral coupling
O = Extension, ipsilateral coupling
```

Figure 6–1B Coupled Movements.

• Combined Motions (not illustrated). A movement is combined when one of the motions in the coupled movement pattern is changed.

6.1   FUNCTIONAL ANATOMY

The cervical spine is the most mobile region of the spinal column. The connection of the cervical spine with the head leads to significant functional consequences in this area. The center of gravity of the head lies relatively forward. This arrangement and the necessity for substantial mobility of the head place a high demand on both the stability and on the mobility of the cervical spine. Thus this section on functional anatomy of the cervical spine particularly illustrates the kinematics of this region. Separate attention is given to the load on the cervical spine in relation to the position of the head.

CERVICAL VERTEBRAL COLUMN

The cervical vertebrae are the smallest vertebrae of the spinal column. They are characterized by small, wide bodies (Figure 6–2). The vertebral foramen is proportionately large and triangular in form. The pedicles project dorsolaterally, and from the articular processes the laminae run in a dorsomedial direction.

The perforated transverse process is typical of the cervical vertebra. Together, these foramina transversaria form a canal through which the vertebral arteries run to the skull. The spinous process lies on the dorsal aspect of the cervical vertebra, which is short and (to a greater or lesser degree) split. Articular processes (superior and inferior) are also found on the vertebra's dorsal aspect. The superior articular process of one cervical vertebra forms a zygapophyseal joint with the inferior articular process of the adjacent cranial vertebra (except for the joints between C1 and the occiput).

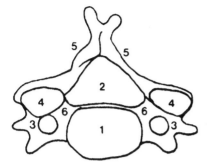

Figure 6–2 Cervical vertebra (C5): cranial view. *1*, Body; *2*, vertebral foramen; *3*, transverse foramen; *4*, superior articular process; *5*, lamina; *6*, pedicle.

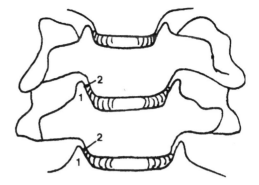

Figure 6–3 Ventral view of two cervical vertebrae (C3-4). *1*, Uncinate process; *2*, uncovertebral joint.

Between the ages of 5 and 10 years, the so-called uncinate processes form at the dorsolateral sides of the third to the seventh cervical vertebral bodies. These uncinate processes extend in a cranial direction (Figure 6–3). During this age period, the uncinate processes form a joint line, which initially is bordered medially by the intervertebral disc. At approximately 10 years of age, these lines lengthen, extending into the intervertebral disc. Töndury[1] describes that an actual split in the disc takes place. Ingrowth of a synovial membrane then occurs, and thus a true synovial joint is formed. According to Töndury, meniscoid structures are also found in these joints (Figure 6–4).

A number of longitudinal ligamentous structures run along the ventral and dorsal aspects of the cervical vertebral column. These ligaments run from the cervical spine, all the way to the lumbar spine. (See Chapter 4, Lumbar Spine, Functional Anatomy.) At the level of the atlas, the posterior longitudinal ligament becomes the tectorial membrane (membrana tectoria) (Figure 6–5).

Occiput, Atlas, and Axis

The atlas, the bearer of the head, is different from the other vertebrae in that it does not have a vertebral body. A true spinous process is also absent. On each side of the lateral cranial aspect of the vertebra are two oval facets, covered with cartilage—the joint surfaces for the condyles from the occiput. In the middle, the joint surfaces are relatively narrow; sometimes the cartilage here is absent, in which case the joint surface then consists of two separate parts (Figure 6–6).

The transverse processes are very long and, as with the other cervical vertebrae, are perforated for the passage of the vertebral arteries. On each cranial side of the posterior arch is a groove (and in some instances a "tunnel") for the vertebral artery. Here the vertebral artery makes a second loop; the first loop is between C1 and C2 and is considerably smaller.

The axis, the second cervical vertebra, forms the pivot around which the atlas and thus also the head turn (Figure 6–7). For this purpose, the axis possesses a large tooth-shaped structure, the dens, which forms almost a right angle to the pedicles. On its ventral side, the dens (also called the odontoid process) forms a joint with the atlas. This part of the dens is covered with cartilage, as is its dorsal aspect, where it articulates with the transverse ligament. On each side of the cranial aspect of the axis, joint surfaces for the atlas are found. These joint facets are convex in a cranial direction.

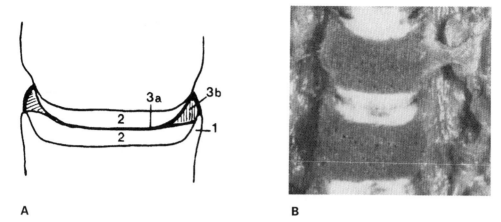

Figure 6–4 The uncovertebral joint. **A**, Schematic section. The synovial membrane grows medially into the disc, ultimately dividing the intervertebral disc into two pieces. **1**, Uncinate process; **2**, intervertebral disc; **3a**, capsule of the uncovertebral joint; **3b**, uncovertebral joint cavity. **B**, Section of the midcervical spine in a 27-year-old patient.[2] The intervertebral disc of C5-6 is in two separate parts.

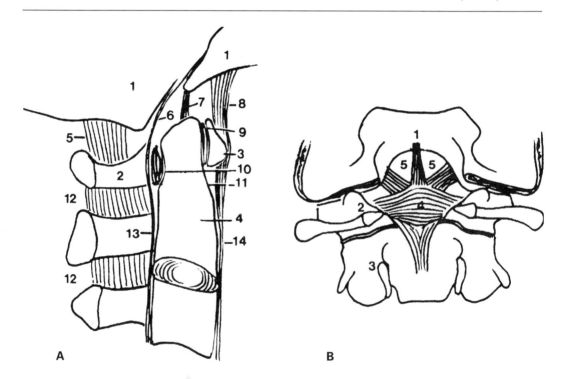

Figure 6–5 Cervical ligaments. **A**, Median sagittal section through the occiput and the first three cervical vertebrae. **1**, Occiput; **2**, posterior arch of the atlas; **3**, anterior arch of the atlas; **4**, dens axis (odontoid process); **5**, posterior atlanto-occipital membrane; **6**, tectorial membrane; **7**, apical ligament of the dens; **8**, anterior antlanto-occipital membrane; **9**, joint between the dens axis and the anterior arch of the atlas; **10**, joint between the dens axis and the transverse ligament of the atlas; **11**, transverse ligament; **12**, ligamentum flavum; **13**, posterior longitudinal ligament; **14**, anterior longitudinal ligament. **B**, Cruciform ligament. **1**, Occiput; **2**, posterior arch of the atlas; **3**, posterior arch of the axis; **4**, cruciform ligament; **5**, alar ligament.

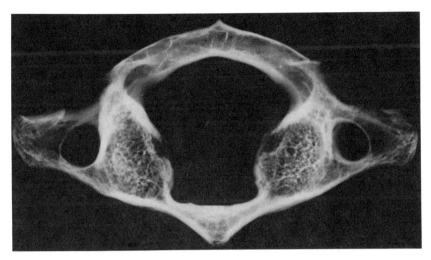

A

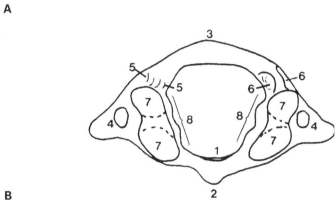

B

Figure 6–6 Atlas. **A**, Cranial view X-ray. **B**, Illustration of the cranial view. **1**, Facet for the dens; **2**, anterior tubercle; **3**, posterior tubercle; **4**, foramen transversarium; **5**, groove for vertebral artery; **6**, vertebral artery canal (when the groove is enclosed); **7**, cartilage-covered part of the superior articular facet (joint surfaces for the condyles of the occiput); **8**, lateral mass.

Joints

Between the occiput and the atlas (C0-1), bilaterally, lie joints with two axes. They are ellipsoid joints by which flexion-extension and sidebend of the head occur. Besides the joint capsule, the anterior atlanto-occipital membrane and the posterior atlanto-occipital membrane connect the head to the atlas.

The atlas and the axis (C1-2) are connected to each other in two ways, in the median plane and laterally. The median connection is called the median atlantoaxial joint, and the lateral connection is the lateral atlantoaxial joint (there are two of these). The median atlantoaxial joint consists of a ventral and a dorsal component. Ventrally, the dens has a connection with the ventral arch of the atlas by means of a synovial joint. On the dorsal side, the dens articulates with the transverse ligament, which is the lower part of the cruciform ligament. The lateral atlantoaxial connections are synovial joints. Both joint partners are biconvex in the parasagittal plane. In the frontal plane, however, the bony configura-

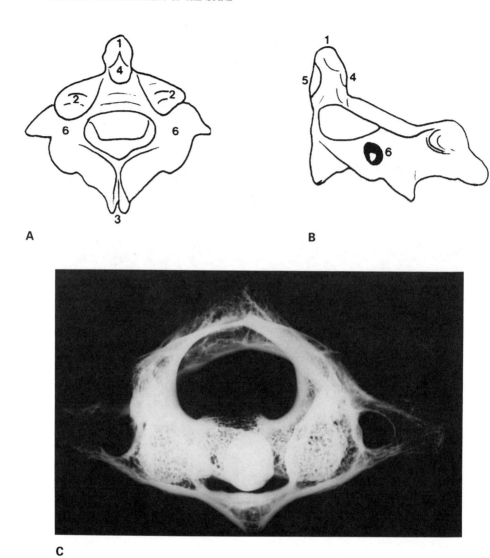

Figure 6–7 Axis. **A**, Cranial view. **B**, Lateral view. **1**, Dens (odontoid process); **2**, superior articular facet (joint surface for the atlas); **3**, spinous process; **4**, groove for the transverse ligament of the atlas (joint surface for the transverse ligament); **5**, facet for the anterior arch of the atlas (joint surface for the atlas); **6**, foramen transversarium. **C**, Cranial view X-ray of the atlas and the axis.

tion demonstrates a slight biconcavity (Figure 6–8).

Strictly speaking, there is no joint between the dens and the occiput. However, there are four strong ligamentous connections: the apical ligament, the tectorial membrane, and the two alar ligaments (Figure 6–5B).

Muscles

Accessory muscles from the large longitudinal muscle system (the longissimus, semispinalis, and splenius capitis) run between the first two cervical vertebrae and the head, along with a number of short muscles (the rectus capitis posterior minor and major and the superior oblique). All of the muscles are involved in maintaining the upright orientation of the head (Figure 6–9) The inferior oblique muscle connects the axis and the atlas; this muscle has a significant (ipsilateral) rotatory effect. The rectus capitis posterior major and minor and the superior and inferior oblique muscles are all innervated by the suboccipital nerve (the dorsal ramus from C1).

Kinematics

In discussing the movement of C0 to C2, didactically it is convenient to differentiate between C0-1 and C1-2. Although each of these segments never moves in isolation, the contribution of the two segments to the total movement is different. The following discussion is based on radiological examinations.[2–6]

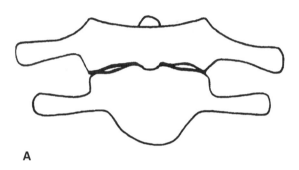

A

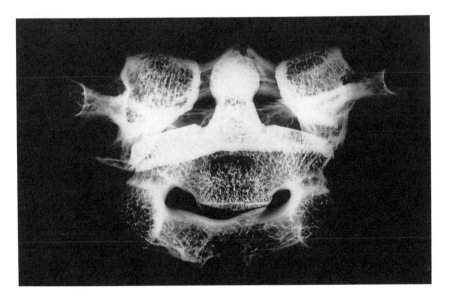

B

Figure 6–8 Atlantoaxial joints. **A**, Illustration of the ventral view; **B**, ventral view X-ray.

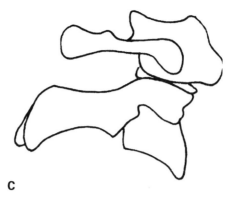

C

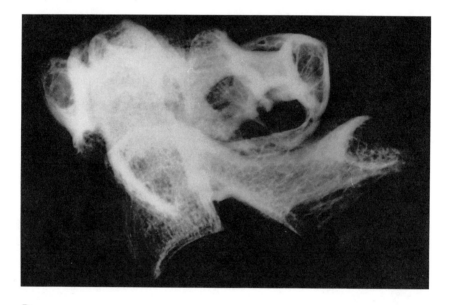

D

Figure 6–8 *C*, Illustration of the lateral view; *D*, lateral view X-ray.

C0-1. In normal movement, the range of motion of C0-1 is the greatest in the sagittal plane. Fielding[3] mentions a range of motion of 10° for flexion and 25° for extension. According to Schmorl and Junghanns,[7] approximately half the flexion-extension movement in the entire cervical spine takes place in the atlanto-occipital joint. The other half occurs in the general area of C1 to C7 (with the least

between C5 to C7). The movement between the head and the atlas is still not completely understood.

During forward bending of the head and the cervical spine, a remarkable phenomenon occurs.[5] Although one expects that the occiput and the dorsal aspect of the atlas arch should move away from each other during forward flexion, the opposite occurs. The occiput and

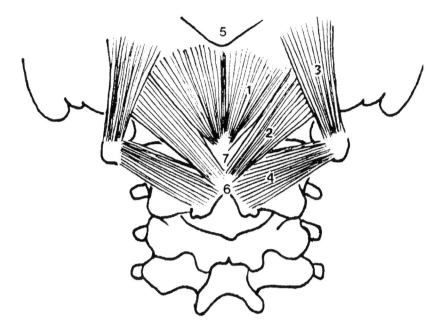

Figure 6–9 The short neck muscles. *1*, Rectus capitis posterior minor; *2*, rectus capitis posterior major; *3*, superior oblique; *4*, inferior oblique; *5*, occiput; *6*, axis; *7*, atlas.

atlas approach each other. This appears to happen in almost every normal vertebral column. Arlen[5] calls this phenomenon the "paradoxical tilt of the atlas" (Figure 6–10).

C1-2. In C1-2 only a small amount of flexion takes place (approximately 15°); however, the chief motion here is the rotation. Schmorl and Junghanns[7] indicate that of the total possible rotation in the cervical spine, approximately 50% occurs in the C1-2 segment. This is reinforced by White and Panjabi.[8] In 26 normal subjects varying between 21 and 26 years of age, Penning and Wilmink[9] found an average amount of rotation of 72.2° between C0 and T1 (the extremes varied from 61° to 84°). They also conclude that an average rotation of 40.5° between C1 and C2 occurs (varying from 29° to 47°); that is 55% of the total cervical rotation. The axis of rotation runs through the dens.[9]

The ventral surface of the dens has contact with the dorsal aspect of the anterior arch of the atlas. During flexion, this contact is disrupted; the dens and the atlas move away from each other. In adults, this distance is not larger than 3 mm, and in children not greater than 4 to 5 mm. In instances where a greater distance is present, one speaks of a "craniovertebral instability."

Kinematic Coupling in the C0 to C2 Region. In the region of C0 to C2, no isolated axial rotation can take place. Axial rotation is always coupled with sidebending. When the head performs a sidebending to the right in the C0 to C2 region, the spinous process of C2 turns left. In other words, C2 performs a right rotation. Because axial rotation of a segment is determined by the movement of the *cranial* vertebra of that segment, the coupled axial rotation is opposite to the initial sidebending.

In axial rotation of the head to the right, the head and atlas initially (during the first 30°) move together to the right in relation to the stable axis.[3] After the first 30°, however, the axis also rotates to the right (the spinous process moves to the left). The axial rotation of the axis to the right results in a coupled ipsilateral sidebending in the C2-3 segment. In order to maintain a pure axial rotation of the head, a left sidebending in C0 to C2 occurs. At the end of the movement, the occiput also rotates very slightly to the right in relation to the atlas.

The specific movement pattern of the occiput in relation to the atlas and the axis is based on tension of the alar ligaments. Because of these ligaments, the kinematic coupling C0-1, C1-2, and C0-2 is not ipsilateral (as in the remainder of the cervical spine), but contralateral.

C2 to C7

Intervertebral Discs

From the C2-3 segment caudally, the vertebral column has intervertebral discs. It is the disc particularly that makes movement in the spine possible. In the cervical spine, the discs amount to approximately one quarter of the total length. In adults, it is assumed that the discs in the cervical vertebral column have minimal to no vascularization. In any case, the nucleus is avascular. It has long been assumed that the discs are not innervated. However, Bogduk et al[10] found that bifurcations of the vertebral nerve and the sinuvertebral nerve (recurrent nerve) penetrate the cervical disc annulus from lateral and dorsal, re-

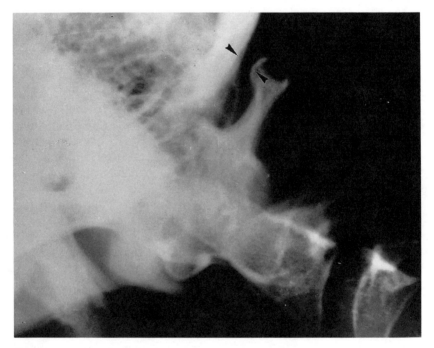

A

Figure 6–10 "Paradoxical tilt" of the atlas. **A**, Maximal flexion. The distance between the posterior arch of the atlas and the occiput is small (arrowheads), while the distance between the atlas and the spinous process of the axis (difficult to see) has increased.

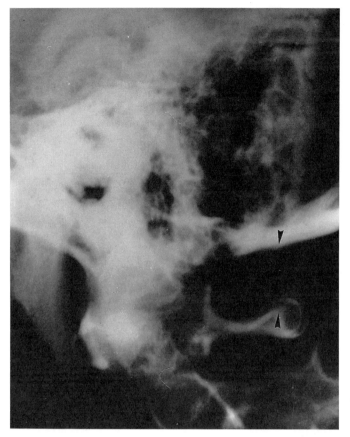

B

Figure 6–10 B Maximal extension. The distance between the posterior arch of the atlas and the occiput is large *(arrowheads),* while the distance between the atlas and the spinous process of the axis is small.

spectively. These branches innervate the outer third of the annulus. Thus according to Bogduk et al, disc lesions can be a primary cause of pain.

Zygapophyseal Joints

On the posterior aspect of the cervical vertebrae lie two superior articular processes and two inferior articular processes. They form joints with the adjacent cranial and caudal vertebrae, respectively (Figure 6–11). The capsule of these joints is rather loose except at the caudal aspect where the laxity of the capsule decreases.

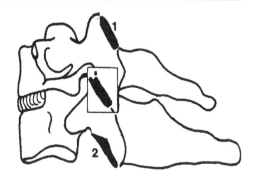

Figure 6–11 Zygapophyseal joint between two cervical vertebrae. The joint lies within the box. *1*, Superior articular process; *2*, inferior articular process.

The position of the joint surfaces in the frontal plane is nearly horizontal. In the parasagittal plane, the joint facets are oriented in such a way that when an imaginary line is drawn parallel to the joint surface, these lines converge cranially in the direction of the eyes. The facets of the upper disc-containing segments are oriented approximately 40° in relation to the transverse plane. The facets of the lower disc-containing segments are inclined approximately 65° in relation to the transverse plane. To a great extent, the position of these articular surfaces determines the movement possibilities of the cervical spine from C2 to C7.

The zygapophyseal joints contain so-called meniscoid folds, which have grown into the joint from the capsule. (This is similar to the presence of the alar plica in the knee joint.) It is still not clear whether or not these structures are innervated and thus can cause pain. Bogduk and Engel[11] state that pain does not occur through damage to the meniscus itself, but rather, for instance, because of a tearing of the meniscus from the capsule.

Uncovertebral Joints

The uncovertebral joints develop after birth.[12] They are fissures that form in the cervical intervertebral discs at the end of the first decade. The uncinate processes, which are present embryologically, are very flat in the first years of life. After approximately the age of 10, these processes become more prominent. At the same time, the lateral sides of the intervertebral discs between the uncinate processes fold in a lateral direction. Here, the fissures occur. (See also Figure 6–4.)

The uncovertebral joints are the most developed in the segments C2-3, C3-4, and C4-5. They are the least (and sometimes not at all) developed in the segments C5-6 and C6-7. As in the zygapophyseal joints, meniscoid structures are also found in the uncovertebral joints.

Kinematics

Penning and his colleagues[9,13] examined the rotation movement in 26 healthy subjects between the ages of 20 and 26. They found the following average amount of rotation per segment:

- C0-1   1.0°
- C1-2   40.5°
- C2-3   3.0°
- C3-4   6.5°
- C4-5   6.8°
- C5-6   6.9°
- C6-7   5.4°
- C7-T1   2.1°

The total amount of unilateral rotation averaged 72.2°. According to Penning and Wilmink, the instantaneous axis of rotation of the various movement segments lies in a plane perpendicular to the joint surfaces of the zygapophyseal joints. Although it is usually assumed that the coupling between rotation and sidebend is determined by the zygapophyseal joints, not only Hall[14] but also Penning and Wilmink[9] are of the opinion that the discs and the "uncovertebral joints" play a large role as well (Figure 6–12).

The uncinate processes are found on the dorsolateral aspect of the vertebral bodies. During sidebend one would expect a translation to occur in the same direction as the sidebend. On the ventral aspect of the cervical segment, this indeed happens. However, on the dorsal aspect this motion is hindered by the uncinate processes. Since the translation at the ventral aspect takes place without hindrance, the dorsal aspect translates in the opposite direction. The combination of these translations induces a rotation in the same direction as the sidebend.[9,14]

The uncinate processes also play a role in the flexion-extension motion of the cervical spine. According to Penning,[13] the axes for

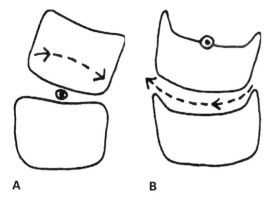

A   **B**

Figure 6–12 The uncinate process in kinematic coupling. **A**, On the ventral side of the cervical vertebrae, the uncinate processes are very small or nonexistent. In sidebend, a minimal translation occurs in the direction of the arrows. **B**, The uncinate processes are found chiefly on the dorsolateral aspects of the vertebrae. A kind of ball-and-socket situation occurs in which the upper vertebra translates in relation to the lower vertebra. This induces an ipsilateral rotation.

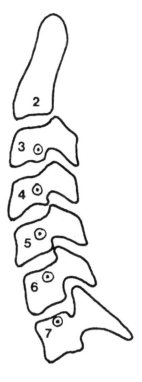

Figure 6–13 The centers of motion in C2-3 to C6-7.

flexion and extension are situated in different locations depending on the segment. The flexion-extension axis for C2-3 is located in the dorsocaudal part of C3; in C6-7 it is located in the middle of the cranial end-plate of C7 (Figure 6–13).

The values for the amount of flexion and extension vary with different age groups. In Table 6–1, the results of research performed by Markuske[15] and Buetti-Bauml[16] are represented.

Table 6–1 Average Amounts of Flexion-Extension in Different Age Groups

Flexion-Extension	3–6 Years[15]	11–14 Years[15]	20–38 Years[16]
C2-3	17°	17°	10.5°
C3-4	21°	22°	17°
C4-5	22°	26°	21°
C5-6	22°	26°	22.5°
C6-7	21°	23°	18°

Penning[13] constructed a mathematical "center of motion" from the (changing) instantaneous axes of rotation during flexion and extension. According to Penning, the fact that the "centers of motion" in the various segments are situated at different points is related to the difference in the movement patterns. At the level of C2-3, a kind of translation motion occurs, whereas between C6-7 there is more a rocking motion.

Here again the uncinate processes play a role. In Penning's opinion, a translation motion needs much more stability. This stability is achieved through larger uncinate processes. Indeed, generally speaking, the uncinate processes of C2-3 have the largest ventral-dorsal dimensions. Töndury[12] equates the uncinate processes to rails that guide the translation motion.

VASCULARIZATION

The vertebral arteries arise from the subclavian artery. From here both arteries run perpendicularly upward through the foraminae transversaria of C6 to C1. At the levels of C2-1 and C1-0, the arteries make a large loop in order to perforate the posterior atlanto-occipital membrane and then enter the skull via the foramen magnum. Ventral to the brain stem the vertebral arteries join together before reaching the basilar artery. Two vessels again arise from the basilar artery: the posterior cerebral arteries. The basilar artery drains into an arterial ring structure (the circle of Willis), which is also joined by the internal carotid arteries.

The vertebral arteries vascularize the cervical vertebral column along with the nerve structures in that area. The basilar artery is responsible for vascularization of the brain stem. In particular, the posterior cerebral arteries vascularize the occipital cortex (which has a function in the visual system).

Branches from the vertebral artery run dorsally to supply the zygapophyseal joints directly. The zygapophyseal joints are also indirectly vascularized by the vertebral artery through branches coming from the radicular arteries. The radicular arteries are segmentally organized vessels that also vascularize the spinal cord. On the dorsal and ventral aspects of the spinal cord, the radicular arteries anastomose with the vertically running anterior and posterior spinal arteries. Research from Dommisse[17] indicates that vascularization via the radicular arteries is significantly varied.

The venous drainage runs via the internal and external vertebral venous plexuses. From this plexus, the vertebral veins arise, which also run through the foramina transversaria of C1 to C6, and via the subclavian vein drain into the brachiocephalic vein.

INNERVATION

In the two upper cervical segments, the spinal nerves exit the vertebral column from directly dorsal of the zygapophyseal joints. In the other segments, they exit ventral to the zygapophyseal joints. In the cervical region, the nerve roots do not run as close to the intervertebral discs as in the lumbar spine. Instead, in the intervertebral foramina, the roots lie just ventromedial to the zygapophyseal joints and just dorsolateral to uncovertebral joints.

The nerve supply for the spinal column itself is organized in the form of networks, which include somatic nerves as well as branches from the autonomic ganglia. Together with afferent somatic nerves, efferent autonomic nerves form the so-called sinuvertebral nerve (also named the recurrent nerve or meningeal nerve). The sinuvertebral nerve runs back into the foramen and innervates structures in the vertebral canal, to include the dura mater, the posterior longitudinal ligament, and the capsules of the zygapophyseal joints. Each motion segment receives nerve fibers from approximately three adjacent segments.[18]

The autonomic innervation of the cervical spine is supplied by the three sympathetic cervical ganglia and by the parasympathetic fibers from the various cranial nerves.

LOAD ON THE CERVICAL SPINE IN RELATION TO POSITION OF THE HEAD

In upright standing, the spinal column forms three curves in the sagittal plane. At the levels of the cervical and lumbar spines, there is a ventral convexity (lordosis). At the level of the thoracic spine, there is a dorsal convexity (kyphosis).

Mechanically, it can be understood why the cervical lordosis is the optimal position for the upright head. The center of gravity of the head is located in front of the flexion-extension axis for the head. Thus the head has the tendency to topple forward. In order to prevent this, the neck muscles have to have a leverage moment in the extension direction.

This muscle activity becomes even more important as the head bends farther forward. As the head bends forward, the flexion moment of the head increases. Because of the neck muscles, the leverage moment then also increases. In a kyphosed position of the cervical spine, this leverage moment becomes even greater, significantly increasing the intradiscal pressure.

The cervical lordosis with an upright head results in the least load on the neck muscles and thus also on the cervical discs. In this position, one is able to look straight ahead.

In activities that require eye-hand coordination, people generally look down. During these activities, most people bend their entire spine into a kind of "complete kyphosis." This position requires—in the lumbar as well as in the cervical region—significant muscle activity and leads to an increase in the intradiscal pressure.[19] Therefore, ergonomically speaking one should strive for working postures and positions whereby the individual does not have prolonged periods of looking downward (see Chapter 12, Prevention of Back and Neck Pain by Improving Posture).

6.2   EXAMINATION

OVERVIEW OF THE EXAMINATION

General Inspection

In the general inspection, the position of the head is particularly important. Various head postures can indicate certain pathology. Sometimes the patient holds the head sidebent and rotated away from the painful side. This indicates a completely different cause than when the patient's head is deviated toward the painful side, but rotated away from the painful side. Interpreting the different head positions is discussed in detail in the section on specific inspection.

History

Age

Pathology of the cervical spine is often age related. For instance, the typical primary disc-related problems are usually seen between the ages of 30 and 50. The cervical postural syndrome is most common in younger people and is encountered frequently. In children, an acute torticollis can occur based on an intradiscal protrusion.

Occupation, Hobby (Sport)

Traumatic subluxations (or dislocations) of the zygapophyseal joints are seen in contact sports, but of course they can also be the result of other trauma. In some occupations, cervical postural syndromes occur because of poor head posture. This is particularly true for people who sit or stand with the head bent forward for prolonged periods.

Chief Complaints

Does the patient complain of pain, paresthesia, weakness, loss of sensation, or dizziness (and/or ringing in the ear)? Often combinations of these complaints are involved.

Onset

It is very important, not only for the diagnosis but also for planning the appropriate treatment, to know whether the symptoms had a sudden or a gradual onset. Also, it is necessary to find out whether the symptoms occurred as the result of a trauma or whether the patient is unaware of the cause. The time of day when the symptoms were first noticed can also give significant information. For instance, symptoms with an acute onset upon getting up in the morning are primarily disc-related.

Duration

Generally, the chance for therapeutic success is greater the shorter the symptom duration. The duration of the symptoms can also be of interest in making the prognosis, because many disorders are self-limiting. For instance, symptoms due to an acute torticollis in children usually do not last longer than 1 week to 10 days at the most, and a patient with a nerve root compression syndrome generally does not have symptoms much longer than 1 year.

Localization of Symptoms

Some patients have only headaches; others have only local cervical pain. In many instances, the pain caused by cervical pathology is also referred into the upper thoracic area. Often the patients experience pain radiating down the arm and/or into the hand. It is important to encourage the patient to localize the symptoms as precisely as possible. Usually the dermatome indicates the segmental location of the lesion.

One should also note whether the symptoms originated in the cervical region or whether they were first felt more distally in the upper extremity. For instance, in a cervical neurinoma the paresthesia usually starts distally (in the fingers) and then gradually spreads in a proximal direction.

Factors That Influence Symptoms

Pain at night can indicate a benign discogenic (segmental) problem. However, if the symptoms occur exclusively at night, one should consider the possibility of malignant pathology. Specific blood tests should be run, and a bone scan is indicated.

Prior History

Recurrence is frequently seen in primary disc-related disorders, especially if the patient has had insufficient explanation regarding the lesion and thus takes too little or no preventive measures. Patients with secondary disc-related disorders usually have a long history of neck problems.

Medication

Note whether the patient is taking any of the following:

- analgesics
- antiphlogistics (anti-inflammatories)
- antihypertensives
- anticoagulants
- cytostatics
- antidepressants.

Patient's Reactions to Symptoms

Does the patient try to function normally for as long as possible, or does he or she immediately call in sick in order to go on bed rest and/or medications?

Specific Inspection

The patient is inspected from behind, from the front, and from both sides. In so doing, the position of the head is noted, as well as the position of the scapulae and the entire spinal column. The hands should also be inspected for swelling and color; in instances of cervicobrachial complaints, the differential diagnosis of thoracic outlet compression syndrome should always be considered. Note any atrophy of shoulder, arm, or hand muscles. Sometimes the position of the head can give significant information.

Sternocleidomastoid Posture

If the patient holds the head in a position of flexion, a sidebend toward the painful side and a contralateral rotation, then one speaks of the so-called sternocleidomastoid posture. This is usually a sign of non–disc-related pathology. It may indicate a traumatic upper- or midcervical zygapophyseal joint subluxation (or dislocation)—particularly when observed in children—as the result of an inflammation in the cervical region. Of course, this posture can also be due to a congenital or perinatal torticollis.

Discogenic Posture

In cervical pathology, the most frequently seen position of the head is slight flexion with a sidebend and rotation away from the painful side. This is the so-called discogenic posture, because this posture is almost always the result of a disc protrusion or prolapse.

Conversion

If the patient demonstrates a sidebend toward the painful side combined with an ipsilateral elevation of the shoulder, then in many cases this indicates a so-called conversion torticollis. Often in the literature, this disorder is defined as a "hysterical torticollis." In such cases, it is necessary to treat not only with psychotherapy but also somatically. (See Chapter 17, Integrative Approach to Diagnosis and Treatment.)

Scoliosis

If the patient has a cervicothoracic scoliosis, then the head is held in the opposite direction of the scoliosis in order to keep a reasonable balance in the vertebral column.

Sprengel's Deformity

In a Sprengel's deformity, the shoulder on one side is elevated while the head is held in its normal position.

Klippel-Feil Syndrome

In the rare Klippel-Feil syndrome, there is an apparent elevated position of both shoulders. It appears as if the patient has no neck. These changes in contour are mostly based on deformities in the shoulder girdle.

Palpation

If swelling is present, it is palpated to determine its consistency and movability. The painful region is never palpated before performing the functional examination. Localization of the pain rarely corresponds to the actual location of the lesion. One does not want to begin the functional examination with misleading information.

Functional Examination

Before beginning the functional examination, note whether the patient is experiencing symptoms *at that moment*. If so, the patient should indicate any changes in the symptoms as a result of the various tests performed during the functional examination.

The affected side is always compared with the nonaffected side.

During the functional examination, attention is given to the following:

- *articular signs* (which motions are painful and/or limited, hypermobile, or unstable)
- *root signs* (mobility test for the cervical nerve roots, muscle strength, sensation, and reflexes)
- *central neurological signs* (for instance, spastic gait, Babinski foot sole reflex)
- *alternative causes for the pain* (thoracic outlet compression syndrome, lesions of the shoulder, elbow, or hand)
- *pain behavior of the patient*

The basic functional examination is performed with the patient in standing or in sitting, and the specific circulation tests are performed in lying.

The segmental functional examination is performed only when the basic functional examination provides insufficient information, or when the interim evaluation indicates that the appropriate treatment brought minimal to no results. Here, the local segmental tests are described under Tests for Supplementary Examination.

TESTS FOR BASIC FUNCTIONAL EXAMINATION

Active Motions

Note the range of motion (normal or limited) and pain (localization).

6.1.   Flexion

6.2.   Left rotation

6.3.   Right rotation

(If pain is provoked during the rotation, the test is repeated in flexion and in extension.)

6.4.   Left sidebend

6.5.   Right sidebend

6.6.   Extension

Passive Motions

Note the range of motion (normal or limited, capsular pattern or noncapsular pattern) and pain (localization).

6.7   Left rotation

6.8   Right rotation

6.9   Left sidebend

6.10   Right sidebend

6.11   Extension

Resisted Tests

Note muscle strength (if there is weakness, severe pathology is indicated) and pain (localization). If only weakness, without pain, is found in the following six tests, generally a very rare lesion of the C1 and/or C2 nerve root(s) should be suspected.

6.12.   Flexion

6.13.   Left rotation

6.14.   Right rotation

6.15.   Left sidebend

6.16.   Right sidebend

6.17.   Extension

TESTS FOR REMAINING FUNCTIONAL EXAMINATION

The remainder of the functional examination includes the tests for muscle strength, sensation, and reflexes. The examination is also performed to find causes of the complaints that might lie outside the cervical region.

Elevation of the Scapulae and the Arms

6.18.   Active bilateral scapular elevation

6.19.   Resisted bilateral scapular elevation (C2 to C4)

6.20.   Active simultaneous elevation of both arms

Resisted Shoulder Tests

6.21/22.   Shoulder abduction, left/right (C5)

6.23/24.   Shoulder adduction, left/right (C7)

6.25/26.   External rotation of the shoulder, left/right (C5, C6)

6.27/28.   Internal rotation of the shoulder, left/right (C5, C6)

Resisted Elbow Tests

6.29/30.   Elbow flexion, left/right (C5, C6)

6.31/32.   Elbow extension, left/right (C7)

Resisted Wrist Tests

6.33/34.   Wrist extension, left/right (C6)

6.35/36.   Wrist flexion, left/right (C7)

Resisted Finger Tests

6.37/38.   Radial abduction (extension) of the thumb, left/right (C8)

6.39/40.   Little finger adduction, left/right (T1)

Sensory Tests

6.41/42. Sensation of thumb and index finger, left/right (C6)

6.43/44. Sensation of the index, middle, and ring fingers, left/right (C7)

6.45/46. Sensation of the ring and little fingers, left/right (C8)

Cervical Reflexes

6.47/48. Brachioradialis reflex, left/right (C5)

6.49/50. Biceps brachii reflex, left/right (C5, C6)

6.51/52. Triceps reflex, left/right (C7)

Remaining Neurological Examination

6.53/54. Patellar tendon reflex, left/right

6.55/56. Achilles tendon reflex, left/right

6.57/58. Foot sole reflex, left/right

Other Tests

6.59/60. Foramina compression test, left/right

6.61. Axial separation test

PALPATION

After the functional examination, if it is accessible, the suspected affected structure is palpated for local tenderness.

TESTS FOR SUPPLEMENTARY EXAMINATION

Tests for Segmental Mobility

Upper Cervical (C0 to C3)

6.62. Flexion test

6.63. Rotation test

6.64. Atlanto-occipital traction test

6.65. Atlantoaxial rotation test

Midcervical and Lower Cervical (C2 to C7)

6.66. Coupled movement

6.67. Coupled movement in flexion

6.68. Coupled movement in extension

6.69. Ventrodorsal and dorsoventral segmental translation

Upper Thoracic

6.70. Coupled movement in flexion

6.71. Coupled movement in extension

Tests for Cervical Spine Stability

6.72. Lateral shift of the atlas in relation to the occiput and the axis

6.73. Ventral shift of the atlas in relation to the axis

TESTS FOR EXAMINATION OF THE BLOOD VESSELS

6.74. Modified DeKleyn and Nieuwenhuyse test

TESTS FOR EXAMINATION OF BALANCE

Romberg standing test
Modified Romberg standing test
Unterberger "walking in place" test
Babinski and Weil "star walk" test
Hautant test

TESTS FOR EXAMINATION OF COORDINATION

Barré arm test
Barré leg test
Finger-to-nose test
Heel-to-knee test

EXAMINATION OF HEARING, VISION, AND EYE MOVEMENTS

Flexion can be painful and/or limited in a number of cervical disorders, but particularly in the instance of disc pathology.

ACCESSORY EXAMINATIONS

In some cases, further imaging techniques are indicated, such as a radiological examination (to include functional views), computed tomography (CT), or magnetic resonance imaging (MRI). Moreover, there may be an indication for other examinations such as the following:

- electromyography
- laboratory tests
- spinal tap
- psychological testing

DESCRIPTION OF TESTS FOR BASIC FUNCTIONAL EXAMINATION

For specific types of tests and indications, see Tests for Basic Functional Examination, according to matching number.

TESTS FOR BASIC FUNCTIONAL EXAMINATION: ACTIVE MOTIONS

The examination of the active motions is performed in order to determine the range of motion and the pattern of movement. When a limitation of motion is present, the examiner should differentiate between a capsular pattern or a limitation that is in a noncapsular pattern. The provocation of pain, paresthesia, or dizziness is noted as well.

6.1 Flexion

Position of the Patient

The patient either sits or stands with the spinal column in its physiological position. If possible, the cervical spine should be in neutral position: this is determined through an optimal occlusion, or in general when the anterior nasal spine and the external acoustic meatus lie in the transverse plane.

Position of the Examiner

The examiner observes the patient during the movement, at first from behind and then, at the end of the motion, from lateral.

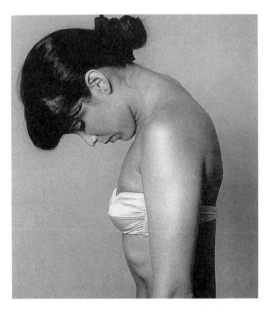

Test 6.1

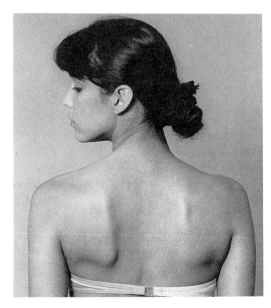

Test 6.2A

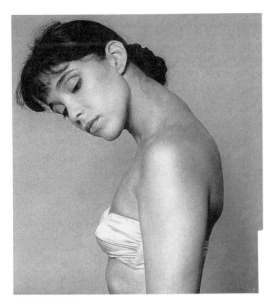

Test 6.2B Left rotation in flexion

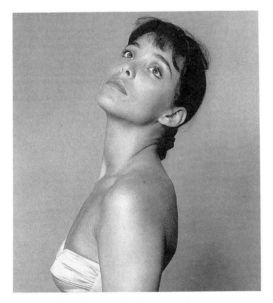

Test 6.2C Left rotation in extension

Performance

The patient brings the chin as far as possible in the direction of the sternal manubrium. The jaw muscles should remain as relaxed as possible. Although generally the distance between the sternal notch and the

chin is approximately 2 cm, the individual variance is great.

6.2 Active Left Rotation

6.3. Active Right Rotation

Position of the Patient

Same as for test 6.1.

Position of the Examiner

The examiner stands behind the patient.

Performance

The patient turns the head as far as possible to the left and then to the right, while the examiner notes the range of motion. There is almost always asymmetry in the cervical spine rotations, without clinical significance. An asymmetrical rotation is of clinical importance only when pain is provoked during one or both rotations. Many disorders of the cervical spine can show limited and/or painful rotations. However, the most striking is limited rotation in the different types of torticollis.

If pain is provoked during rotation, the test can be repeated in flexion and in extension (tests 6.2B and 6.2C.).

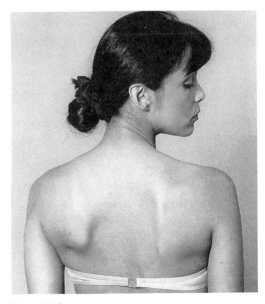

Test 6.3A

6.4. Left Sidebend

6.5. Right Sidebend

Position of the Patient

Same as for test 6.1.

Position of the Examiner

The examiner stands behind the patient.

Performance

Without making a visible rotation, the patient brings the head as far as possible in sidebend to the left and then to the right. As in the rotations, there is almost always asymmetry in cervical sidebend, and the most striking is in the various types of torticollis.

6.6. Extension

Position of the Patient

Same as for test 6.1.

Position of the Examiner

The examiner stands next to the patient.

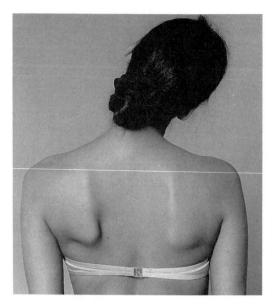

Test 6.5

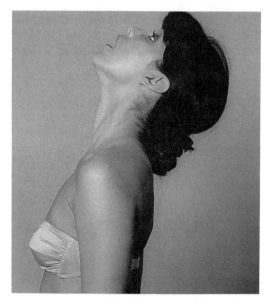

Test 6.6

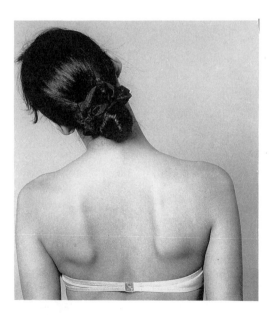

Test 6.4

Performance

The patient brings the head as far as possible backward (in extension). No motion should occur in the lumbar spine, and only minimal motion should be allowed in the thoracic spine. The patient holds the mouth open in a relaxed way, to take tension off the platysma muscle and allow for maximal range of motion in the cervical spine. Normally, the nose and forehead can be brought into the horizontal plane. Of course, one should also consider individual differences. With limitations in a capsular pattern, the extension motion is the most limited. Furthermore, the extension is limited in almost all disc lesions.

TESTS FOR BASIC FUNCTIONAL EXAMINATION: PASSIVE MOTIONS

In examining the passive motions, the range of motion is compared with that found in the active tests. Often one observes more mobility in passive than in active motions. Determining the end-feel is very important. As with active motions, provocation of the symptoms is also noted.

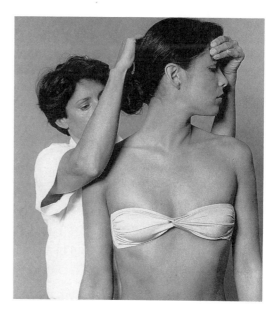

Test 6.7

6.7. Left Rotation

6.8. Right Rotation

Position of the Patient

Same as for test 6.1.

Position of the Examiner

The examiner stands behind the patient, opposite to the side being tested.

Performance

If the left rotation is being tested, the examiner grasps the patient's forehead with the left hand, placing the volar aspect of the elbow against the dorsal aspect of the patient's left shoulder. The examiner's right hand grasps the back of the patient's head on the left side with the volar aspect of the elbow placed against the front of the patient's right shoulder. In this position, trunk rotation is prevented. Using both hands, the examiner brings the patient's head as far as possible into left rotation, and the end-feel is tested by

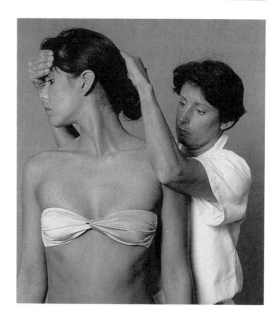

Test 6.8

applying overpressure. In the same manner, the right rotation is tested.

As mentioned in the active rotation tests, many disorders of the cervical spine show limited and/or painful rotations. However, the most striking is limited rotation in the different types of torticollis. With passive rotations, it is particularly important to test the end-feel. The normal end-feel is firm.

6.9. Left Sidebend

6.10. Right Sidebend

Position of the Patient

Same as for test 6.1.

Position of the Examiner

The examiner stands behind the patient.

Performance

If the left sidebend is being tested, the examiner places the volar aspect of the left elbow against the posterolateral aspect of the patient's left shoulder. The left hand grasps the top of the patient's head with the fingertips facing to the right. The right hand fixes the patient's right shoulder at its lateral aspect. Using the left hand, the examiner now brings the patient's head into a left sidebend.

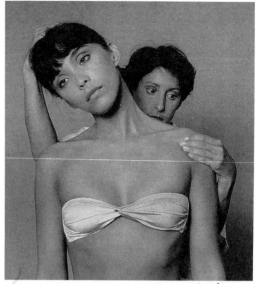

Test 6.10   *look at it*

The end-feel is tested by exerting overpressure at the end of the motion in the direction of the clavicle. In the same manner, the right sidebend is tested.

If the patient complains only of a pulling sensation on the opposite side, the examiner brings the right shoulder girdle into elevation. In this way, the trapezius muscle is no longer on a stretch, and in many cases the pain also disappears. If this is not the case, the pain is likely coming from the cervical spine itself.

As previously mentioned in the active tests, there is almost always asymmetry in cervical sidebend, and the most striking is in the various types of torticollis. Of importance in this test is the end-feel, which is normally firm; usually it is firmer than in the rotations.

6.11. Extension

Position of the Patient

Same as for test 6.1.

Position of the Examiner

The examiner stands next to the patient.

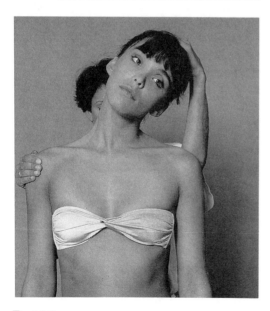

Test 6.9

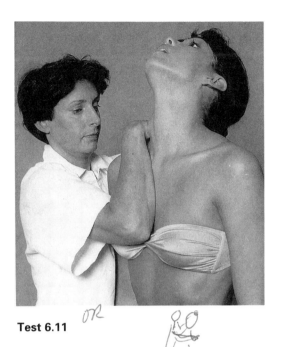

Test 6.11

Performance

To fix the patient's trunk, the examiner places the volar aspect of the forearm against the patient's sternum, and with the hand grasps the shoulder in the area of the trapezius muscle. The other hand is placed on top of the patient's head with the fingertips just resting on the forehead. The patient holds the mouth open. Cautiously, the examiner now extends the patient's cervical spine by tilting the patient's head backward. End-feel is tested by exerting gentle overpressure.

As already mentioned in active extension, in a capsular pattern of limitations this motion is the most limited. Also, the extension is limited in almost all disc lesions. In this test, the normal end-feel is firm.

TESTS FOR BASIC FUNCTIONAL EXAMINATION: RESISTED TESTS

The following six resisted tests are particularly directed toward determining C1 or C2 pathology that manifests itself through muscle weakness (sometimes in combination with pain). The examiner estimates the patient's strength (roots C1 and C2). If pain and weakness are exhibited, serious pathology is usually indicated. Further examination by a specialist is necessary (including CT scan, MRI, and laboratory tests).

6.12. Flexion

Position of the Patient

Same as for test 6.1.

Position of the Examiner

The examiner stands next to the patient.

Performance

The examiner places the heel of one hand against the patient's forehead. The other hand supports the patient's cervical lordosis. The patient is instructed to pull the chin in slightly and push the forehead against the examiner's hand. The examiner exerts isometric resistance.

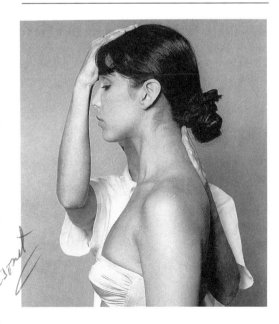

Test 6.12

6.13. Left Rotation

6.14. Right Rotation

Position of the Patient

Same as for test 6.1.

Position of the Examiner

The examiner stands behind the patient.

Performance

In testing the left rotation, the examiner's volar aspect of the left elbow is placed against the anterolateral aspect of the patient's left shoulder. The volar aspect of the right elbow is placed against the posterolateral aspect of the patient's right shoulder. With the left hand, the examiner grasps the patient's forehead from ventrolateral. The thenar and hypothenar eminences of the other hand rest on the dorsolateral aspect of the back of the patient's head. The patient is instructed to turn the head to the left, while the examiner exerts isometric resistance. In the same manner, the right rotation is tested.

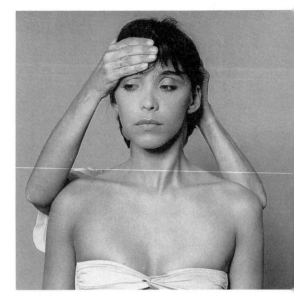

Test 6.14

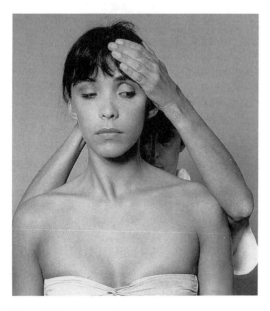

Test 6.13

6.15. Left Sidebend

6.16. Right Sidebend

Position of the Patient

Same as for test 6.1.

Position of the Examiner

The examiner stands obliquely behind the patient on the side to be tested.

Performance

When testing the left sidebend, the examiner places the volar aspect of the left elbow against the lateral aspect of the patient's left shoulder, while the hand rests against the lateral side of the patient's head. With the right hand, the examiner stabilizes the patient's right shoulder from lateral. The patient is now asked to bend the head sideways while the examiner exerts isometric resistance.

In the same manner, the right sidebend is tested.

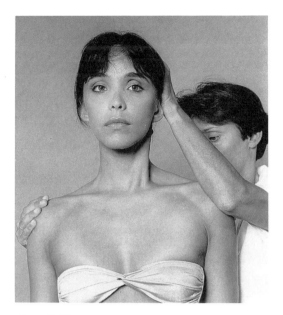

Test 6.15

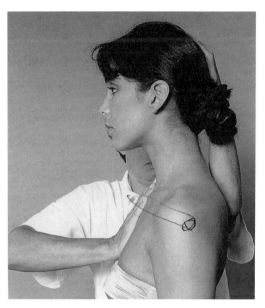

Test 6.17

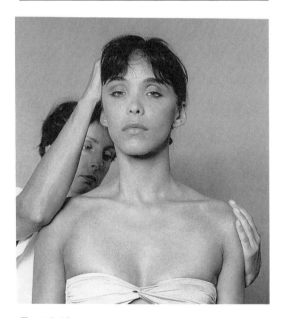

Test 6.16

6.17. Extension

Position of the Patient

Same as for test 6.1.

Position of the Examiner

The examiner stands next to the patient.

Performance

The volar aspect of the examiner's elbow is placed against the patient's upper thoracic spine, with the hand resting flat against the back of the patient's head. The other hand is placed on the patient's sternum with the forearm held horizontally. The patient is instructed to push the back of the head into the examiner's hand, and the examiner exerts isometric resistance.

DESCRIPTION OF TESTS FOR REMAINING FUNCTIONAL EXAMINATION

For specific types of tests and indications, see Tests for Remaining Functional Examination, according to matching number.

TESTS FOR ELEVATION OF THE SCAPULAE AND THE ARMS

Tests 6.18 and 6.20 are directed at ruling out shoulder girdle and shoulder problems.

Test 6.19 is specifically for pathology of the nerve roots C2 to C4.

6.18. Active Bilateral Scapular Elevation

Position of the Patient

Same as for test 6.1.

Position of the Examiner

The examiner stands behind the patient.

Performance

The patient is instructed to pull both shoulders up as high as possible. If scapular elevation has full range of motion and is not painful, the scapulothoracic motion is normal and there is (usually) no lesion of the acromio-and/or sternoclavicular joints. This test is performed particularly to rule out shoulder girdle pathology. If there is any doubt about the presence of pathology here, the entire shoulder examination should be performed.

6.19. Resisted Bilateral Scapular Elevation (C2 to C4)

Position of the Patient

Same as for test 6.1.

Position of the Examiner

The examiner stands behind the patient. From behind, the examiner places both hands on top of the patient's shoulders.

Performance

After the patient pulls both shoulders up as high as possible, the examiner tries to pull the patient's shoulders into depression. Normally, this is impossible. In instances of weakness, the patient is unable to hold the affected side in elevation. In this test, the nerve roots of C2 to C4 are tested. Weakness almost always indicates serious pathology.

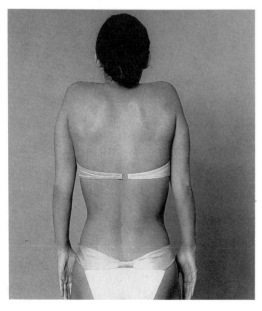

Test 6.18

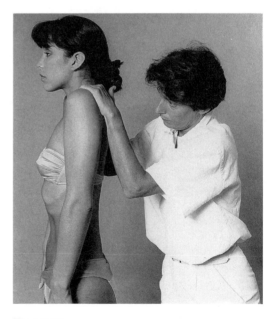

Test 6.19

6.20. Active Simultaneous Elevation of Both Arms

Position of the Patient

Same as for test 6.1.

Position of the Examiner

The examiner observes the patient from behind.

Performance

The patient is instructed to raise both arms slowly. This test generally rules out shoulder pathology. However, in rare instances, active arm elevation can be painful and/or limited as a result of a cervical lesion. In this case, it usually concerns a fracture of one spinous process or of one transverse process. Active arm elevation can also be painful and limited in the presence of a stress fracture of the first rib.

TESTS FOR FUNCTIONAL EXAMINATION: RESISTED SHOULDER TESTS

Resisted shoulder tests are performed to test the roots of C5 through C7. If pain is elicited, shoulder pathology is usually suspected. In this instance, the pain is usually localized only in the shoulder and not at all in the cervical region.

6.21/22. Shoulder Abduction, Left/Right (C5)

Position of the Patient

The patient stands or sits with arms resting alongside the body.

Position of the Examiner

The examiner stands next to the patient on the side being tested.

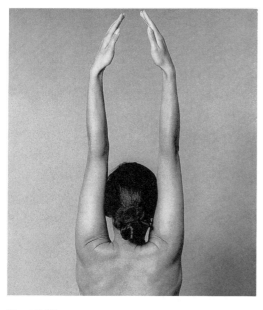

Test 6.20

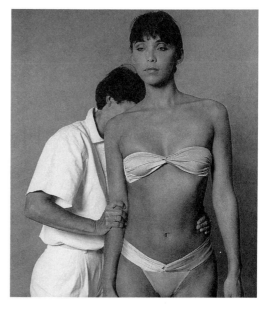

Test 6.21/22

Performance

If the right side is being tested, the examiner's right hand grasps the lateral aspect of the patient's distal upper arm. The other hand stabilizes either the patient's pelvis or shoulder on the opposite side. The patient is now instructed to push the arm away from the body (to abduct the arm), while the examiner exerts isometric resistance. The test is performed on both sides. This test examines the C5 nerve root in particular. If pain is elicited in the shoulder, one should suspect shoulder pathology such as of the supraspinous muscle and/or the subacromial-subdeltoid bursa.

6.23/24. Shoulder Adduction, Left/ Right (C7)

Position of the Patient

The patient stands or sits with arms resting alongside the body.

Position of the Examiner

The examiner stands next to the patient on the side being tested.

Performance

The examiner grasps the medial aspect of the patient's distal upper arm. The other hand stabilizes the patient at the lateral aspect of the patient's pelvis on the same side being tested. The patient is now instructed to hold the arm against the body (adducting the arm), while the examiner applies isometric resistance. Both sides are tested. In this way, the C7 nerve root in particular is tested. In the case of shoulder pathology, the various adductors are tested.

6.25/26. External Rotation of the Shoulder, Left/Right (C5, C6)

Position of the Patient

The patient stands or sits with arms resting alongside the body. The elbow of the side be-

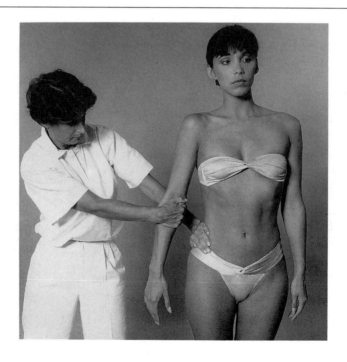

Test 6.23/24

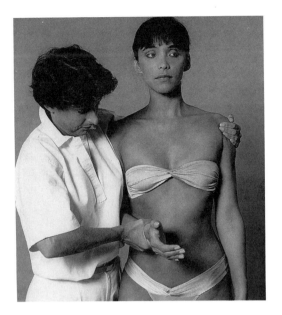

Test 6.25/26

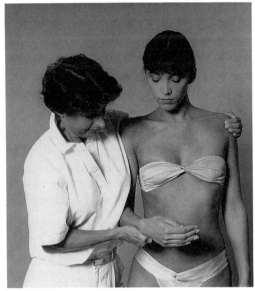

Test 6.27/28

ing tested is positioned in 90° flexion, and the shoulder is brought into the physiological zero position.

Position of the Examiner

The examiner stands next to the patient on the side being tested.

Performance

If the right side is being tested, the examiner's right hand grasps the distal aspect of the patient's forearm. The other hand stabilizes the patient at the opposite shoulder. The patient is now asked to rotate the forearm away from the body (externally rotate the arm), while the examiner exerts isometric resistance. The test is performed on both sides. In this way, particularly the C5 and C6 roots are tested. In the case of shoulder pathology, pain can be provoked due to a lesion of the infraspinous muscle.

6.27/28. Internal Rotation of the Shoulder, Left/Right (C5, C6)

Position of the Patient

Same as for test 6.25/26.

Position of the Examiner

The examiner stands next to the patient on the side being tested.

Performance

If the right side is being tested the examiner places the fingers of the right hand against the volar aspect of the patient's distal forearm, just proximal to the patient's wrist. The other hand stabilizes the patient at the opposite shoulder. The patient is now asked to rotate the forearm toward the body (internally rotate the arm), while the examiner applies isometric resistance. Both sides are tested. This tests particularly the roots of C5 and C6. In the case of shoulder pathology, pain that is provoked can be due to a lesion of the subscapularis muscle.

TESTS FOR FUNCTIONAL EXAMINATION: RESISTED ELBOW TESTS

Resisted elbow tests, as in resisted tests of the shoulder, are directed at the nerve roots C5 through C7. If pain is provoked—depending on the localization of the pain—one should suspect a lesion of the shoulder or elbow musculature.

6.29/30. Elbow Flexion, Left/Right (C5, C6)

Position of the Patient

Same as for test 6.25/26.

Position of the Examiner

Same as for test 6.25/26.

Performance

If the right side is being tested, the examiner places the right hand on the volar aspect of the patient's forearm, just proximal to the wrist. The examiner's forearm is positioned vertical to the patient's forearm. The other hand stabilizes the patient's arm at the elbow. The patient is now asked to bend the elbow while the examiner applies isometric resistance. Both sides are tested. This test examines the C5 and C6 nerve roots. If pain is provoked, there may be pathology of the biceps brachii muscle.

6.31/32. Elbow Extension, Left/Right (C7)

Position of the Patient

Same as for test 6.25/26.

Position of the Examiner

Same as for test 6.25/26.

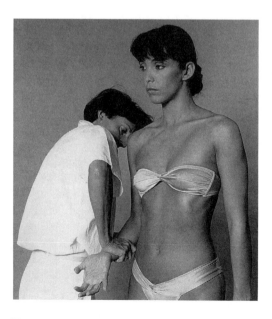

Test 6.29/30

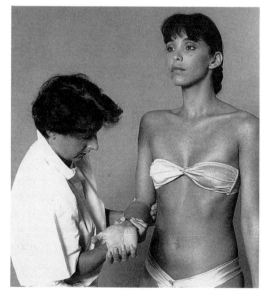

Test 6.31/32

Performance

If the right side is being tested, the examiner places the right hand on the dorsal aspect of the patient's forearm, just proximal to the wrist. If the patient and the examiner are approximately the same height, the examiner can place the dorsal aspect of the patient's distal forearm against the examiner's iliac crest. If the patient is taller than the examiner, the examiner stabilizes his or her own elbow against the iliac crest (as pictured). The other hand stabilizes the patient's arm at the elbow. The patient is now asked to straighten the elbow, and the examiner applies isometric resistance. Both sides are tested. This test examines the C7 nerve root. If pain is provoked, one should consider subacromial pathology.

TESTS FOR FUNCTIONAL EXAMINATION: RESISTED WRIST TESTS

Resisted wrist tests are directed at testing the nerve roots C6 and C7. If pain is pro-voked—depending on the localization of the pain—one should suspect a lesion of the wrist or elbow musculature.

6.33/34. Wrist Extension, Left/Right (C6)

Position of the Patient

The patient stands with the arms relaxed at the sides.

Position of the Examiner

The examiner stands next to the patient on the side to be tested.

Performance

In testing the right side the examiner places the right hand against the dorsum of the patient's right hand. The left hand grasps the patient's forearm from radial. The patient's elbow is supported in extension, resting on the distal part of the examiner's left upper arm. The patient is instructed to push the hand up (extend the wrist), while the ex-

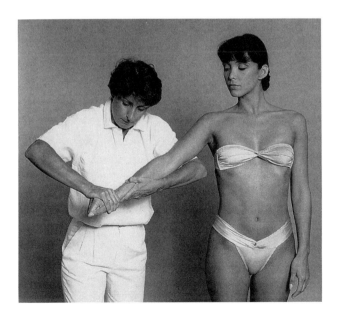

Test 6.33/34.

aminer exerts isometric resistance. Both sides are tested. This test examines the C6 nerve root. If pain is elicited at the lateral aspect of the elbow, one should suspect a lateral epicondylitis (tennis elbow).

6.35/36. Wrist Flexion, Left/Right (C7)

Position of the Patient

Same as for test 6.33/34.

Position of the Examiner

Same as for test 6.33/34.

Performance

In testing the right side the examiner's right hand grasps the patient's right hand from palmar. The examiner's left hand stabilizes the patient's forearm from dorsal, just proximal to the patient's wrist. The patient's elbow is supported in extension, resting on the distal part of the examiner's left upper arm. The patient is instructed to push the hand down (flex the wrist), and the examiner

exerts isometric resistance. Both sides are tested. This test examines the C7 nerve root. If pain is elicited at the medial aspect of the elbow, there may be a medial epicondylitis (golfer's elbow).

TESTS FOR FUNCTIONAL EXAMINATION: RESISTED FINGER TESTS

Resisted finger tests are directed at testing the C8 and T1 nerve roots. If pain is provoked—depending on the localization of the pain—one should suspect a lesion of the thumb muscles or of the third palmar interosseus muscle.

6.37/38. Radial Abduction (Extension) of the Thumb, Left/Right (C8)

Position of the Patient

Same as for test 6.33/34.

Position of the Examiner

The examiner stands next to or in front of the patient on the side to be tested.

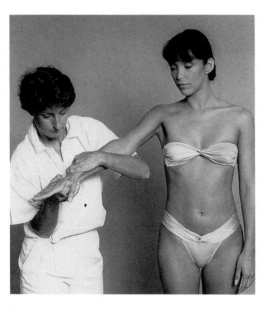

Test 6.35/36

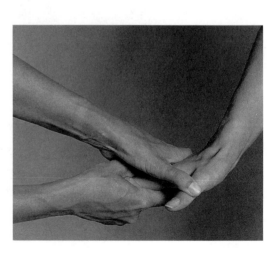

Test 6.37/38

Performance

The examiner grasps the fingers of the patient and places the thumb of the other hand against the interphalangeal joint of the patient's thumb. The patient is instructed to radially abduct (extend) the thumb while the examiner applies isometric resistance. In the same manner the other side is tested. This test examines the C8 nerve root. If the test is painful, there is likely a lesion of one of the extensor tendons of the thumb.

6.39/40. Little Finger Adduction, Left/ Right (T1)

Position of the Patient

Same as for test 6.33/34.

Position of the Examiner

Same as for test 6.33/34.

Performance

The patient abducts the little finger, and the tip of the examiner's index finger is placed

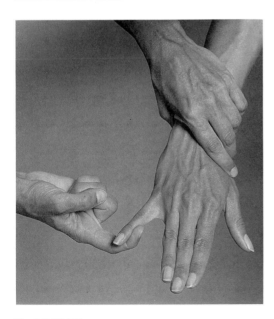

Test 6.39/40

against the radial aspect of the little finger's distal interphalangeal joint. With the other hand, the examiner stabilizes the patient's wrist from dorsal. The patient is asked to bring the extended little finger toward the ring finger, while the examiner applies isometric resistance. The test is then repeated on the other side. This test examines the T1 nerve root. If the patient indicates pain during the test, there may be a lesion of the third palmar interosseus muscle.

TESTS FOR FUNCTIONAL EXAMINATION: SENSORY TESTS

Sensation is tested to differentiate between the roots of C6 to C8. Attempting to differentiate sensory disturbances at higher levels is of little use because the overlap of the dermatomes is too great.

6.41/42. Sensation of Thumb and Index Finger, Left/Right (C6)
(not illustrated)

6.43/44. Sensation of the Index, Middle, and Ring Fingers, Left/Right (C7) (not illustrated)

6.45/46. Sensation of the Ring and Little Fingers, Left/Right (C8)
(not illustrated)

Position of the Patient

In either sitting or standing, the patient holds both arms extended in front of the body.

Position of the Examiner

The examiner stands in front of the patient.

Performance

Manually, by stroking over the patient's skin with slight pressure, the examiner tests the sensation of both sides at the same time. If a sensory disturbance is suspected in another nerve root, the corresponding dermatome should also be tested.

TESTS FOR FUNCTIONAL EXAMINATION: CERVICAL REFLEXES

Examining the cervical reflexes is aimed at gaining information about the C5 to C7 nerve roots. All tests are performed on both sides. Keep in mind that a general hyper-reflexia can indicate either nervousness or a central nervous system lesion. If a disturbance in the reflex is noted, this usually gives a definite localization of the cervical problem.

6.47/48. Brachioradialis Reflex, Left/ Right (C5)

Position of the Patient

The patient stands or sits with the arms relaxed. The arm being tested is positioned in 90° elbow flexion with the forearm resting in the neutral position.

Position of the Examiner

The examiner stands obliquely in front of the patient at the side to be tested.

Performance

With one hand, the examiner grasps the ulnar aspect of the patient's forearm just proximal to the wrist. Using the other hand, the examiner tests the brachioradialis tendon just proximal to its insertion on the radius (approximately 3 cm proximal to the styloid process of the radius). Instances of a hyper- or hyporeflexia generally indicate a C5 nerve root irritation.

6.49/50. Biceps Brachii Reflex, Left/ Right (C5, C6)

Position of the Patient

The patient stands or sits with the arms relaxed. The arm being tested is positioned in 90° elbow flexion with the forearm in supination.

Position of the Examiner

The examiner stands obliquely in front of the patient on the side to be tested.

Performance

With one hand, the examiner grasps the patient's elbow from ulnar so that the thumb

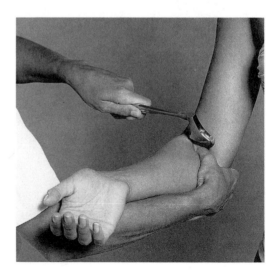

Test 6.47/48   **Test 6.49/50**

rests upon the tendon of the biceps brachii. The patient's forearm rests on the examiner's forearm. Using the other hand, the examiner performs the test by tapping the reflex hammer against the thumb lying on the biceps tendon. Instances of a hyper- or hyporeflexia generally indicate a C5 or C6 nerve root irritation.

6.51/52. Triceps Reflex, Left/Right (C7)

Position of the Patient

The patient stands or sits with the arms relaxed.

Position of the Examiner

The examiner stands next to the patient on the side being tested.

Performance

With one hand, the examiner grasps the patient's forearm just distal to the elbow, po-sitioning the elbow in 90° flexion. One can also grasp the upper arm and let the forearm hang in a relaxed position with the elbow flexed 90°. The reflex is tested just proximal to the olecranon on the triceps tendon. Instances of a hyper- or hyporeflexia generally indicate an irritation of the C7 nerve root.

TESTS FOR FUNCTIONAL EXAMINATION: NEUROLOGICAL EXAMINATION

The remaining neurological tests are performed to rule out the possibility of central neurological pathology. All tests are performed on both sides.

6.53/54. Patellar Tendon Reflex, Left/Right

Position of the Patient

The patient sits on the treatment table with the lower legs hanging over the edge.

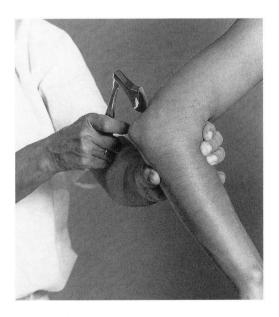

Test 6.51/52

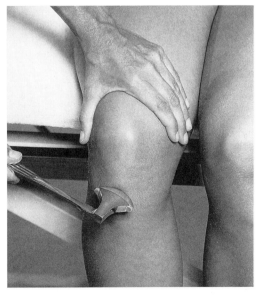

Test 6.53/54

Position of the Examiner

The examiner stands or sits obliquely in front of the patient on the side to be tested.

Performance

The patellar tendon reflex is tested via the patellar ligament, which is between the tibial tuberosity and the apex of the patella. This test is particularly significant in patients with a cervical myelopathy.

6.55/56. Achilles Tendon Reflex, Left/Right

Position of the Patient

Same as for test 6.53/54.

Position of the Examiner

The examiner squats in front of the patient.

Performance

With one hand, the examiner brings the patient's foot into extension (dorsiflexion). The other hand tests the Achilles tendon.

This test is particularly significant in patients with cervical spinal cord pathology.

6.57/58. Foot Sole Reflex, Left/Right

Position of the Patient

Same as for test 6.53/54.

Position of the Examiner

The examiner squats in front of the patient.

Performance

The examiner moves the pointed end of the reflex hammer along the sole of the patient's foot, beginning at the heel on the lateral side to the head of the fifth metatarsal and then medially over to the base of the great toe. Normally, the patient pulls the foot away and flexes the toes. However, other reactions are also possible. The pathological Babinski reflex is extension of the great toe, spreading of the other toes, and flexion of the knee and hip. The presence of a pathological Babinski reflex indicates a serious central neurological disturbance.

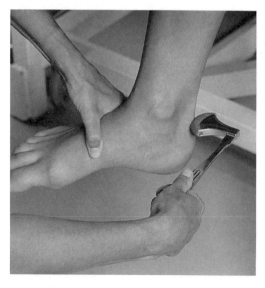

Test 6.55/56

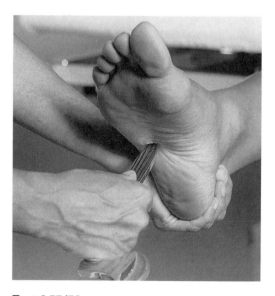

Test 6.57/58

OTHER TESTS

6.59. Foramina Compression Test, Left

6.60. Foramina Compression Test, Right *(Spurling)*

Position of the Patient

The patient sits on a stool or on the long side of the treatment table with the spine in its physiologically neutral position.

Position of the Examiner

The examiner stands behind the patient.

Performance

The examiner places one hand on the lateral aspect of the patient's head and moves the head in slight ipsilateral rotation and sidebend with simultaneous extension. The other hand either reinforces the first hand or stabilizes the patient at the shoulder. The examiner then performs slight, abrupt, axial pressure. If a root in the intervertebral foramen does not have adequate space, this test

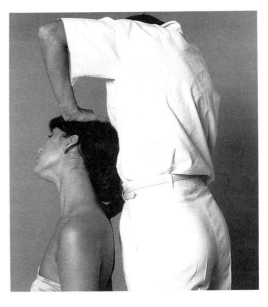

Test 6.60

will result in root compression. *arm pain* In some cases pain may not be elicited even though obvious compression has occurred. This can happen in patients in whom the sensation is already severely disturbed. *Can be false (−)*

6.61 Axial Separation Test

Position of the Patient

Same as for tests 6.59 and 6.60.

Position of the Examiner

Same as for tests 6.59 and 6.60.

Performance

The examiner grasps the patient's head with both hands, ensuring that pressure is not exerted over the patient's ears. In slight extension, in the neutral position, and in slight flexion, the examiner performs slight axial separation and holds this for several seconds.

This test is helpful in determining the appropriate treatment in instances when axial separation (continuous traction) is indicated.

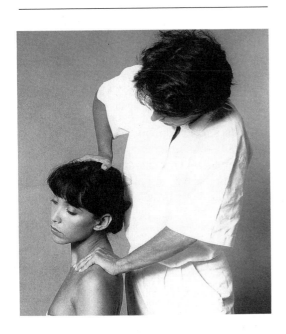

Test 6.59

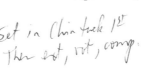
Workbook p. 72-75
Modify Spurling: Set in chin tuck 1st
Then ext, rot, comp.

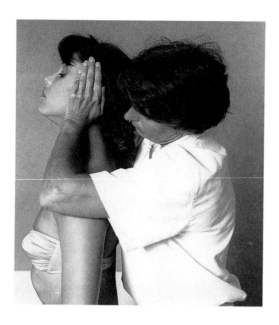

Test 6.61A Axial separation test in slight extension

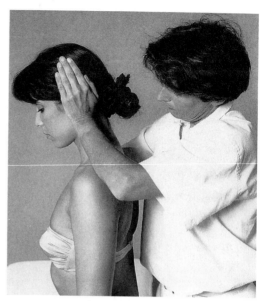

Test 6.61C Axial separation test in slight flexion

The position in which the pain decreased during the axial separation is later used in the treatment. However, axial separation should never be applied for a long period of time or with much force with the cervical spine in the flexed position.

DESCRIPTION OF TESTS FOR SUPPLEMENTARY EXAMINATION

For specific types of tests and indications, see Tests for Supplementary Examination, according to matching number.

A supplementary examination is necessary when the basic functional examination is either negative or provides insufficient information.

TESTS FOR SEGMENTAL MOBILITY: UPPER CERVICAL (C0 TO C3)

The following tests are performed to determine segmental mobility. Hypomobility without neurological deficits can be an indication for manual mobilization. If a hypermobility or

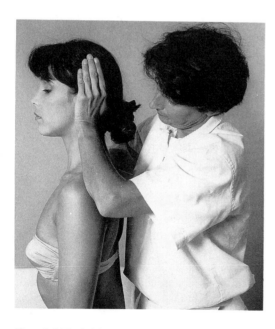

Test 6.61B Axial separation test in neutral position

instability is found, then depending on the severity of the problem, treatment may consist of stabilizing exercises, wearing a cervical collar, or even surgery. In order to be able to perform and interpret the functional examination, considerable experience is required.

6.62 Flexion Test

Position of the Patient

The patient sits upright on a stool or with the back supported against the chair. The spinal column is in its physiologically neutral position.

Position of the Examiner

The examiner stands next to the patient.

Performance

The examiner palpates the cranial and caudal aspects of the C2 spinous process between the tips of the index and middle fin-

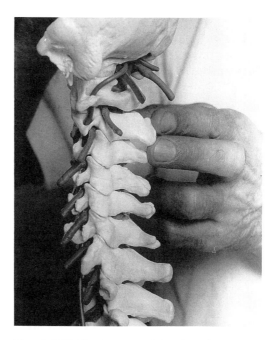

Test 6.62B Flexion test: skeletal model

gers. The other hand is placed on the patient's head and performs an upper cervical flexion (short nod). The palpating hand registers the movement of the spinous process of the axis. During the flexion movement, the axis makes an extension motion with the resulting palpable movement of the spinous process in a caudal and slightly dorsal direction. If this dorsocaudal motion of the spinous process of the axis does not occur, an atlanto-occipital, an atlantoaxial, or a C2-3 limitation of motion may be present or there may be a hypermobility or instability in any one of these segments. In the last instance, the apical ligament is especially affected.

6.63 Rotation Test

Position of the Patient

The patient sits upright on a stool or with the back supported against the chair. The spinal column is in its physiologically neutral position.

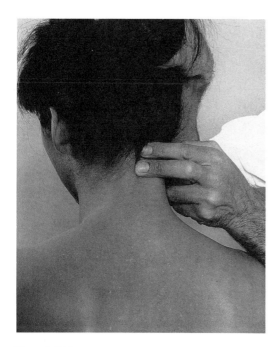

Test 6.62A

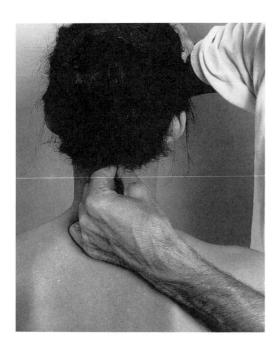

Test 6.63A Initial position of the rotation test.

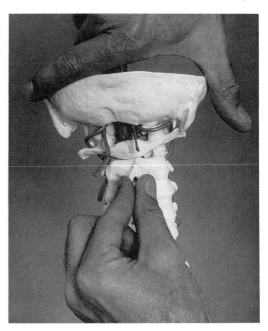

Test 6.63C Rotation test: skeletal model

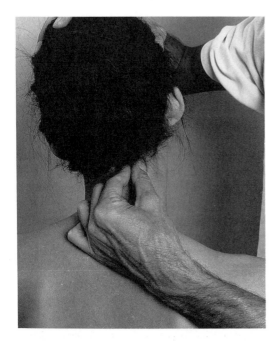

Test 6.63B End position of the rotation test

Position of the Examiner

The examiner stands next to the patient.

Performance

The examiner palpates the lateral aspects of the C2 spinous process between the thumb and index finger. The other hand is placed on the patient's head. While the fingers fix the C2 spinous process, the other hand passively brings the patient's head into a very slight (upper cervical) sidebend. During this sidebend, the axis rotates immediately. Thus, the spinous process moves in the contralateral direction. The sidebend is performed on each side. If the examiner feels immediate pressure against the fixing fingers, the alar ligaments are likely to be intact (or there may be a hypomobility in the atlanto-occipital joints that mimics the intact ligaments). If the examiner is able to make a slight sidebend of the patient's head without feeling immediate pressure against the fixing fingers, it is likely that the alar ligament, occipital portion, has a certain degree of laxity. Thus, there is a laxity in the upper cervical segments of C0 to C2.

6.64 Atlanto-Occipital Traction Test

Position of the Patient

The patient sits upright on a stool or with the back supported against the chair with the hands resting in the lap. The spinal column is in its physiologically neutral position.

Position of the Examiner

The examiner stands next to the patient opposite the side being tested. The examiner keeps the knees slightly flexed.

Performance

If the left side is being tested, the examiner's right hand grasps the patient's head and stabilizes it against the sternum. The little finger has contact with the mastoid process. The tip of the index finger of the other hand is placed between the cranial aspect of the transverse process of the atlas and the mastoid process. The patient's head is passively brought into slight (approximately 4°) upper cervical flexion with coupled left sidebend and right rotation. By extending the knees, the examiner performs a separation in the left atlanto-occipital joint. The separation motion is performed several times. The palpating finger registers the amount of separation; the examiner compares it with that of the other side.

6.65. Atlantoaxial Rotation Test

Position of the Patient

Same as for test 6.64.

Position of the Examiner

The examiner stands next to the patient, opposite the side being tested.

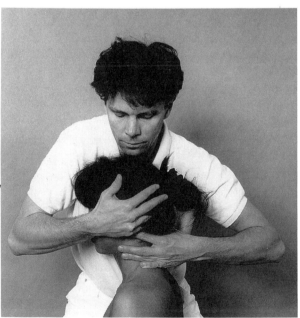

Test 6.64A

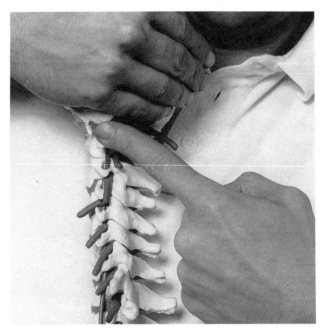

Test 6.64B Atlanto-occipital traction test: skeletal model

Performance

If the left side is being tested, the examiner grasps the patient's head in such a way that the little finger lies against the dorsolateral aspect of the posterior arch of the atlas. With the other hand, the examiner fixes the dorsal aspect of the axis between the thumb and index finger. Four movements are now performed during which the amount of motion and the end-feel are determined. The examiner stands on the patient's right side (to test the left atlantoaxial joint) and performs the following:

1. upper cervical flexion with left rotation and right sidebend (Figure 6.65)
2. upper cervical extension with right rotation and left sidebend

Then the examiner stands on the patient's left side (to test the right atlantoaxial joint) and performs the following:

3. upper cervical flexion with right rotation and left sidebend

4. upper cervical extension with left rotation and right sidebend

TESTS FOR SEGMENTAL MOBILITY: MIDCERVICAL AND LOWER CERVICAL (C2 TO C7)

6.66 Coupled Movement

Position of the Patient

The patient lies supine with the head in a neutral position.

Position of the Examiner

The examiner stands at the head of the treatment table.

Performance

The examiner supports the lateral aspect of the patient's head with one hand. The testing hand is placed at the caudal vertebra of the segment being tested, with the radial side of

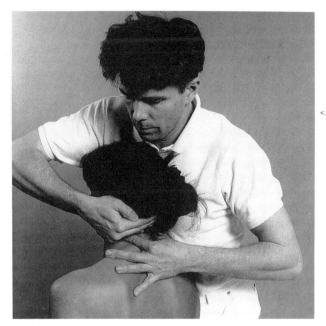

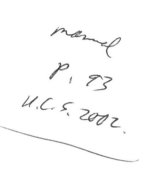

Test 6.65

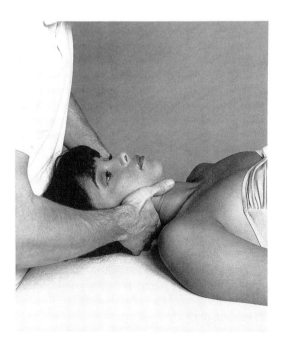

Test 6.66A Coupled movement C2–3

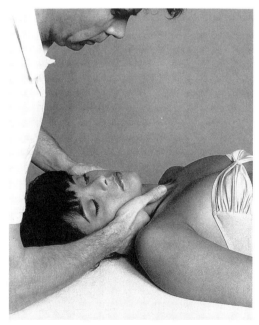

Test 6.66B Coupled movement C6–7

the index finger resting against the lamina and the posterior aspect of the superior articular process. The index finger is parallel to the joint line (in the direction of the orbita). The forearm is in line with the index finger. By performing a movement in a ventromedio-cranial direction (perpendicular to the position of the forearm), the segment being tested is brought into an ipsilateral sidebend and rotation. Segment by segment, the movement is tested, first on one side and then on the other. Not only is the amount of motion in the segment assessed, but more importantly, the end-feel is determined. This is a fast and simple way to obtain information about segmental mobility.

6.67. Coupled Movement in Flexion

Position of the Patient

The patient sits upright on a stool or with the back supported against the chair with the hands resting in the lap. The spinal column is in its physiologically neutral position.

Position of the Examiner

The examiner stands next to the patient opposite the side to be tested.

Performance

If the left side is being tested, the examiner grasps the patient's head with the right hand. The index finger of the other hand palpates the segment being tested between the dorsal aspect of both adjoining articular processes. The thumb and index or middle finger fix the segment's caudal vertebra. The examiner now brings the patient's head simultaneously into a coupled (ipsilateral) sidebend and rotation with flexion. The movement is performed away from the side being tested (in this instance, right sidebend, right rotation, and flexion). At the same time, the fingers at the caudal vertebra fix and register when the caudal vertebra begins to move with the cranial segments. If the caudal vertebra is fixed with

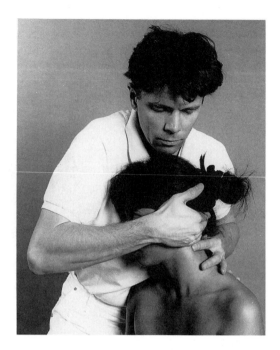

Test 6.67 Coupled movement in flexion, C2–3, left zygapophyseal joint

the thumb and middle finger, the index finger can palpate the zygapophyseal joint of the segment being tested (see test 6.68). In this way all the segments from C2-3 to C6-7 are tested, first on one side and then on the other side. Generally (in a normal cervical spine), the total range of motion gradually increases the more caudally one tests.

6.68. Coupled Movement in Extension

Position of the Patient

Same as for test 6.67.

Position of the Examiner

The examiner stands next to the patient, opposite the side being tested.

Performance

If the left side is being tested, the examiner grasps the patient's head with the right hand.

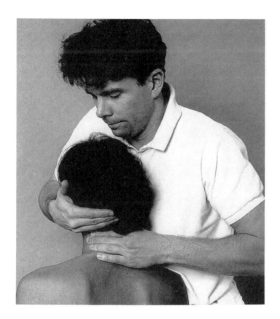

Test 6.68 Coupled movement in extension, C3–4, left zygapophyseal joint

The index finger of the other hand palpates the segment being tested between the dorsal aspect of both adjoining articular processes. The thumb and index or middle finger fix the segment's caudal vertebra. The examiner now brings the patient's head simultaneously into a coupled (ipsilateral) sidebend and rotation with extension. The movement is performed toward the side being tested (in this instance, left sidebend, left rotation, and extension). At the same time, the fingers at the caudal vertebra fix and register when the caudal vertebra begins to move with the cranial segments. If the caudal vertebra is fixed with the thumb and middle finger, the index finger can palpate the zygapophyseal joint of the segment being tested. In this way all the segments from C2-3 to C6-7 are tested, first on one side and then on the other side. Generally (in a normal cervical spine), the total range of motion gradually increases the more caudally one tests.

6.69. Ventrodorsal and Dorsoventral Segmental Translation

Position of the Patient

The patient is positioned in sidelying as close to the edge of the table as possible, with the hips and knees in approximately 70° flexion. The spinal column should be in its physiologically neutral position.

Position of the Examiner

The examiner stands in front of the patient at the level of the patient's sternum. The patient's head rests on the volar aspect of the examiner's cranial forearm. The patient's forehead has contact with the front of the examiner's upper arm. With the hand, the examiner grasps the back of the patient's head in such a way that the ulnar side of the hand has contact with the dorsal aspect of the segment's cranial vertebra. With the other forearm, the examiner stabilizes the patient's trunk in a neutral position; the thumb and index finger of that hand fix the caudal vertebra of the segment being tested.

Performance

The cranial hand is the testing hand, while the caudal hand fixes. First the head is positioned in upper cervical flexion. The cranial hand then moves the head and the cranial vertebra of the segment being tested as one unit from dorsocaudal to ventrocranial and back. The motion is repeated several times. The direction of motion is specified by the position of the zygapophyseal joints. In general, when one moves in the direction of the orbita this corresponds to the position of the zygapophyseal joints. (Keep in mind that, in general, the angle that the zygapophyseal joints make to the horizontal is larger in the lower cervical region than in the midcervical region. However, because of the large variability in the position of the zygapophyseal joints and the actual posture of the cervical spine—flattened lordosis versus hyper-

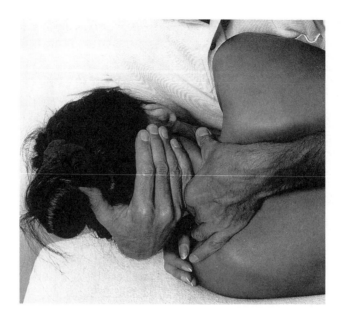

Test 6.69

lordosis—the direction of motion can vary.) In this manner, the motion segments from C2-3 to C7-T1 are tested. Hypomobility, limitation of motion, hypermobility, and/or instability can be palpated by the experienced examiner. Hypermobility, as well as hypomobility, can be present without causing any symptoms. If there is an instability or a limitation of motion, then in many instances this test provokes the patient's symptoms.

TESTS FOR SEGMENTAL MOBILITY: UPPER THORACIC

6.70. Coupled Movement in Flexion

Position of the Patient

The patient sits upright on a stool or with the back supported against the chair with the hands resting in the lap. The spinal column is in its physiologically neutral position.

Position of the Examiner

The examiner stands next to the patient.

Performance

With one hand, the examiner grasps the patient's head and cervical spine whereby the

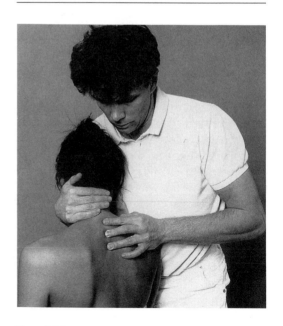

Test 6.70

ulnar aspect of the little finger lies against the dorsal aspect of C7. The patient's head is stabilized between the examiner's forearm and the ventral aspect of the trunk. The examiner places the index, middle, and ring fingers between and just lateral to (on the side farthest away) the spinous processes of C7 to T3. Now the examiner performs a simultaneous flexion, sidebend, and ipsilateral rotation in a direction toward the examiner. (In other words, if the examiner is standing on the right side of the patient, simultaneous flexion, right sidebend, and right rotation are performed.) The palpating fingers register the amount of upper thoracic movement and the end-feel. In this manner, the segments C7-T1 to T3-4 are tested. The examiner then tests the coupled movements in the opposite direction by standing on the patient's other side.

6.71. Coupled Movement in Extension

Position of the Patient

Same as for test 6.70.

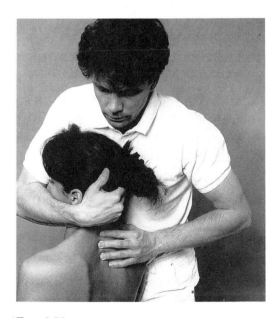

Test 6.71

Position of the Examiner

Same as for test 6.70.

Performance

The examiner grasps the patient's head in such a way that the little finger lies just caudal to the occiput. The examiner's upper arm rests against the patient's forehead. The patient's head is stabilized between the examiner's arm and the ventral aspect of the trunk. The fingers of the other hand are placed between, and just lateral to (on the side closest to the examiner), the spinous processes of C7 to T3. The patient's head first is brought into an upper cervical flexion, then the coupled movements of extension, sidebend, and ipsilateral rotation are performed in a direction away from the examiner. (In other words, if the examiner is standing on the patient's right side, a simultaneous extension, left sidebend, and left rotation are performed.) The palpating fingers register the amount of upper thoracic movement and the end-feel. In this manner, the segments C7-T1 to T3-4 are tested. The examiner then tests the coupled movements in the opposite direction by standing on the patient's other side.

TESTS FOR CERVICAL SPINE MOBILITY

In the segmental mobility examination, various tests have already been described in which stability can be determined. The following upper cervical stability tests concern specific movements that cannot be performed actively. (These tests are similar to the varus and valgus tests for the knee and elbow joints.) The tests discussed here are the most reliable tests in determining an upper cervical instability.

Warning: It is possible that an instability can be masked by a limitation of motion at the same level, for instance due to muscle splinting or articular pathology. Particularly in the cervical spine, this fact is very important because mobilization, to include manipulations, in such cases can cause severe neurological complications. A very thorough basic functional examination (which also includes patient history) usually leads to an understanding of the pattern of the patient's symptoms and signs. Every deviation from this needs further special examination.

6.72. Lateral Shift of the Atlas in Relation to the Occiput and the Axis

Position of the Patient

The patient lies supine with the head in a neutral position and the arms relaxed alongside the body.

Position of the Examiner

The examiner stands or sits at the head of the treatment table.

Performance

The mobility of the atlas is tested both to the right and to the left. The following de-

scription is for testing the lateral shift to the left. With the left hand, the examiner fixes C2 as well as the occiput. First, the tip of the index finger localizes the spinous process of C2. Next, the examiner rests the radial aspect of the index finger's proximal phalanx against the left lamina of the axis. By bringing the wrist into extension, the thenar eminence is now placed against the mastoid process. The ulnar side of the forearm rests on the treatment table. The tip of the right thumb is placed on the radial aspect of the proximal interphalangeal joint of the right index finger whereby the entire index finger is flexed. The flat tip of the thumb is now placed against the transverse process of the atlas (located between the mastoid process and the mandibular ramus). With the right thumb, the examiner carefully exerts pressure against the transverse process of the atlas (pushing it to the left). Normally, almost no movement should occur. Thus, interpreting the amount of mobility of the atlas in this direction is practically impossible. Usually in instances of

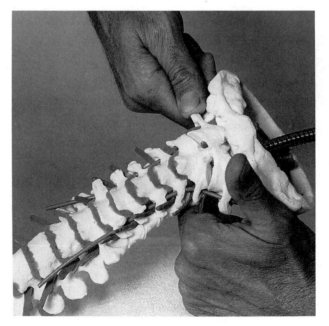

Test 6.72A Skeletal model

Upper C. — manual 2002, p. 82
for sitting

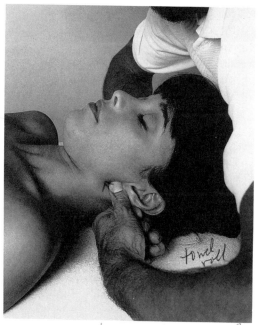

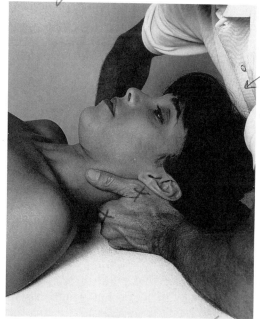

lean on head,

Test 6.72B Lateral shift to right *Thumb on C-1, push lat. ghtb pad & hold 10-30 sec.*

Test 6.72C Lateral shift to left *thenar on mastoid index on C-2 T proces & sp. proces.*

pathological hypermobility, the patient's symptoms are provoked immediately. In particular, the transverse ligament is tested.

6.73. Ventral Shift of the Atlas in Relation to the Axis

Position of the Patient

The patient lies supine with arms relaxed alongside the body. The head is in the neutral position. *— Bk of head on towel to get upper C- flexion,*

Position of the Examiner

The examiner stands or sits at the head of the treatment table.

Performance

The examiner localizes the spinous process of C2 with the tips of both index fingers and then shifts the fingertips slightly cranially (to the space between the occiput and the C2 spinous process) and laterally (just medial to

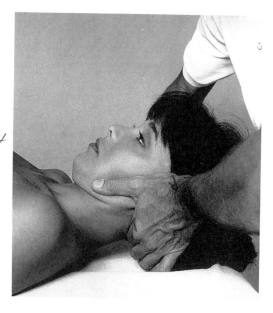

Test 6.73

Ck P at dens. → M or Neuro Sx ↑ in Bk or arms is a Red Flag!

the mastoid process). Without moving the index fingers, the examiner now grasps the patient's head and fixes it against the table. By bringing both wrists into ulnar deviation, the patient's head is positioned into slight upper cervical flexion. The examiner then flexes both index fingers pushing the altas in a ventral direction. Normally, almost no movement should occur. Possible hypermobility or instability usually is not palpable because in most cases the patient immediately experiences his or her symptoms. Here, particularly the transverse ligament is tested.

TESTS FOR EXAMINATION OF THE BLOOD VESSELS

Examination of the blood vessels is particularly important in diagnosing vertebrobasilar disorders. If one is considering treating the patient with rotatory manual therapy techniques, it is imperative that the following tests be performed. During the testing, the test is discontinued as soon as the patient experiences his or her symptoms or if the patient's symptoms are reproduced immediately on positioning the head and do not disappear within 15 seconds. If one or more tests are positive, further examination should be conducted by a specialist.

6.74. Modified DeKleyn and Nieuwenhuyse Test

Position of the Patient

The patient lies supine with the head over the edge of the treatment table. The eyes should remain open.

Position of the Examiner

The examiner sits at the head of the treatment table, supporting the patient's head with both hands.

Performance

The following passive movements of the cervical spine are performed:

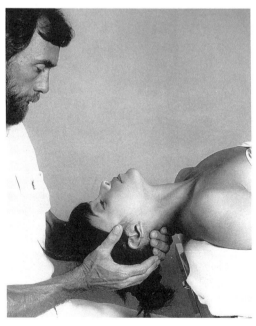

Test 6.74A Extension

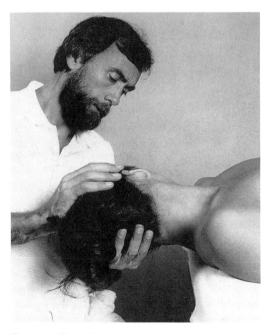

Test 6.74B Left rotation

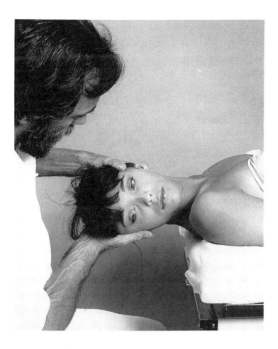

Test 6.74C Right rotation

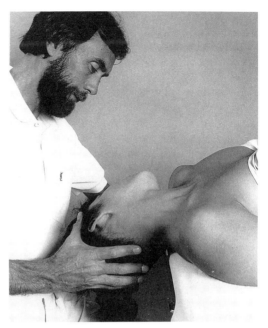

Test 6.74D Extension with left rotation and left sidebend

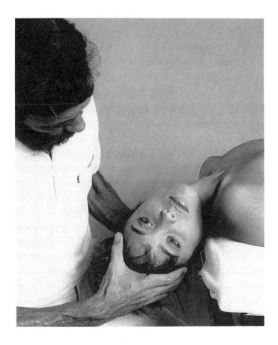

Test 6.74E Extension with right rotation and right sidebend

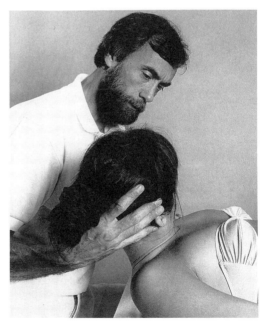

Test 6.74F Flexion with left rotation and right sidebend

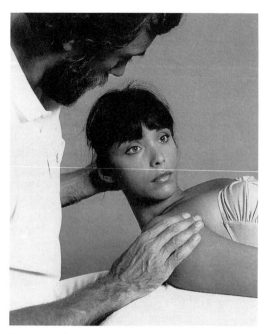

Test 6.74G Flexion with right rotation and left sidebend

- extension
- right and left rotation
- extension with ipsilateral rotation and sidebend, to both sides
- flexion with rotation and contralateral sidebend, to both sides

Each position is held for a maximum of 2 minutes (or shorter if the patient's symptoms are reproduced immediately on positioning the head and do not disappear within 15 seconds). After each test, the cervical spine is returned to the neutral position and held there for approximately 1 minute. Although in the literature it is stated that extension of the cervical spine has no influence on the flow of the vertebral arteries, it is striking that in one research group with suspected vertebrobasilar insufficiency, the extension produced their recognizable symptoms in 35% of the patients.[20]

The following factors play a role in the determination of a vertebrobasilar insufficiency:

- the types of symptoms
- the moment at which the symptoms arise and disappear again
- the course of the symptoms during the test

If the symptoms remain present during or after the test, or have an increasing character, and are recognized by the patient as his or her particular symptoms, the test is positive. However, if the symptoms decrease during the test, there is a good possibility that there is no vertebrobasilar insufficiency syndrome. Instead, the symptoms are likely due to a disturbance in the cervical function. When one test is found to be positive, the other tests are not performed.

The combined movement of extension with rotation appears to be a very reliable and valid test for the flow of the vertebral arteries and the basilar artery. Thus it can be considered a pathognomonic test for the vertebrobasilar insufficiency syndrome.[20]

If the patient complains of dizziness during the rotation test in the basic functional examination, the examiner cannot be certain whether this is due to a dysfunction of one or both vertebral arteries (or of the basilar artery) or due to an aberration in the vestibular system. If so the following test can be performed: The patient is instructed to look straight ahead while actively performing trunk rotations as quickly and as largely as possible (alternating left and right). In this way, in principle, the same rotation has occurred as in rotating the head, but the difference is that the patient's head does not move. If the patient is not dizzy with this maneuver, the symptoms are likely due to an aberration in the vestibular system.

DESCRIPTION OF TESTS FOR EXAMINATION OF BALANCE

In complaints of dizziness and in coordination disturbances, both balance and coordination are examined. If one or more tests are positive, further examination by a specialist is indicated. The following summary is taken from Oostendorp.[20]

Romberg Standing Test

Position of the Patient

The patient stands with the feet together. If this is not possible, the patient should stand with the minimal distance necessary between the feet, whereby the patient is still to be able to maintain balance.

Position of the Examiner

The examiner observes the patient.

Performance

The patient closes the eyes. The test is positive when the patient loses his or her balance in the position in which balance was maintained with the eyes open.

Modified Romberg Standing Test (Kirby)

Position of the Patient

The patient stands with the feet successively as follows:

Class 1: 30 cm apart
Class 2: 15 cm apart
Class 3: together
Class 4: 30 cm apart in stride (one foot in front of the other), with a side-to-side distance between the two feet of 10 cm
          4A—left foot in front
          4B—right foot in front
Class 5: 30 cm apart in stride (one foot in front of the other), and also in line
          5A—left foot in front
          5B—right foot in front
Class 6: standing on one foot
          6A—left foot
          6B—right foot

Class 7: class 5 and class 6 are repeated, but now on a balance beam at a height of 30 cm

Position of the Examiner

The examiner observes the patient.

Performance

With eyes open, the patient maintains the position in each class for 3 minutes. If the patient needs more than five corrections to maintain balance, then one class lower is tested again.

Unterberger "Walking in Place" Test

Position of the Patient

The patient stands with eyes closed.

Position of the Examiner

The examiner observes the patient.

Performance

The patient is instructed to walk in place. For every 50 steps, a rotation of the body of up to 45° is normal. The test is positive if the patient turns more than 45°.

Babinski and Weil "Star Walk" Test

Position of the Patient

The patient stands with the eyes closed.

Position of the Examiner

The examiner observes the patient.

Performance

The patient is instructed to take five steps forward, followed by five steps backward; this is repeated 10 times. The test is positive if the patient makes a star figure in performing the test (*marche en étoile*). In a disturbance of the balance, the direction of turning is the same as observed in the "walking in place" test.

Hautant Test

Position of the Patient

The patient sits on a stool with the back and head supported. The arms are extended in front of the body with the forearms in pronation and the palms facing downward.

Position of the Examiner

The examiner stands in front of the patient. The tips of the examiner's index fingers are placed opposite to the tips of the patient's middle fingers.

Performance

The patient closes the eyes. The examiner notes whether the arms move in a sideward direction. The patient is instructed to bring the head (and cervical spine) into extension and rotation, while the examiner holds the patient's hands to prevent a physiological synkinetic movement of the arms. The patient then holds the head in this position and tries not to move the arms.

The test is judged in two stages. If there is already sideward movement of the arm(s) when the patient first closes the eyes, and if the direction of this movement corresponds to the direction in which the patient tended to fall during the Romberg standing test, a disturbance in the vestibular system may be indicated. During or directly after the patient moves the head into extension and rotation, if one arm manifests a sideward deviation, a disturbance in the vascularization in the vertebrobasilar supply area is indicated. Because such disturbances are often based on upper cervical dysfunction, extra attention should be given to the upper cervical examination.

DESCRIPTION OF TESTS FOR EXAMINATION OF COORDINATION

If the patient complains of dizziness or coordination disturbances, not only balance but also coordination is examined. If one or more tests are found to be positive, then further examination by a specialist is indicated. The following summary is largely taken from Oostendorp.[20]

Barré Arm Test

Position of the Patient

The patient either stands or sits with the arms extended forward in the horizontal plane. The forearms are supinated with the palms up.

Position of the Examiner

The examiner observes the patient.

Performance

The patient closes the eyes. The test is positive if the arms slowly sink and, at the same time, pronate. See the following test, Barré leg test, for the interpretation.

Barré Leg Test

Position of the Patient

The patient lies prone with both knees flexed 45°.

Position of the Examiner

The examiner observes the patient.

Performance

The patient closes the eyes. The test is positive if one leg slowly sinks (particularly in a jerky manner). If one or both Barré tests are positive, there is likely to be a lesion of the central nervous system. Generally, one or more pathological reflexes are also present.

Finger-to-Nose Test

Position of the Patient

The patient either sits or stands.

Position of the Examiner

The examiner observes the patient.

Performance

With eyes open, the patient brings the tip of the index finger to a specific point (for instance, the nose). The same movement then is repeated with the eyes closed. The test is positive when a deviated movement occurs.

Heel-to-Knee Test

Position of the Patient
The patient lies supine.

Position of the Examiner

The examiner observes the patient.

Performance

With open eyes, the patient brings the heel of one leg to the knee of the other leg, slides it down the shin to the foot and brings it back again. The test is repeated with the eyes closed. The test is positive if deviated movements occur.

INDICATIONS FOR EXAMINATION OF HEARING, VISION, AND EYE MOVEMENTS

With symptoms from the cervico-occipital region during which the patient complains of hearing or vision disturbances, examination by a specialist is necessary. The same holds true for a patient with a nystagmus.

6.3   PATHOLOGY

PRIMARY DISC-RELATED DISORDERS

In this book, primary disc-related disorders are considered to be disorders whereby the impression is that the patient's signs and symptoms are caused by a lesion of a disc. In some cases, the causal role of the disc is not yet scientifically proven. However, in our view the evidence is convincing enough to consider these primary disc-related disorders nonetheless.

Various cervical syndromes are the direct or indirect result of traumatic or degenerative changes of the cervical intervertebral disc. Of all disc pathology, 36% is localized in the cervical spine.[21]

Cervical Posture Syndrome

Strictly seen, the cervical posture syndrome does not yet belong to the primary disc-related disorders; however, the relation with the local cervical syndrome is so close that it is discussed under this category.

The cervical posture syndrome arises as a result of an imbalance of the cervicothoracic musculature. When the head is positioned too far forward in relation to the thorax (anterior position), the cervical muscles, particularly the levator scapulae, are overloaded. This syndrome, also called the tired neck syndrome, is seen three times more often in women than in men. Patients' ages vary from very young (after the age of 6 years as a result of "hanging" the head over the school desk) to approximately the age of 40 years.

Although the cause is usually poor posture, bifocal glasses, for instance, can also force the patient to hold the head in an anterior position. Prolonged sitting with both arms forward, such as when driving a car, also leads to the cervical posture syndrome. Overload of the cervical musculature can also occur when the shoulders are held (forced) in prolonged depression, such as when carrying heavy objects on or off the shoulders.

The cervical posture syndrome can be part of the so-called total body syndrome; in this instance, the patient complains not only of neck pain, but also of back pain, with or without radiating pain into the legs.

Differential Diagnosis

For differential diagnosis, see Local Cervical Syndrome.

Clinical Findings

- The patient complains of pain and a tired feeling in the neck, the upper thoracic region, and the head. Usually there is local pain and tenderness in the region of the attachments of the levator scapulae at the linea nuchae and the superior angle of the scapula.

- Many patients have a stiff neck and in some cases also complain about discomfort in the temporomandibular joint. Most likely, because of the abnormal position of the head, the occlusion is not optimal and the patient experiences symptoms in this joint.

- Sometimes, a thoracic outlet compression syndrome is also present. This is seen particularly in patients with sloping shoulders. In women with heavy breasts, this is occasionally the case.

- Besides thoracic outlet compression syndrome, neuralgic pain in the distribution of the ulnar and/or radial nerve is often noted. Patients frequently have a cervical postural syndrome in conjunction with a subacromial/subdeltoid bursitis or tennis elbow.

- In many instances, the cervical posture syndrome develops into a local cervical syndrome.

- The functional examination yields few, if any, findings. Sometimes there is a slight limitation of motion. Usually all cervical motions have full range of motion, but the patient complains of a "pulling" in the end-ranges. In instances of a thoracic outlet syndrome, the Roos elevated arm stress test is positive. (The Roos el-

evated arm stress test is performed with the shoulders in 90° abduction and the scapulae in retraction. The elbows are flexed to 90° and the patient is asked to open and close the hands forcefully for a period of 3 minutes.)

Treatment

Treatment is focused primarily on correcting and maintaining the proper head posture. Thorough explanation regarding the disorder, along with ergonomic advice, is given. In principle, the optimal position of the head corresponds to an optimal occlusion. During the exercises described below, the patient should keep the craniomandibular muscles relaxed.

Along with improving the work posture, strengthening the cervical and thoracic musculature is very important. The strengthening exercises emphasize muscles that bring the head from its anterior position into a neutral position whereby the chin is pulled in. Another effective exercise is the so-called cervicothoracic bridge exercise: the patient lies supine with the knees flexed and the feet flat on the floor. The head rests on a small pillow, and the arms are relaxed alongside the body. Without help from the hands and the arms, the patient puts the cervicothoracic spine into lordosis and holds this position for 6 seconds, while continuing to breathe in a relaxed manner.

When consequences of a posture syndrome include thoracic outlet compression syndrome, a subacromial/subdeltoid bursitis, or a tennis elbow, it is best first to treat the postural syndrome. Improvement of the posture can lead to a spontaneous recovery of the other disorders. If that is not the case, then the patient is treated more locally for the bursitis or tendinitis.

In stubborn cases, good results can be achieved with an infiltration of a local anesthetic at both insertions of the levator scapula muscle. If the levator scapula muscle causes symptoms bilaterally, both sides can be treated simultaneously. If there is also tenderness in the interspinal ligament, this area can be injected as well; in instances of residual pain, a corticosteroid can be injected, but only into the ligament.

Local Cervical Syndrome

The local cervical syndrome is seen mostly in patients between the ages of 30 and 45. In many cases, there is a history of one or multiple incidences of an acute torticollis. This disorder is seen twice as often in women as in men. In the past, the cause of this nonspecific posture-related cervical syndrome was always a topic of discussion. Since the improvement of imaging diagnostics (CT scan and more recently MRI), the presence of a disc protrusion at the level of the symptomatic segment has been demonstrated in many patients with a local cervical syndrome.

The symptoms can have either an acute or a gradual onset. If the disc is the primary cause of the symptoms, they can best be explained as coming from an irritation of the recurrent nerve and of the dorsal ramus. Pain at the base of the skull, which often accompanies this syndrome, can be explained by the fact that the trapezius muscle (pars descendens) almost always has increased tension. This leads to an irritation of the greater occipital nerve, which causes radiating pain into the back of the head. In many patients who go untreated, a chronic recurring cycle develops with intervals of pain relief that may last for months and sometimes years.

Most of the lesions originate in C5-6 (41%) or in C6-7 (33%),[2] because this is where most of the motion takes place. Moreover, at these two levels the intervertebral disc is the least protected because the uncinate processes are almost absent. In addition, the lower cervical region undergoes greater loads due to the transition into the relatively rigid thoracic spine (Figures 6–14 to 6–20).

Initially, the symptoms arise after prolonged sitting with the cervical spine in kyphosis (such as during writing, typing, reading, etc). Rotation movements are usually the first to be painful. Often the patients attribute the symptoms to sitting for a prolonged period in a draft. In reality, the combination of prolonged sitting with a poor posture is responsible for the symptoms. Increased tension in the musculature occurs (also due to the cold), which increases the pulling force of the muscles and thereby leads to increased intradiscal pressure.

Characteristically, in many instances, the symptoms worsen at night. This is due to the often unfavorable position of the neck during lying. Irritation of the nerve roots along with muscle tension arises, which causes the patient to wake up. Sometimes the pillow is either too thick or too thin, giving inadequate support to the cervical spine.

Cervical disc protrusions or prolapses give rise to an acceleration of the physiological discosis (disc degeneration). Bony contact of

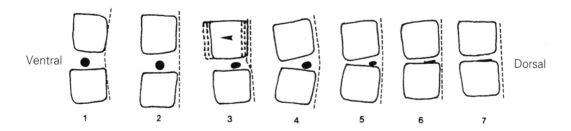

Ventral   Dorsal

1   2   3   4   5   6   7

Figure 6–14 The radiological stages of cervical disc degeneration as described by Jenkner.[22] *1*, Normal; *2*, post-traumatic edema with a loss of lordosis; *3*, slight anterolisthesis; *4*, kyphotic kink; *5*, dehydration of the disc; *6*, diminished kink; *7*, end-stage.

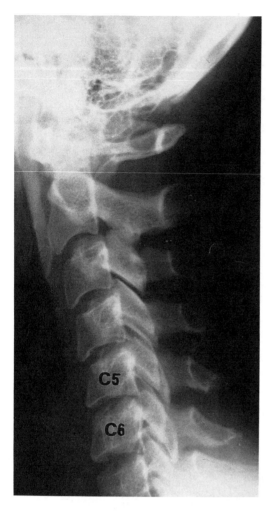

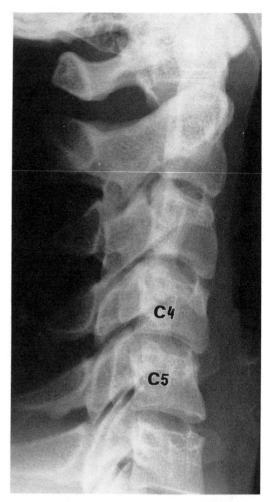

Figure 6–15 Conventional lateral X-ray of the cervical spine in a 25-year-old woman. There is an obvious kyphotic kink of the C5-6 segment. Clinically, the woman demonstrated a C6 nerve root syndrome without neurological signs. The patient was treated with a dorsoventral mobilization. After two treatment sessions, she had complete relief of her pain, even though the symptoms had been present for 14 months.

Figure 6–16 Conventional lateral X-ray of the cervical spine in a 42-year-old man. There is an obvious kyphotic kink of the C4-5 segment. Clinically, the man demonstrated a C5 nerve root syndrome without neurological signs. The patient was treated with dorsoventral mobilizations. Even though the patient had experienced these symptoms for several years, the pain was completely relieved after three treatments.

the uncinate processes occurs because of the loss of disc height. This in turn leads to arthrotic changes of the uncinate processes and later also of the zygapophyseal joints (spondylarthrosis). Because of this, a narrowing of the intervertebral foramen occurs as well as irritation of the spinal nerve and pressure on the vertebral artery. Finally, a painless limitation of the cervical spine occurs (capsular pattern). To a great extent, the mobility of the first two cervical segments remains unchanged.

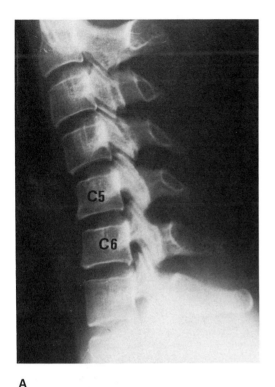

A

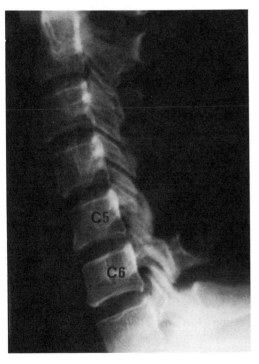

B

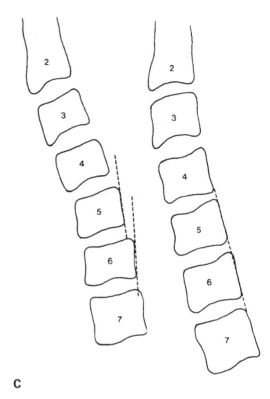

C

Figure 6-17 The cervical spine of a 39-year-old woman, who had complaints of cervical pain for 13 years. Clinically, she demonstrated a C6 nerve root syndrome without neurological signs. **A**, Lateral X-ray. There is a loss of lordosis in the C5-6 segment. The patient was treated with dorsoventral mobilizations and had complete relief of her pain after two treatments. **B**, Three weeks after the second treatment. The normal physiological lordosis is again present. **C**, Schematic illustration of the X-rays from **A** and **B**. The drawing on the left is the situation before and, on the right, the situation after treatment.

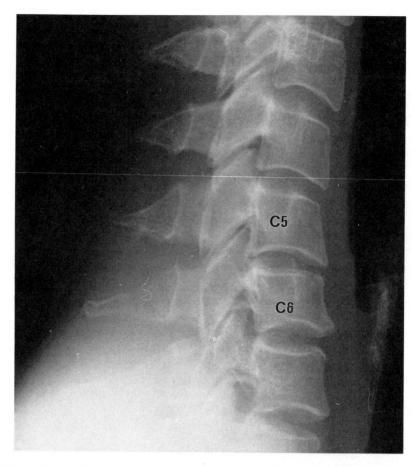

Figure 6–18 Lateral view of the cervical spine in a 38-year-old patient with a C6 nerve root syndrome. There is a kyphotic kink in the C5-6 segment.

Jenkner[22] describes disc edema in patients in the acute stages. Radiologically, an *increase* in the disc height is visible. In the later stages, to a greater or lesser degree, the cranial partner in the segment slides ventrally—an anterolisthesis. The nucleus shifts dorsally and very gradually, a kyphotic kink occurs in the affected segment. Thereafter, the accelerated discosis takes place, leading to the frequently seen loss of lordosis (Figure 6–14).

Differential Diagnosis

Metastases, generally from cancerous bronchial, thyroid, breast, or kidney tumors, can create symptoms similar to those of a be-nign cervical syndrome. This is the case particularly when the primary tumor has gone undiagnosed. The resisted tests are then both painful and weak. Primary tumors in the cervical spine are rare. Imaging techniques (X-ray, bone scan, CT scan, and/or MRI) confirm the diagnosis. In addition, a neurinoma of one of the cervical nerve roots or a spondylitis sometimes can cause symptoms similar to those of a local cervical syndrome.

Clinical Findings

- When the problem lies in the midcervical spine (C3 to C5), the patient usually

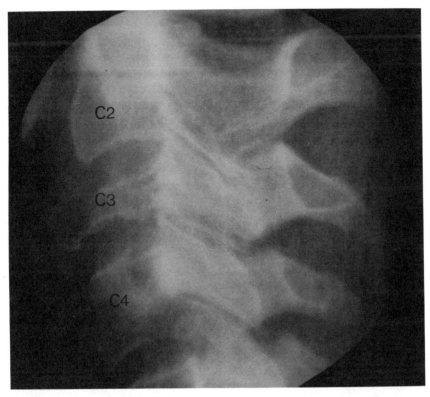

Figure 6–19 Conventional lateral X-ray of C2 to C4 in a 48-year-old patient with a C3 cervical syndrome. Ten years earlier, the patient underwent surgery for breast cancer. There is vertebra plana (flattened vertebra) of C3 as the result of metastases from the breast cancer.

complains of unilateral neck pain with pain in the region of the trapezius muscle, pars descendens. If the lesion is localized in the lower cervical region (C5 to C7), then the patient often has pain between the scapulae. These patients usually have referred tenderness in the area of the rhomboid muscles and the levator scapula. In both instances, pain can be experienced at the back of the head. Sometimes there is a vague radiation of the symptoms into the posterior aspect of the upper arm.

- Some patients demonstrate an antalgic position; the head is held in slight flexion with a minimal sidebending and slight rotation away from the painful side.

- There are no neurological signs.

- Coughing, sneezing, and straining do not provoke the symptoms.

- In the functional examination, one or more motions of the neck are painful and limited in a noncapsular pattern. Despite the often present marked muscular tension, resisted tests are negative.

- In many cases, the standard radiological examination shows a loss of cervical lordosis, often with a slight kyphotic kink in one segment. The segments most often affected are C5-6 or C6-7. The kinked position of the segment results from a dorsal shift of the center of the intervertebral disc. Even though the nucleus pulposus has practically disappeared in this age

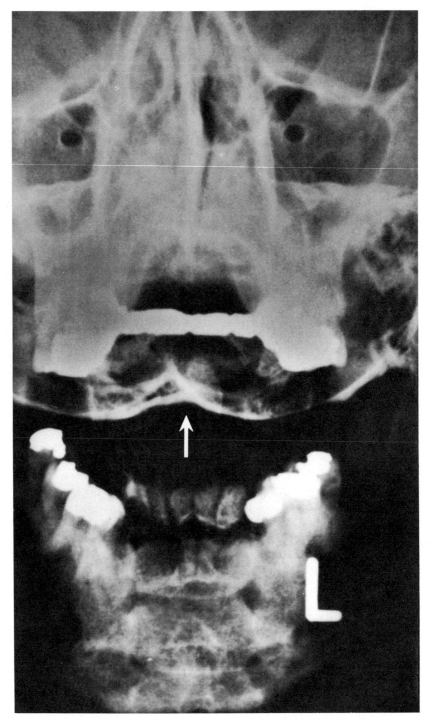

Figure 6–20 Conventional anterior-posterior X-ray in a man with an apparent benign local cervical syndrome. Within a few weeks, the patient developed a capsular-pattern limitation of motion. As demonstrated on the X-ray, the dens has "disappeared" due to a tumor. (An **_arrow_** indicates where the dens should be.)

group, a rather large shift of disc material is still possible.

- Due to the weight of the head, the cervical discs sustain a significant amount of load. To a large extent, this is compensated for by the cervical musculature. Thus, in a normal posture (with the cervical spine in its physiological lordosis), with normal tension in the muscles, the pressure in the lower cervical discs is 5.6 kg/cm^2. Without the muscles, the pressure in the discs increases to approximately 40 kg/cm^2.

Treatment

First, a thorough explanation is given to the patient regarding the lesion and its natural progression. The patient should be aware of the consequences of poor cervical posture. In the physiological position, the load on the cervical structures is the least. Treatment also consists of manual traction, mobilization, and/or manipulation. In very acute cases, when the manual treatment techniques cannot be applied because of pain, medication may be indicated. In addition, a cervical collar can be worn. Stabilizing exercises should always be given if the problem recurs. The patient is encouraged to perform these exercises daily at home.

Acute (Discogenic) Torticollis

Acute torticollis is most often seen in children and young adults. It is an early form of the cervical primary disc-related disorders. In many instances, the problem arises during the night as a result of lying with the cervical spine in a flexed and sidebent position. Unfavorable influences act upon the cervical discs when the head remains in the same position over a long period of time. Usually, a person changes positions frequently during sleep. Due to sleeping pills, alcohol, or extreme fatigue, a person may maintain a certain position much longer than normal, causing an extreme *intradiscal* shift of the central disc material (Figure 6–21). Upon waking, the patient has the feeling of a stiff neck. Then, while making a (usually minor) movement, a click is heard with subsequent severe unilateral neck pain.

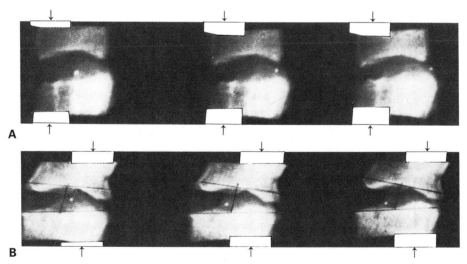

Figure 6–21 Shifting of the disc material during asymmetrical compression (50 to 100 kg) of the C4-5 disc in an 18-year-old subject. The shift is marked by a metal pin. *Source:* Reprinted from *Bandscheibenbedingte Erkrankungen* by J. Krämer with permission of Georg Thieme Verlag, © 1978. **A**, Load on the anterior aspect of the segment (kyphosis); **B**, load on the posterior aspect of the segment (lordosis).

Differential Diagnosis

Post-Traumatic (See Traumatic Lesions).

- Grisel's disease
- Traumatic atlantoaxial subluxation
- Unilateral or bilateral subluxation/dislocation

Nontraumatic (See Other Pathology).

- Spastic torticollis (a condition of cramping in the sternocleidomastoid muscle in which the head is pulled into slight flexion, ipsilateral sidebending, and contralateral rotation)
- Spasmodic torticollis
- Congenital torticollis. In newborn babies with this disorder, the head is in ipsilateral sidebend and contralateral rotation. The exact cause is unknown. Klippel-Feil syndrome should be considered in the differential diagnosis. In these congenital disorders, deformations of the cervical vertebrae are present, such as fused vertebrae. In many cases, the neck is strikingly short.
- Conversion torticollis

Clinical Findings

- The patient complains of severe unilateral pain and holds the head sidebent and rotated away from the painful side, along with simultaneous cervical flexion. The intradiscal protrusion causes irritation of the nocisensoric fibers of the recurrent nerve in the posterior longitudinal ligament and the dura mater. Through the specific forced position of the head, the pressure on the spinal nerve and the recurrent nerve is kept as low as possible; the intervertebral foramen increases in size on the affected side.
- The functional examination shows a severely limited and painful rotation and sidebend toward the painful side. The extension motion is also very limited and painful. When performed correctly, the resisted tests cause minimal to no discomfort.
- There are no neurological deficits.
- Coughing, sneezing, and straining are either negative or only mildly positive.
- Imaging diagnostics (CT scan or MRI) are indicated only if the history or examination reveals atypical findings.

Treatment

Without treatment, the symptoms usually last approximately 2 to 3 weeks. After 1 week, there is such drastic improvement that the patient again can function normally. With treatment, the symptoms usually last only a few days.

The patient should be given a thorough explanation about the problem as well as the necessary ergonomic advice. The treatment of preference is manual axial separation in the antalgic position of the cervical spine. Usually the neutral position is achieved within a few minutes. From this position, considerable improvement can be achieved by bringing the head slightly into the painful rotation and supporting it there with a sandbag for approximately 5 to 10 minutes. The head is then brought farther into the rotation and supported for another several minutes. This procedure is repeated several times. When no further improvement is reached with the rotation, the repositioning technique is performed for the sidebend. In addition, either before or after the repositioning technique, axial separation with rotation can be performed. This should occur first in the rotation that is the least painful. When no further improvement is noted with this technique, axial separation with rotation is performed cautiously in the direction of the painful rotation.

After treatment, the patient is given a cervical collar to wear until the next treatment session. The patient initially should be seen daily for treatment. At the same time, the patient should be constantly aware of his or her posture to ensure that the head does not return to the antalgic position. Wearing the cervical collar at night is also necessary. The pillow should not be too thick, but also not too thin. It should be firm, and when the patient lies on the side it should bridge the gap between the shoulder and the head.

Cervicobrachial Syndrome

The cervicobrachial syndrome is caused by a posterolateral disc protrusion or prolapse. To a large degree, the severity of the symptoms is dependent on the size of the spinal canal. For instance, a small disc protrusion in a small spinal canal can lead to severe symptoms, while a disc prolapse in a very large canal sometimes causes only mild problems (Figure 6–22).

This disorder is seen mostly in people younger than 45 years of age. In one epidemiological study,[23] the youngest patient with a disc prolapse was 20 and the oldest patient was 64 years old. The ratio of men to women in this study was 1.4 to 1. In many cases, these patients have already experienced several episodes of a local cervical syndrome.

The symptoms can have an acute as well as a gradual onset. The biggest difference between a local cervical syndrome and the cervicobrachial syndrome is that in the latter the symptoms are not only localized in the neck and scapula region, but they also radiate down the arm and often into the fingers.

Frequently there is a trauma in the history. Such a trauma, either direct or indirect, may have taken place years earlier. Sometimes a cervical disc prolapse occurs as a result of repeated lifting of heavy objects. In the study by Kelsey et al,[23] 28% of the subjects had symptoms after a traffic accident.

By far, most cervical disc protrusions and prolapses occur in the C5-6 and/or C6-7 segments. In instances of root compression at levels above and below these two segments, serious pathology should first be ruled out.

Differential Diagnosis

In patients over 45 years of age with a long history of cervical problems, one should think primarily of a cervical nerve root compression

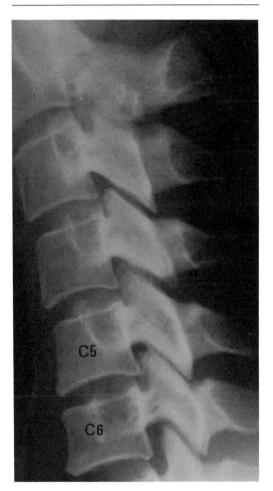

A

Figure 6–22 Cervical spine in an adult man with a slight cervicobrachial syndrome on the left. **A**, Conventional lateral view X-ray. The C5-6 disc is minimally narrowed and the cervical lordosis is diminished. Clinically the patient is considered to have a slight C6 nerve root syndrome. **B**, CT scan at the level of the C5-6 disc. There is a large posterolateral disc prolapse on the left (**arrowheads**), with compression of the left C6 nerve root and deformation of the dural sac. The spinal canal is large enough that the symptoms are mild.

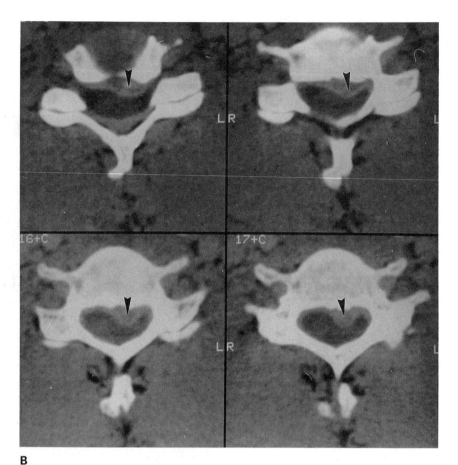

B

Figure 6–22 continued

syndrome. A neurinoma can cause similar symptoms, except that in this disorder the paresthesia generally begins distally and then spreads proximally. For further differential diagnosis, refer to Local Cervical Syndrome.

Clinical Findings

- Most patients complain of neck pain that radiates into the shoulders and is predominately on one side. At the same time, in almost all cases, pain is also referred to the interscapular region. Al-

though symptoms in the arm and hand can be the first to appear, more often the symptoms start with pain in the cervical region. However, if the symptoms do originate in the hand and/or arm, other pathology, such as a cervical neurinoma, should be ruled out.

- Usually pain radiating into the arm is localized in the C6 or the C7 dermatomes and less frequently in the C5 or C8 dermatomes. Disc-related lesions in the other segments are rare. In addition, the patient may have complaints of sensory disturbances or loss of strength. Sympathetic reactions can also arise, such as acrocyanosis (Raynaud's sign) and cold, clammy hands. Often the patient also describes a swollen feeling of the hand; however, this swelling cannot be confirmed objectively.

- In the functional examination, limited range of motion in a noncapsular pattern is evident. Rotation and sidebending to the affected side are painful and limited. In most patients, extension is also limited and painful. The limitation in rotation increases when it is tested in extension.

- Whenever motor and/or sensory deficits are found, the presence of a disc prolapse is very likely. In this instance, coughing, sneezing, and straining provoke pain in the neck, shoulder, and arm regions.

- In a posterolateral disc prolapse, the foraminal compression test can be positive.

- Root compression of T1 to T4 as a result of a disc prolapse is rarely seen. If the patient has symptoms particularly from the T1 nerve root, serious pathology should be considered (Figure 6–23).

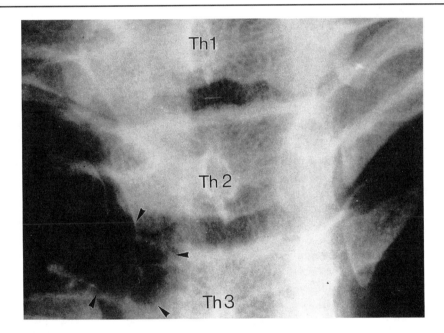

A

Figure 6–23 Cervicothoracic spine of a patient who was referred to the physical therapist with a "right cervicobrachial syndrome." There were symptoms of a root irritation of T2 and T3. The patient was sent back immediately with the request for further imaging examination. **A**, Conventional AP X-ray. There is a defined interval in the right upper pole of the T3 vertebral body. The right pedicle is destroyed, and a soft tissue mass is visible.

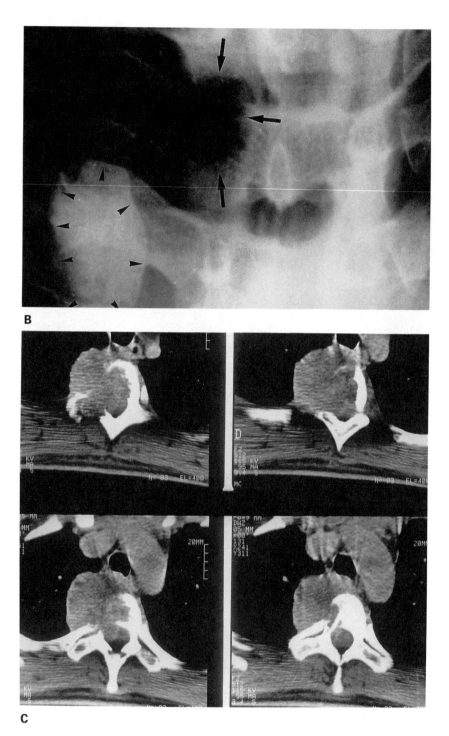

Figure 6–23 B, Conventional AP X-ray, taken 3 months after the first one (**A**). Under the destroyed right pedicle (**arrows**), the soft tissue mass is even more visible (**arrowheads**). **C,** CT scan of T3. There is an extensive bony defect. The bone is replaced by a tumorous soft tissue mass on the right.

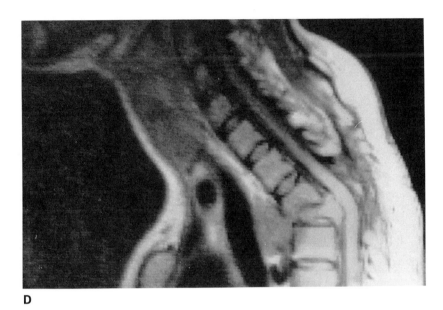

D

Figure 6–23 D, MRI, sagittal view. There is severe destruction with wedge-shaped flattening of the T3 vertebral body.

Treatment

If the patient has never experienced root symptoms before, the brachial (arm) symptoms usually resolve in a period of 3 to 4 months. If the problem is recurrent, then especially after repeated incidences, the pain in the arm and hand can ultimately become chronic. If there are motor deficits, the symptoms disappear faster than when there are no deficits.

As with all disorders, it is very important to give the patient thorough information about the lesion. Because the ultimate prognosis is favorable in most cases, the patient should be reassured. Ergonomic advice is also necessary.

Cervical mobilization is generally indicated if there are no neurological findings, and the lesion is considered to be a protrusion (in-stead of a prolapse) (Figures 6–24 to 6–27). Refer to Indications and Contraindications for cervical mobilization in section 6.4, Treatment. Particularly in the acute phase, heat modalities, soft tissue techniques, nonsteroidal anti-inflammatories, and rest are indicated. In chronic cases, paravertebral injections with a local anesthetic can offer pain relief. Surgery is seldom necessary.

Cervicomedullary Syndrome

The cervicomedullary syndrome is the most severe form of cervical disc prolapse. It involves a posterocentral disc prolapse in which compression of the spinal cord occurs.

This rare syndrome can have a traumatic as well as gradual onset. In the latter instance, it is particularly important to rule out other pa-

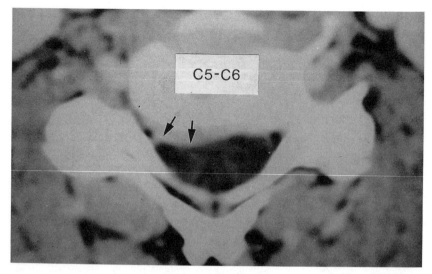

A

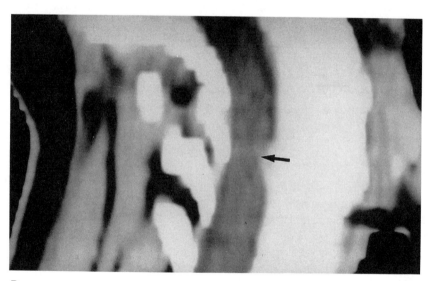

B

Figure 6–24 CT scan at the level of the C5-6 disc in a 37-year-old man with a right C6 cervicobrachial syndrome. **A**, Normal technique after intravenous injection of contrast medium. There is mild postero-lateral bulging of the disc (***arrows***). The dural sac is compressed and pushed away on one side. **B**, Paramedian reconstruction, right. A disc prolapse is obvious (***arrow***).

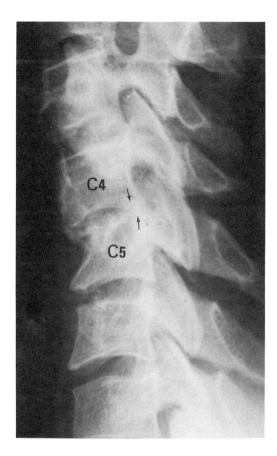

Figure 6–25 There is a partial fusion of the C4 and C5 vertebral bodies. However, clinically the patient has a C6 root syndrome. General manual mobilization is contraindicated. This patient was treated with local segmental dorsoventral mobilization of C5-6. In addition, the patient wore a cervical collar. After 3 weeks (four treatments), the patient reported complete relief of pain.

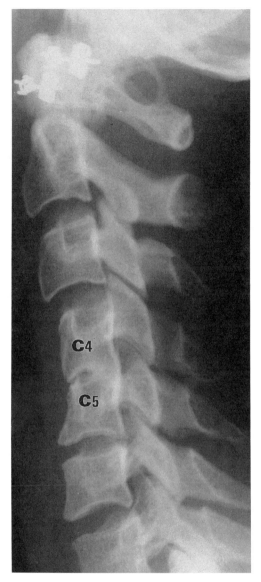

Figure 6–26 In this 34-year-old patient, the C4-5 segment is fused. Clinically the patient presented with a C7 nerve root syndrome. General manual mobilization is contraindicated. This patient was treated with local segmental dorsoventral mobilization of C6-7. In addition, the patient wore a cervical collar. After 4 weeks (five treatments), the patient reported complete relief of pain.

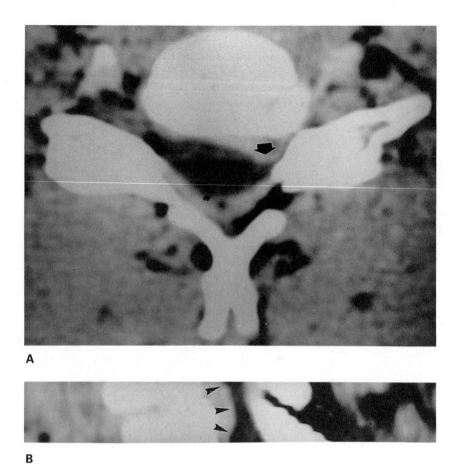

A

B

Figure 6–27 CT scan at the level of the C6-7 disc in a 48-year-old woman with a left C7 cervicobrachial syndrome. **A**, Normal technique after intravenous contrast medium injection. There is a large disc prolapse (**arrow**), which protrudes into the intervertebral foramen and compromises the C7 nerve root. **B**, Paramedian reconstruction, left. There is pronounced compression of the neural structures. The protrusion, both cranial and caudal, is obvious (**arrowheads**).

thology that can compress the spinal cord, such as tumors (Figures 6–28 and 6–29). However, the most frequent causes of spinal cord compression are fractures with dislocation of part of the vertebra. (See Traumatic Lesions.) In rare cases, degenerative changes such as dorsal bone spurs can compress the spinal cord. Although this syndrome, as well as all other disc-related syndromes, is seen mostly in patients between the ages of 35 and 55, exceptions do occur (Figures 6–30 and 6–31).

Clinical Findings

- In the most pronounced form of the cervicomedullary syndrome, the patient has primarily neurological symptoms

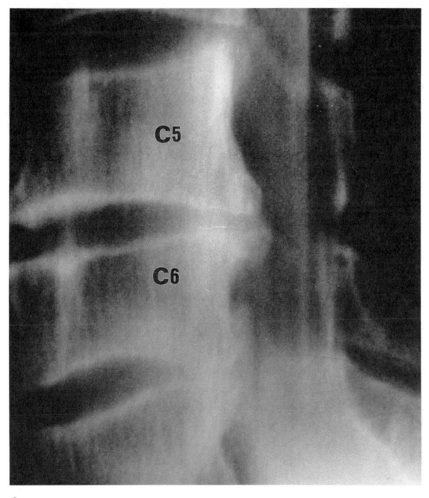

A

Figure 6–28 The cervical spine in a 56-year-old patient with a very gradually occurring spinal cord compression. **A**, Lateral tomogram, C4 to C7. **B**, CT scan at the level of C5. There is severe dorsal bony spurring with a reduction in the cross section of the spinal canal and resultant compression of the spinal cord.

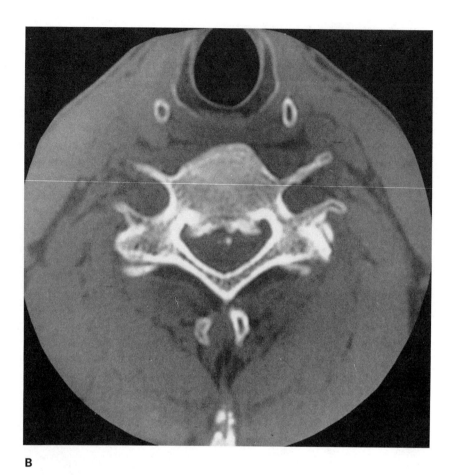

B

Figure 6–28 continued

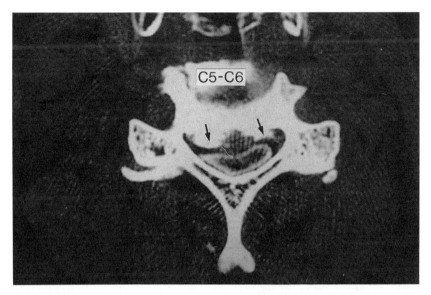

A

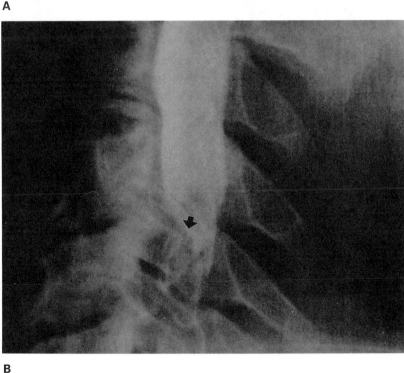

B

Figure 6–29 The cervical spine in a 52-year-old patient with a very gradually occurring cervicomedullary syndrome. **A**, Myelo-CT scan at the level of C5-6. There is very severe dorsal spurring (**arrows**) with significant compression of the spinal cord. **B**, Myelogram of the cervical spine. There is a complete stop (**arrow**) of the contrast medium at the level of C4-5.

and very little pain. The patient complains of an "electric current" feeling that can occur in different places either spontaneously or dependent on movements in the cervical spine (particularly flexion). These electric current sensations can be experienced in the whole body, but also only in the legs and/or in the arms.

- Because of the pressure on the spinal cord, pyramidal tract disturbances initially cause abnormal reflexes. In particular, the lower extremities are affected. For instance, an abnormal Babinski foot sole reflex is present. Later, spastic hemiparesis and paraparesis can develop. In even later stages, ataxia and pronounced gait disturbances appear.

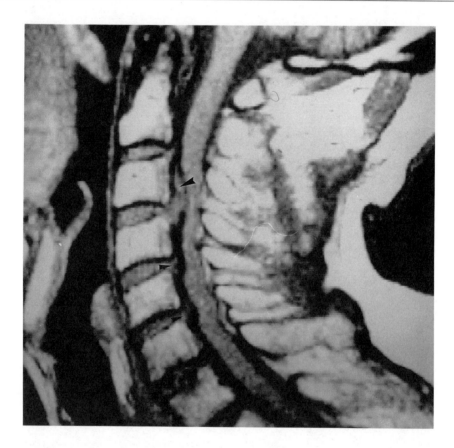

Figure 6–30 MRI of the cervical spine in a man with an acutely occurring cervicomedullary syndrome. There is a severe disc prolapse at the C3-4 level with a fragment that dislocated cranially behind the vertebral body of C3 (**large arrowhead**). Less extensive disc protrusions are demonstrated at the C4-5 and C5-6 levels (**small arrowheads**).

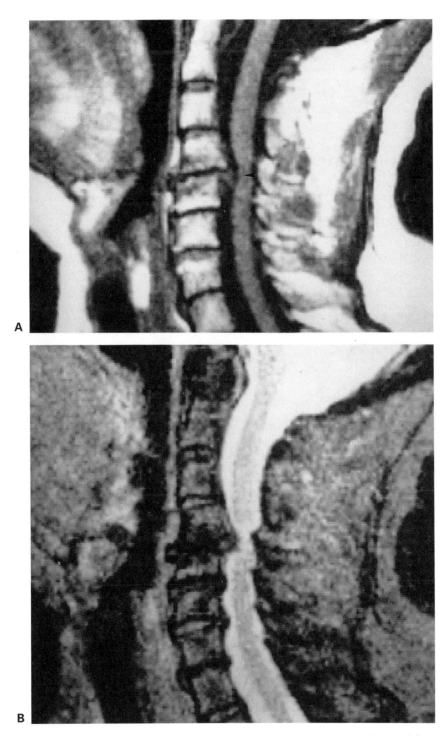

Figure 6–31 MRI of the cervical spine in a 67-year-old woman with a cervicomedullary syndrome. **A**, Normal technique. There is a disc prolapse at C4-5 (***arrowhead***) with severe spinal cord compression. **B**, Technique making the spinal cord especially visible. The severity of the compression is best seen in this view.

- CT scan and/or MRI examinations are indicated (Figures 6–32 and 6–33).

Treatment

Treatment consists of immediate surgery. Otherwise, there is danger that the symptoms will become irreversible.

SECONDARY DISC-RELATED DISORDERS

In this book, secondary disc-related disorders are disorders in which one of the following has occurred:

- A primary disc lesion was experienced earlier.

- The normally occurring physiological degeneration of the segment is accelerated.
- Due to trauma, the normal adaptation to the degeneration is made impossible.

Thus, secondary discogenic disorders always involve situations in which extreme disc degeneration is later coupled with changes in the zygapophyseal joints. This leads to narrowing of the spinal canal and the intervertebral foramen. In some cases, the causal role of an earlier primary disc-related problem is not (yet) confirmed. However, in our view the evidence is convincing enough to consider these as secondary disc-related disorders nonetheless.

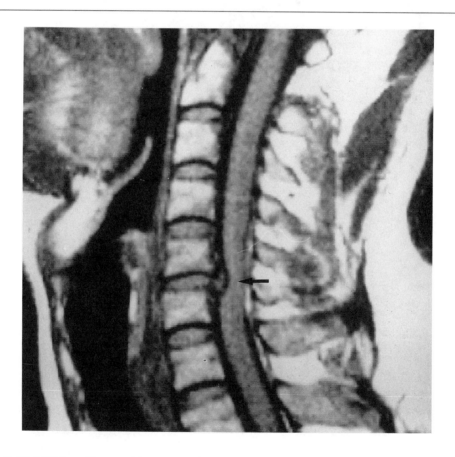

Figure 6–32 MRI in a 30-year-old woman with a cervicobrachial syndrome. There is a central disc prolapse (**arrow**) with medullary compression.

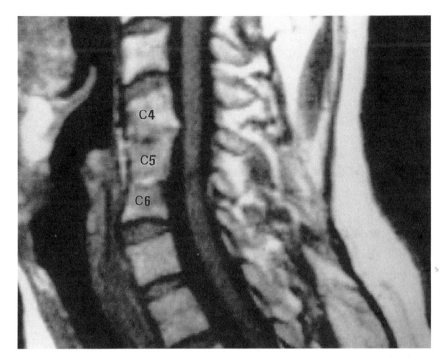

Figure 6–33 MRI of the cervical spine in a 45-year-old man who had a disc prolapse at two levels. A spondylosyndesis was performed of C4-5 and C5-6. In this procedure, the intervertebral discs were replaced with a bone chip.

Nerve Root Compression Syndrome

A nerve root compression syndrome can occur in patients who already have a long history of neck pain, either with or without radicular symptoms. After a period of minimal to no symptoms, without experiencing a trauma, the symptoms very gradually begin again, and are felt especially in the arm.

Because of an acceleration of the discosis (physiological disc degeneration), osteophytes on the uncinate processes and the zygapophyseal joints develop. Initially, the nerve root has sufficient room. However, because of the accelerated course of the discosis, a segmental hypermobility occurs. This leads to an increase in the osteophytosis and the reserve space for the root in the intervertebral foramen is ultimately "consumed" (Figure 6–34).

After a fracture a loose fragment occasionally compromises the nerve in the intervertebral foramen. (See Figure 6–56).

Differential Diagnosis

Nondiscogenic pathology, such as tumors, can also cause radicular pain. For further differential diagnosis, refer to Local Cervical Syndrome. If the patient also has neurovascular symptoms and complains of unilateral headache, then one should differentiate between a migraine and other disorders that can cause headaches, dizziness, and ringing in the ears. Often an examination by a specialist is necessary (such as a neurologist, an otolaryngologist, or an ophthalmologist).

Clinical Findings

- The local cervical pain is usually minimal. The patient has pain in the arm that is dependent on certain positions and movements, particularly those that cause a decrease in the size of the intervertebral foramen. Such movements include extension and ipsilateral side-bending, possibly in combination with the ipsilateral rotation.

- Often the patient wakes up at night because of the pain and paresthesia in the corresponding dermatome of the affected segment.
- If the osteophytosis extends laterally, then compression of the vertebral artery may result (Figure 6–35). In this instance, the patient also experiences neurovascular symptoms. (Refer to Vertebrobasilar Insufficiency.) These symptoms include headache, dizziness, ringing in the ears, and swallowing and hearing disturbances as well as vision disturbances.

- The functional examination is dependent on the severity of the symptoms at the time. Ipsilateral sidebending can be painful, along with one or both of the rotations. Extension is almost always limited and painful. At the end-range of every motion, the end-feel is hard.

- In rare instances, there are neurological deficits.

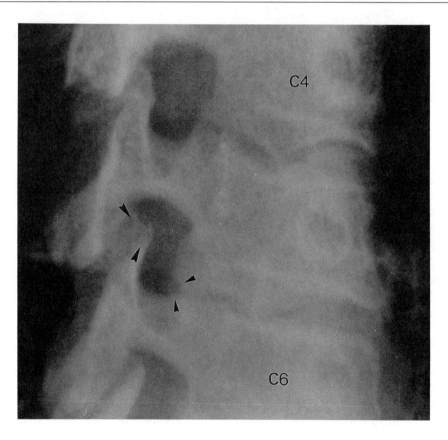

Figure 6–34 Conventional oblique X-ray of C4-6 in a 57-year-old man with a nerve root compression syndrome of C6. There is narrowing of the C5-6 intervertebral foramen as a result of the moderate uncarthrosis (**small arrowheads**), and the significant zygapophyseal joint arthrosis (**large arrowheads**).

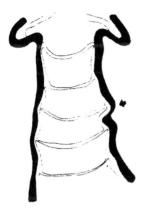

Figure 6–35 Compression of the vertebral artery as the result of lateral osteophytes extending from the uncinate processes. *Source:* Reprinted with permission from *Bandscheibenbedingte Erkrankungen* by J. Krämer with permission of Georg Thieme Verlap, © 1978.

- In many cases the foramina compression test is positive. In instances of neurovascular symptoms, the DeKleyn and Nieuwenhuyse test is positive. (For performance of the DeKleyn and Nieuwenhuyse test, refer to section 6.2, Examination.)

Treatment

Usually there is a chronic recurring course to the symptoms, with intervals of pain relief lasting months to years. As the physiological fibrosing of the affected motion segment ultimately resolves the relative segmental hypermobility, the symptoms generally disappear. The patient should be thoroughly informed about the self-limiting nature of this disorder. Ergonomic advice is also necessary. Particular attention should also be given to using the proper pillow at night.

In severe cases, heat modalities, a cervical collar, or nonsteroidal anti-inflammatories can provide some relief of pain (Figures 6–36 and 6–37). In therapy-resistant cases, paravertebral blocks, facet denervations, or possibly rhizotomy is considered. Surgery is rarely indicated.

Mobilization of the cervical spine is contraindicated. In so doing, the physiological fibrosing process is disturbed.

Limitation of Motions in the Capsular Pattern

As a result of the progressive degenerative process, a nonpainful capsular pattern limitation of motion evolves. This limitation is found particularly at the level of C5 to C7 and to a lesser degree from C2 to C5. The upper cervical segments remain the most mobile. However, here also—usually after a trauma—degenerative changes can occur, which then lead to a severe limitation of motion in the capsular pattern (Figures 6–38 to 6–40).

Differential Diagnosis

A capsular pattern of limitation in younger patients, as well as a sudden spontaneous capsular pattern of limitation in older patients, always indicates an inflammatory process or a tumor. Refer also to Rheumatoid Arthritis of the Cervical Spine.

Clinical Findings

- Most patients have no complaints. Because the upper cervical spine remains mobile, the function of the cervical spine as a whole is not significantly disrupted. Some patients, more often men than women, complain of a stiff neck and headache upon waking in the morning. Generally the pain disappears in the course of the day.

- The functional examination indicates the capsular pattern limitation of motion: a symmetrical limitation of rotation and sidebending; extension is the most limited and flexion is the least limited.

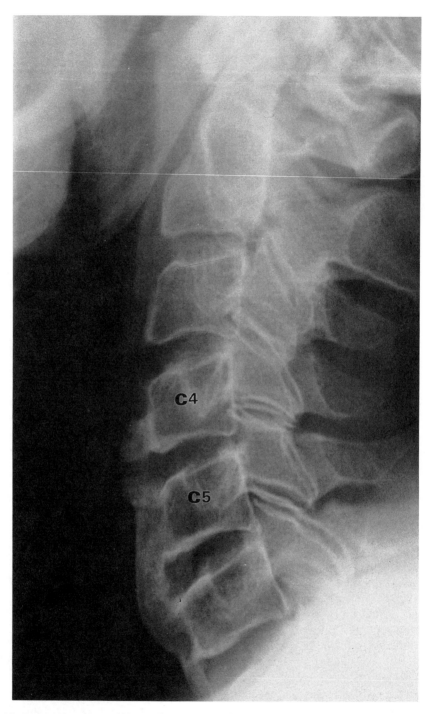

Figure 6–36 Conventional lateral X-ray of a 50-year-old man with a nerve root compression syndrome of C5. There is a pronounced ankylosing osteophytosis and hyperostosis on the ventral aspects of C4 to C7. The patient is a dock worker and has carried 75-kg sacks of coffee for many years. The symptoms consist of mild radiating pain in the C5 dermatome and local neck pain. After 2 weeks of wearing a cervical collar, the pain resolved.

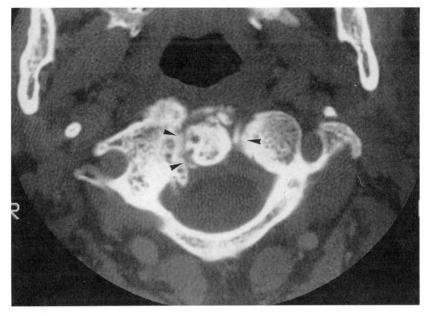

A

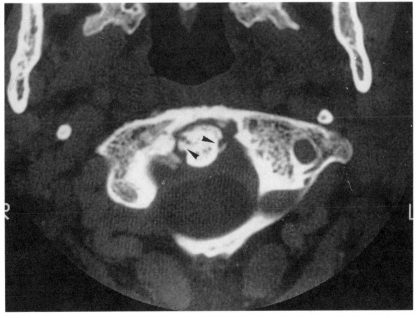

B

Figure 6–37 CT scan of a 41-year-old man with a severe, gradually occurring limitation of motion in the capsular pattern as a result of a trauma experienced years earlier. *A* and *B*, Degenerative changes between the atlas and the dens (***arrowheads***), right more obvious than left.

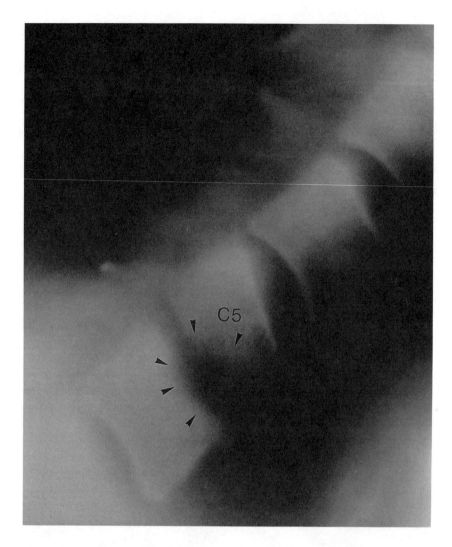

Figure 6–38 Lateral tomogram of the cervical spine (C3 to C7) in a 34-year-old man who presented with a capsular pattern limitation of motion. There is spondylodiscitis at C5-6.

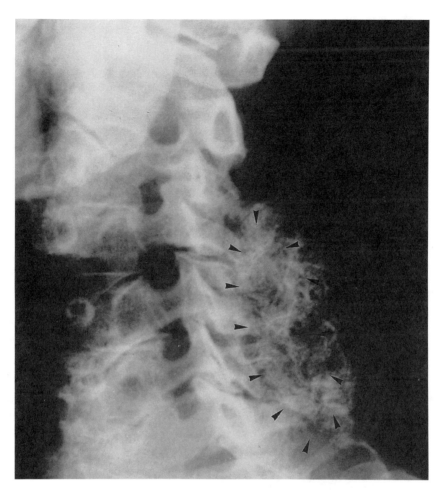

Figure 6–39 Conventional X-ray of a 47-year-old man with a sudden onset of a capsular pattern limitation of motion. There is a large osteochondroma at the level of the spinous processes of C3 to C7.

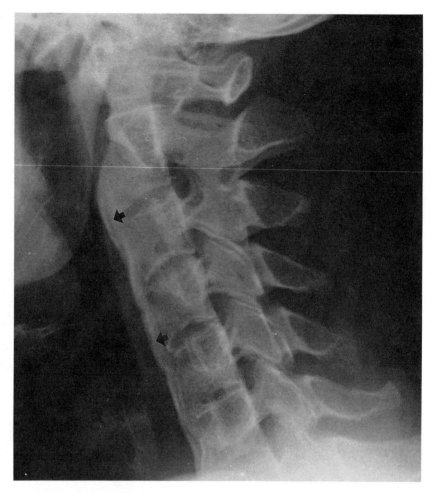

Figure 6–40 Conventional lateral X-ray in a patient with ankylosing spondylitis. Clinically the patient presented with a severe limitation of motion in the capsular pattern. Ossification of the anterior longitudinal ligament is clearly visible (**arrows**).

Treatment

If the individual has no pain, the limitation of motion should go untreated. The patient should be given thorough information regarding the problem. Patients with typical occipital pain can generally be helped by treatment with gentle manual traction. Other manual mobilization is contraindicated.

TRAUMATIC LESIONS

In this book, traumatic disorders include not only lesions of which the patient is aware of the traumatic onset, but also lesions such as "spontaneous" fractures in which a prolonged degenerative process has been present. Also included in this category are the non–disc-related disorders that *can*, but do not necessarily, have a traumatic onset.

Post-Traumatic Cervical Syndrome

In the post-traumatic cervical syndrome, trauma is central to the problem. However, in many cases the symptomatology and treatment are the same as in primary disc-related disorders. Thus, after a trauma one can differentiate between a *local cervical* syndrome and a *cervicobrachial* syndrome, and in severe cases a *cervicomedullary* syndrome. Joint subluxations (or dislocations) and fractures can also occur. In these instances, there is almost always a simultaneous rupture of the capsuloligamentous structures.

Various types of trauma can be differentiated:

- hyperflexion trauma
- hyperextension trauma
- acceleration trauma
- combination trauma
- rotation trauma

Depending on the type of accident, injuries to the head, brain, shoulder, and/or arm must also be considered when there has been a trauma to the cervical spine (Figures 6–41 to 6–46).

Clinical Findings

Hyperflexion Trauma. In most cases, the hyperflexion trauma is the result of a sports

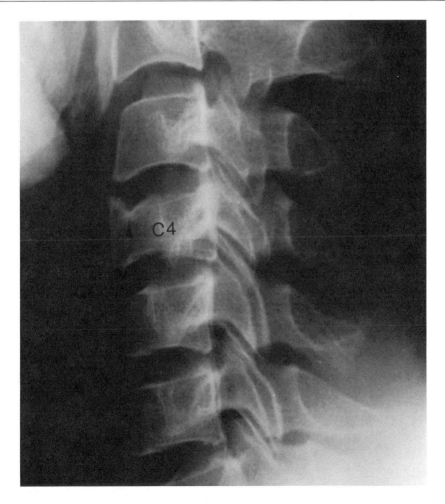

Figure 6–41 Conventional lateral X-ray of the cervical spine of a 32-year-old woman who sustained a hyperflexion trauma. There is a compression fracture (***arrowhead***) of the C4 vertebral body.

injury, such as a failed somersault or a bad fall during judo or wrestling. The possible consequences are classified into ventral and dorsal.

Ventral Consequences. In hyperflexion trauma, compression fractures of the vertebral bodies can occur. One of the most serious consequences of a hyperflexion trauma is rupture of the transverse ligament of the atlas. As a result of the ruptured ligament, the dens of the axis compromises the spinal cord. The dens itself sometimes fractures (see Traumatic Atlantoaxial Subluxation/Dislocation).

Vertebral dislocations can occur at every level of the cervical spine (see Bilateral Zygapophyseal Joint Subluxation/Dislocation).

These dislocations are usually paired with fractures.

Dorsal Consequences. Hyperflexion trauma can also lead to an overstretch or tear of the zygapophyseal joint capsules, with or without fractures of the facets. Sprains or tears of various other ligamentous connections in the dorsal part of the cervical spine can also occur. Sometimes an avulsion fracture of a spinous process occurs. Fractures of the posterior arch of the atlas are rare. In addition, severe sprains of the dorsal musculature can occur.

Almost every injury is accompanied by a disc lesion. Usually the lesion involves a rupture of

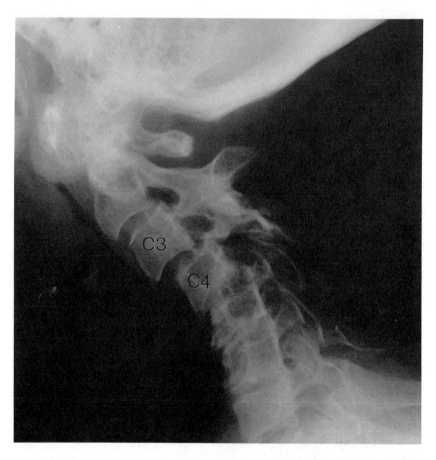

Figure 6–42 Conventional lateral X-ray of the cervical spine of a 50-year-old woman who sustained a hyperflexion trauma. There is a ventral dislocation of C3-4, which is more pronounced than at C4-5. In addition, there are significant degenerative changes visible.

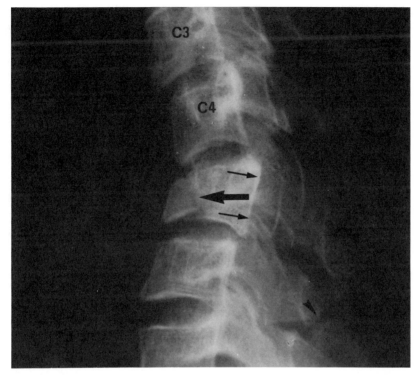

A

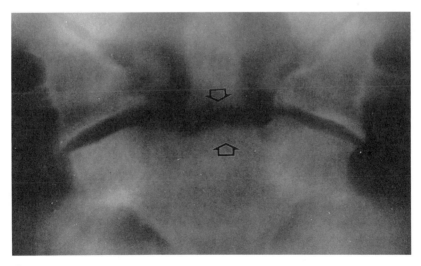

B

Figure 6–43 Cervical spine of a 24-year-old patient who already had had several serious motorcross accidents. After this trauma, severe compression of the spinal cord resulted. **A**, Conventional lateral X-ray. There is a ventral compression fracture of C5 (**large arrow**) with a dorsal shift of the back wall of the vertebral body (**small arrows**). In addition, there is a fracture of the C6 spinous process (**arrowhead**) and an old fracture of the C7 spinous process (**lower arrowheads**). **B**, AP tomogram at the level of C0 to C3. There is a fracture of the base of the dens (**arrows**).

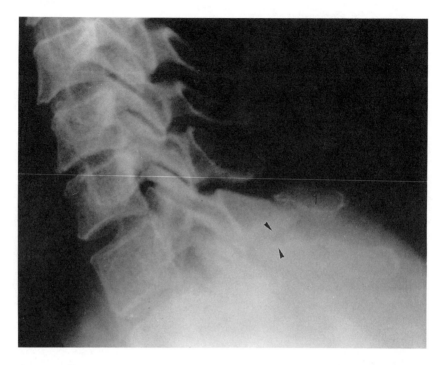

Figure 6–44 Conventional lateral X-ray of the cervical spine in a 46-year-old man. Clinically he presented with a C6 cervicobrachial syndrome. There is an old fracture of the C7 spinous process (***arrowheads***) with a free fragment (***1***), as the result of a hyperflexion trauma from years earlier. Now it is of no clinical significance.

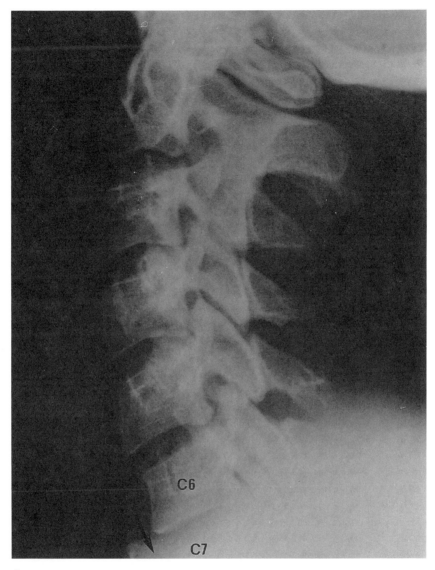

A

Figure 6–45 Cervical spine of a 38-year-old man who sustained a hyperflexion trauma. **A**, Conventional lateral functional X-ray, extension. There is a compression fracture of C7 (**arrow**).

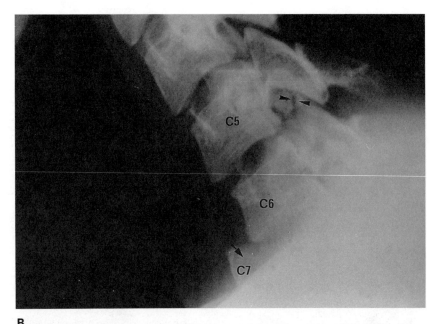

Figure 6–45 B, Conventional lateral functional X-ray, flexion. There is an additional fracture of the pedicle and the C5 facet (***arrowheads***). ***C***, CT scan. A CT scan best indicates the severity of the fracture, in this instance a "burst" fracture.

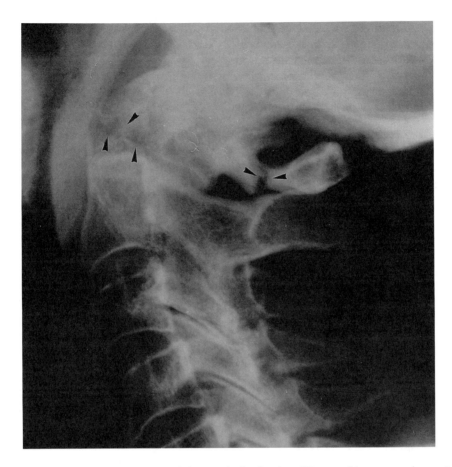

Figure 6–46 Conventional lateral X-ray of the cervical spine in a 56-year-old woman who sustained a severe hyperextension trauma. A fracture dislocation of the dens is noted (***left arrowheads***). In addition, the posterior arch of the atlas has fractured against the spinous process of the axis (***right arrowheads***).

the annulus fibrosus through which disc material prolapses. Injuries to the vertebral artery are seldom seen in hyperflexion traumas.

Prognosis. The prognosis of a hyperflexion trauma is good, as long as there were no fractures or disc prolapses. In the absence of fractures and disc prolapses, the patient is treated as if there were a local cervical syndrome. To support the treatment, the appropriate physical therapy or medication is provided to aid in the resorption of the usually present hematoma.

Hyperextension Trauma. A hyperextension trauma occurs in various contact sports, for example, by a punch on the chin during boxing. Of course, a hyperextension trauma can also occur during a car accident and in diving accidents, due to shallow water. The possible consequences are classified into ventral and dorsal.

Ventral Consequences. A hyperextension trauma can lead to an overstretch of the disc, the anterior longitudinal ligament, and the anterior neck muscles. Because of this, a retropharyngeal hematoma can develop, causing disturbances in swallowing. The swallowing disturbances are significant in making the diagnosis. In general, if there are no swallowing disturbances, severe traumatization can be ruled out.

Dorsal Consequences. Due to compression, subluxations, or dislocations of the zygapophyseal joints, severe disc lesions can also occur. Occasionally, a fracture of one of the spinous processes occurs. A fracture of the dens is also rare, but often leads to significant compression of the spinal cord. If the dens dislocates, this can lead to death.

Injury of the vertebral artery is often seen as a consequence of a hyperextension trauma. Patients who already have degenerative changes in the immediate area of the vertebral artery are particularly susceptible.

Acceleration Trauma. Acceleration trauma, also called whiplash, is a combination of a hyperextension trauma and a hypertraction trauma (Figure 6–47). Most often it occurs as a result of a rear-end collision. At first, the cervical spine undergoes a hyperextension because of the slowness of the mass: the head remains relatively behind while the trunk moves forward. Then, due to a stretch on the anterior structures, a hypertraction occurs. In this way, the head is thrown forward and upward. If the chin ultimately hits against the sternum, a second hypertraction mechanism occurs. If a seat belt is not worn, a hyperflexion trauma occurs when the individual collides against an object from the front. In many cases, there is also a component of cervical sidebending and/or rotation to the trauma. This is termed a combination trauma.

Sances et al[24] state that when someone is hit from behind with a velocity of 20 km/h, a 5-cm lengthening of the spinal cord occurs. This leads to injury of the medulla oblongata, the brain stem, and the thalamus (Figure 6–48).

Macnab[25] writes that during an acceleration trauma, the disc can tear loose from the vertebral body, resulting in a severe instability. In addition, Webb and Terrett[26] propose that the anterior neck muscles can tear along with the anterior and posterior longitudinal ligaments. At the same time, a vascular spasm of the vertebral artery can occur.

The severity and the duration of the symptoms are dependent on the following factors:

- the position of the head during the trauma
- the type of car
- the type of car seat
- whether or not a shoulder restraint is used
- whether or not a seat belt is used
- the velocity of the car coming from behind
- the weight of the head

In the mildest of cases, the patient initially has no symptoms. The symptoms start several hours later or sometimes even a few days afterward. At first, the individual pays little attention to the symptoms, considering them to be a matter of course. A study performed in the United States[26] with 1200 patients, all of whom had sustained acceleration traumas, found that the first visit to the physician regarding the symptoms was an average of 9 months after the initial injury. Of course, in instances of severe trauma, such as vertebral fractures and/or spinal cord compression, the symptoms are experienced immediately.

Furthermore, as the result of an acceleration trauma all of the various disc-related cervical syndromes can occur. At the same time, the patient may experience various symptoms also seen in a functional vertebrobasilar insufficiency. These symptoms include the following:

- headache
- dizziness
- ringing in the ears
- neck pain
- pain between the scapulae
- pain, sometimes also paresthesia, in one or both arms
- cervical nystagmus

For many insurers, the acceleration trauma is a significant problem. In many cases,

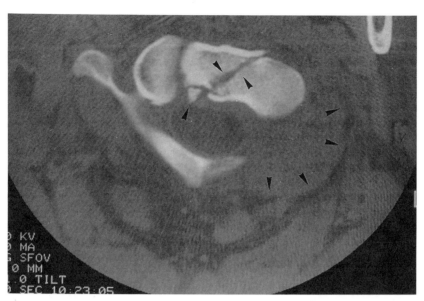

Figure 6–47 CT scan of C2 in a patient who sustained a severe whiplash injury. There is an oblique fracture through the vertebral body of C2 (***two arrowheads*** in the middle) with a loose fragment (***left arrowhead***). This is a rare consequence of an injury. At the same time, there is significant soft tissue swelling (***four arrowheads*** at the right).

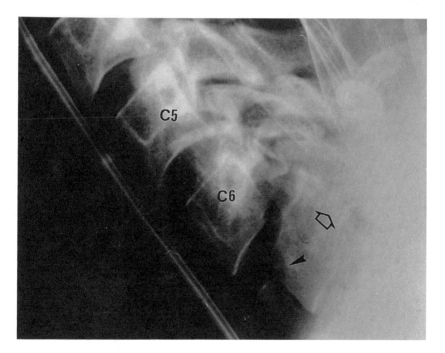

Figure 6–48 Conventional lateral X-ray of a 40-year-old patient who was involved in a serious auto accident. A compression fracture of C7 is noted (***arrowhead***), with significant dorsal displacement (***open arrow***), causing severe compression of the spinal cord. The lines on the X-ray are from an inflatable immobilizing splint.

months pass before the patient visits the physician. Moreover, in the physical examination there is usually very little in terms of demonstrable objective findings. Because of this, the patient is considered to be exaggerating the symptoms in order to attain a large settlement from the insurance company. However, Macnab[25] performed a follow-up study on patients 2 years after they received payment from the insurance company. The majority of the group still had their symptoms.

Actually, a cervical nystagmus is the only symptom that can be objectified. Oosterveld et al[27] found that 70% of all patients with an acceleration trauma had cervical nystagmus. Thus, for insurance companies, this could be an important standard (measurable by use of nystagmography).

Combination Trauma. A combination trauma occurs when rotation and/or sidebending of the cervical spine is combined with a hyperflexion and/or hyperextension trauma (Figure 6–49). The consequences are the sum of all the lesions described above.

Rotation Trauma. The seldom-seen rotation trauma usually occurs as the result of a forced rotation that was performed in order to improve a dysfunction in the cervical spine. If the therapist carefully questions and examines, it is almost impossible to do harm to the patient. Manipulation in spite of contraindications (due to the pathology, age of the patient, etc.) can lead to serious consequences, ranging from temporary neurological deficits to death. Usually this involves patients with an upper cervical instability or pathology

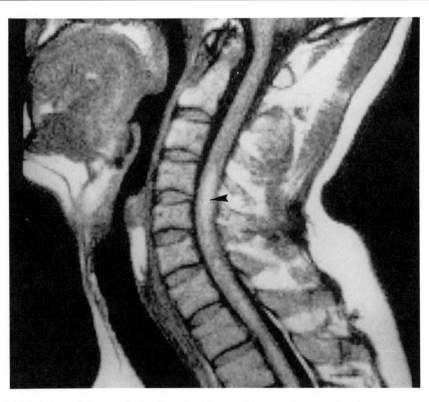

Figure 6–49 MRI view of the cervical spine of a 46-year-old man who sustained a severe combination trauma. The hyperintense zone in the medulla (***arrowhead***) indicates bleeding in the spinal cord due to the trauma.

of the vertebral artery (Figure 6–50). (Refer also to Vertebrobasilar Insufficiency.)

Treatment

For all post-traumatic lesions, one should accurately differentiate between the possible consequences. If a discogenic disorder is determined, treatment consists of the same procedures as described under the various primary disc-related syndromes. If a fracture is demonstrated, treatment depends on the severity and the localization of the fracture. Sometimes immobilization in a hard cast is indicated, and in other cases surgery must be performed. Some severe dislocations can be repositioned manually with the patient under general anesthesia, followed by continuous traction. It is almost always beneficial to support the treatment with nonsteroidal anti-inflammatory medications.

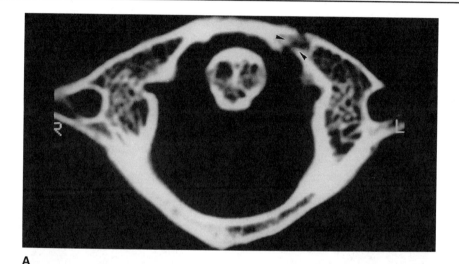

A

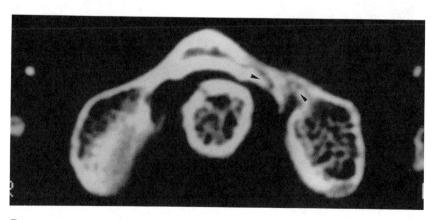

B

Figure 6–50 CT scan of the atlas in a young patient who had a severe rotation trauma. Clinically the patient had symptoms from an upper cervical instability due to a rupture of the transverse ligament. ***A***, and ***B***, In both views, a fracture of the anterior arch of the atlas is visible (***arrowheads***), however, without significant displacement.

Particularly in whiplash traumas, prevention is of great importance. Of course, wearing a three-point seat belt is a significant safety measure, as well as the construction of so-called crush zones in the vehicle itself. Unfortunately, too little attention is given to the following points:

- The proper position of the head rest. A head rest that is positioned lower than the level of the neck can make the consequences of a whiplash trauma even worse. The ideal height of the head rest is slightly higher than the level of the eyes, which is the position of the center of gravity of the head. On the average, it is about 7 cm above the level of the eyes.
- The use of air bags. Today, air bags are automatically being built into many of the automobiles on the market. They prevent severe trauma to the skull when the head is thrown forward. In fact, air bags should be included in every vehicle.

Traumatic Atlantoaxial Subluxation/Dislocation

Traumatic atlantoaxial subluxation/dislocation can occur at every age in both males and females. Usually the lesion occurs as the result of a serious trauma, such as a collision. In some cases, a sports injury is involved, for instance, from a fall during skiing, judo, wrestling, or pole vaulting (Figures 6–51 and 6–52).

Generally, a rotation subluxation (or dislocation) is involved, sometimes in combination with a dens fracture. A spondylolisthesis of the axis can also occur; this almost always happens in conjunction with a dens fracture (hangman's fracture).

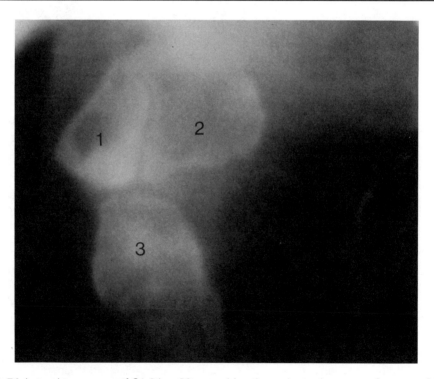

Figure 6–51 Lateral tomogram of C1-2 in a 23-year-old patient who took a very unfortunate fall during judo. There is a fracture of the dens with a ventral dislocation of the caudal part. *1*, Anterior arch of the atlas; *2*, cranial fragment of the dens; *3*, caudal part of the dens.

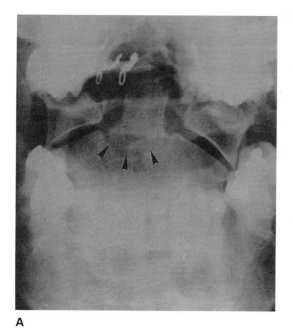
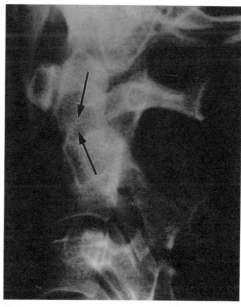

A   **B**

Figure 6–52 Conventional AP *(A)*, and lateral *(B)*, X-rays of the cervical spine in a 50-year-old woman who was in a traffic accident several years earlier. On the AP view, there are the remains of a fracture (***arrowheads***). The lateral view demonstrates an angulation of the dens (***arrows***).

Clinical Findings

- If the patient survives the trauma, the resulting symptoms and signs are severe, encompassing every possible consequence of injury to the spinal cord, including vertebrobasilar problems. There is almost always a spastic paraparesis or quadriparesis, such as ataxia.

- The patient holds the head in a forced position of flexion. In instances of a rotatory subluxation (or dislocation), the flexion is combined with an ipsilateral sidebending and a contralateral rotation.

- Of course, in such cases a functional examination cannot be performed. Extreme caution must be used in transporting the patient. The head and neck must be supported in the same position as directly after the accident.

- Extensive imaging examinations are indicated, preferably CT and/or MRI.

Treatment

Treatment is operative. However, in many cases the patients are left with permanent consequences of the partial transverse spinal cord lesion.

Unilateral Zygapophyseal Joint Dislocation and Fracture Dislocation

Unilateral zygapophyseal joint dislocation and fracture dislocation always occur as the result of a severe rotation trauma or a combination trauma. The type of injury is determined particularly by the direction of the rotation and the accompanying sidebend (Figures 6–53 to 6–55). For instance, in a left rotation trauma, an automatic left sidebend also occurs, thus causing a dislocation of the zygapophyseal joint on the right side. However, if the left rotation is paired with a right sidebend (against the automatic coupling pattern), then not only will there be a dislocation of the right zygapophyseal joint, but there also will be a fracture of the lamina, the

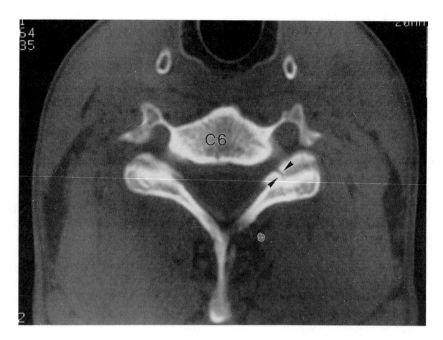

Figure 6–53 CT scan of C6 in a 44-year-old man after a traffic accident. There is a fracture of the left cranial facet of C6 (***arrowheads***).

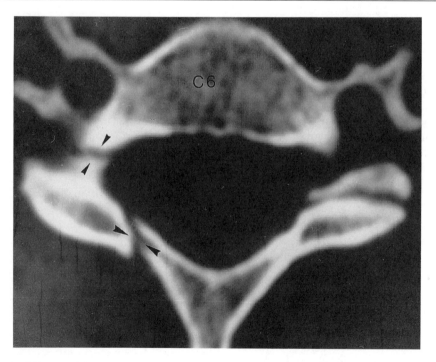

Figure 6–54 CT scan of C6 in a 42-year-old man after a serious fall. There is a fracture of the pedicle (***small arrowheads***) and of the lamina (***large arrowheads***).

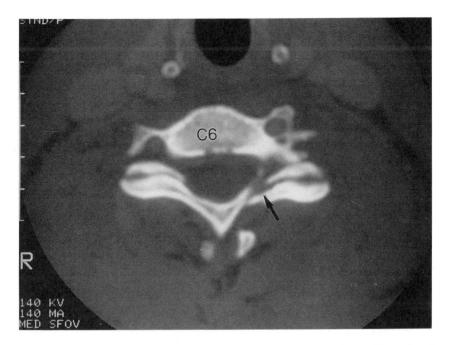

Figure 6–55 CT scan of C6 in a 21-year-old man after a severe skiing accident. There is a fracture of the left lamina (***arrow***).

pedicle, or the articular process. On the other hand, in a right rotation trauma, the left zygapophyseal joint dislocates. Again, the right rotation combined with a left sidebend results in both a dislocation and a fracture on the left side.

Clinical Findings

- Besides the local pain, there are almost always radicular symptoms. The most frequently affected segments are C5-6 and C6-7. Depending on the dislocation, the head is usually held in a forced position. For instance, in a right dislocation, the head is held in left sidebend and left rotation. In this case, the cranial vertebra is subluxated (or dislocated) anteriorly.
- Performing a functional examination is impossible. All movements away from the antalgic posture are very painful and limited.

- Neurological signs are present, especially when there is a simultaneous fracture. In this case, coughing, sneezing, and straining are painful.
- Imaging diagnostics, preferably CT scan or MRI, are necessary.

Treatment

Treatment depends on the severity of the lesion. Usually, reduction of the dislocation can be accomplished by manual traction under general anesthesia.

Bilateral Zygapophyseal Joint Subluxation/Dislocation

Although rare, the bilateral zygapophyseal joint subluxation/dislocation occurs as the result of a trauma involving symmetrical flexion with a component of minimal axial compression (Figures 6–56 to 6–59). The dislocation can occur at all levels, including the upper thoracic region (Figures 6–60 and 6–61).

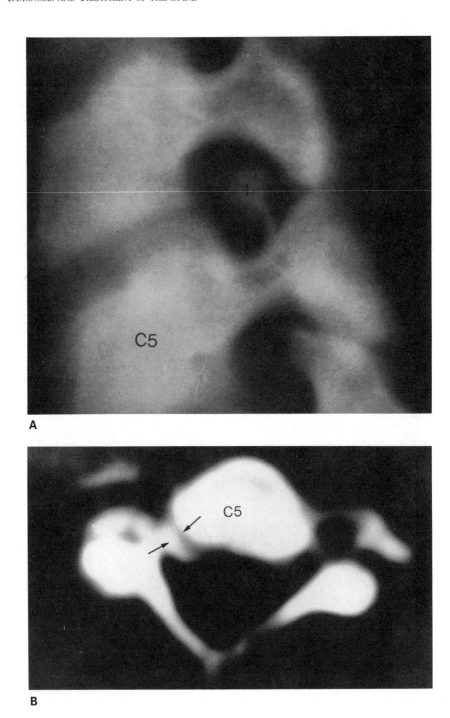

Figure 6–56 Cervical spine (C3-5) of a 22-year-old man after a traffic accident. Clinically, he presents with severe right C5 radicular pain. **A**, Tomogram, lateral view. There is a fracture of the left C5 cranial facet with a dislocation of this fragment in the intervertebral foramen **(1)**. **B**, Old CT scan at the level of C5. The right intervertebral foramen is no longer visible because it is filled with the fragment (**arrows**).

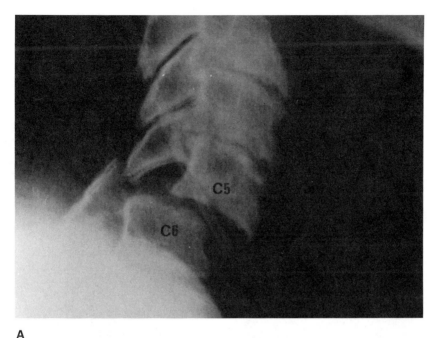

A

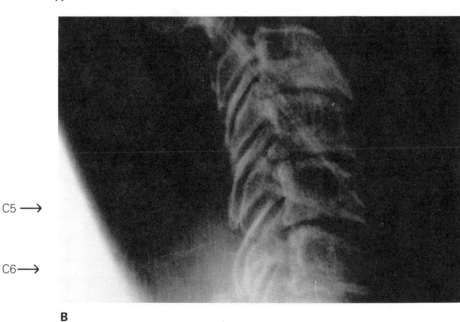

C5 $\longrightarrow$

C6 $\longrightarrow$

B

Figure 6–57 Conventional lateral X-ray of the cervical column in a 65-year-old woman. **A**, There is a traumatic fracture dislocation of C5-6 with significant signs of spinal cord compression. There are also severe degenerative changes from C3 to C7, from which the patient never reported symptoms. **B**, The same patient, several weeks later, after manual reduction under general anesthesia and continuous traction. There is proper position of the cervical spine. The patient still has minimal symptoms of spinal cord compression.

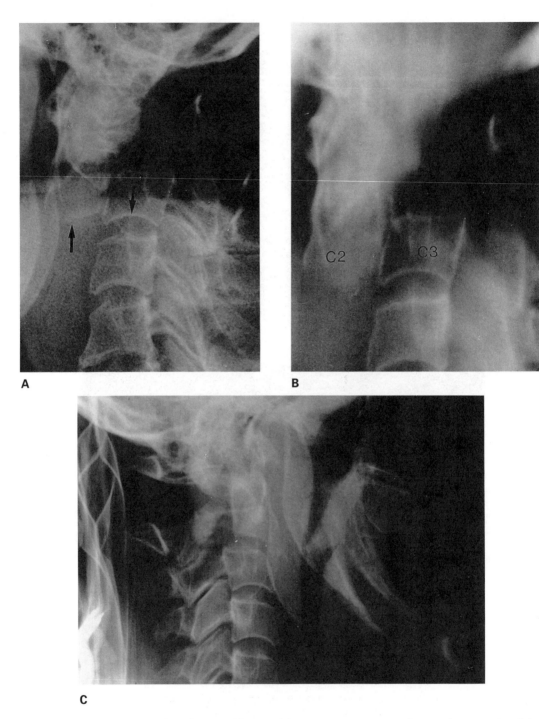

Figure 6–58 Cervical spine in a 50-year-old man with a very severe traumatic complete anterior dislocation of C2-3. **A**, Conventional lateral X-ray. The lower edge of C2 (**left arrow**) lies at the level of the lower edge of C3 (**right arrow**). **B**, Tomogram. **C**, Conventional lateral X-ray after manual reduction under general anesthesia and continuous traction. The patient had almost no complaints.

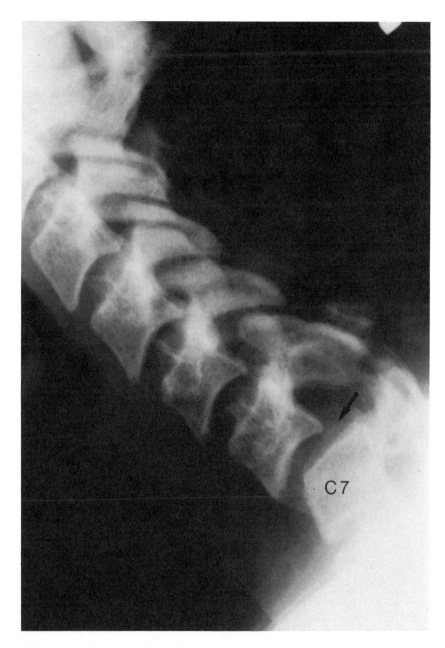

Figure 6–59 Conventional lateral X-ray of the cervical spine in a 26-year-old woman after a serious traffic accident. There is a ventral dislocation of C6 in respect to C7, with fractures of the articular facets and the lamina. Clinically, she had severe medullary compression: quadriplegia.

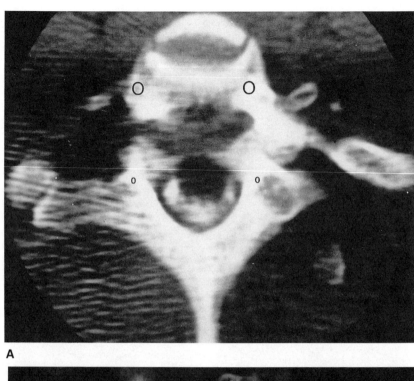

A

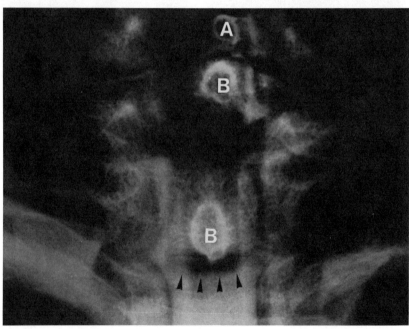

B

Figure 6–60 Upper thoracic spine in a 19-year-old man after a serious traffic accident. **A**, CT scan of T1-2. There is a very severe ventral dislocation of T1 (**large circles**), over T2 (**small circles**). **B**, Myelogram, AP view. There is a complete stop of the contrast medium at the level of the dislocation (**arrowheads**). The large distance between the spinous processes of T1 (**B**) and T2 (**B**) and the small distance between T1 and C7 (**A**) is striking.

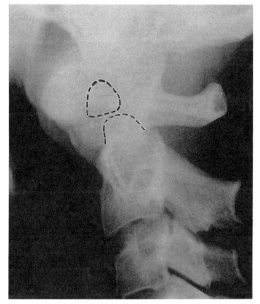

A

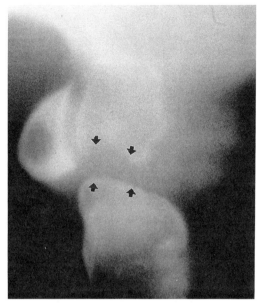

B

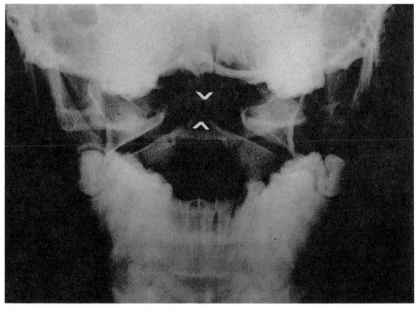

C

Figure 6–61 Upper cervical spine in an 18-year-old patient with clinical symptoms of an upper cervical instability. **A**, Conventional lateral X-ray of the upper cervical spine. There is an os odontoideum; the cranial part of the dens does not have a bony connection to the caudal part. This can be congenital or the result of an old fracture. **B**, Lateral tomogram of C0-1. The free fragment of the dens is more obvious on this view. **C**, Conventional AP X-ray of C0-1 (through the opened mouth). There is an obvious disruption between the two parts of the dens.

Clinical Findings

- All the signs and symptoms of a severe ligament rupture and damage to the disc are demonstrated. Occasionally, there are also symptoms from pressure on the spinal cord. In severe cases, the spinal cord itself is injured.
- The cervical spine is held in flexion. If the patient is still conscious, movement is impossible.
- Usually there is bilateral root irritation, often without neurological deficits.
- Coughing, sneezing, and straining are almost always painful.
- Imaging diagnostics are necessary. In conventional X-rays, the lateral view is of particular diagnostic importance. CT and MRI best indicate the extent of the injury.

Treatment

Treatment consists of manual reduction under general anesthesia, followed by continuous traction or spondylosyndesis (fusion).

Grisel's Syndrome

Grisel's syndrome can occur at any age, in both men and women. It involves a congenital or acquired weakening of, in particular, the transverse ligament of the atlas (Figures 6–62 and 6–63). In individuals with this disorder, a normal movement or a minor trauma can cause a dislocation of the dens from the axis. This disorder is seen especially in the patients with

- rheumatoid arthritis
- ankylosing spondylitis

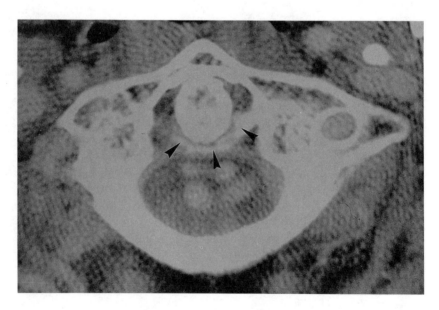

Figure 6–62 CT scan of the atlas-dens connection in a 64-year-old man with complaints of severe headache. Clinically, an upper cervical instability is suspected because the stability tests provoked the patient's symptoms. There is calcification of the transverse ligament of the atlas (**arrowheads**). This is an absolute contraindication for manual mobilization. By means of a functional CT examination, an instability could not be confirmed.

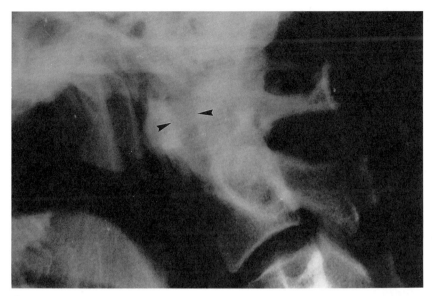

A

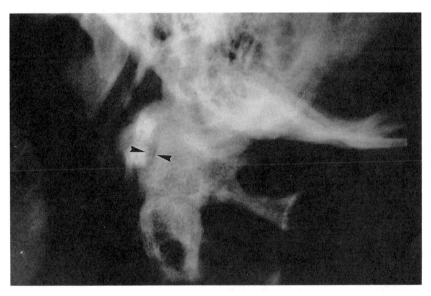

B

Figure 6–63 Conventional lateral X-ray of the upper cervical spine in a 52-year-old patient with atlantoaxial instability due to psoriatic arthritis. **A**, Unstable in flexion; **B**, stable in extension.

- psoriatic arthritis
- regional infections such as lymphangitis
- nose and throat infections

Furthermore, it can arise in instances of

- primary tumors or metastases
- congenital dens anomalies
- congenital ligamentous laxity, such as in Down syndrome

Due to an earlier trauma, the transverse ligament of the atlas may also be weakened and later rupture with a subsequent minor trauma. In the presence of severe degenerative changes in the upper cervical segments, a seemingly minor trauma can also lead to an instability.

Clinical Findings

- Headaches in the occipital region are the chief complaints in this disorder. Neck and/or shoulder pain is less pronounced. There are symptoms of spinal cord damage, as well as vertebrobasilar problems.
- Often the head is held in forced flexion. All movements are very painful and limited. Due to muscle splinting, they are almost impossible to perform.
- Depending on the severity of the lesion, the following signs of spinal cord compression can be found:
  1. abnormal reflexes
  2. spastic hemi-, para-, or quadriparesis
  3. ataxia
- Imaging diagnostics in conjunction with the history (infection, etc) are the most important guides to reaching a diagnosis.

Treatment

Treatment depends on the severity of the lesion. In many cases, surgery is necessary.

Stress Fracture of the C7 or T1 Spinous Process

Stress fractures of the C7 or T1 spinous processes seldom occur. They can occur in

people who have spent many unaccustomed hours spading, raking, or shoveling snow.

Clinical Findings

- The patient complains of local pain.
- Functional examination of the cervical spine elicits pain in both flexion and extension. Active elevation of the shoulder girdle is painful, and active elevation of the arm is very limited and painful. Passive arm elevation is painful, but only slightly limited. There is significant tenderness to palpation of the affected area.
- Coughing, sneezing, and straining provoke local pain.
- The radiological examination demonstrates the stress fracture.

Treatment

The injury is self-limiting and heals within 2 months. Pain medication can be administered as necessary.

Stress Fracture of the First Rib

Stress fractures of the first rib are seen much more often in men than in women. Usually the patients are between 20 and 40 years old. The cause is an overload, generally during sports such as Olympic handball, water polo, other throwing sports, and sometimes in the contact sports (Figures 6–64 and 6–65).

As a differential diagnosis, contracture of the costocoracoid fascia and an arthritis of the first costotransverse joint should be considered.

Clinical Findings

- Patients complain of unilateral pain at the base of the neck.
- Although neurological signs are absent, some patients develop a thoracic outlet syndrome with resultant paresthesia in the fingers.
- The functional examination of the cervical spine indicates a painful flexion and pain on sidebending away from the affected side. Resisted sidebending to-

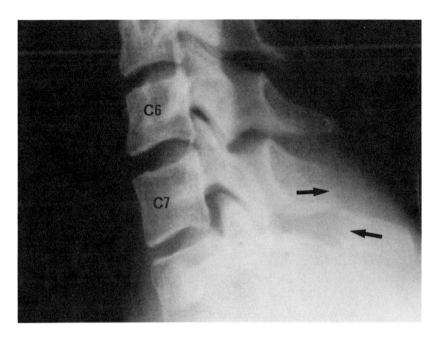

Figure 6–64 Conventional lateral X-ray of the cervical spine in a 17-year-old young man with a stress fracture and dislocation of the C7 spinous process. The fracture (***arrows***) occurred as the result of very heavy digging and lifting.

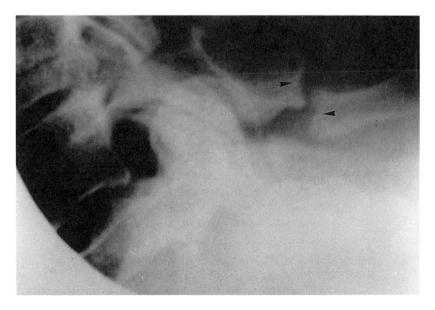

Figure 6–65 Conventional lateral X-ray of the lower cervical spine in a 56-year-old woman with a C6 cervicobrachial syndrome. There is an old fracture of the C7 spinous process (***arrowheads***), which occurred while jumping on the bed with her children 25 years earlier. The fracture is an incidental finding and no longer has clinical significance.

ward the affected side is extremely painful. Active and passive elevation of the shoulder girdle provokes pain on the affected side. Active and passive elevation of the arm also provokes the pain.

- Coughing, sneezing, and straining increase local pain.
- Radiological examination indicates the stress fracture.

Treatment

Treatment consists of reassuring the patient; the fracture heals within 2 months.

FORM ABERRATIONS OF THE SPINAL COLUMN

In discussing form aberrations of the spinal column, the disorders primarily characterized by abnormal kyphosis/lordosis/scoliosis are considered, along with the chronic disorders that affect the morphology of the spinal column as a whole. More localized chronic disorders are discussed under Other Disorders.

See Chapter 5, Thoracic Spine section 5.3, for more information on kyphosis, scoliosis, and osteoporosis–related disorders.

Rheumatoid Arthritis of the Cervical Spine

In 85% of patients with rheumatoid arthritis, aberrations of the cervical spine develop (Figures 6–66 and 6–67). Usually this involves softening of the ligament and the synovial joints. Erosion of the joints as well as the dens can also occur. In principle, this can lead to subluxations (or dislocations) at every level. The most serious consequences arise as a result of softening of the upper cervical ligaments. In particular, when the transverse ligament of the atlas is affected, the atlas can sublux anteriorly in relation to the axis, resulting in compression of the spinal cord from the dens. In erosion of the dens, a posterior subluxation can arise. Caudal to C2, espe-

cially at the level of C5-6 and C6-7, the danger of spinal cord compression is great because of the smaller diameter of the spinal canal.

Clinical Findings

- In most patients, rheumatoid arthritis has already been diagnosed. The cervical symptoms usually begin with gradually increasing pain in the neck and in the back of the head, which worsens during flexion of the cervical spine.
- Because of compression of the vertebral artery during cervical spine extension and/or rotation, functional disturbances of the brain stem and the cerebellum arise. (Refer to Vertebrobasilar Insufficiency for more detailed information.)
- If there is already an anterior subluxation (or dislocation) of the atlas, symptoms of spinal cord compression can also occur. (Refer to Cervicomedullary Syndrome and Bilateral Zygapophyseal Joint Subluxation/Dislocation.)
- During the functional examination, the passive motions in particular should be performed very carefully. (See also Grisel's Syndrome.) Almost all of the passive motions are painful. Often there is a limitation of motion in the capsular pattern. In addition, the resisted tests are usually painful. Performing the upper cervical stability test should be done with extreme caution. Localizations must be precise and minimal force should be exerted.
- Extensive imaging examinations are necessary.

Treatment

In the nonacute phase, an analgesic effect can be achieved with gentle massage and physical therapy modalities. The patient should be thoroughly informed about the disorder. Particular attention should be paid to maintaining good posture and to avoiding abrupt movements of the head. If there is al-

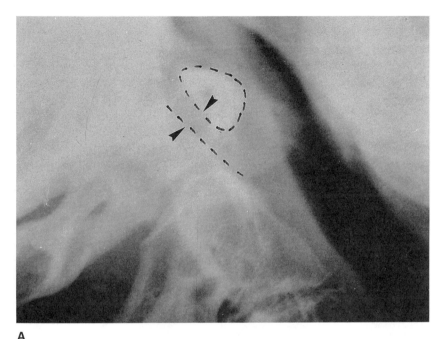

A

B

Figure 6–66 Conventional lateral X-ray of the upper cervical spine in a patient with rheumatoid arthritis and an atlantoaxial instability. **A**, Flexion. The distance between the dens and the anterior arch of the atlas (***arrowheads***) is abnormally large. Clinically, the patient manifests symptoms of spinal cord compression. **B**, Extension. The distance between the dens and the anterior arch of the atlas (***arrowheads***) is normal.

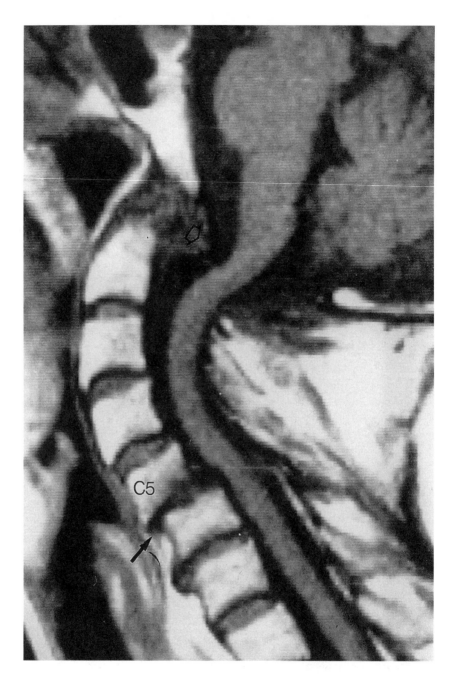

Figure 6–67 MRI of the cervical spine in a patient with rheumatoid arthritis and clinical signs of a severe upper cervical instability. There is destruction of the cranial part of the dens with a posterior subluxation (***open arrow***) pushing into the spinal cord and the distal part of the medulla oblongata. In addition, there is an anterolisthesis of C5 (***lower arrow***).

ready an instability, then a stabilizing (hard) cervical collar should be worn. In severe cases, surgical treatment (fusion) is indicated.

Every form of manual mobilization is absolutely contraindicated. This is also the case even when the patient has neck pain in conjunction with only a monarthritis in a joint lying far from the cervical spine.

OTHER DISORDERS

The fact that the pathology discussed under "Other Disorders" does not fall under the categories of primary disc-related disorders, secondary disc-related disorders, traumatic lesions, and postural deviations of the vertebral column does not imply that these disorders are less important. In a number of cases, there is a partial overlap with the earlier types of pathology. For instance, cervical posture syndrome is discussed under Primary Disc-Related Disorders.

Spastic Torticollis

Spastic torticollis is seen in children as well as adults and is found equally frequently in males and females (Figure 6–68). There are various causes for the muscle tension in the sternocleidomastoid muscle, including the following:

- epidemic encephalitis
- otitis media
- mastoiditis
- juvenile polyarthritis

Especially in children with a spastic torticollis, the presence of tumors should be considered.

Examination by a specialist is necessary to differentiate a spasm of the sternocleidomastoid from a spontaneous atlantoaxial subluxation (or dislocation), which is seen particularly in patients with congenital or acquired weakening of the atlanto-occipital and atlantoaxial ligamentous complex (see Grisel's Syndrome).

Clinical Findings

- The pain is unilateral and usually localized in the neck-shoulder region. The severity of the pain varies, depending on the cause and depending on the patient.
- The head is held in the so-called sternocleidomastoid position: flexion, ipsilateral sidebending, and contralateral rotation of the cervical spine.
- In the functional examination, contralateral sidebending, extension, and ipsilateral rotation are limited and/or painful.
- Generally, X-rays in patients older than 35 years indicate misleading "degenerative changes."
- Especially if the cause is not obvious, examination by a specialist is indicated.

Treatment

Treatment depends on the cause and should be determined by the appropriate specialist.

Spasmodic Torticollis

In most cases, spasmodic torticollis manifests itself as a tic. At involuntary moments, the patient's head moves briefly to one side. The same side is always involved. Occasionally the disorder is due to an extrapyramidal lesion. However, in an extrapyramidal lesion, the head unwillingly moves very slowly in a certain direction.

Clinical Findings

- There are no complaints of pain.
- The position of the head is normal, except at the instant that the involuntary movement occurs.
- The functional examination is negative.
- If an obvious tic is not manifested, then examination by a neurological specialist is indicated.

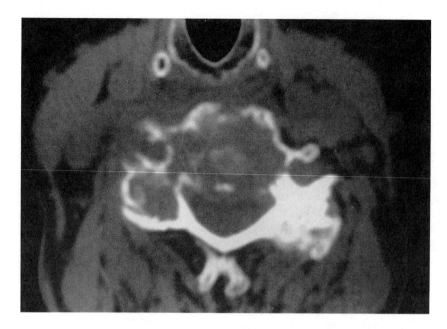

Figure 6–68 CT scan at the level of C5 in an adult patient with a spastic torticollis. The onset was very gradual. There is severe destruction of the vertebral body and the vertebral structures on the right side due to a tumor.

Treatment

If the disorder is due to an extrapyramidal problem, then the appropriate treatment is determined by the neurological specialist. Most of the patients with a tic do not require treatment. If treatment is desired, psychotherapy is indicated.

Conversion Torticollis

Primarily, the conversion torticollis ("hysterical torticollis") should be dealt with by a psychotherapist, possibly in combination with physical therapy. Seldom do people over 50 years of age present with this disorder; it is most often seen in adolescents and younger adults.

Clinical Findings

- Patients complain of diffuse pain in the head, neck, and shoulders, whereby the pain is predominantly on one side.

- The position of the head is characteristic: there is a sidebending toward the painful side and the patient holds the shoulder girdle on the same side in elevation.

- The functional examination indicates limitations of motion in every direction. The end-feel appears to be caused by muscle spasm. However, when slowly performing the passive motions, one can easily conquer the muscle contractions.

- There are no neurological signs.

- Coughing, sneezing, and straining do not increase the pain.

- When performed, the radiological examination indicates the known "degenerative changes" if the patient is older than 35 years.

Treatment

Treatment consists of psychotherapy, whereby support through physical therapy (massage, cautious stretching, heat modalities) often brings good results.

Retropharyngeal Tendinitis

Retropharyngeal tendinitis is a rare lesion that is seen equally frequently in men and women between the ages of 25 to 80 years. The cause is unknown.

In the differential diagnosis, a retropharyngeal abscess should be considered.

Clinical Findings

- Patients complain of an acute onset of head and neck pain. Sometimes the cervical spine is held in slight flexion.
- In the functional examination, rotations are symmetrically limited and painful. Extension is also limited and painful. Resisted flexion and resisted rotations are also painful.
- There are no neurological signs; however, coughing and sneezing are so painful that the patient has to hold the head still with both hands. Swallowing is painful.
- The radiological examination indicates a calcium deposit ventral to the vertebral body of the axis. An MRI demonstrates a thickening of the longus colli muscles. The normal thickness of 3 mm has increased to 10 to 15 mm.

Treatment

Treatment consists of pain medication to relieve the symptoms. The disorder is self-limiting and heals within 2 to 3 weeks.

Contracture of the Costocoracoid Fascia

The etiology behind the contracture of the costocoracoid fascia is unknown. Cyriax[28] describes a number of cases of contractures of the costocoracoid fascia in patients with a long-standing tuberculosis in the apex of the lung. The disorder is rare and is seen mostly in the age group between 25 and 50 years.

Clinical Findings

- There is a characteristic localization of the pain. The patient complains of unilateral pain in the region of the pectoralis minor and in the scapula, as well as at the base of the neck.
- The most striking finding in the functional examination is a slightly limited and painful elevation of the shoulder on the affected side. Contralateral side-bending of the cervical spine is painful. Resisted ipsilateral sidebending is painful. Protraction of the shoulder on the affected side is also painful. All resisted tests of the shoulder provoke pain at the base of the neck.
- There are no neurological signs.
- Coughing, sneezing, and straining are not painful.
- The radiological examination is negative, except for the usual physiological degenerative changes in patients older than 35 years.

Treatment

Treatment consists of surgical excision of the fascia from the pectoralis minor. Physical therapy, such as stretching, is fruitless.

Subacute Atlantoaxial Arthritis

The rare subacute atlantoaxial arthritis is seen exclusively in men between the ages of 25 and 40 years. The disorder is a nonspecific inflammation of the atlantoaxial capsuloligamentous complex. The history is usually unremarkable.

In the differential diagnosis, other arthritides and tumors are considered.

Clinical Findings

- The patient complains of a gradual increase, over several weeks, of pain and stiffness in the mid- and upper cervical region. The patient does not have a fever.

- In the functional examination, rotations are severely and symmetrically limited and painful. The other motions are normal.
- There are no neurological signs.
- Coughing, sneezing, and straining are negative.
- The erythrocyte sedimentation rate (ESR) is normal.
- The radiological examination demonstrates no aberrations. The diagnosis is determined based on the functional examination.

Treatment

This disorder is best treated with nonsteroidal anti-inflammatory medications. If there is not complete relief of pain within a few weeks of beginning the medication, further blood tests and imaging diagnostics are indicated.

Arthritis of the First Costotransverse Joint

The symptoms of this rare arthritis of the first costotransverse joint are similar to those experienced in a stress fracture of the first rib. It can be caused by overload as well as by systemic illness. In the latter case, the patient has already probably had incidents of arthritis in other joints.

In the differential diagnosis, a stress fracture of the first rib and contracture of the costocoracoid fascia should be considered.

Clinical Findings

- The patient complains of pain at the base of the neck. Sometimes the head is held slightly sidebent toward the painful side.
- In the functional examination, sidebending of the cervical spine away from the affected side is the most painful mo-

tion. Contraction of the scaleni muscles against resistance is painful: ipsilateral sidebending with contralateral rotation and flexion. Sometimes active arm elevation is very painful and limited. Passive arm elevation is not limited and causes minimal discomfort.

- There are no neurological signs.
- Coughing, sneezing, and straining sometimes provoke local pain.
- The radiological examination is negative, except for the normal physiological degenerative changes of the cervical spine.
- An intra-articular injection with a local anesthetic confirms the diagnosis.

Treatment

Generally an intra-articular injection of corticosteroid cures the problem.

Vertebrobasilar Insufficiency

Vertebrobasilar insufficiency consists of recurrent periods of relative ischemia in the vertebrobasilar supply area due to a temporary decrease in, or "blockage" of, the flow of the vertebral and the basilar arteries and their branches[29] (Figure 6–69).

Oostendorp[20] describes a "functional" vertebrobasilar insufficiency as a form of vertebrobasilar insufficiency in which the signs and symptoms are provoked through movements of the cervical spine. This occurs in the absence of organic aberrations, such as arteriosclerosis. Vertebrobasilar insufficiency can occur with any cervical disorder and also as a solitary disorder.

In the differential diagnosis, other disorders of the cervical spine in which the vertebral artery can be compromised should *always* be considered. For instance, vertebrobasilar insufficiency can be seen as a result of severe degenerative changes of the zygapophyseal joints and the uncovertebral joints, in subluxations or dislocations, and in tumors.

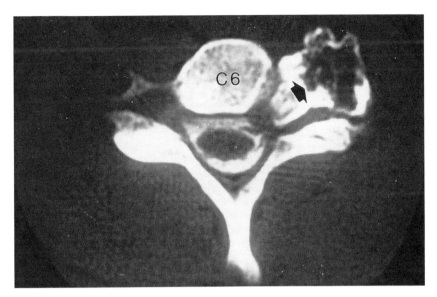

A

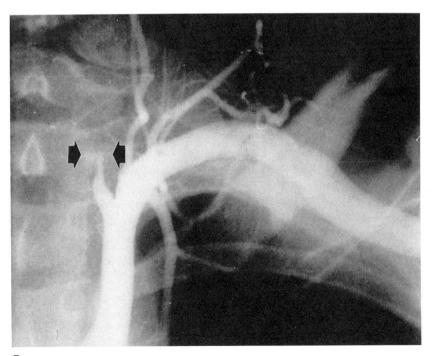

B

Figure 6–69 The cervical spine of a 42-year-old man with complaints of dizziness and left neck pain with C6 radicular symptoms. **A**, Myelo-CT scan at the level of C6. There is a large osteochondroma on the left (**arrow**), with subsequent significant compression of the vertebral artery and the C6 nerve root. **B**, Angiogram. Complete obstruction (**arrows**) of the vertebral artery.

Clinical Anatomy

The vertebral and basilar arteries and their branches vascularize structures in both the cervical and the intracranial regions. Intracranial structures supplied by these arteries include the following:

- medulla oblongata
- pons
- mesencephalon (midbrain)
- parts of the cerebellum

Function of the reticular formation and the vestibular core complex are dependent on these structures. The cerebellum is sensitive to vascular disturbances because there are no anastomoses from other blood supplies. The same is true for the equilibrium system.

Clinical Findings

Oostendorp[20] describes the clinical picture of a functional vertebrobrasilar insufficiency as a "kaleidoscope-like pattern of signs and symptoms connected with the multitude of functional centers of the brain which are localized in the vertebrobasilar supply area." Based on his observations, Oostendorp classifies the symptoms into four categories:

1. cervicocephalic signs and symptoms, which include referred "sensations" and referred pain from the upper cervical region, headaches, dizziness in conjunction with movement of the cervical spine, face pain, and disturbances in hearing and vision
2. neurological signs and symptoms, which include "drop attacks," attacks of syncope, and paresthesia in the lower extremities
3. vegetative signs and symptoms, such as swallowing disturbances, nausea, perspiration, anxiety, and heart palpitations
4. cervicobrachial signs and symptoms, such as referred "sensations" and referred pain from the mid- and lower

cervical region, neck pain, shoulder-arm pain, paresthesia in the upper extremities, and an antalgic position of the cervical spine.

In a functional vertebrobasilar insufficiency, there is no underlying organic lesion. To a large degree, the diagnosis of a functional vertebrobasilar insufficiency is determined based on the history. The signs and symptoms of the actual vertebrobasilar insufficiency syndrome are well described in neurology. The actual vertebrobasilar insufficiency syndrome is usually more easily identified and objectified than the functional vertebrobasilar insufficiency syndrome.

The DeKleyn and Nieuwenhuyse test[30] provokes the patient's symptoms in both forms of vertebrobasilar insufficiency. (See section 6.2 for performance of this test.)

Treatment

Oostendorp[20] suggests the following physical therapy measures in the treatment of a functional vertebrobasilar insufficiency:

- transcutaneous electrical nerve stimulation (TENS)
  1. paravertebral, C2 to C5 and C8 to T5
- mechanical vibration
  1. paravertebral, C1 to T8
  2. costotransverse joints T1 to T8
- movement therapy
  1. mobilization of the cervical and thoracic spines
  2. mobilization of the costotransverse and costovertebral joints, T1 to T8
  3. stretching of the cervico-occipital muscles, as well as the sternocleidomastoid and pectoralis major muscles
- postural instruction
- balance exercises.

Neurinoma

Although a neurinoma in the cervical spine can occur without a known cause, it is seen

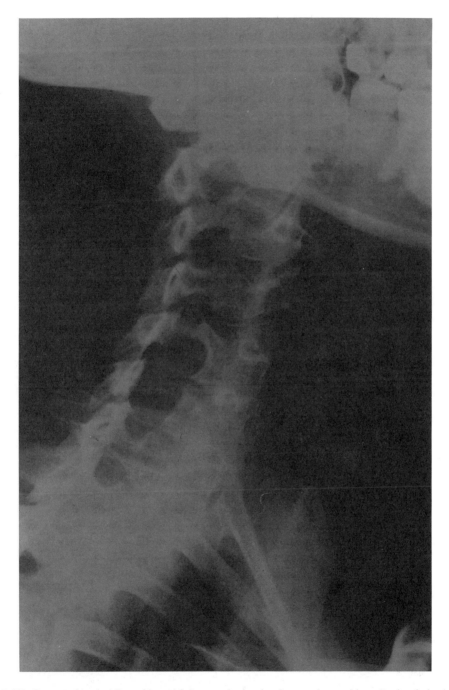

Figure 6–70 Conventional oblique X-ray of the cervical spine in a patient with paresthesia in the right hand and arm. Together, the intervertebral foramina of C5-6 and C6-7 form one large opening due to the cervical neurinoma.

mostly in patients with neurofibromatosis (Figures 6–70 and 6–71). The lesion is rare in both men and women and is usually seen in individuals over 20 years of age.

Clinical Findings

- The most significant symptoms consist of paresthesia and pain, which starts distally (in the hand) and from there slowly extends proximally. In severe cases, paresthesia is also experienced unilaterally in the upper half of the thorax. The paresthesia and pain exist in several dermatomes.
- The functional examination is normal except for flexion of the cervical spine: the paresthesia increases. Gradually, motor and sensory deficits also occur, initially from one and later from several nerve roots. In an even later stage, symptoms from spinal cord irritation may also arise.
- Coughing, sneezing, and straining provoke pain in the arm and the hand.
- If the symptoms have been present for a long period, the oblique view X-ray often demonstrates an abnormally large intervertebral foramen. The size of the foramen increases through erosion due to the expansive growth of the neurinoma. CT scan and MRI clearly indicate the tumor.

Treatment

Treatment is symptomatic. In severe cases, the neurinoma is removed surgically. For a summary of cervical spine pathology, see Appendix A, Differential Diagnosis of the Spine.

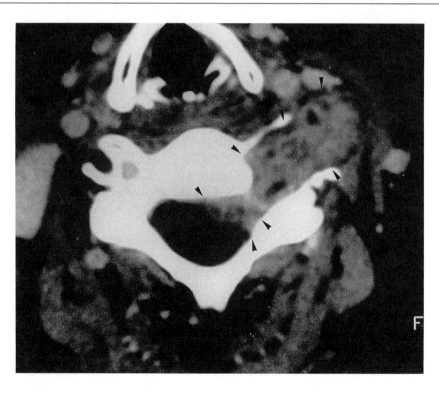

Figure 6–71 CT scan at the level of C5 in a patient who complains of paresthesia in the left hand and arm. The left intervertebral foramen is enlarged as the result of a neurinoma of the C5 nerve root that has extended into the spinal canal.

6.4 TREATMENT

INTRODUCTORY OVERVIEW

Information

After the patient history, inspection, and functional examination, a diagnosis can usually be determined. Further examination is necessary if a diagnosis cannot be reached. As soon as the diagnosis is definite, the patient should be thoroughly informed regarding the disorder. The explanation should include significant anatomical and clinical facts regarding the lesion.

In addition to the anatomical and clinical information, ergonomic advice should also be given. This advice includes instruction in posture and body mechanics. The patient should know exactly how to sit, stand, lie down, and lift. (For more detailed information, refer to Chapter 12, Prevention of Back and Neck Pain by Improving Posture.)

Mobilization

Indications

Manual mobilization and/or manipulation of the cervical spine is indicated in primary discogenic disorders in patients younger than 45 years of age. This age limit is not absolute. Occasionally, patients who are older than 45 years can also have primary disc-related problems and will benefit from treatment with mobilization. Most primary disc-related disorders are seen in the age group 35 to 40 years.

In limitations of motion in the upper cervical spine, mobilization is indicated only when instability in that area has been specifically ruled out. Instances in which an upper cervical instability can arise are discussed under contraindications.

Mobilization is also indicated in a functional disturbance of the cervical column, even without the presence of a disc lesion. Of course, all contraindications must first be ruled out.

The mobilization and manipulation techniques shown in the following pages include the following:

- axial separation, with or without "extra pull"
- axial separation and rotation, with or without "extra pull"
- axial separation and sidebend, with or without "extra pull"
- dorsoventral mobilization
- upper cervical segmental techniques, with or without axial separation
- midcervical and lower cervical segmental techniques, with or without axial separation

The number of possibilities for manual therapeutic treatment for a limitation of motion in the cervical spine is enormous. In this chapter, very limited numbers of these mobilizations/manipulations are discussed. Only the safest of all the techniques are described.

Particularly in regard to the separation manipulation techniques, some manual therapists suggest that the techniques are not very specific and therefore can be dangerous. However, the nonspecific effect has never been proven. In discogenic disorders (in which the axial separation techniques are indicated), the results are far better when techniques with axial separation are used than when techniques without separation are performed. These techniques have been performed by many therapists, over many years, without complications ever arising. Of course, it is absolutely imperative that all contraindications are cleared and that the stability, vascular, and neurological tests are negative.

In the authors' experience, the short-term and long-range effects of the axial separation techniques offer better results in primary disc-related problems than the local segmental techniques. (To date, there are no well-controlled studies to confirm this.)

Postural and other forms of ergonomic advice, together with the patient's home exercises, are the most important components in treating the majority of cervical spine complaints.

Absolute Contraindications: General

- Upper cervical instability can arise as a result of the following systemic disorders:
    1. osteogenesis imperfecta
    2. Ehlers-Danlos syndrome
    3. Down syndrome
    4. Marfan syndrome
    5. rheumatoid systemic diseases, such as rheumatoid arthritis, gout, Reiter's syndrome, etc
- Upper cervical instability can also be seen
    1. after an accident
    2. in patients with "drop attacks" (the patients fall down without losing consciousness)
    3. in patients with dizziness
    4. during or directly after a throat infection, especially in children (one should be wary of an atlanto-occipital and atlantoaxial instability)
    5. if there is a history of septic arthritis (the stability examination should be carefully performed)
- Limitation of motion in the capsular pattern, without known cause
- Torticollis with splinting of the sternocleidomastoid muscle
- Presence of spinal cord signs (for example, electric current sensations in the hands and/or feet, positive Babinski foot sole reflex, etc)
- Neurological deficits
- (Functional) vertebrobasilar insufficiency

- Unexplainable pain during the night
- Use of anticoagulants
- If symptoms are elicited, or already existing symptoms increase, during the treatment

Precautions

- Pregnancy, after the third month
- Use of birth control pills
- Prolonged use of corticosteroids
- General hypermobility
- Osteoporosis (techniques with rotation are particularly contraindicated)
- Anomalies and fusions of the vertebrae (for instance, in block or wedge vertebrae)
- Negative functional examination

Contraindications: Specific

Most of the just-mentioned contraindications do not apply to the dorsoventral mobilization technique. This technique has only the following contraindications:

- Limitation of motion in the capsular pattern, in which the capsular pattern is caused by a local inflammation or tumor
- If symptoms are elicited, or already existing symptoms increase, during the treatment

Continuous (Mechanical) Traction

As already mentioned, most of the mobilization techniques are performed with axial separation. Continuous (mechanical) traction is seldom necessary. Some patients react well to continuous traction. However, these patients will almost always respond just as well, or even better, to manual axial separation (with or without extra pull).

Indications

Continuous traction is indicated in the following:

- Primary discogenic disorders

- Headache in elderly patients, which decreases during a trial of manual axial separation; after this, the duration of the traction can be gradually increased

Contraindications

Contraindications for continuous traction include the following:

- In principle, the same contraindications listed for mobilization/manipulation
- If symptoms are elicited, or already existing symptoms increase, during the treatment

Cervical Collar

Various types of cervical collars exist: soft, firm, and hard. The most important function of a soft cervical collar is to keep the cervical region warm. Although some patients feel comfortable with a soft collar, rarely does their pain decrease. Thus, the soft collar is seldom used. Besides keeping the cervical region warm, the firm collar also functions to immobilize the cervical spine partially. Choosing the proper type of firm cervical collar is important. The appropriate collar ensures the proper position of the head, and at the same time provides a continuous slight cervical axial separation (Figure 6–72). This separation occurs only when the collar supports both the back of the head and the chin.

The firm collar is frequently used for patients with a cervical syndrome, in the acute phase. After the first mobilization treatment, it is often beneficial for the patient to wear the collar for the remainder of the day (and night). Many patients benefit from wearing the collar for several days or weeks. If the patient has pain mainly at night, the collar should be worn at night. Some patients have pain only during certain activities during the day. In this instance, it is recommended that they wear the collar only at those times.

In patients over 45 years of age, mobilization of the cervical spine is much less often indicated. Good results are often achieved

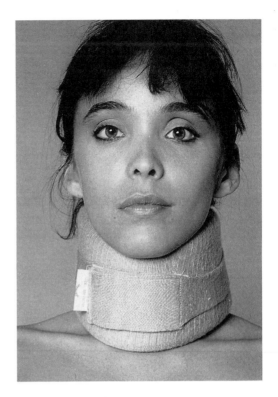

Figure 6–72 A firm cervical collar provides warmth, partial immobilization, and slight axial separation.

when these patients wear a firm cervical collar in conjunction with taking nonsteroidal anti-inflammatory medication.

A hard cervical collar is applied only in instances of cervical instability. In this way, the cervical spine is completely immobilized and the amount of axial separation can be controlled.

Exercise

Manual therapy should always be supplemented by an exercise program. Patients should perform only a few effective motions, in order to maintain the improvement attained during the treatment. It is important to perform the exercises several times per day. The program may include active motions and/or stretching exercises.

In instances of a segmental instability, stabilization exercises should be performed in addition to wearing a cervical collar. Patients with cervical complaints due to a postural syndrome or disc pathology also benefit from stabilization exercises.

There are many exercises for achieving better functional stability of the cervical spine. Initially, only the simplest stabilizing exercises should be given. In this way, every patient is able to perform the exercise program. Most important, the exercises should be performed daily. Furthermore, the patient should not experience pain either during or after the exercises.

The patient stabilizes the head with one or both hands. In each direction, the patient exerts isometric resistance, pushing the head into the hand. Per direction, the exercise is repeated 10 times: holding 6 to 10 seconds, and relaxing 6 to 10 seconds. During the exercises, the patient must continue to breathe in a regular and relaxed manner. The following motions should be included in the exercise program:

- right sidebend (Figure 6–73)
- left sidebend (Figure 6–74)
- extension (Figure 6–75)
- left rotation (Figure 6–76)
- right rotation (Figure 6–77)
- flexion (Figure 6–78)

For the flexion exercise, the chin is first pulled in before the head is pushed against the hand in a ventral direction.

MANUAL PAIN-RELIEVING TECHNIQUES

Soft tissue techniques are generally applied before performing the local segmental examination and in preparation for treatment with mobilization. These soft tissue techniques have a strong analgesic, and usually relaxing, effect. With decreased cervical muscle tension, or spasm, it is much easier for the therapist to palpate and register movement. During treatment with mobilization, the techniques will be more effective.

There are a number of sites in the cervical region where transverse friction can be performed. In principle, every tender site can be treated, even though it usually involves areas of referred pain or tenderness. Temporary pain relief results, allowing for more effective performance of the segmental examination and/or segmental treatment.

Transverse Friction of Insertions of the Suboccipital Muscles
(Figure 6–79)

Position of the Patient

The patient lies in a prone position on the treatment table with the forehead resting on the hands. The head is positioned in slight flexion, without rotation.

Position of the Therapist

The therapist stands opposite the side to be treated, at the level of the patient's cervical spine.

Performance

By means of palpation, the most tender area is localized. The most tender area is often located just caudal to the lateral third of the inferior linea nuchae. The therapist places the index finger, reinforced by the middle finger, directly lateral from the tender spot. The thumb rests on the other side of the patient's head, at a level slightly cranial to the index finger. During the "friction" phase, the index finger moves from laterally to medially and slightly cranially. At the same time, pressure is exerted in a ventromediocranial direction (toward the thumb). Pain arising during this technique is likely due to pressure on the greater occipital nerve. In this instance, the transverse friction is performed in an area just medial or lateral to that spot.

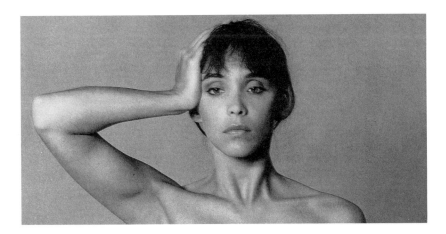

Figure 6–73 Right sidebend.

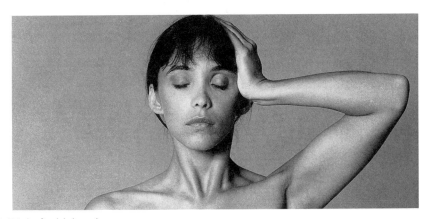

Figure 6–74 Left sidebend.

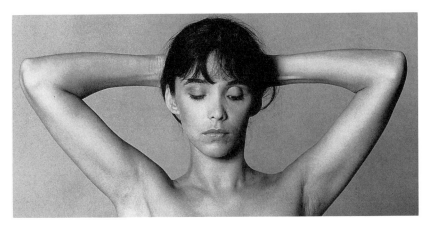

Figure 6–75 Extension.

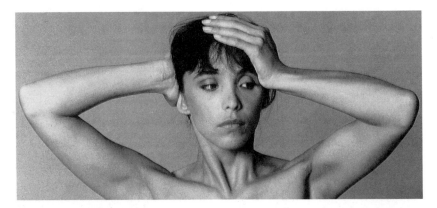

Figure 6–76 Left rotation.

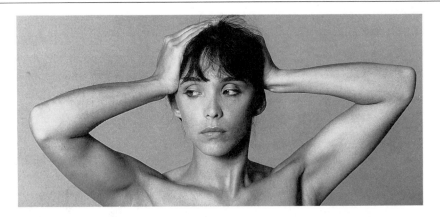

Figure 6–77 Right rotation.

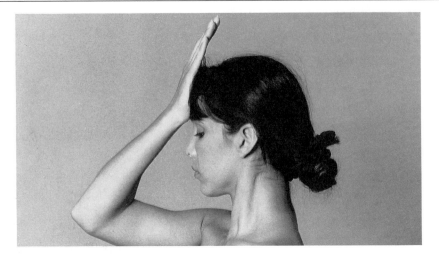

Figure 6–78 Flexion.

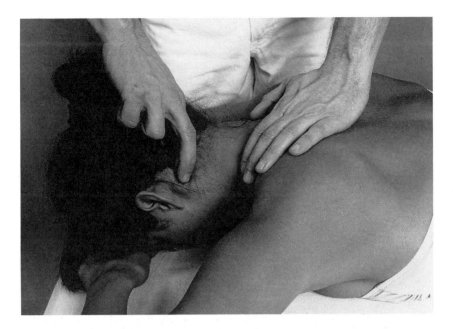

Figure 6–79 Transverse friction of the insertion of the suboccipital muscles at the linea nuchae.

Segmental Vibration and Rhythmic Movement: Traction, C2 to C7

(Figure 6–80)

Position of the Patient

The patient sits on a chair and rests against the chair back.

Position of the Therapist

The therapist stands next to the patient, with both knees slightly flexed.

Performance

With the hand and forearm, the therapist grasps the patient's head from a ventral approach. The hand rests against the lateral side of the head while the fingers grasp the occiput. In this instance, the ulnar side of the hand is placed on C2. When treating other segments, the ulnar side of this hand is placed against the cranial vertebra of the segment being treated. Without bringing the head into a rotation or sidebend, the therapist fixes the head between his or her arm and sternum. Care is taken not to exert pressure against the ears. The thumb and index finger of the other hand are placed against the transverse process of the caudal vertebra, in this instance C3.

To perform slight segmental axial separation, as well as to stabilize the cervical spine, the therapist extends both knees. With the caudal hand, the therapist then performs gentle vibration or oscillations in a direction that is perpendicular to a line connecting the segment to the orbita.

This treatment can also be performed unilaterally. In this instance, the vibration or oscillation is performed only on one side. The technique is an effective mobilization as well.

MANUAL SOFT TISSUE TECHNIQUES

Paravertebral Transverse Stretch during Cervical Flexion of C2 to C7

Figure 6–80 also illustrates this technique. The only difference here is that the dorsal arm is now positioned in the direction of the orbita.

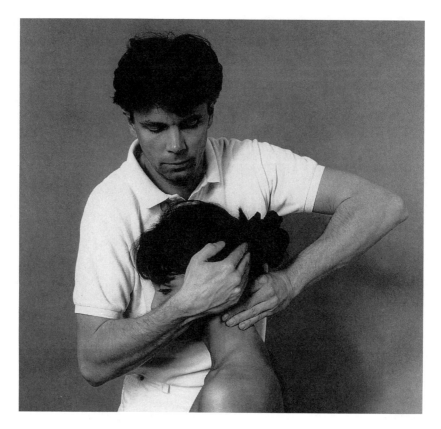

Fig 6–80 Traction, vibration, of C2-3.

Position of the Patient

The patient sits on a chair, resting against the chair back.

Position of the Therapist

The therapist stands next to the patient.

Performance

With the hand and forearm, the therapist grasps the patient's head from a ventral approach. The hand rests against the lateral side of the head while the fingers grasp the occiput. Without bringing the head into a rotation or sidebend, the therapist fixes the head between his or her arm and sternum. Care is taken not to exert pressure against the ears. From each side, the thumb and fingers grasp the dorsal aspect of the neck, at the level of the transverse processes. The therapist's thumb and index finger (and subsequently, the forearm) point in the direction of the orbita.

After first performing an upper cervical flexion, a flexion movement in the rest of the cervical spine is performed. At the same time, the thumb and fingers push toward each other, through the musculature, and simultaneously pull in a dorsal direction. The therapist begins at the level of C2-3, and the flexion motion is performed no further than this point. The end position is held for approximately 1 second, before returning to the initial position. The therapist repeats this technique several times in a rhythmic manner.

The same procedure can then be performed per segment, by shifting the dorsal hand caudally. As the successive caudal segments are emphasized, increasingly more flexion is performed. This technique can be used to treat the segments C2-3 to C6-7.

In the same way, coupled movements in flexion can also be performed. After first performing an upper cervical flexion, the therapist brings the patient's head simultaneously into flexion, ipsilateral rotation, and sidebending. In this instance, pressure is emphasized on the convex side of the cervical spine.

Paravertebral Transverse Stretch during Coupled Movement of C0 to C1 (Figure 6–81)

Position of the Patient

The patient lies supine with the arms relaxed alongside the body.

Position of the Therapist

The therapist sits or stands at the cranial end of the table.

Performance

With one hand, the therapist stabilizes the patient's head at the forehead. If the right side is to be treated, the therapist positions the patient's head (and upper cervical spine) in slight left sidebending. With the index and/or middle fingers of the right hand, the therapist "hooks" the suboccipital paravertebral musculature. The musculature is then "pulled" in a lateral and ventral direction while the head is simultaneously rotated slightly toward the side being treated. In this example, the rotation is to the right. The end position is held for approximately 1 second before returning to the initial position. The therapist repeats this

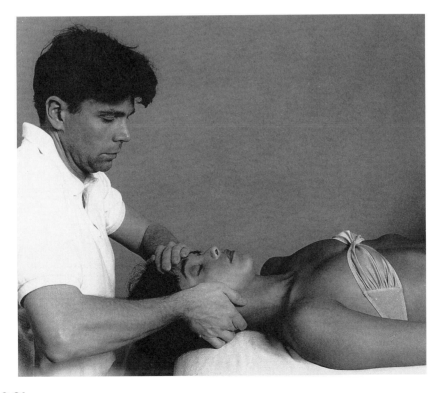

Figure 6–81

technique for several seconds, or minutes, in a rhythmic manner.

Paraverthebral Transverse Stretch during Coupled Movement of C1 to C2 (Figure 6–82)

Position of the Patient

The patient lies in a supine position with the arms relaxed alongside the body.

Position of the Therapist

The therapist sits or stands at the cranial end of the table.

Performance

With one hand, the therapist stabilizes the patient's head at the forehead. If the right side is to be treated, the therapist positions the patient's head (and upper cervical spine) in slight left sidebending. With the index and/or middle fingers of the right hand, the therapist "hooks" just medial to the paravertebral musculature between the atlas and axis. The musculature is then "pulled" in a lateral and ventral direction. At the same time, the hand on the patient's forehead rotates the patient's head toward the side being treated. In this example, the rotation is to the right. (In this technique, the rotation is considerably greater than in the previous technique. Between C0 and C1, the amount of rotation is minimal, whereas between C1 and C2 there is a significant degree of rotation.) The end position is held for approximately 1 second before returning to the initial position. The therapist repeats this technique for several seconds, or minutes, in a rhythmic manner.

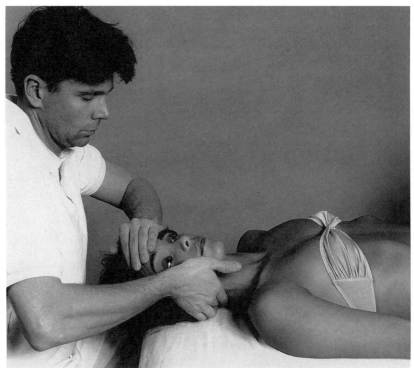

Figure 6–82

For Discs
More toward nonpainful rotation,   stroke over C2/C3...C-67

Paraverterbal Transverse Stretch during Coupled Movement of C2 to C7 (Figure 6–83)

Position of the Patient

The patient lies in a supine position with the arms relaxed alongside the body.

Position of the Therapist

The therapist sits or stands at the cranial end of the table.

Performance

If the right side is to be treated, the therapist places the index and middle fingers of the right hand against the medial edge of the paravertebral musculature at the level of C2. The other fingers lie against C1 and the occiput. The index and middle fingers of the left hand are placed on the opposite (in this case, the left) side, against the spinous process of C3.

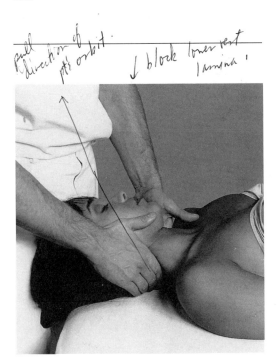

Figure 6–83 Transverse stretch of the right paravertebral musculature, during coupled left sidebending and left rotation of C2-3.

With the right hand, the therapist now pulls the musculature in a lateral and ventral direction, along a line connecting the segment with the orbita. At the same time, the left hand stabilizes the caudal vertebra. In this way, a coupled movement in flexion, left side-bending, and left rotation occurs in the C2-3 segment. The end position is held for approximately 1 second before returning to the initial position. The therapist repeats this technique for several seconds, or minutes, in a rhythmic manner.

The same procedure can then be performed per segment, by shifting the hands caudally. As the successive caudal segments are emphasized, increasingly more movement is performed. This technique can be used to treat the segments C2-3 to C6-7.

GENERAL MOBILIZATION TECHNIQUES

During the following axial separation techniques, it is very important that the therapist not wear a watch or any other jewelry. Because of increased pressure of these objects against the patient's skin, discomfort and subsequent muscle splinting can result. If the patient wears dentures, either they should be removed or a small piece of foam rubber should be placed between the teeth.

General Axial Separation

(Figures 6–84A–H)

Position of the Patient

The patient lies in a supine position on the treatment table, with the head in a neutral position and the arms resting alongside the body.

Position of the Therapist

The therapist stands cranially to the patient. The treatment table is brought to a height of the therapist's greater trochanter.

Position of the Assistant

The assistant stands next to the patient at the level of the pelvis. Once the patient lies down, the assistant places his or her hands bilaterally at the lateral, superior aspect of the patient's shoulders. Later, as the therapist applies the axial separation, the assistant ensures that the patient is completely stabilized (Figure 6–84C).

Performance

First, the patient is asked to sit on the treatment table with the legs on the table, whereby the hips and knees are flexed. The patient holds the spine in a neutral position. The therapist places one hand against the patient's neck and the other hand at the level of the upper thoracic spine. If the therapist is right-handed, the left hand is placed against the patient's neck. The patient is then instructed to lie down slowly without flexing the spinal column. At the same time the therapist supports the patient as much as possible (Figures 6–84A and 6–84B).

If the patient has severe pain, or if the patient also has back pain, it is recommended that the patient first move from sitting at the edge of the table to a sidelying position. From there, the patient can then move into supine.

As soon as the patient is lying supine, the therapist determines the best position to perform the axial separation. This depends on the weight of the therapist and the weight of the patient. To achieve sufficient axial separation, if the therapist is light, the patient should lie with the head over the edge of the table. If the therapist is heavier than the patient, the patient's head can remain on the table. In this instance, it may be necessary to place a thin pillow or wedge at the level of the upper thoracic spine (Figure 6–84D).

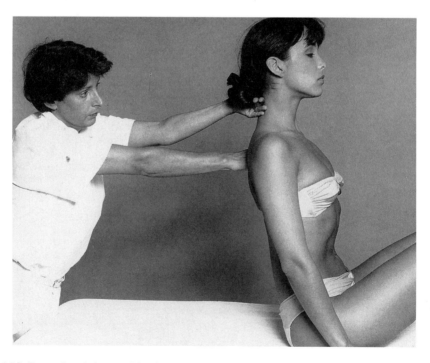

Figure 6–84A From the sitting position, the therapist slowly supports the patient into the lying position.

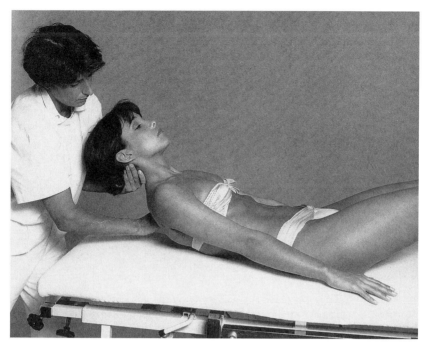

Figure 6–84B The therapist supports the patient the entire way from sitting to lying.

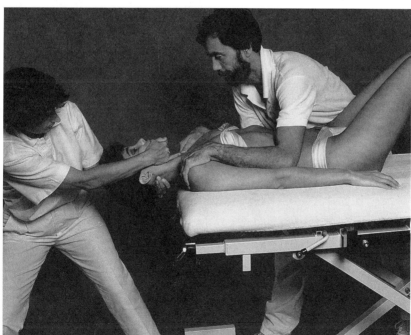

Figure 6–84C Application of axial separation.

If deviated,
head on bed,
foot less
under
head.

stand in stride

Foot draw
cephalin slightly
head.

Lower hand hooks
lat. edge on
occiput.
Chin hand holds, supports
position $\bar{c}$ $\bar{p}$

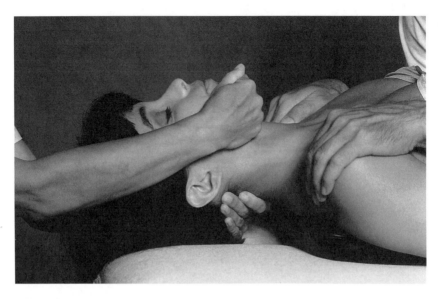

Figure 6–84D A thin pillow may be placed under the upper thoracic spine, in instances when the therapist is heavier than the patient and the patient's head remains on the table.

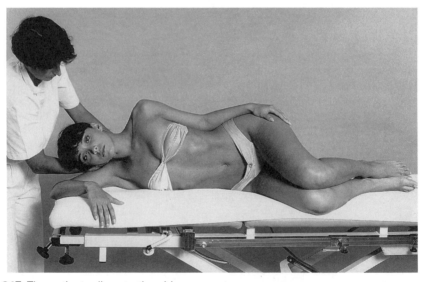

Figure 6–84E The patient rolls onto the side.

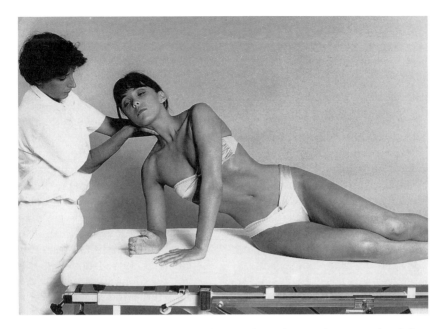

Figure 6–84F After tightening the abdominal muscles, the patient pushes up to the sitting position. At the same time, the therapist supports the patient's neck.

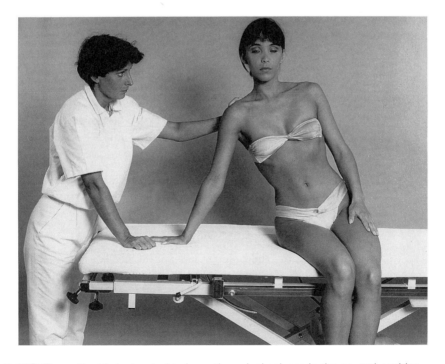

Figure 6–84G The patient is instructed to keep the spinal column in the neutral position.

In the functional examination, a trial axial separation is applied in three different positions of the cervical spine:

1. in the neutral position
2. in slight flexion
3. in slight extension

In supine, this procedure is again repeated. Most patients have the most comfort when the axial separation is given in the neutral position. However, if the patient has an antalgic deviation in flexion, the axial separation should be performed initially in (as minimal as possible) flexion.

The axial separation must never cause pain and/or muscle splinting. The axial separation can be maintained for several seconds or for several minutes, after which the separation is gradually released.

The therapist grasps the patient's head from the dorsal aspect, so that the ulnar side of the little finger has contact with the base of the occiput. The patient's cervical spine rests in the palm of the therapist's hand. The other hand is placed at the patient's chin, avoiding pressure against the ventral structures of the neck. Sometimes it is necessary to use only two or three fingers at the patient's chin.

The therapist places the left foot against the bottom rung of the treatment table, if the cranial edge of the table lies vertically above the lower rung. If a similar table is not available, then the therapist can stabilize the left foot against the foot of the assistant, which is then placed directly underneath the cranial edge of the table. If this is not possible, the therapist must absolutely ensure that the feet do not slip on the floor while performing the technique.

With the feet fairly wide apart, the therapist slowly releases the weight from the back foot, thereby slowly increasing the axial separation. Depending on the patient's tolerance and the weight of the therapist, the therapist can also slowly extend the elbows to increase further the axial separation. (This sequence can also be performed in the reverse order.)

The axial separation occurs primarily in the mid- and lower cervical segments. Research has indicated that minimal to no separation occurs between the segments C0-1 and C1-2.[29]

In order to get up when the treatment is over or when re-examining the painful cervical motions, the patient first rolls onto the side (Figure 6–84E). After tightening the abdominal muscles, the patient pushes up to the sitting position. At the same time, the therapist supports the patient's neck (Figures 6–84F and 6–84G).

This treatment can also be performed as a manipulation. One has to be certain that the diagnosis is correct and that there are no contraindications. Treatment with axial separation is indicated in patients with primary disc-related pathology who are younger than 45 years of age. The best indications are

- unilateral neck-scapular pain
- bilateral scapular pain

This treatment is also recommended for patients older than 45 years of age who complain of headaches upon waking in the morning.

After every axial separation, the patient is retested. As long as there is improvement, the technique can be repeated.

General Axial Separation with Rotation (Figures 6–85A and 6–85C)

The nonpainful or least painful rotation is performed first. Initially, the rotation is performed to approximately one-third of the available range of motion. (Figure 6–85A).

Position of the Patient

The patient lies in a supine position on the treatment table, with the head in a neutral position and the arms resting alongside the body.

Position of the Therapist

The treatment table is brought to a height of the therapist's greater trochanter. The

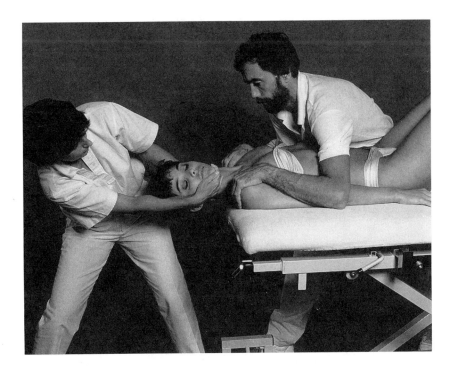

Figure 6–85A Axial separation with approximately one-third of the available rotation.

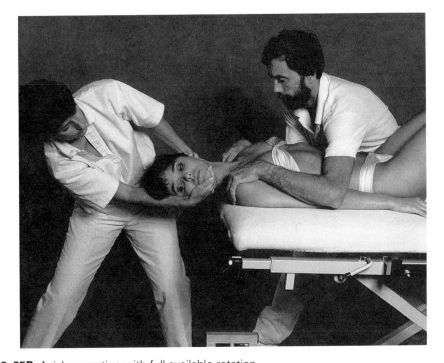

Figure 6–85B Axial separation with full available rotation.

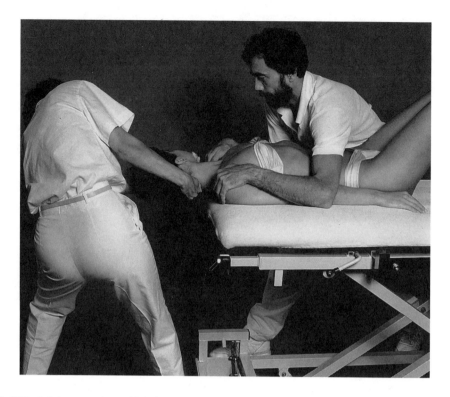

Figure 6–85C Axial separation with left rotation.

therapist stands cranially to the patient. The patient slides cranially, until the head lies over the edge of the table. The therapist supports the patient's head in the neutral position.

Position of the Assistant

The assistant stands next to the patient at the level of the pelvis. Once the patient lies down, the assistant places his or her hands bilaterally at the lateral, superior aspect of the patient's shoulders. Later, as the therapist applies the axial separation, the assistant ensures that the patient is completely stabilized (Figure 6–85A).

Performance

The performance of this technique is similar to that for General Axial Separation. Here the therapist first applies the axial separation and then slowly rotates the head. When rotating the patient's head to the right, the therapist grasps the patient's chin with the right hand (Figure 6–85B). In left rotation, the left hand grasps the chin (Figure 6–85C).

It is extremely important that during the rotation, pain and/or muscle splinting do not occur. For this reason, the nonpainful or least painful rotation is always performed first.

If a click is heard during the rotation, the head is not brought farther into rotation. After every rotation technique, the patient is rechecked. If improvement is noted, then the technique is repeated.

If there is no improvement (but also no increase in pain), after rotating to one-third in the nonpainful or least painful direction, the axial separation with rotation technique is repeated, but this time rotating to two-thirds the available range of motion. The progression in the rotations for the axial separation with rotation technique is as follows:

1. one-third the available rotation in the nonpainful or least painful direction
2. two-thirds the available rotation in the nonpainful or least painful direction
3. full available rotation in the nonpainful or least painful direction
4. one-third the available rotation in the painful direction
5. two-thirds the available rotation in the painful direction
6. full available rotation in the painful direction

When the patient does not demonstrate improvement, only then does the therapist progress to the next sequence in rotations. The therapist continues to perform the same technique as long as the patient continues to improve (ie, less pain and/or increased range of motion).

This treatment can also be performed as a manipulation. The therapist has to be certain that the diagnosis is correct and *that there are no contraindications*. The indications for general axial separation with rotation are the same as described under General Axial Separation. However, if the patient has bilateral neck-scapular pain, the amount of rotation performed should be minimal.

The manipulation is performed in the direction of the axial separation. In this instance, the therapist first applies axial separation, then rotates the patient's head. After rotating the head to the desired degree, the therapist exerts an abrupt "extra pull." The initial amount of axial separation must be maintained both before and after the "extra pull." Finally, the head is returned slowly to the neutral position, and the axial separation is slowly released.

General Axial Separation with Sidebend (Figures 6–86A and 6–86B)

Position of the Patient

The patient lies in a supine position on the treatment table, with the head in a neutral

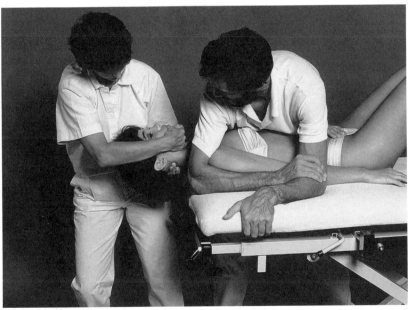

Figure 6–86A

fixate 1 side across.
diag across body,
+ fixates body c̄ ōr's body

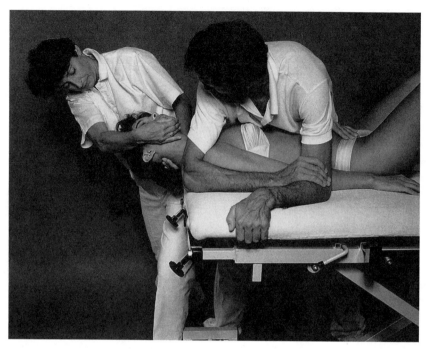

Figure 6–86B Axial separation with sidebend.

[handwritten notes] DeeDee Circles (R) foot around + touches it to floor to stabilize c̄ (L)SB, Avoid any (R) rotation. Try to keep neutral,

position and the arms resting alongside the body. The patient lies as close as possible to the edge of the treatment table, at the side toward which the mobilization will be performed.

Position of the Therapist

The therapist stands cranially to the patient. If the sidebend is going to be performed to the left, then the therapist places the left foot underneath the corner of the treatment table. As mentioned in the description for General Axial Separation, the therapist must ensure that the feet do not slip during this technique.

The patient now slides cranially, until the head lies over the edge of the table. The therapist supports the patient's head in the neutral position. If the sidebend is going to be performed to the left, then the therapist grasps the patient's chin with the right hand. The forearm rests against the right side of the

patient's head. Both of the therapist's elbows are flexed (Figure 6–86A).

Position of the Assistant

The assistant stands next to the patient at the level of the thorax. If a left sidebend is going to be performed (Figure 6–86B), the assistant stands on the left side of the patient and fixes the right shoulder with his or her right arm such that the right forearm rests on the table. The left elbow is placed against the patient's right side; the hand grasps the edge of the table. With his or her right hand, the assistant grasps his or her left elbow from ventral.

Performance

The therapist grasps the patient's head and applies axial separation, in the same manner as described under General Axial Separation. After taking the weight off the leg farthest from the table, the therapist slowly shifts this leg dorsally and then in the direction of the assistant. To a greater or lesser degree, a half circle is made with the foot. During the entire movement, the therapist's hands and arm maintain contact with the patient's head. In so doing, a sidebend is made under axial separation.

As mentioned under General Axial Separation with Rotation, the initial technique should be performed to approximately one-third of the available movement. Thus, in this example the therapist performs one-third of the patient's left sidebending range of motion.

If a click is heard during the sidebend, the head is not brought farther into sidebend. After every sidebending technique, the patient is rechecked. If improvement is noted, the technique is repeated. If there is no improvement (but also no increase in pain), after sidebending to one-third, the axial separation with sidebend technique is repeated, but this time going to two-thirds the available range of motion. If still no improvement is noted, the therapist repeats the technique to end range of the available painless range of motion. Only when the patient does not demonstrate improvement does the therapist progress to the next sequence in sidebend. The therapist continues to perform the same technique as long as the patient continues to improve (ie, less pain and/or increased range of motion).

This treatment can also be performed as a manipulation. The manipulation is performed in the direction of the axial separation. In this instance, the therapist first applies axial separation and then sidebends the patient's head. After laterally flexing the head to the desired degree, the therapist exerts an abrupt "extra pull" in the direction of the axial separation. The initial amount of axial separation must be maintained both before and after the "extra pull." Finally, the head is slowly returned to the neutral position, and the axial separation is slowly released.

The sidebend is always performed away from the painful side. For instance, if the patient's pain is localized on the right side, then the sidebend mobilization is performed to the left. This is the case even if the left sidebend is more painful and limited than the right. This is in contrast to the rotation mobilization, where one first performs the nonpainful or least painful rotation.

The patient returns to sitting as described under General Axial Separation.

Lateral Shifting with Slight General Axial Separation (Figures 6–87A and 6–87B)

This mobilization is particularly effective after an axial separation with sidebend performed earlier. Also, this technique is very effective in relieving treatment soreness.

Position of the Patient

The patient lies in a supine position on the treatment table. The head is in a neutral position and the arms rest alongside the body.

Position of the Therapist

The therapist stands cranially to the patient.

Performance

The therapist grasps the patient's head with both hands, ensuring not to cover the ears. The patient is then instructed to slide upward, bringing the head over the edge of the table. The therapist exerts slight axial separation and shifts body weight from right to left in alternating movements, without causing a rotation of the patient's head.

Manual Treatment for an Acute (Discogenic) Torticollis

Position of the Patient

With support from the therapist, the patient is brought from sitting on the treatment table to a supine lying position. The head is held in an antalgic position and should be supported as much as possible in this position.

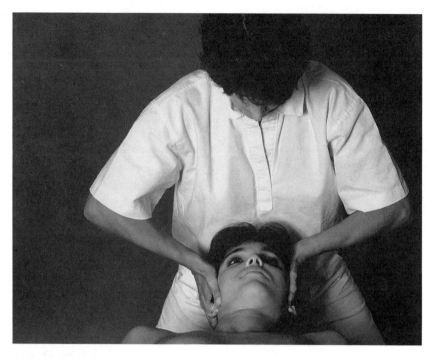

Figure 6–87A Lateral shift to the left.

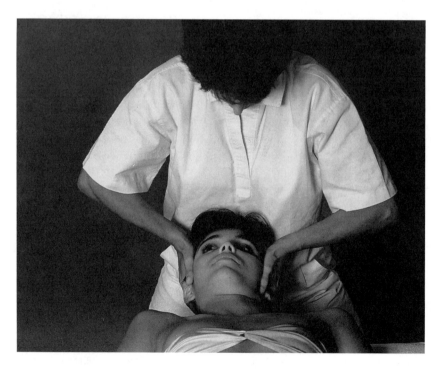

Figure 6–87B Lateral shift to the right.

Position of the Therapist

The therapist stands cranially to the patient.

Performance

From the antalgic position, the therapist performs slight axial separation for a duration of approximately 30 seconds. If the patient notes relief of pain during the technique, the amount of axial separation can be increased. After each technique, the patient is rechecked. If improvement is noted and the antalgic position can be slightly corrected, the therapist repeats the axial separation in the new position. The therapist progresses in this manner until the neutral position has been reached.

If no improvement is noted and the patient still demonstrates an antalgic posture in lying, then the therapist applies axial separation in line with the antalgic posture. Under this axial separation, the therapist now performs a small amount of rotation away from the antalgic position. The head is first returned to the initial position before releasing the axial separation. The same can be performed with the sidebend. After each technique, the patient is rechecked. As long as there is improvement, the therapist progresses in this manner until the neutral position has been reached.

Once the neutral position has been reached, the patient is treated with general axial separation. As long as improvement is noted, the therapist continues with this technique. If the neutral position has been reached and the patient no longer demonstrates improvement, then the axial separation techniques are progressed as follows:

1. general axial separation
2. general axial separation with "extra pull"
3. general axial separation with rotation in the nonpainful or least painful direction
   (a) one-third rotation
   (b) one-third rotation with "extra pull"
   (c) two-thirds rotation
   (d) two-thirds rotation with "extra pull"
   (e) full rotation
   (f) full rotation with "extra pull" in the axial separation
4. general axial separation with rotation in the painful direction
   (a) one-third rotation
   (b) one-third rotation with "extra pull"
   (c) two-thirds rotation
   (d) two-thirds rotation with "extra pull"
   (e) full rotation
   (f) full rotation with "extra pull" in the axial separation
5. general axial separation with sidebend away from the painful side
   (a) one-third sidebend
   (b) one-third sidebend with "extra pull"
   (c) two-thirds sidebend
   (d) two-thirds sidebend with "extra pull"
   (e) full sidebend
   (f) full sidebend with "extra pull" in the axial separation

Only when the patient does not continue to demonstrate improvement does the therapist progress to the next technique in the sequence. The progression listed above generally takes place over several days of treatment. The therapist continues to perform the same technique as long as the patient continues to improve (ie, less pain and/or increased range of motion).

In the treatment of the acute discogenic torticollis, considerable improvement can be achieved with a repositioning technique. This *HGP*

H.E.P

repositioning technique is applied in the following instances:

- during the initial treatment, if improvement cannot be gained with the axial separation in the antalgic position as well as with attempts at correcting the rotation or sidebending under axial separation
- at the end of the first few treatments, when the range of motion is still significantly limited
- as a home program for the patient in the acute phase of the torticollis (The patient should perform the program two to three times per day.)

The patient's head is brought slightly into the direction of the painful rotation and is supported there with a sandbag for approximately 5 minutes. The therapist then checks to see whether the rotation can be performed slightly farther. Again, the head is supported in this position for another few minutes. The procedure is repeated several times. When no further improvement is reached with the rotation, the repositioning technique is performed for the sidebend.

Usually the patient also benefits from wearing a firm cervical collar for the first 3 days. This collar should be worn not only during the day, but also at night. Initially, the patient should be seen daily for treatment.

LOCAL SEGMENTAL MOBILIZATION TECHNIQUES

Dorsoventral Mobilization

Jenkner

(Figures 6–88A–H)

The dorsoventral mobilization is an ideal treatment technique for patients with primary disc-related pathology, in whom the lateral view X-ray indicates a kyphotic kink at the level of the symptomatic segment. (Refer to section 6.3, Pathology: Primary Disc-Related Disorders.)

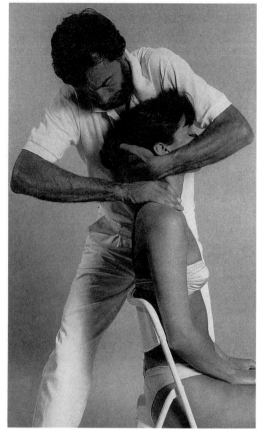

Figure 6–88A Dorsoventral mobilization of C5-6.

When treatment is indicated in instances of primary disc pathology, the mobilization techniques are always performed with axial separation. Sometimes, the axial separation should not be applied generally through the entire cervical spine; in these instances, the dorsoventral mobilization is the treatment of preference. For instance, occasionally patients with primary discogenic problems also have symptoms such as dizziness or tinnitus. In cases of block vertebrae, either above or below the symptomatic segment, the general axial separation techniques are contraindicated. However, the local segmental dorsoventral mobilization can be applied instead (Figure 6–88A).

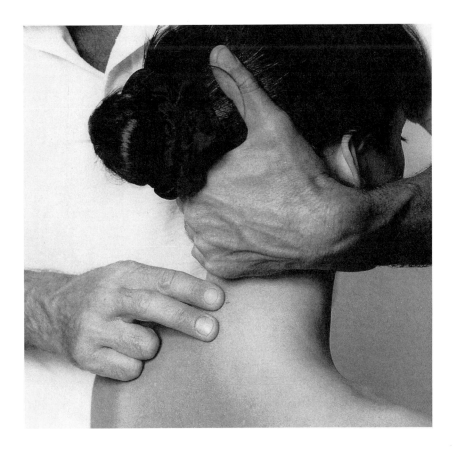

Figure 6–88B Localization of the C7 spinous process.

A lateral view X-ray can be performed to determine the affected segment. However, an experienced therapist can obtain the same information from the local segmental examination. In most instances, there is a functional disturbance in the C5-6 segment. Frequently the C6-7 segment is affected; of the lower cervical segments, the C4-5 segment is the least often affected. Primary discogenic lesions of the other cervical segments are very rare.

Position of the Patient

The patient sits on a chair, with the back supported by the back of the chair.

Position of the Therapist

The therapist stands next to the patient.

Performance

The therapist localizes the spinous process of C7. From this reference point, depending on the localization of the affected segment, the spinous processes of C6, C5, or C4 can be localized. The therapist grasps the head of the patient in such a way that the little finger rests against the cranial vertebra of the segment being treated. The therapist places the web space of the other hand at the level of the caudal vertebra's spinous process (Figures 6–88B and 6–88C).

While fixing with the caudal hand, the therapist performs a local axial separation in the segment with the cranial hand (Figure 6–88D). Next, the therapist extends the

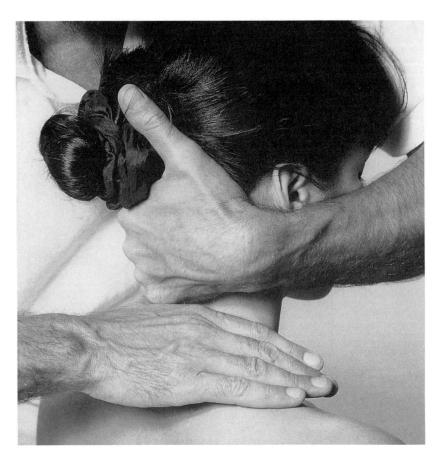

Figure 6–88C The therapist places the web space of one hand at the level of the caudal vertebra's spinous process.

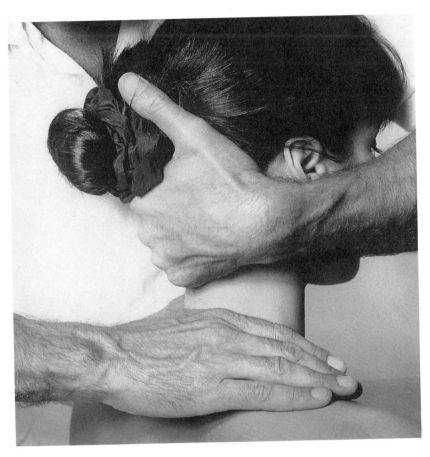

Figure 6–88D With the cranial hand, the therapist performs a local axial separation in the segment.

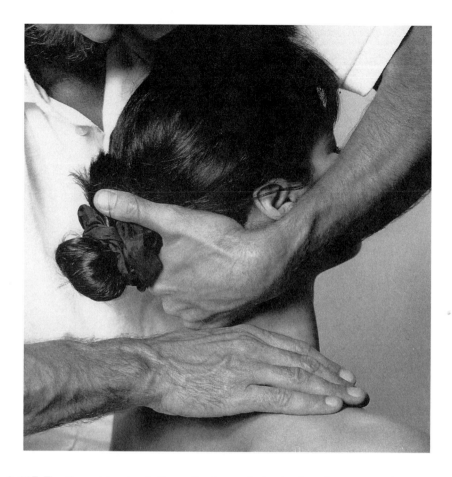

Figure 6–88E The therapist extends the patient's cervical spine into the segment being treated.

patient's cervical spine into the segment being treated (Figure 6–88E). The actual mobilization now occurs when the therapist pushes the caudal vertebra horizontally in a ventral direction (Figure 6–88F). At the same time, the cranial hand maintains both the extended position and the local axial separation.

Respecting pain and end-feel, the caudal vertebra is held in this ventral position for 8 to

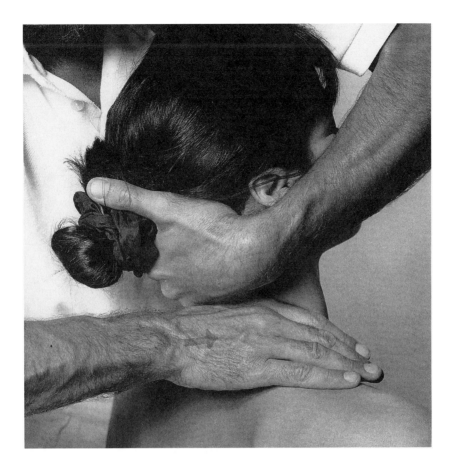

Figure 6–88F The therapist pushes the caudal vertebra horizontally in a ventral direction.

10 seconds. After the 8 to 10 seconds, the pressure is reduced slightly for a few seconds, before performing the ventral mobilization once more. The therapist then slowly releases the ventral pressure, returns the patient's head to the neutral position, and gradually releases the axial separation.

The patient is rechecked. If the cervical range of motion has increased, the mobilization technique can be repeated.

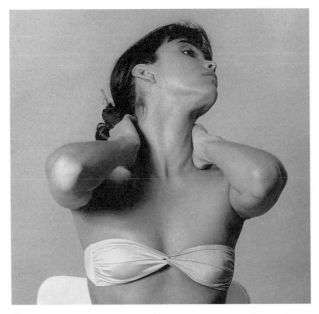

G

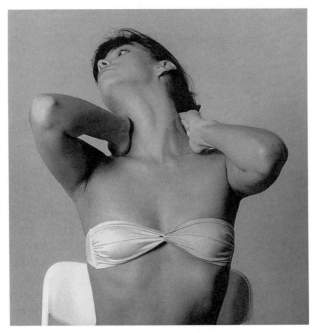

H

Figures 6–88G and 6–88H Home exercise after the dorsoventral mobilization.

Home Exercise for the Patient
(Figures 6–88G and 6–88H)

After two or three mobilizations, the patient is instructed in a home exercise program in order to maintain the increased mobility. The patient is taught how to find the C7 spinous process, and from there the appropriate spinous process of the affected segment's caudal vertebra (C6, C7, or C5). The patient places the tips of the index and/or middle fingers of both hands on this spinous process and exerts slight pressure in a ventral direction.

The patient is instructed to tuck the chin in. From the neutral position, the patient extends the cervical spine as far as possible, without pain, while maintaining the ventral pressure with the fingers. Then in a slow and relaxed way, the patient rotates the head, alternating left and right. (Some patients have much more rotation than do other patients.)

This exercise should be performed without pain. The patient should perform the exercise daily, at least five to ten times throughout the day.

MOBILIZATION TECHNIQUES, C0 to C1

The following techniques are especially effective in patients with postural- or movement-related headaches due to a functional disturbance of the atlanto-occipital joint.

Traction Mobilization of C0 to C1
(Figure 6–89)

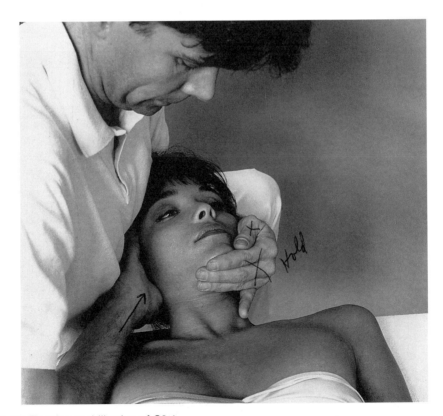

Figure 6–89 Traction mobilization of C0-1.

Position of the Patient

The patient lies on the treatment table with the arms resting alongside the body.

Position of the Therapist

The therapist stands next to the treatment table, at the level of patient's head, on the side to be treated.

Performance

If the right side is to be treated, the therapist holds the patient's head with the left arm in such a way that the patient's head rests on the forearm. The fingers grasp the patient's chin. The patient's head is supported between the therapist's arm and trunk.

The therapist places the radial aspect of the right metacarpophalangeal II joint (MCP II) against the dorsal aspect of the patient's mastoid process. The thumb lies ventral to

the patient's ear. The therapist now brings the patient's head into an upper cervical ipsilateral sidebend and contralateral rotation. In other words, when treating the right side, the head is brought into slight upper cervical right sidebend and left rotation. From this position, the traction is performed. The direction of the traction is cranial and slightly toward the midline.

The technique can be performed in an oscillatory way for pain relief, it can be held for several seconds as a mobilization, or it can be performed as a manipulation.

Flexion Mobilization of C0 to C1
(Figure 6–90)

Position of the Patient

The patient sits on a stool or a chair. If there is not a chair back to support the patient, the

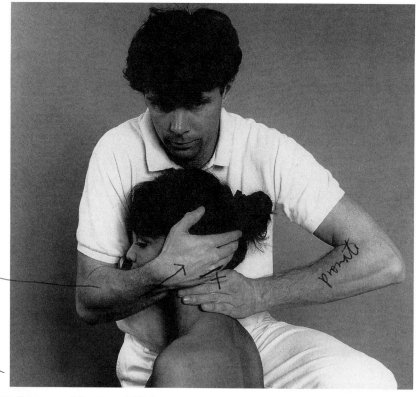

Figure 6–90 Flexion mobilization of C0-1.

therapist supports the patient's back with the leg (as pictured).

Position of the Therapist

The therapist stands next to the patient.

Performance

If the left side is being treated, the examiner uses the right arm to grasp the patient's head from ventral. Without exerting pressure against the ears, the patient's head is held between the therapist's right hand and sternum. The little finger has contact with the mastoid process and occiput. The other hand stabilizes the atlas from dorsal, with the thumb on one side and the index finger on the other side.

While the caudal hand fixes, the therapist brings the patient's head into an upper cervical flexion. At the same time, the therapist shifts the occiput in a dorsocranial direction in relation to the atlas. After holding this end position for approximately 1 second, the patient's head is brought back to the initial position. This technique is performed in a slow, rhythmic manner for several seconds or minutes.

Unilateral Flexion Mobilization of C0 to C1 (Figure 6–91)

Position of the Patient

The patient sits on a stool or a chair. If there is not a chair back to support the patient, the therapist supports the patient's back with the leg (as pictured).

Position of the Therapist

The therapist stands next to the patient, opposite the side to be treated.

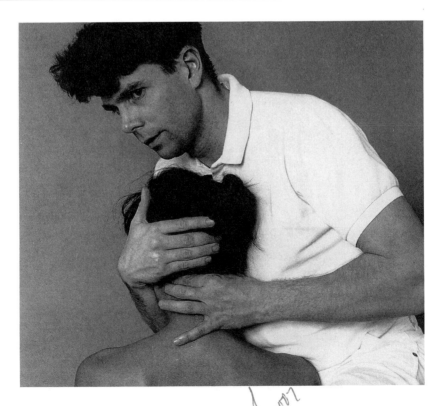

Figure 6–91 Unilateral flexion mobilization of C0-1.

Performance

If the left side is being treated, the examiner uses the right arm to grasp the patient's head from ventral. Without exerting pressure against the ears, the patient's head is held between the therapist's right hand and sternum. The little finger has contact with the mastoid process and occiput. The left hand stabilizes the atlas. The index finger is placed on the dorsolateral aspect of the left C1 transverse process, and the thumb is placed on the dorsolateral aspect of the right C1 transverse process.

While fixing the atlas with the caudal hand, the therapist slightly flexes the patient's head, shifting the occiput in a dorsocranial direction. At the same time, the patient's head is brought into an ipsilateral rotation and contralateral sidebend. (In other words, if the left side is being treated,

the head is brought into a left rotation and right sidebend.) After holding this end position for approximately 1 second, the patient's head is brought back to the initial position. This technique is performed in a slow, rhythmic manner for several seconds or minutes.

MOBILIZATION TECHNIQUES, C2 TO C7

The next three mobilizations are especially indicated for patients in whom pain and/or limited range of motion was found during the local segmental functional examination. Patients who did not have complete recovery or did not have any improvement with the general mobilization techniques may also benefit from these techniques, providing the functional examination gives the proper indications.

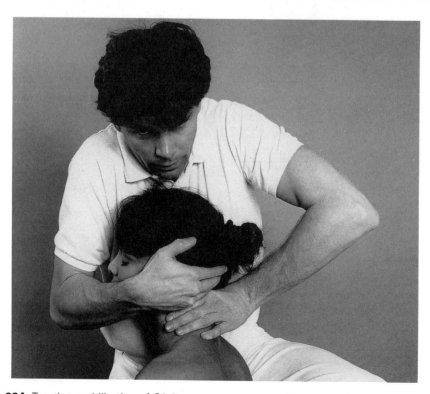

Figure 6–92A Traction mobilization of C2-3.

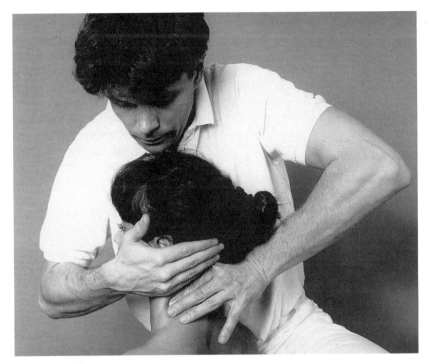

Figure 6–92B Traction mobilization of C4-5 in prepositioned left sidebend and left rotation.

Traction Mobilization of C2 to C7

(Figures 6–92A and 6–92B)

Position of the Patient

The patient sits on a stool or a chair. If there is not a chair back to support the patient, the therapist supports the patient's back with the leg.

Position of the Therapist

The therapist stands next to the patient.

Performance

With one arm, the examiner grasps the patient's head from ventral. Without exerting pressure against the ears, the patient's head is stabilized between the therapist's hand and sternum. The therapist grasps the head of the patient in such a way that the little finger rests against the cranial vertebra of the segment being treated.

The index finger and thumb of the other hand are placed against the dorsal aspect of the caudal vertebra's zygapophyseal joints.

From cranial, the therapist fixes the patient's head, the cranial segments, and the cranial vertebra of the segment being treated. With the caudal hand, the therapist then exerts pressure in a ventrocaudal direction; this direction is perpendicular to a line connecting the affected segment with the orbita.

The traction can be performed bilaterally by exerting equal pressure with both thumb and index finger. Unilateral traction can also be emphasized by pushing mainly with either the thumb or index finger. For pain relief, the traction can be performed in an oscillatory manner. For a mobilization effect, the traction is held for several seconds.

The technique can be performed with the affected segment in its physiological resting position. However, it can also be applied with the segment pre-positioned in the limited direction. After positioning the segment as far as possible in the limited direction, traction is performed with either a bilateral or a unilateral emphasis (see the following technique).

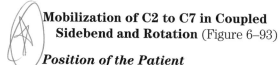

Mobilization of C2 to C7 in Coupled Sidebend and Rotation (Figure 6–93)

Position of the Patient

The patient sits on a stool or chair. If there is not a chair back to support the patient, the therapist supports the patient's back with the leg (Figure 6–93).

Position of the Therapist

The therapist stands next to the patient.

Performance

With one arm, the therapist grasps the patient's head from a ventral approach. Without exerting pressure against the ears, the patient's head is held between the therapist's hand and sternum. The therapist grasps the head of the patient in such a way that the little finger rests against the cranial vertebra of the segment being treated.

The index finger and thumb of the other hand are placed against the dorsal aspect of the caudal vertebra's zygapophyseal joints.

The therapist positions the patient's head in rotation and sidebend, in a direction away from the therapist. (In other words, if the therapist stands on the patient's right side, the patient's head is brought into a left rotation and left sidebend.) The head is rotated and laterally flexed just to the point where the segment being treated is reached. Thus, this segment is pre-positioned in coupled rotation and sidebend. The head is then stabilized in this position.

From this position, the therapist can perform two different mobilization techniques.

1. With the caudal hand, the therapist exerts bilateral pressure in a traction direction: perpendicular to a line connecting the affected segment with the orbita. If pressure is exerted unilaterally, against the zygapophyseal joint opposite to the therapist (in the pictured example, the left side), then em-

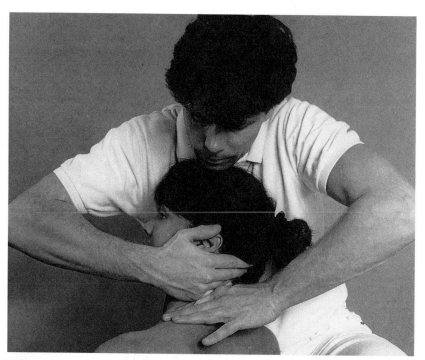

Figure 6–93 Mobilization of the left C5-6 zygapophyseal joint in pre-positioned left rotation and coupled left sidebend.

Can do ext. on 1 side - rhymira × 5 min.   Retest   If no Δ,
then flex " other side

phasis is placed on traction with a pre-positioned extension component. If pressure is exerted unilaterally, against the zygapophyseal joint closest to the therapist, then emphasis is placed on traction with a pre-positioned flexion component.

2. In this pre-positioned position, the therapist brings the patient's head further into rotation with the cranial hand. The caudal hand fixes the caudal vertebra of the segment being treated. In this way, rotation is specifically mobilized.

Mobilization of C2 to C7 with Locking in Sidebend and Combined Rotation
(Figure 6–94)

Position of the Patient

The patient sits on a stool or a chair. If there is not a chair back to support the patient, the therapist supports the patient's back with the leg (Figure 6–94).

Position of the Therapist

The therapist stands next to the patient.

Performance

With one arm, the therapist grasps the patient's head from a ventral approach. Without exerting pressure against the ears, the patient's head is held between the therapist's hand and sternum. The therapist grasps the head of the patient in such a way that the little finger rests against the cranial vertebra of the segment being treated.

The index finger and thumb of the other hand are placed against the dorsal aspect of the caudal vertebra's zygapophyseal joints.

The therapist positions the patient's cervical spine in a sidebend away from the therapist and a combined (contralateral) rotation. *This positioning occurs only in the segments cranial to the segment being treated.*

The therapist performs an axial separation in the segment's zygapophyseal joints by

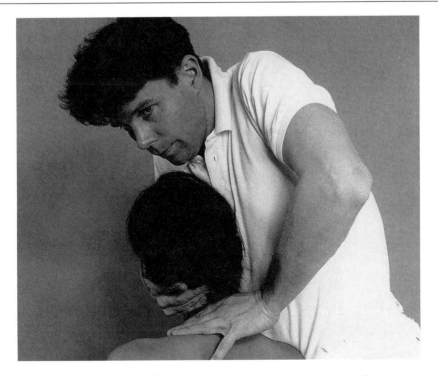

SB –
see Manual
p. 111

Figure 6–94 Mobilization of the left C5-6 zygapophyseal joint during right rotation.

slightly extending the knees. With the caudal hand, the therapist exerts pressure in a ventral and slightly caudal direction, perpendicular to a line connecting the affected segment with the orbita.

This technique is indicated for functional disturbances of the cervicothoracic junction and/or the upper thoracic spine. Problems are seen in these two areas, particularly in patients with a thoracic outlet syndrome.

General Axial Separation Manipulation for the Cervicothoracic Junction and the Upper Thoracic Segments: In Sitting (Figures 6–95A–H)

Position of the Patient

The patient sits transversely on the treatment table, as close as possible to the edge.

Position of the Therapist

The therapist stands behind the patient (Figure 6–95A).

Performance

The patient is instructed to lift both arms up, so that the therapist can reach, with both arms, underneath the patient's axillae (Figure 6–95B). From this position, the therapist flexes the elbows, placing the index and middle fingers of both hands on the spinous processes of the upper segments in the area to be treated (Figure 6–95C). The patient is then asked to place the fingertips on top of the therapist's hands (Figure 6–95D). The therapist grasps the patient's thumbs between thumb and index finger (Figure 6–95E).

The patient is instructed to relax completely and hang back against the therapist's thorax (Figure 6–95F). In order to support

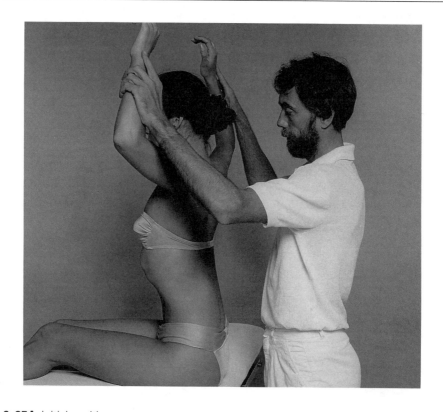

Figure 6–95A Initial position.

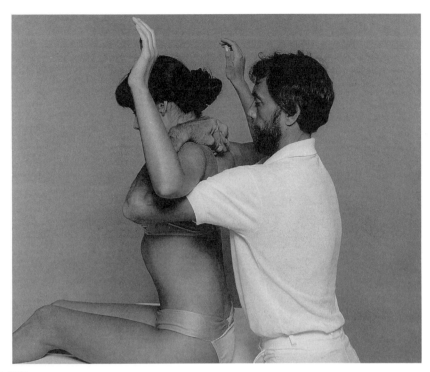

Figure 6–95B

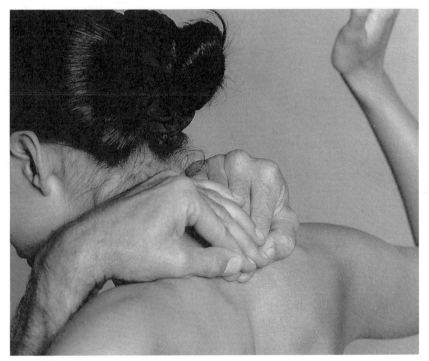

Figure 6–95C The therapist places the fingers against the cranial spinous processes of the area to be treated.

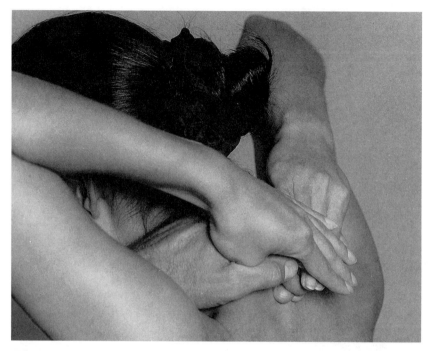

Figure 6–95D

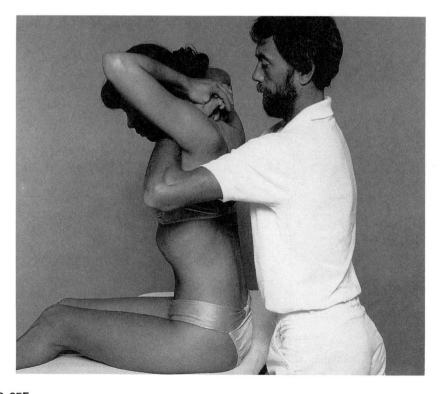

Figure 6–95E

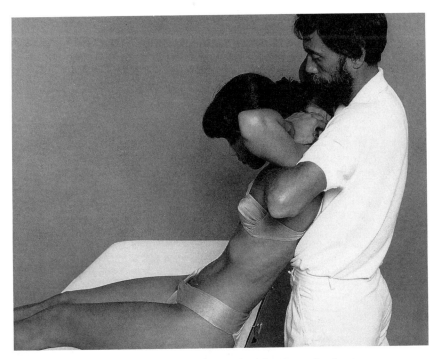

Figure 6–95F The patient relaxes, bringing the thoracic spine into a kyphosis.

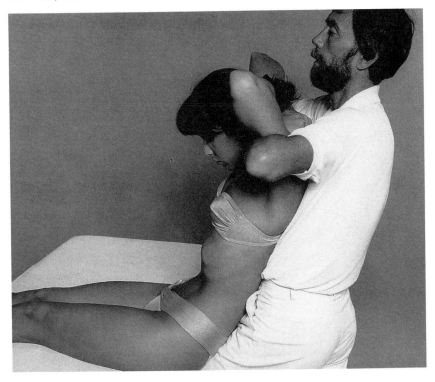

Figure 6–95G The therapist supports the patient's lumbar spine.

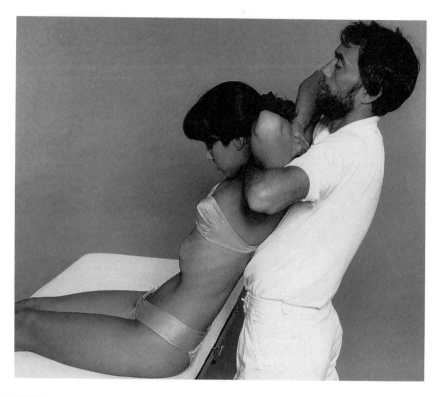

Figure 6–95H The therapist exerts overpressure by extending his or her own thoracic spine.

the patient's lumbar spine, the therapist brings one leg forward (Figure 6–95G). The therapist places the manubrium of the sternum against the spinous processes of the lower segments in the area to be treated.

The patient is asked to take a deep breath. During the exhalation, the therapist takes up the pre-tension by exerting pressure in a ventral and caudal direction with the fingers. At the same time, the therapist exerts pressure in a ventral and cranial direction with the sternum.

Just at the end of the exhalation and before the patient begins to inhale again, a short overpressure is given, both with the fingers (in a caudal direction) and with the sternum (in a cranial direction). In order to perform this overpressure, the therapist performs an abrupt extension of his or her thoracic spine (Figure 6–95H).

Although the therapist places the affected segment between the fingers and sternum, this technique generally has an effect on several segments. This effect is never harmful.

REFERENCES

1. Töndury G. *Angewandte und Topographische Anatomie.* Stuttgart: Georg Thieme Verlag; 1981.
2. Lewit K, Krausova L. Beitrag zur Flexion der Halswirbelsäule. *Fortschr Roentgenstr.* 1962;97:38.
3. Fielding JW. Cineroentgenography of the normal cervical spine. *J Bone Joint Surg [Am].* 1954; 39:1280.
4. von Gutman G. X-ray diagnosis of spinal dysfunction. *Man Med.* 1982;5:73.

5. Arlen A. Die Paradoxale Keppbewegung der Atlas in der Funktionsdiagnostik der Halswirbelsäule. *Man Med.* 1977;1:16.

6. Arlen A. Roentgenologische Funktionsdiagnostik der Wirbelsäule. *Man Med.* 1979;2:24.

7. Schmorl G, Junghanns H. *The Human Spine in Health and Disease.* 2nd ed. New York: Grune & Stratton; 1971.

8. White AA, Panjabi MM. *Clinical Biomechanics of the Spine.* Philadelphia: JB Lippincott Co; 1978.

9. Penning L, Wilmink JT. Rotation of the cervical spine: a CT study in normal subjects. *Spine.* 1987;12:732.

10. Bogduk N, Windsor M, Inglis A. The innervation of the cervical discs. *Spine.* 1988;13:2.

11. Bogduk N, Engel R. The menisci of the lumbar zygapophyseal joints: a review of their anatomy and clinical significance. *Spine.* 1984;9:454.

12. Töndury G. *Entwicklungsgeschichte und Fehlbildungen der Halswirbelsäule.* Stuttgart: Hippokrates Verlag; 1958.

13. Penning L. Differences in anatomy, motion development and aging of the upper and lower cervical disc segments. *Clin Biomech.* 1988;3:37.

14. Hall MC. *Luschka's Joint.* Springfield, Ill: Charles C Thomas; 1965.

15. Markuske H. *Untersuchung zur Statik und Dynamik der Kindlichen Halswirbelsäule: Der Aussagewert Seitlicher Röntgenaufnahmen.* Stuttgart: Hippokrates Verlag; 1971.

16. Buetti-Bauml C. *Funktionelle Roentgendiagnostik der Halswirbelsäule.* Stuttgart: Georg Thieme Verlag; 1954.

17. Dommisse GF. The blood supply of the spinal cord. *J Bone Joint Surg [Br].* 1974;56:225.

18. Wyke BD. Neurology of the cervical spinal joints. *Physiotherapy.* 1979;65:72.

19. Andersson BJG, Ortengren R, Nachemson AL, Elfstrom G, Branon H. The sitting posture: an electromyographic and discometric study. *Orthop Clin North Am.* 1975;6:105.

20. Oostendorp RAB. *Funktionele Vertebrobasillaire Insufficiëntie: Onderzoek en Behandeling in de Fysiotherapie.* Nijmegen: Catholic University; 1988. Dissertation.

21. Krämer J. *Bandscheibenbedingte Erkrankungen.* Stuttgart: Georg Thieme Verlag; 1978.

22. Jenkner FL. *Das Cervikalsyndrom: Manuelle und elektrische Therapie.* Vienna: Springer Verlag; 1982.

23. Kelsey JL, et al. An epidemiological study of acute prolapsed cervical intervertebral disc. *J Bone Joint Surg [Am].* 1984;66:907–914.

24. Sances A, Weber RC, Larson SJ, Cusick JS, Myklebust JB, Walsh PR. Bioengineering analysis of head and spine injuries. *CRC Crit Rev Bioeng.* 1981;6:79–122.

25. Macnab IMB. The whiplash syndrome: symposium on disease of the intervertebral disc. *Orthop Clin North Am.* 1971;2:389–403.

26. Webb MN, Terrett AFJ. Whiplash: mechanisms and patterns of tissue injury. *J Aust Chirop Assoc.* 1985;15(2):60–69.

27. Oosterveld WJ, Kortschot HW, Kingma GG, de Jong HAA, Saatchi MR. Electronystagmographic findings following cervical injuries. In: *Neck Injury in Advanced Military Aircraft Environments.* Conference Proceedings No. 471, Advisory Group for Aerospace Research and Development. NATO 1991;7:1–74.

28. Cyriax J. *Textbook of Orthopaedic Medicine.* Volume 1: *Diagnosis of Soft Tissue Lesions.* 7th ed. London: Baillière Tindall; 1979.

29. Ausman JI, Shrontz CE, Pearce JE, Diaz FG, Crecelius JL. Vertebrobasilar insufficiency: a review. *Arch Neurol.* 1985;42:803–808.

30. Kleyn A de, Nieuwenhuyse AC. Schwindelanfälle und Nystagmus bei einer bestimmten Stellung des Kopfes. *Acta Otolaryngol.* 1927;11:155–157.

SUGGESTED READING

Altongy JF, Fielding JW. Combined atlanto-axial and occipito-atlantal rotatory subluxation. *J Bone Joint Surg [Am].* 1990;72:923.

Andrew T, Piggot H. Growth arrest for progressive scoliosis: combined anterior and posterior fusion of the convexity. *J Bone Joint Surg [Br].* 1985;67B:193–197.

Archer IA, Dickson RA. Stature and idiopathic scoliosis: a prospective study. *J Bone Joint Surg [Br].* 1985;67:185–188.

Barker ME. Manipulation in general medical practice for thoracic pain syndromes. *Br Osteopath J.* 1983;15:95–97.

Biemond A, Jong JMBV de. On cervical nystagmus and related disorders. *Brain.* 1969;92:437–458.

Bohlman HH, Zdeblick TA. Anterior excisions of herniated thoracic discs. *J Bone Joint Surg [Am].* 1988;70:1038–1047.

Bolender NF, Schönström NSR, Spengler DM. Role of computed tomography and myelography in the diagnosis of central spinal stenosis. *J Bone Joint Surg [Am].* 1985;67:240–246.

Bywaters EGL. Rheumatoid and other diseases of the cervical interspinous bursae, and changes in the spinous processes. *Ann Rheum Dis.* 1982;41:360–370.

Cats A. De aandoeningen van de rug (1): juvenile Kyfose (Morbus Scheuermann). *Reuma Wereldwijd.* 1984;8(2):1–4.

Cats A. De aandoeningen van de rug (2): osteoporose. *Reuma Wereldwijd.* 1984;8(4):1–4.

Cats A. De aandoeningen van de rug (3): spondylosis hyperostotica. *Reuma Wereldwijd.* 1984;8(4):1–4.

Citron N, Edgar MA, Sheehy J, Thomas DGT. Intramedullary spinal cord tumors presenting a scoliosis. *J Bone Joint Surg [Br].* 1984;66:513–517.

Daruwalla JS, Balasubramaniam P. Moiré topography in scoliosis: its accuracy in detecting the site and size of the curve. *J Bone Joint Surg [Br].* 1985;67:211–213.

Daruwalla JS, Balasubramaniam P, Chay SO, Rajan U, Lee HP. Idiopathic scoliosis: prevalence and ethnic distribution in Singapore schoolchildren. *J Bone Joint Surg [Br].* 1985;67:182–184.

Davidson RI, Dunn EJ, Metsmaker JN. The shoulder abduction test in the diagnosis of radicular pain in cervical extradural compressive monoradiculopathies. *Spine.* 1981;6:441–444.

Deacon P, Berkin CR, Kickson RA. Combined idiopathic kyphosis and scoliosis: an analysis of the lateral spinal curvatures associated with Scheuermann's disease. *J Bone Joint Surg [Br].* 1985;67:189–192.

Deacon P, Flood BN, Dickson RA. Idiopathic scoliosis in three dimensions: a radiographic and morphometric analysis. *J Bone Joint Surg [Br].* 1984;66:509–512.

Defesche HFHG, Broere G. Het spinale hematom. *Ned Tijdschr Geneeskd.* 1980;124:157–160.

Dvorak J. Weichteilverletzungen der Halswirbelsäule: Möglichkeiten der funktionellen Computertomographie. *Man Med.* 1987;25:111–115.

Edgar MA. To brace or not to brace? *J Bone Joint Surg [Br].* 1985;67:173–174.

Ernst WK. Angeborene und konstitutionelle Fehlformierungen im Thoraxbereich im Kindesalter. *Krankengymnastic.* 1988;40:379–382.

Fisk JW, Baigent ML, Hill PD. The incidence of Scheuermann's disease: preliminary report. *Am J Phys Med.* 1982;61:32–35.

Flatley TJ, Anderson MH, Anast GT. Spinal instability due to malignant disease: treatment by segmental spinal stabilisation. *J Bone Joint Surg [Am].* 1984;66:47–52.

Fredrickson BE, Baker D, McHolick WJ, Yuan HA, Lubicky JP. The natural history of spondylolysis and spondylolisthesis. *J Bone Joint Surg [Br].* 1984;66:699–707.

Georgopoulos G, Pizzutillo PD, Myung SL. Occipito-atlantal instability in children. *J Bone Joint Surg [Am].* 1987;69:429–436.

Hayashi K, Yabuki T. Origin of the uncus and of Luschka's joint in the cervical spine. *J Bone Joint Surg [Am].* 1985;67:788–791.

Heywood AWB, Learmonth ID, Thomas M. Cervical spine instability in rheumatoid arthritis. *J Bone Joint Surg [Br].* 1988;70:702–707.

Hsu LCS, Lee PC, Leong JCY. Dystrophic spinal deformities in neurofibromatosis: treatment by anterior and posterior fusion. *J Bone Joint Surg [Br].* 1984;66:495–499.

Jarzem PF, Kostuik JP, Filiaggi M, Doyle DJ. Spinal cord distraction: an in vitro study of length, tension, and tissue pressure. *J Spinal Disord.* 1991;4:177–192.

Johnson DP, Fergusson CM. An early diagnosis of atlanto-axial rotatory fixation. *J Bone Joint Surg [Br].* 1986;68:698–701.

Ker NB, Jones CB. Tumors of the cauda equina: the problem of differential diagnosis. *J Bone Joint Surg [Br].* 1985;67:358–362.

Kikuchi S, Macnab I, Moreau P. *Localization of the Level of Symptomatic Cervical Disc Degeneration.* Edinburgh: E & S Livingstone.

Kleinrensink, GJ, Anatomist. Department of Anatomy. Rotterdam: Erasmus University; Personal conversation.

Koes BW et al. Effectiviteit van manuele technieken bij nekklachten. *Med Contact.* 1989;44:1181–1184.

Lewit K, Krausova L. Beitrag zur Flexion der Halswirbelsäule. *Fortschr Roentgenstr.* 1962;97:38.

Lysell E. Motion in the cervical spine: an experimental study on autopsy specimens. *Acta Orthop Scand Suppl.* 1969;123:5.

Maigne R. Low back pain of thoracolumbar origin. *Arch Phys Med Rehabil.* 1980;61:389–394.

Muller JWTh. Klinische lessen: rugpijn. *Ned Tijdschr Geneeskd.* 1980;124,44:1857–1860.

Nicholson MW. Whiplash: fact, fantasy or fakery. *Hawaii Med J.* 1974;33:168–170.

Nötges A. Differentialdiagnose und Therapie des Thoraxschmerzes aus kardiologischer Sicht. *Krankengymnastik.* 1988;40:377–378.

Panjabi M, Dvorak J, Crisco J III, Oda T, Hilibrand A, Grob D. Flexion, tension, and lateral bending of the upper cervical spine in response to alar ligament transections. *J Spinal Disord.* 1991;4(2):157–167.

Papaioannou T. Scoliosis associated with limb-length inequality. *J Bone Joint Surg [Am].* 1982;64:59–62.

Pennie BJ, Agambar LJ. Whiplash injuries: a trial of early management. *J Bone Joint Surg [Br].* 1990;72:277–279.

Perret E. Neuropsychologische Folgen von Schleudertraumen der Halswirbelsäule. *Man Med.* 1987;25:120–123.

Pincott JR, Davies JS, Taffs LF. Scoliosis caused by section of dorsal spinal nerve roots. *J Bone Joint Surg [Br].* 1984;66:27–29.

Roberts AP, Connor AN, Tolmie JL, Connor JM. Spondylothoracic and spondylocostal dysostosis. *J Bone Joint Surg [Br].* 1988;70:123–126.

Sachs B, Bradford D, Winter R, Lonstein J, Moe J, Willson S. Scheuermann kyphosis: follow-up of Milwaukee-brace treatment. *J Bone Joint Surg [Am].* 1987;69:50–57.

Savini R, Gherlinzoni F, Morandi M, Neff JR, Picci P. Surgical treatment of giant-cell tumor of the spine: the experience at the Istituto Ortopedico Rizzoli. *J Bone Joint Surg [Am].* 1983;65:1283–1330.

Schwartz H. Zur konservativen Behandlun frischer Weichteilverletzungen der Halswirbelsäule. *Man Med.* 1987;25:116–119.

Siegal T, Tiqva P. Vertebral body resection for epidural compression by malignant tumors: results of forty-seven consecutive operative procedures. *J Bone Joint Surg [Am].* 1985;67:357–382.

Slätus P et al. Cranial subluxation of the odontoid process in rheumatoid arthritis. *J Bone Joint Surg [Am].* 1989;71:189–195.

Vortman BJ. Kinesiologie der Halswirbelsäule vor und nach Manipulation. *Man Med.* 1984;22:49–53.

Waddell G, Reilly S, Torsney B, et al. Assessment of the outcome of low back surgery. *J Bone Joint Surg [Br].* 1988;70:723–727.

Welter HF, Thetter O, Schweiberer L. Kompressionssyndrome der oberen Thoraxapertur. *Meunch Med Wochenzeitschr.* 1984;126:1122–1125.

Wyke B. The neurological basis of thoracic spinal pain. *Rheumatol Phys Med.* 1970;10:356–367.

Wyke B. Morphological and functional features of the innervation of the costovertebral joints. *Folia Morphol.* 1975;23:296–305.

Yates O, Jenner J. Lage rugpijn—Welke oorzaak? *Mod Med.* January 1980:42–45.

Yoganandan N, Pintar FA, Sances A Jr, Maiman DJ. Strength and motion analysis of the human head-neck complex. *J Spinal Disord.* 1991;4(1):73–85.

CERVICAL SPINE REVIEW QUESTIONS

1. What is the cause of an acute torticollis in children and adolescents whereby the head is held in a contralateral sidebend and rotation?
2. A congenital torticollis is due to a contracture of which muscle in the neck?
3. Name two differential diagnosis possibilities for a discogenic acute torticollis in children.
4. How can one immediately differentiate a hysterical torticollis from other types of torticollis?
5. What is the typical antalgic posture for an individual with Grisel's syndrome?
6. Which fractures are most commonly seen in traumatic atlantoaxial dislocations?
7. What kinds of spinal cord compressions can be expected in Grisel's syndrome?
8. When one suspects a possible high cervical subluxation or dislocation after a trauma, is a thorough functional examination indicated before a radiological examination?
9. How does a spasmodic torticollis present itself?
10. What are the determining factors for the localization of a unilateral facet subluxation or dislocation?
11. What is the treatment of choice for a bilateral facet dislocation?
12. What are the findings in the functional examination when a patient has a subacute atlantoaxial arthritis?
13. What are the typical radiological (X-ray) findings in a patient with retropharyngeal tendinitis?
14. What is the treatment of choice for cervical posture syndrome?
15. Describe the pain localization in a local cervical syndrome.
16. What is the most painful passive test in the cervical spine when one has a stress fracture of the first rib?
17. What is the treatment of choice for a traumatic arthritis of the first costotransverse joint?
18. What is the most painful and limited motion in a stress fracture of the spinous process of C7?
19. What is the most significant finding in the functional examination in a contracture of the costocoracoid fascia?
20. What is the cause of a cervical nerve root compression syndrome?
21. In a cervical nerve root compression syndrome, what is the most commonly affected nerve?
22. Which nerve(s) is/are most commonly affected in a cervicobrachial syndrome?
23. Which differential diagnosis deserves to be considered with a cervicobrachial syndrome lasting longer than 5 months?
24. A cervical neuroma is seen primarily in patients with which specific neurological disease?
25. Which test in the functional examination reproduces the typical complaints of a patient with a cervical neuroma?
26. At which levels in the cervical spine are the uncinate processes least developed?
27. How can one best differentiate whether cervicobrachial complaints are caused by a thoracic outlet syndrome or by cervical pathology?
28. Which muscle groups can show a weakness when the C7 root is compromised?
29. Name the neurological levels of the biceps, triceps, and brachioradialis reflexes.
30. Which fingers are a part of the sixth cervical dermatome?

CERVICAL SPINE REVIEW ANSWERS

1. Disc protrusion.
2. Sternocleidomastoid muscle.
3. Spastic torticollis and Grisel's syndrome.
4. The patient holds the head in an ipsilateral sidebend and holds the shoulder in elevation.
5. Flexion, ipsilateral sidebend, and contralateral rotation of the cervical spine.
6. Dens fracture and hangman's fracture.
7. Disturbances of the tendon reflexes, spastic hemi- and paraparesis, ataxia, and positive Babinski.
8. Radiological examination is necessary. Functional examination is contraindicated.
9. The patient involuntarily and intermittently turns the head to the same side.
10. The determining factors are the coupling patterns and the amount of axial compression.
11. Fusion (spondylodesis).
12. Severely and symmetrically limited and painful cervical spine rotations.
13. A calcium deposit ventral to the body of the axis.
14. In the first instance, improve the head and cervical spine posture, as well as the working conditions. In the second instance, treat the musculature.
15. Unilateral pain in the neck and the area of the trapezius muscle, pars descendens; sometimes also pain between the scapulae.
16. Sidebending of the cervical spine away from the affected side.
17. Intra-articular injection with a corticosteroid.
18. Active abduction-elevation of the arm.
19. Slightly limited active and passive elevation of the shoulder on the affected side.
20. Narrowing of an intervertebral foramen through uncovertebral osteophytes.
21. C5.
22. C6 and C7.
23. A cervical neuroma.
24. Neurofibromatosis (Recklinghausen's disease).
25. Flexion of the cervical spine.
26. C5 to C6 and C6 to C7.
27. By performing the Roos test. (See thoracic outlet compression syndrome diagram.)
28. Shoulder adductors, triceps brachii muscle, and the wrist flexors.
29. Respectively, C5 to C6, C7, and C5.
30. Thumb and index finger.

7

Temporomandibular Joint

7.1 CRANIOMANDIBULAR DYSFUNCTION

INTRODUCTION

Over the past few years, craniomandibular dysfunction (CMD) has become a concern of physical therapists. Traditionally, CMD belongs to the realm of dentistry. In dentistry, gnathologists specialize in the treatment of dysfunctions of the masticatory system. Patients with specific complaints and etiological findings are usually treated by gnathologists.

Physical therapists are interested in CMD because their diagnostic and technical treatment skills can be applied to the symptoms associated with this disorder. In treatment by a physical therapist, the patient's posture and musculoskeletal system need to be addressed; abnormalities may result in complaints and dysfunctions of the masticatory system. When evaluating a patient with chronic complaints, a multidisciplinary approach is recommended.

OVERVIEW

Costen, an ear, nose, and throat (ENT) specialist, originally described several symptoms that are seen in CMD.[1] Based on findings from 11 patients, symptoms include decreased hearing capacity; numb feeling in the ear; clicking noise during chewing; ringing in the ear; pain in and around the ear; dizziness; headache; and a burning feeling in the tongue, throat, and/or the side of the nose. This combination of symptoms is known as the Costen syndrome. In Costen's opinion, these complaints are a result of the mandible's closing too far because of missing teeth and/or molars. Normalizing the occlusion would reduce the complaints. Costen attributed the onset of symptoms to irritation of the chorda tympani nerve, the auriculotemporal nerve, and the meninges as a result of changes in the temporomandibular joint (TMJ).[2]

Schwarz[3] introduced the TMJ pain dysfunction syndrome, in which he emphasized the total function of the masticatory system (TMJ and its related muscles). Primary etiological events were considered to be psychological factors (stress related) and muscle spasms.

Laskin[4] described the myofascial pain dysfunction syndrome. Myofascial pain dysfunction syndrome is diagnosed if the complaints are unilateral, there are no radiological changes, and the TMJ is not painful on palpation at its dorsal aspect.

Generally, CMD is diagnosed by the presence of one or more of the following symptoms[5,6]:

- pain and sensitivity in the area of the masticatory muscles and the TMJ
- TMJ noises
- limitation of motion and deviations of the motion pattern of the mandible

The patient population has a heterogeneous character with diverse complaints. In addition, the symptoms of CMD are similar to symptoms stemming from other regions. For example, cervicocephalic syndrome has symptoms that include dizziness, headache, earache, and swallowing disturbances.[7] (See Vertebrobasilar Insufficiency in Chapter 6). Also, symptoms of CMD syndrome can be similar to those of disorders with a completely different pathogenesis, such as tumors or infections.

For the purposes of this book, CMD is considered a dysfunction of the musculoskeletal system, located in the masticatory system, with respect for the arthrogenic and myogenic chains and the influences of neurogenic structures, the viscera, and the psyche.[8]

The traditionally used evaluation techniques from dentistry, such as active range of motion and palpation, limit the ability to gain precise information about CMD. Therefore, additional evaluation techniques of the masticatory system are described in the following sections. These can help to differentiate CMD from problems that are caused by something other than CMD.

During evaluation and treatment of patients with CMD, the importance of the dentist is obvious in regard to the etiology of this disorder. By examining the relationship between the teeth and the molars of the upper and lower jaws, insights as to the reasons for the onset of signs and symptoms in the TMJ region can be gained. This approach is attributed to Costen's publication. Relation, occlusion, and articulation are purely dental factors.

In addition to dentists, other medical specialists (ENT physician, neurologist) and other disciplines (psychologist, speech pathologist) also evaluate and treat CMD. Because of the wide range of symptoms in CMD, physical therapists, with their knowledge of musculoskeletal dysfunctions, should also be involved in the care of patients with CMD. Cooperation between dentist and therapist is essential.

TERMINOLOGY

In this section, several relevant dental terms are defined. These terms are used within dentistry to describe etiological factors involved in CMD. In addition, the terms are necessary for optimal communication and cooperation among the various disciplines.

Parafunctions

Within clinical dentistry, there is a difference between parafunctions (nonphysiological functions) and physiological functions of the masticatory system. Parafunctions include grinding (bruxism), clenching the jaw, and all other habits that patients have regarding their natural teeth or dentures, such as nail biting, chewing on pencils, etc.

Derksen[9] described bruxism as a semi- or subconscious parafunction that occurs at night and/or during the day. It involves static and/or dynamic contact between the chewing surfaces of the mandible and maxilla. Lip and cheek biting are also parafunctions but do not fall under the definition of bruxism. Parafunctions are seen quite often and do not necessarily require treatment. Treatment is considered only when a relationship is found with other aberrations. However, in severe cases of wear and tear of the teeth, dental interference is indicated.

Occlusion and Relation

Occlusion is defined as a situation in which there is static contact between one or more dentition elements of the mandible with one or more dentition elements of the maxilla.

The amount of contact between mandible and maxilla, as well as the position of the mandible in relation to the skull, defines the term *occlusion* even more precisely. Maximal occlusion is the position with the most points of contact. Normally, this is the position the patient demonstrates when asked to bite down (Figure 7–1).

In maximal occlusion, the relief of the chewing surface complexes of the mandible and maxilla has the best fit. Reproducibility is great (to within 0.015 mm) because of the presence of ridges and grooves.[11] Because of this reproducibility, the position of the mandible in relation to the skull can be determined uniformly. Because the condylar processes are an integral part of the mandible, their position in relation to the mandibular fossae is also defined.

The position of the mandible in relation to the skull is termed *relation*. A special position is the centric relation. Centric relation is the position of the mandible in relation to the skull when the Frankfort plane is horizontal (represented in profile by an imaginary line between the lowest point on the margin of the orbit and the highest point on the margin of the auditory meatus) (Figure 7–2A). In this position, the mandibular heads are in the most "unforced" dorsal position in relation to the articular fossae. *Unforced* means that, in determining the position of the mandible, the examiner does not apply a dorsal force on the chin. (Compare with Occlusion and Articulation in section 7.2, Examination.)

In earlier dental literature, the lateral temporomandibular ligament was considered to be responsible for the limitation of motion in the dorsal direction. However, recent research from Savalle on the function of this ligament proved this hypothesis to be incorrect.[12]

When the mandible is in the centric relation and there is simultaneous contact between the mandible and maxilla (occlusion), the position is called *centric occlusion*. If the mandible is in maximal occlusion during this

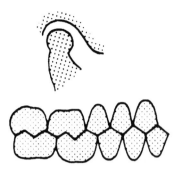

Figure 7–1 Illustration of maximal occlusion. *Source:* Reprinted from *Inleiding to de Bouw en Functie van het Kauwstelsel* by A.A.D. Derksen with permission of Bohn, Scheltema and Holkema, © 1997.

position, it is called *centric maximal occlusion.*

In Figure 7–2A, the graphic representation of the range of motion of a point located at the lower incisors is depicted. The form of the most cranial part of this figure (Figure 7–2B) is largely determined by the form of the dentition elements, the maximal range of motion in anterior and posterior positions, and other anatomical structures.

Maximal occlusion is shown by position 1, centric occlusion by position 2. To determine a more dorsal position of the mandible, pressure can be applied to the chin in a dorsal direction.[11] In Figure 7–2B, this is position 3, the *retruded contact position.*

In earlier dental literature,[13,14] it was postulated that positions 1, 2, and/or 3 should match one another to increase the chance of proper physiological functioning. This view has been abandoned. A difference in anterior-posterior direction of 1 mm between positions 1 and 3 is now considered acceptable.[15]

Because of morphological changes (of the dentition and/or joints), it is possible for the mandible to be in the centric relation without a maximal occlusion. In this case, there is only contact between one or several dentition elements from the maxilla and mandible. To bring the dentition elements into maximal occlusion, the mandible has to slip in a certain direction. Usually, the direction of this slip is ventral, occasionally combined with a lateral component. Sometimes this direction is purely lateral. A ventrally directed slip is called a *procentric* maximal occlusion; a lat-

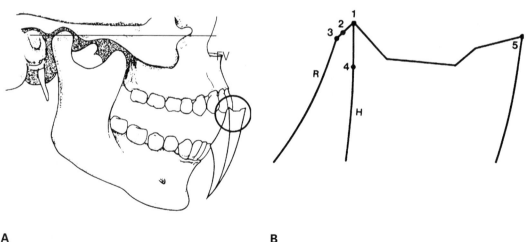

A   **B**

Figure 7–2 A, Maximal range of motion of the mandible in the sagittal plane.[15] FV = FP Frankfort horizontal plane. **B**, Most cranial part of **A. 1**, Maximal occlusion; **2**, centric occlusion; **3**, retruded contact position; **4**, resting position; **5**, protruded contact position; **R**, rotation; **H**, habitual opening and closing motion, according to Steenks.[15]

eral slip is called a *laterocentric* maximal occlusion. In this situation, the initial contact location between the dentition elements of mandible and maxilla is called an *occlusion disturbance* (Figure 7–3A). These contact points are often located at the canine teeth and premolars.[15]

In Figure 7–3B, the contact points in maximal occlusion are illustrated. Clinically seen, even if an occlusion disturbance is present, the patient still bites down directly into a maximal occlusion. Thus, the habitual closing motion of the mandible is adapted to the maximal occlusion (Figure 7–2B). Occlusion

disturbances are traced by moving the mandible passively in oscillations from a slightly open position toward position 2 or position 3[15] (Figure 7–2B).

Resting Position

The resting position is another important jaw relation. It is the position of the mandible in relation to the skull, in which the Frankfort plane runs horizontally and the jaw-related muscles are relaxed. In a standing or sitting position, with the head straight, there is usually no contact between the upper and lower

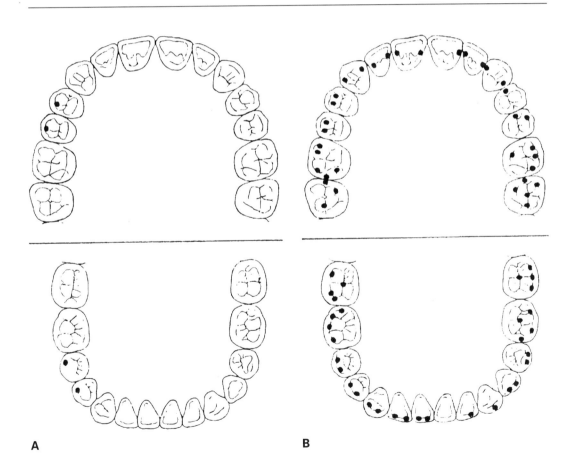

A **B**

Figure 7–3 *A*, Documentation of the occlusion points in centric occlusion; ***B***, maximal occlusion. *Source:* Reprinted from *Inleiding to de Bouw en Functie van het Kauwstelsel* by A.A.D. Derksen with permission of Bohn, Scheltema and Holkema, © 1997.

dentition elements. The space between the teeth and molars of the mandible and maxilla is called the "free way space," or interocclusal clearance. The average free way space measured at the front is about 2 to 3 mm. Variations occur and can be explained by influences such as head and/or body posture, sleeping habits, and psychological and other factors.

The resting position occurs because of the resting activity of the musculature. The supra- and infrahyoid muscles keep the hyolaryngeal complex in position. These muscle groups, in combination with gravity, prevent contact between the chewing surface complexes of the mandible and maxilla. In an anteroposterior direction, there is also balance (to include the dorsal fibers of the temporal muscles and the lateral pterygoid muscles). Besides the greater or lesser amount of muscle activity determining the resting position, the elasticity of the soft tissue structures is also important.[16]

The resting position is located on the trajectory of the habitual closing motion (position 4 in Figure 7–2B).

Articulation

The dynamic contact between the dentition elements of the mandible and maxilla is called *articulation*. When the patient moves the mandible from the maximally occluded position into a lateral direction, in which tooth contact is maintained, three articulation patterns can be observed.

1. *Canine guiding:* At the ipsilateral side, also called the active side, only contact between the canine teeth is demonstrated. At the contralateral side, also called the nonactive side, there is no contact (Figure 7–4).
2. *Unilateral balanced articulation:* At the ipsilateral side, contact remains between all the elements. At the contralateral side, there is no contact (Figure 7–5).
3. *Bilateral balanced articulation:* At the ipsilateral and contralateral side, contact exists between the maximal amount of elements.

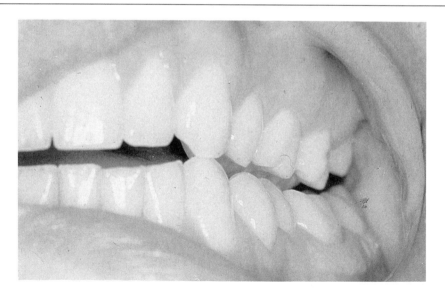

Figure 7–4 Canine guiding. *Source:* Reprinted from *Craniomandibulaire Dysfunctie Vanuit Fysiotherapeutisch en Tandheelkundig Perspectief* by M.H. Steenks and A. de Wijer with permission of DeTijdstroom, © 1989.

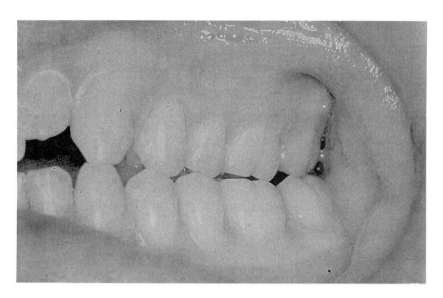

Figure 7–5 Unilateral balanced articulation. *Source:* Reprinted from *Craniomandibulaire Dysfunctie Vanuit Fysiotherapeutisch en Tandheelkundig Perspectief* by M.H. Steenks and A. de Wijer with permission of DeTijdstroom, © 1989.

In the natural dentition, without obvious abrasion (wearing away), the first two types occur. The bilateral balanced articulation is usually the goal for the production of a complete denture.

Disturbances in Articulation

Disturbances in articulation occur when the molar cusps or incisor edges of the teeth disturb the motion of the mandible in a frontal or lateral direction. An articulation disturbance in the proal (forward) movement is determined when contact occurs on one front element or a unilateral contact exists in the molar region during this motion. Articulation disturbances on the active side lead to a disturbance of the local contact. For example, after a restoration, cusps of the elements that previously made contact may be no longer able to do so (Figure 7–6A). This is more likely to happen in a unilateral balance articulation than in a canine guiding. Articulation disturbances at the nonactive side can result in a loss of contact at the nonactive side (Figure 7–6B).

Dentition

The dentition elements are named for their anatomical shape. To allow for documentation, a system was developed on the quadrant indication (first number, 1 to 4) and the anatomical characteristics (second number, 1 to 8). An example of the complete natural dentition is shown in Figure 7–7A. Another form of documentation is shown in Figure 7–7B. With the use of these diagrams, it is possible to indicate missing elements and other specifics, such as parafunctional abrasions, occlusion and articulation disturbances, and increased mobility (Figure 7–8).

EPIDEMIOLOGY

Over the years, significant data have been gathered regarding the incidence of CMD. In the CMD literature, two different kinds of populations are described. Earlier publications were mainly related to patient populations from specialized clinics (clinics to which patients had been referred by their family

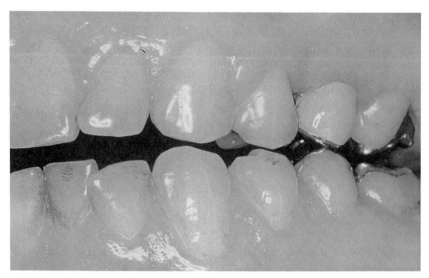

A

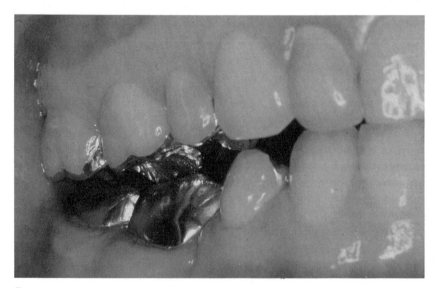

B

Figure 7–6 *A*, Articulation disturbance at the active side, on the left, at the level of 25 to 35. Levels 23 to 33 and 24 to 34 made prior contact evidenced by the abrasion facets. *B*, Articulation disturbance at the nonactive side, on the right, at the level of 17 to 47; at the active side (left, not visible), there is no contact. *Source:* Reprinted from *Craniomandibulaire Dysfunctie Vanuit Fysiotherapeutisch en Tandheelkundig Perspectief* by M.H. Steenks and A. de Wijer with permission of DeTijdstroom, © 1989.

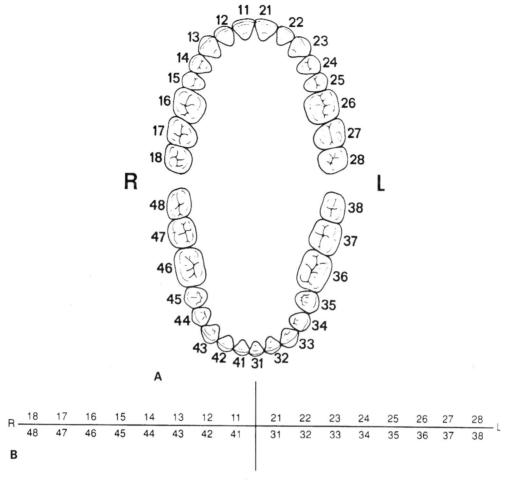

A

R	18	17	16	15	14	13	12	11	21	22	23	24	25	26	27	28	L
	48	47	46	45	44	43	42	41	31	32	33	34	35	36	37	38	

B

Figure 7–7 **A**, Sketch of the dental arches with the documentation codes for the dentition elements of the natural permanent dentition; **B**, diagram used to document dentition status. *Source:* Reprinted from *Craniomandibulaire Dysfunctie Vanuit Fysiotherapeutisch en Tandheelkundig Perspectief* by M.H. Steenks and A. de Wijer with permission of DeTijdstroom, © 1989.

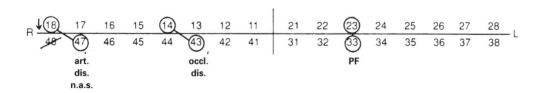

Figure 7–8 Example of dentition status with documented specific findings. **48**, Missing element; **18**, outgrown; **occl. dis.**, occlusion disturbance at the level of 14 to 43; **art. dis. n.a.s.**, articulation disturbance of the nonactive side at the level of 18 to 47; **PF**, parafunctional abrasion at the level of 23 to 33.

physicians). The other populations were researched through questionnaires and clinical examinations.

In studies from specialized outpatient clinics, certain tendencies were found.[9] There was a higher incidence among women than men, and the most often affected age group was 20 to 30 years. A satisfactory explanation for the difference between genders in the CMD population from outpatient clinics has not yet been found.

Population research, which was performed later, originally involved selected populations.[17,18] Helkimo[19] gathered epidemiological data from nonselected groups. This author designed a clinical "dysfunction index" to describe the amount of dysfunction. Based on a point system (0, 1, or 5 points), five symptoms are judged, as follows:

1. limitation of motion of the mandible in different directions
2. decreased joint function, based on movement patterns, joint noises, and/or the existence of subluxations or locking
3. tenderness to palpation of the muscles
4. tenderness to palpation of the joints
5. pain during active movements of the mandible

The most important conclusion from this research indicates that there is no difference in the incidence of symptoms between male and female. In addition, signs and symptoms are equally divided over the age categories researched. Based on the dysfunction index from patient history, 50% of the population mentioned the presence of symptoms. In the same population, the clinical dysfunction index indicated that 80% had some form of dysfunction. In 22%, there was a serious form of dysfunction according to Helkimo's classification.[19] In 20% to 25% of the studied population, treatment should have been necessary. Later studies, from Reider and Martinoff,[20] confirmed the above-mentioned tendencies.

However, based on the research design of these studies, the conclusion regarding the necessity of treatment is questionable. Other aspects should also be considered, such as progressiveness, the natural course, and the complaints of the patient. Treatment necessity can be indicated only by a specific clinical examination.

ETIOLOGY

One of Helkimo's conclusions is that there was no dominant etiological factor.[19] In recent literature, there is a unanimous conclusion that a multifactorial etiology is involved in craniomandibular dysfunction.[8,21] The most important factors are occlusoanatomical, neuromuscular, and psychological. According to DeBoever[21] and DeBoever and Steenks,[5] the chance of developing symptoms is increased if all three factors are involved. However, the presence of these factors is not a guarantee for the onset of symptoms. The degree to which each of the various factors contributes to the problem can vary individually, which may explain the increase and decrease of the complaints within a certain time period. Interaction between these factors also occurs, such as bruxism as a result of occlusion disturbances.

The occlusoanatomical factor is mainly a mechanical one. Because of occlusion and/or articulation disturbances, the mandible is forced to close in a different position or parafunctional motion. This can result in an overuse of the TMJ and/or masticatory muscles. In instances of a significant loss of the dorsal support zone, chewing takes place more in the front (in a more anterior position), causing the likelihood of increased joint force.

Besides the etiological factors, the adaptation capacity (age, general health) and rate at which the occlusion and articulation disturbances develop are important in regard to the occurrence of symptoms. A restoration that suddenly disturbs the existing relationships can have a greater influence on the development of symptoms than an occlusion disturbance based on a change in the growth patterns.

Dibbets[22] describes a population of patients treated by an orthodontist who were followed longitudinally. In the studied time frame (18 years), signs and symptoms (objective, subjective, and radiological changes) appeared to develop and resolve without clear causes.

According to DeBoever[21] and DeBoever and Van Steenberghe,[23] bruxism (grinding and clenching), as well as other parafunctions, should be interpreted as neuromuscular factors. These factors are different from the physiological functions such as chewing, swallowing, and talking in that there is constant muscle activity with significant muscle activation in positions of the mandible. (These positions are not always reproducible during clinical examination.) The three characteristics of bruxism (duration, force, and position) cause a wearing away of the dentition elements, as well as overuse of the TMJ, the masticatory muscles, and sometimes the fixation system of the dentition elements.

The role of the psychological factors is usually translated into stress. Rugh and Solberg[24] state that there is no scientific proof for the concept that CMD is correlated to a certain personality profile. Instead, emotional factors such as anxiety, frustration, and anger result in increased muscle tension. Constant increased muscle tension could result in symptoms similar to those found in CMD, with or without increased parafunctional activities. The constant stress causes a continuous ergotropic situation; thus, the sensitivity to injury increases. As a result, the loadability of the tissue can decrease, after which a normal load can cause symptoms to arise.

In general, unicausal thinking regarding the etiology of functional disturbances has been abandoned, even when the factors are apparently limited to the masticatory system. Especially in chronic symptoms, the accom-panying pain can be similar to other chronic disorders. Thus, in treating CMD the principles of treatment for patients with chronic pain are also applicable.[25] In addition to local factors (ie, factors affecting the masticatory system), external factors can have an influence. These factors include posture,[26–28] disorders of the spine (upper cervical and cervicothoracic junction), and increased orthosympathetic activity (due to stress, nociception, visceral hypersensitivity[29]).

CLINICAL FINDINGS

According to DeBoever and Steenks[5] and Rugh and Solberg,[24] the classic symptoms of CMD are the following:

- pain in the region of the TMJ and the masticatory muscles
- limitation of motion of the mandible and disturbances of the movement pattern
- TMJ noises such as clicking and crepitation

Pain in the TMJ is attributed to irritation of the bilaminar region of the articular disc and/or articular capsule. The articular surfaces are not innervated; therefore, they cannot be responsible for pain originating from the TMJ. Instead, irritation can be caused by overstretching (such as during yawning), ventral and dorsal shifting of the articular disc, or changes in the intra-articular relationships with a loss of the dorsal support zone.

Pain in the masticatory muscles can be due to a decrease in local circulation, the presence of parafunctions, or increased orthosympathetic activity. In chronic disorders, structural changes in the collagen of the muscles can develop. It is also important to locate trigger points in the muscle groups of the throat and neck, because they can refer pain to the head region (Figure 7–9). For the dentist, it is especially important to recognize that referred pain in the dentition elements can come from trigger points in the masticatory muscles. Otherwise, painful dentition el-

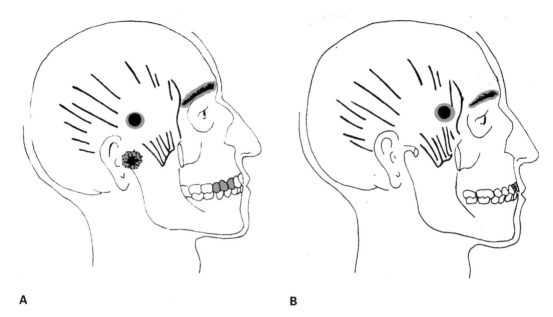

A   B

Figure 7–9 *A*, Zone of referred pain from a trigger point in the temporal muscle (medial part); *B*, zone of referred pain from a trigger point in the temporal muscle (ventral part). *Source:* Reprinted from *Myofacial Pain and Dysfunction: The Trigger Point Manual* by J. Travell and G. Simons with permission of Williams & Wilkins, © 1983.

ements may be treated, for example, with a root canal treatment or extraction, with unsuccessful results. The toothache remains even after extraction.

An important characteristic of musculoskeletal pain is its reproducibility. Similar to other disorders of the musculoskeletal system, symptoms within the masticatory system can be provoked at any time. Usually these symptoms are unilateral, or at least an obvious difference exists in the intensity between each side. Movements of the mandible provoke the symptoms. Typical examples include chewing on hard or tough food, wide opening of the mouth, biting off something, and sometimes talking.

Characteristic locations of pain include the cheek (masseter muscles), the temple (temporal muscles), and the region above the eye.[31] A closely related symptom is fatigue, described by patients as a "heavy feeling" in the mandible. Usually, the patient indicates the cheeks as the location of this heavy feeling. If the symptoms are present upon waking

or the symptoms wake the patient up, the examiner should suspect parafunctional behavior (bruxism). If the TMJ feels stiff and tired in the morning and the symptoms decrease during the day, the examiner should also suspect parafunctional activities.

Short (ie, seconds), sharp, stabbing pain caused by touching the skin or mucous membrane is not an indication for CMD. In these instances, the pain is more likely to be due to a neuralgia.[32]

A limitation of motion can have an arthrogenic cause, but also a myogenic cause. In the latter, structural changes within the muscle can cause pain when the muscle-tendon unit is stretched.

The natural course of CMD shows a typical sequence. First there is a period of clicking of the TMJ, without pain. The clicking can be based on form changes of the TMJ, which may have been present from youth. These changes can be interpreted as signs of adaptation resulting from a change in the loading of the TMJ. The changes are termed "deviation in form."[33]

A specific form of clicking is the reciprocal click. This is a click at the beginning of the opening motion and a click at the very last part of the closing motion (just before the molars contact each other, or at the moment that the patient bites through). This kind of clicking is based on a displacement of the disc.

In the normal TMJ, the relationships of the mandibular head, the articular disc, and mandibular fossa in maximal occlusion are illustrated in Figure 7–10A. The posterior band lies cranial to the mandibular head. In a wide-open mouth, the mandibular head is positioned slightly ventral to the lowest point of the articular tubercle; during this motion, the articular disc moves simultaneously with the articular head (Figure 7–10A, *3*). During closing, the opposite sequence occurs. The coordination of the anterior and posterior movement of the articular disc is performed through activity of the lateral pterygoid muscle.[34] The strong attachments of the articular disc to the lateral and medial pole have a passive contribution as well.

In a ventral translation of the disc, the posterior band of the articular disc lies ventral to the mandibular head when the mandible is positioned in maximal occlusion (Figure 7–10B, *0*). In this situation, the bilaminar region lies cranial to the mandibular head. During opening of the mouth from maximal occlusion, the mandibular head slips over the posterior band at the initial phase of opening. This is accompanied by a clicking sound (Figure 7–10B, *1*). With further opening, the same motions that take place in a normally functioning TMJ occur. Upon closing from a wide-open position, the normal physiological motion pattern is followed, with one exception. Just before the molars contact each other at the end of the closing motion, the mandibular head slips behind the posterior part of the articular disc, or the disc slips in front of the mandibular head. This causes a clicking during closing of the mouth.

One characteristic of the reciprocal click is its reproducibility. Such clicking occurs during motions of the mandible, causing transla-tions in the TMJ: depression, contralateral movement, and the proal movement.[36] This counts only when the entire posterior band (from medial to lateral) is located ventral to the mandibular head. In partial translations (only the lateral part of the disc translated, meaning that a medial ventral translation occurs), the clicking occurs only during some motions.

Another typical observation is the disappearance of the click during opening and closing of the mouth from a slightly proal position of the mandible. In general, this amounts to 1 to 2 mm of proal movement, which is enough to cause a prior clicking. This situation is referred to as a *disc displacement with reduction*.[37] Reduction means the return of the articular disc to its normal position.

If these signs are present over a period of time, it is possible that the next phase, locking, occasionally will occur. This occurs because the mandibular head is temporarily not slipping over the posterior band. Thus, this part of the articular disc forms a blockade for the translating condylar process (Figure 7–10C, *3*). When the locking becomes permanent, it is called *disc displacement without reduction*. Initially it is accompanied by a severe limitation of motion (maximal interincisal mouth opening of 15 to 25 mm), the disappearance of clicking, and usually an onset or increase of pain.

After awhile, the mobility of the TMJ can decrease because of form changes of the articular disc. Finally a situation develops in which opening the mouth is permanently limited (maximal opening of the mouth 35 to 40 mm). The initial configuration of the disc is lost; the biconcave form changes into a biconvex form. To a certain extent, the motion pattern during opening adjusts to the decreased motion of the TMJ. Because the mandibular head now articulates with the eminence via the bilaminar region, changes in this part of the articular disc develop. These changes include perforations and the formation of cartilage.

As a result of the anatomical relationships (strong connections of the articular disc to

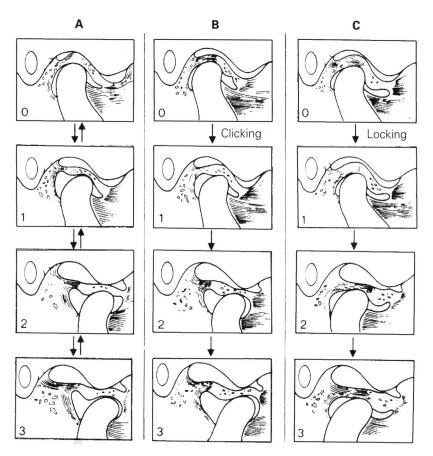

Figure 7–10 A, Diagram of the normal motion sequence (**0** to **3**) in the TMJ during opening and closing of the mouth. **B**, Ventral displacement of the disc with reduction (**0** to **3**); there is clicking in phase **0** to **1** with opening and closing. **C**, Ventral displacement of the disc without reduction (**0** to **3**); the condyle is locked by the disc (**0** to **1**) causing a translation limitation of the condyle. *Source:* Reprinted from Steenk, M.H. and Touw, W.D. *Jaarboek Fysiotherapie*, pp. 314–351, with permission of Bohn, Scheltema and Holkema, © 1987.

the medial and lateral pole), displacements usually take place in a dorsal and/or ventral direction. Clinical experience indicates that ventral displacement occurs more often. When the disc is displaced dorsally, the retrusion motion is especially limited. This is indicated by an inability to perform complete occlusion of the molars at the ipsilateral side (Figure 7–11). The ventral displacement is recognizable to a lesser extent at the contralateral side.

The symptoms resulting from disc displacement are usually so obvious that the history and the examination of the active range of motion offer sufficient information concerning the nature of this disorder. Further clinical examination and an Orthopantomograph should confirm and/or support this diagnosis. Arthrography, arthroscopy, and magnetic resonance imaging (MRI) can provide more information in cases of doubt (Figure 7–12). If a trauma occurred prior to the development of symptoms, fractures should be ruled out in the differential diagnosis.

A thorough clinical examination is the foundation for the diagnosis of functional disorders of the masticatory system.

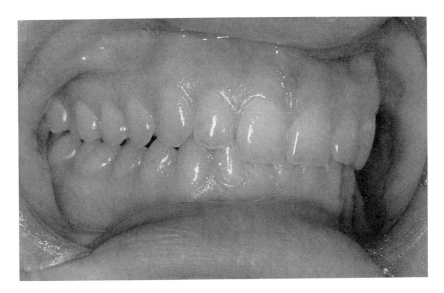

A

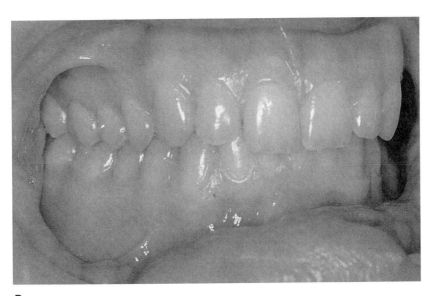

B

Figure 7–11 Dorsal displacement of the disc. **A**, In the acute phase of displacement; **B**, maximal occlusion after reduction.

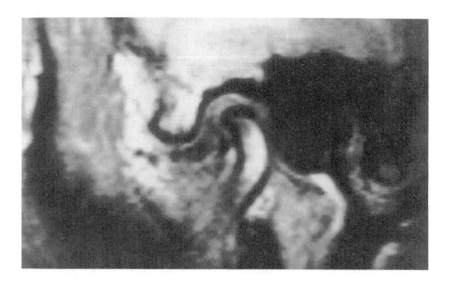

Figure 7–12 MRI of the temporomandibular joint.

7.2 EXAMINATION

INTRODUCTION

The clinical examination of patients with CMD begins with a gnathological examination. In the presence of acute symptoms, such as an occlusion disturbance after receiving a crown that is too high, further medical and/or paramedical examination usually is not indicated. In order to determine the problem in chronic complaints of pain, or in complaints without an obvious cause in the masticatory system, information from the dentist, medical findings from the family physician, and findings from the functional examination by a physical therapist must all be considered.[25,35,38] A standard questionnaire can be helpful here.[8,31] The history is taken in a patient-centered way; in other words, the patient's part in the information exchange is significant.[39]

The dentist is educated in making a gnathological diagnosis. The status of the dentition is determined and the functional examination of the masticatory system is performed. At the same time, the possibility of an underlying disease process is determined. Psychogenic and the viscerogenic (for instance, ears, nose, and throat) influences are also considered. The physical therapist should focus on the functional diagnostics of the musculoskeletal aspect of the masticatory system, including the spinal column, shoulder girdle, and posture of the patient.

Multifactorial Approach

In chronic complaints, a multifactorial approach is necessary. (For more detailed information, see Chapter 2, General Aspects of Examination and Treatment.)

In acute problems, it is likely that there is a monofactorial etiology. In this instance, the influence of the causal factor can be great, such as in the occurrence of a functional disturbance after the placement of a bridge. The masticatory examination and therapy are limited in this case.

GENERAL INSPECTION

The examiner gains a general impression of the patient even before the patient has spoken. For instance, the head posture is very important, as well as the patient's facial expression. In fact, the general inspection also takes place during the history and continues into the specific inspection.

HISTORY

Besides the local aspects, other pathology should also be considered, including disorders of the spinal column, internal organs, and ear; dental problems; and/or an increased orthosympathetic activity.[40] For instance, in regard to endogenous factors, influences from the upper cervical joints[7,27,41–43] and the lungs[29,44–46] are evaluated. The upper cervical joints (occiput-atlas, atlas-axis), C2-3, and the suboccipital muscles are innervated by the spinal nerves C1 to C3. These structures can cause referred pain in the frontal, retro-orbital, temporal, and occipital regions of the head. They also refer pain into the area of the temporomandibular joints. The following signs and symptoms can arise from the upper cervical region: headache, dizziness, facial pain, hearing disturbances, and visual disturbances.[7,40]

In lung pathology, hyperalgesia often arises in the segmental areas of C3, C4, and T1 to T9.[29,44–46] In pathology of the lung and the pleura, the branches of the trigeminal nerve, particularly at their exiting sites, but also in the entire supply area, become hyperalgesic. In these instances, the musculature of the neck and shoulder girdle becomes tender and hypertonic (McKenzie's visceromotor reflex).[44]

Patients may complain of reflexogenic headache, neck, and interscapular stiffness and pain.[27] If these patients visit the clinic for complaints of the masticatory system (for instance, clicking and fatigue of the jaw), it is important to consider and differentiate the reflexogenic influence of the somatogenic and neurogenic factors (particularly cervical, C0 to C3, and thoracic, C8 to T3) and the viscerogenic factor in the final diagnosis.

Medical intervention and earlier treatment and its results are noted, particularly in regard to dental surgery. During the history, the examiner pays attention to habits or abnormal mouth behavior, including locking of the jaw, an abnormal position of the tongue in rest and during speaking and swallowing, and insufficient lip closing. Through observation, other habits can be noted such as biting or sucking the lip, cheek, or tongue.

SPECIFIC INSPECTION

The inspection is concentrated on posture and the upper part of the body. Although the following points are of particular importance:

- position of the cervical spine and head
- position of the scapulae, clavicles, and shoulder joints
- visible changes in the skin, muscles, and joints

The scope of this section is limited to the masticatory system.

Inspection by the physical therapist is directed at noting the normal anatomical structures. Through an orienting inspection, aberrations can be determined and submitted to the dentist. During the inspection, particular attention is paid to symmetry. Important orientation points are the eyes, lips, median lines, the mandibular angle, and the chin. For example, facial asymmetry can be seen in facial paresis, an abscess, Klippel-Feil syndrome, torticollis, congenital deformations, and growth disturbances. Facial movements are observed and the pupils are noted (mydriasis or miosis, Horner's syndrome). Trophic disturbances in conjunction with vegetative influences are also significant findings.[40]

The status of the dentition can be registered on the form presented in Figure 7–7B. In determining the dentition status, loss of support, changes in the dental arches, and migration are also noted. The vestibulum oris and the cavum oris are checked. The vestibulum oris is the part of the oral cavity located between the row of teeth and the cheek. The cavum oris is the space between the dental arches, thus the part where the tongue moves in occlusion. The upper side of the cavum oris is bordered by the roof of the mouth; the osseous anterior three fourths is called the palatum durum (hard palate), and the fleshy posterior one fourth is termed the palatum molle (soft palate). The posterior edge of the palatum molle has two folds on each side. The space between is the tonsillar sinus (Figure 7–13). A tonsil lies on each side of this space.

During the inspection of the tongue (also known as the lingua), the following are observed: the corpus linguae (oral part) and the basis linguae (pharyngeal part). Under the tongue, in the midline, the common discharge areas of the submandibular and the greater sublingual ducts are located. The mucous membrane on the upper side of the corpus linguae (body of the tongue) is characterized by different structures: sulcus medianus, sulcus terminalis, vallate papillae, fungiform papillae, filiform papillae, and foliate papillae (Figure 7–14).

Inspection during Movement

The local inspection can be supplemented with inspection of activities of daily living (ADL), in which particular attention is given to provoking the complaints (ie, inhibiting activities). ADL can be judged to gain insight about the specific activities within the masticatory system. Examples include inspection of chewing, yawning, swallowing, working

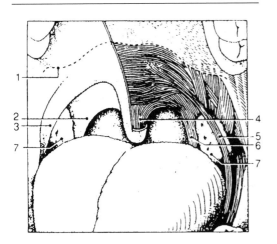

Figure 7–13 Schematic illustration of the course of the muscles in relation to the palatum molle (soft palate). *Source:* Reprinted from DeBaat et al., *Nederlands Tijdschrift voor Tandheelkunde,* Vol. 94, with permission of Tijil Tijdschriften B.V., © 1987. **1**, Junction of the palatum durum and palatum molle with, dorsally, the aponeurosis; **2**, palatopharyngeal fold; **3**, palatoglossal fold; **4**, uvula and muscle of the uvula; **5**, palatoglossus muscle; **6**, palatopharyngeus muscle; **7**, tonsil.

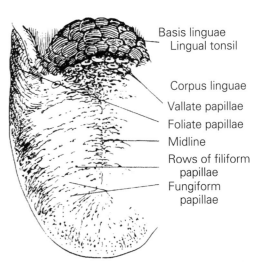

Figure 7–14 The base of the tongue (basis linguae) takes up one third of the total length and is covered with tonsilar tissue. At the border between the corpus and the basis linguae, a V-shaped row of vallate papillae is found. At the same level, a few foliate papillae are located along the side of the tongue. *Source:* Courtesy of Letty Moss-Salentijn and Marlene Klijvert, 1980.

postures, and the playing of musical instruments (ie, blowing instruments).

Occlusion and Articulation

Examination of occlusion and articulation is mainly performed by the dentist. Although the occlusion examination is actually an evaluation of the passive motions of the mandible, because of the involvement of dentition, a dentist's opinion is required. However, this does not mean that the orientating examination by the experienced physical therapist can be forgone. The dentist judges the occlusion regarding the following aspects:

- morphological aspects (curve, general position of the mandible in relation to the maxilla in a sagittal and transverse aspect)
- the moment of contact in the maximal occlusion coming from the right and left chewing surface complexes
- the number of contact points, left and right, in the dental arch in maximal occlusion
- the support in the molar region
- the vertical dimension
- the sliding off from the "retruded contact position" and/or centric occlusion to the maximal occlusion; this concerns the function of the joint (disc displacement, arthrosis)

The centric relation of the mandible is determined by means of the "guided closure" technique, in the dentistry literature termed "moderate chin guidance."[19] According to Steenks,[15] the procedure for judging centric occlusion is performed in three phases:

1. The patient indicates the place of contact between the teeth of the mandible and maxilla in centric occlusion.
2. Examination is performed regarding a possible discrepancy between centric and maximal occlusion: the magnitude

of the trajectory between centric occlusion and maximal occlusion, as well as the direction of the movement that the mandible makes in this trajectory.

3. If discrepancies are found, the precise place of contact between the elements of the upper and lower dental arches is determined in centric occlusion.

This sequence offers the greatest amount of information about this part of the occlusion examination. In addition, it is a simple evaluation procedure that asks a minimal amount of measuring and documentation. In remaining within the scope of this section's objective, the third phase is not discussed. The interested physical therapist is referred to the dentistry literature for more details.[15]

Phase 1

Examination in the first phase (judging the centric occlusion) is performed in the following sequence:

1. The patient is instructed to sit upright, look straight ahead, and relax (particularly the facial muscles and arm and shoulder musculature), allowing the back of the head to rest against the head support,
2. Because the resting position is the starting position, it must be determined that the mandible is in a resting position. Therefore, the patient is asked whether there is room between the teeth of the mandible and the maxilla. If not, the patient is instructed to relax even more (the mandible has to feel heavy). The examiner palpates the masseter muscle to ensure that the patient is relaxed.
3. The examiner moves the mandible from the resting position upward. The force is applied exclusively in a vertical direction and should be as small as possible. In this context, the position of the examiner is important: the forearm and

arm are in the sagittal plane. Movement of the jaw occurs by means of the elbow; the shoulder and arm remain fixed.

4. As soon as the mandible is moved upward, the force is discontinued and the mandible returns to the initial position. The mandible then is again moved upward. In this way, a smooth movement in and out of the resting position is induced, whereby the teeth gently tap against each other. The frequency is approximately four times per second.

5. The patient indicates where incisors and/or molars touch each other: left/right, in the front/back, all at once, etc.

6. The procedure is repeated to be certain of the findings; two successive determinations must have the same results.

Comment. The examiner can be misled if the patient assists in the movement while still giving the impression that the musculature is relaxed. This can be controlled by suddenly interrupting the movement. In complete relaxation, the mandible stops moving at the same instant that the examiner's hand is held still.

Phase 2

The procedure in the second phase (central versus maximal occlusion) is performed in the following sequence:

1. The mandible is moved as described for phase 1. As the mandible approaches the centric relation, the movement is stopped at the instant of first contact: centric occlusion.

2. The examiner parts the patient's lips and instructs the patient to bite; if centric and maximal occlusion are identical, the jaw does not move. If there is a discrepancy between the centric and maximal occlusion, the mandible slides off. Extent and direction of the trajec-

tory are evaluated. In exceptional cases, the mandible does not slide off; in this instance, there is a large deviation between the position of the mandible when the patient first indicates contact and the maximal occlusion. In this way, the occlusion disturbance can be identified.

3. This phase is also repeated to confirm the findings.

It is advisable to practice the bite motion beforehand. Patients have a tendency first to open the mouth and then to bite down. In this case, the habitual closing motion is performed and no sliding off will be detected.

Research by Steenks[15] and Steenks and Bosman[47] demonstrated that in a group of subjects ($N = 26$) without functional disturbances the distance between maximal occlusion and centric occlusion averaged 0.23 mm, measured from a position of a point several millimeters in front of the frontal elements. The distance between maximal occlusion and "retruded contact position" amounts to 0.61 mm. The subjects were evaluated in the upright sitting position.

In evaluating articulation, contact between the chewing surface complexes of the maxilla and mandible is determined by active movement of the mandible to the left, right, ventral, and dorsal. The dentist looks for contact zones during these tests that disturb the motions. Findings are combined with findings from the dental examination: integrity of teeth and periodontium, movability of the teeth, excessive wear and tear of the occlusal surfaces, and migration and development of the elements.

In a patient with suspected CMD, the trained physical therapist notes the morphology of the bite, gross deviations in the vertical dimension (from wearing a full prosthesis over a long period of time), and the support in the area of the molars. Based on information from the patient, the moment and place of the first contact in maximal occlusion can be determined. The aim of this type of orienting examination is to detect any possible etiological factors in the masticatory system that were not considered earlier and to refer this information on to the dentist. Parafunctional abrasion is determined by detecting facets on the incisors or molars (Figure 7–15). Clenching behavior can cause mucous membrane folds on each side of the inside of the cheeks (Figure 7–16). Elements with parafunctional abrasion can be documented on a chart such as shown in Figure 7–7B.

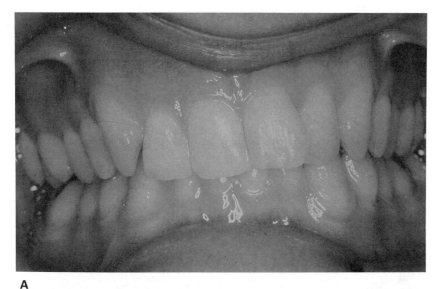

A

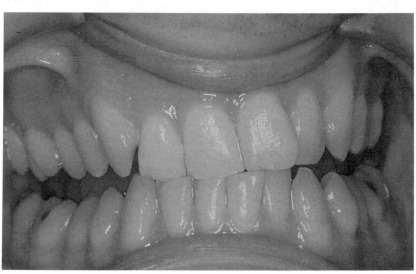

B

Figure 7–15 Parafunctional abrasion on the frontal elements. **A**, Maximal occlusion; **B**, upper and lower front elements brought into contact with each other.

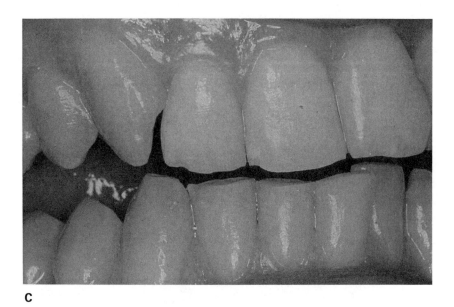

C

Figure 7–15 *C*, detail of the abrasion facets, particularly noted on elements 1.1, 1.2, 3.1, 4.1, 4.2, and 4.3.

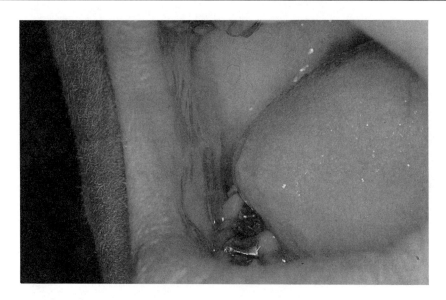

Figure 7–16 Fold in the cheek mucous membrane caused by clenching. Note the impressions on the tongue.

FUNCTIONAL EXAMINATION

After the history and the inspection, the structures of the musculoskeletal part of the masticatory system are examined. Tests include active and passive motions, traction, translation, compression, resisted tests, and the supplementary examination.

The functional examination of the musculoskeletal aspect of the masticatory system consists of the following parts:

- general movement evaluation
  1. active motions
  2. passive motions
  3. resisted provocation tests
- additional movement evaluation
  1. compression
  2. traction
  3. translation
- supplementary examination
  1. palpation (including the segmentally related areas)[40]
  2. specific examination (to include neurological)

3. specific tests, directed at certain structures (for instance, muscles) and/or pathological conditions (electromyelography, radiography, laboratory examination)

The exact performance and integration of these tests are described elsewhere.[8] In this chapter, only selected tests are described.

General Movement Evaluation

Active Motions (Figures 7–17 to 7–20)

- depression (Figure 7–17)
- elevation (Figure 7–18)
- lateral excursion (Figure 7–19)
- protrusion (Figure 7–20A)
- retrusion (Figure 7–20B)

The findings in the movement examination can be reported in a chart similar to that shown as Table 7–1. The measurements are made with a ruler in which the divisions start at 0. Another tool is the caliper. In maximal opening of the mouth, the vertical overbite is

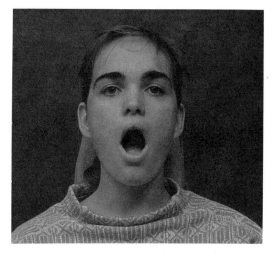

A

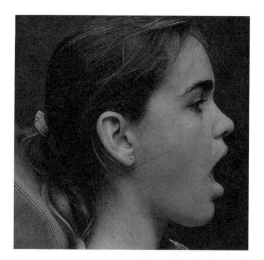

B

Figure 7–17 Active motion: depression of the mandible. ***A***, Frontal view; ***B,*** side view.

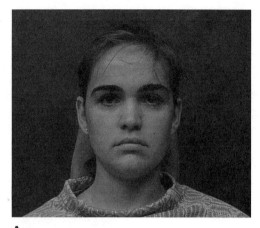

A

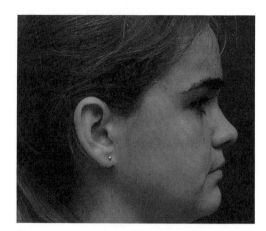

B

Figure 7–18 Active motion: elevation of the mandible. **A**, Frontal view; **B**, side view of the right side of the sitting patient.

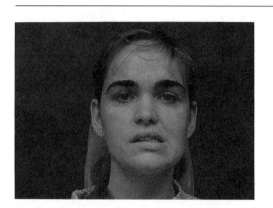

A

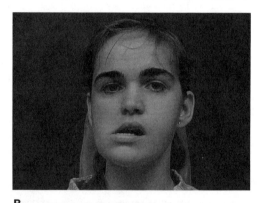

B

Figure 7–19 Active motion: lateral excursion of the mandible. **A**, To the left; **B**, to the right.

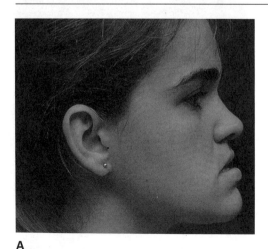

A

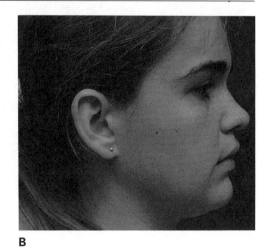

B

Figure 7–20 Active motion. **A**, Protrusion of the mandible; **B**, retrusion of the mandible.

Table 7-1 Chart for Reporting Findings during the Movement Examination

Test	Range of Motion	Trajectory of Motion	Signals	Instant of Appearance	Location	Reproducibility	End-Feel	Particular Details (eg, willingness to move)
Active motions	+	+	+	+	+	+	o	+
Passive motions	+	+	+	+	+	+	+	+
Resisted tests	o	o	+	+	+	+	o	+
Compression	o	o	+	+	+	+	o	+
Traction/ translation	+	+	+	+	+	+	+	+

measured; in protrusion, the sagittal overbite (Figures 7–21 and 7–22). In the retrusion motion, the resulting value is subtracted from the sagittal overbite (Figure 7–23). These corrections are made in order to have an idea about the range of motion.

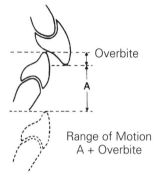

Figure 7–21 Measuring the range of motion in opening.

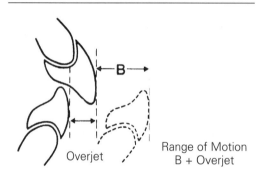

Figure 7–22 Measuring the range of motion in the protrusion motion.

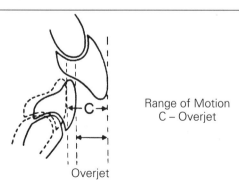

Figure 7–23 Measuring the range of motion in the retrusion motion.

Active Motions (Figures 7–24 to 7–26)

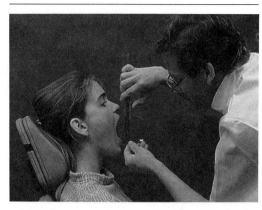

Figure 7–24 Active motion examination measurements: measuring the maximal mouth opening by means of a caliper, according to Steenks and deWijer.[8]

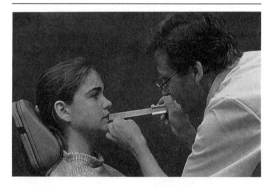

Figure 7–25 Active motion examination measurements: measuring the maximal protrusion and retrusion by means of a caliper.

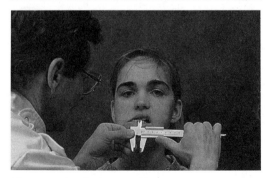

Figure 7–26 Active motion examination measurements: measuring the maximal lateral excursion motion by means of a caliper.

Passive Motions (Figures 7–27 to 7–33)

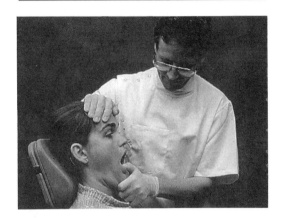

Figure 7–27 Passive motion examination: depression of the mandible and determining the end-feel by exerting slight overpressure against the incisal aspects of the lower elements. The cervical spine is stabilized by the fixing hand at the forehead.

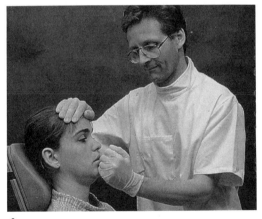

A

Figure 7–28 Passive motion examination: depression of the mandible, demonstrated in phases. **A,** Initiating the depression.

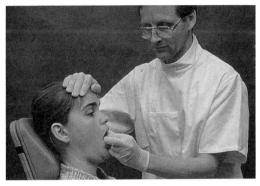

B

Figure 7–28 B, The examiner places the index and middle fingers against the cutting edges of the lower incisors; the thumb is placed against the cutting edges of the upper incisors. The depression is performed through a scissors motion of the fingers.

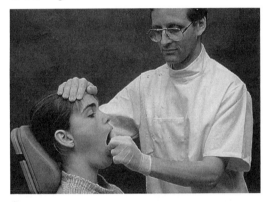

C

Figure 7–28 C, Testing end-feel.

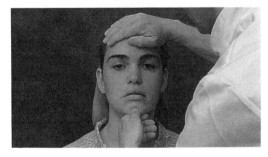

Figure 7–29 Passive motion examination: elevation of the mandible. The index finger lies underneath the mandible; the thumb of the examiner is placed against the front of the chin. The mandible is moved upward until the elements contact each other. This is a form of occlusion examination.

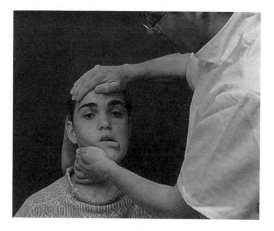

Figure 7–30 Passive motion examination: lateral excursion of the mandible. The examiner fixes firmly and with the thumb moves the mandible in a lateral direction.

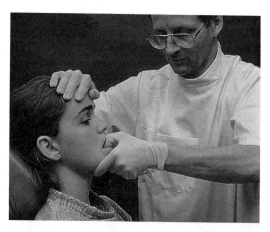

Figure 7–32 Passive motion examination: protrusion of the mandible. The examiner protrudes the jaw by flexing the interphalangeal joint of the thumb and supporting it against the upper front elements.

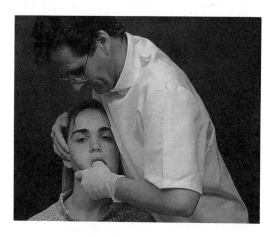

Figure 7–31 Passive motion examination: intraoral technique for the lateral excursion of the mandible. The palpating fingers lie against the lateral pole of the TMJ. The thumb of the moving hand is placed on the occlusal surfaces of the lower elements; the index and middle fingers rest along the mandible.

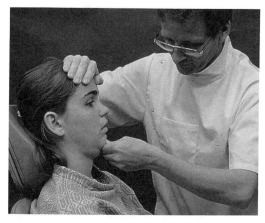

Figure 7–33 Passive motion examination: retrusion of the mandible. The moving thumb and index finger are placed against the chin. From a slightly protruding position a retrusion-push is given in a dorsocranial direction.[48]

Traction and Translation (Figures 7–34 and 7–35)

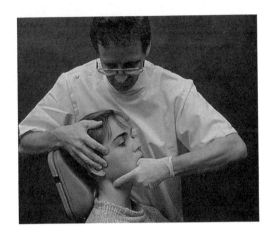

A

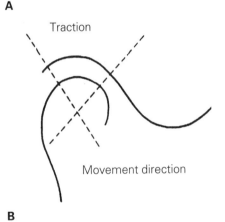

Traction

Movement direction

B

Figure 7–34 Passive motion examination.
A, Traction of the TMJ; **B**, direction of traction.

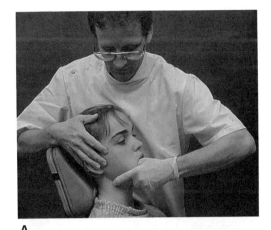

A

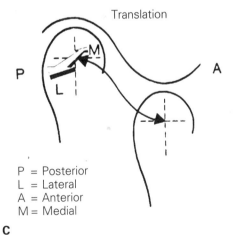

B

Translation

P = Posterior
L = Lateral
A = Anterior
M = Medial

C

Figure 7–35 Passive motion examination.
A, Translation in an anterior direction;
B, translation in a medial direction;
C, illustration of the possible translation directions.

Compression (Figure 7–36)

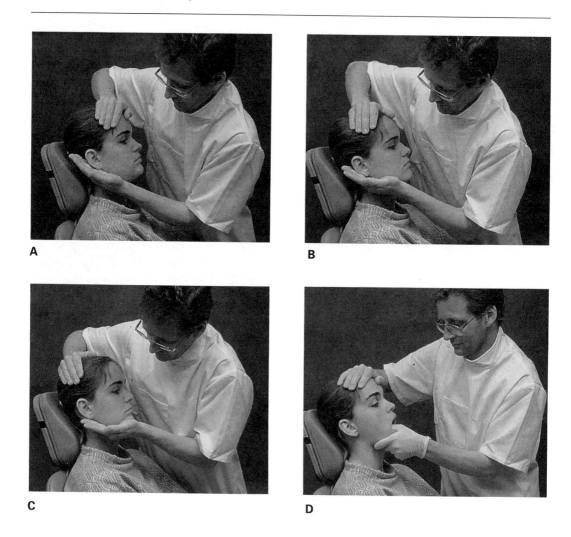

A

B

C

D

Figure 7–36 Compression directions: **A**, Ventrocranial. **B**, cranial. **C**, dorsocranial. The fixing hand stabilizes the head and the spine. Note the various positions of the fixing and the moving hands. **D**, For the intraoral techniques, the thumb from the moving hand is placed on the occlusal surfaces; the index and middle fingers rest against the mandible. During the opening motion, compression is given in a dorsocranial, more cranial, and ventrocranial direction.

Resisted Tests (Figure 7–37)

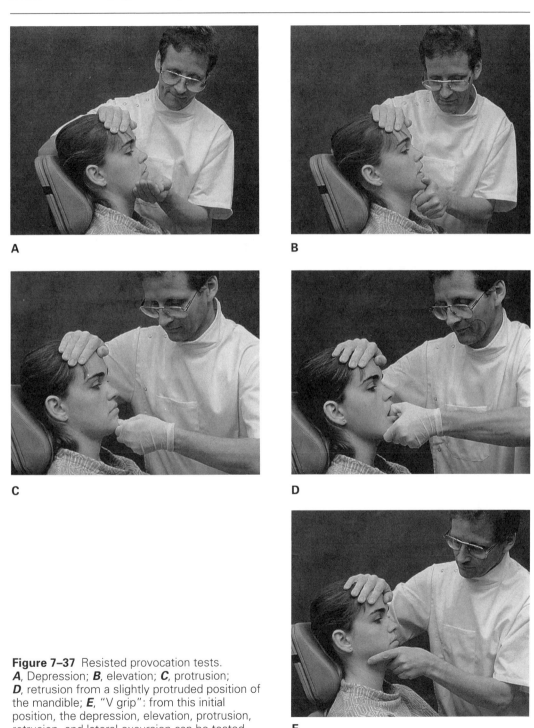

Figure 7–37 Resisted provocation tests.
A, Depression; ***B***, elevation; ***C***, protrusion;
D, retrusion from a slightly protruded position of
the mandible; ***E***, "V grip": from this initial
position, the depression, elevation, protrusion,
retrusion, and lateral excursion can be tested.

Coordination (Figure 7–38)

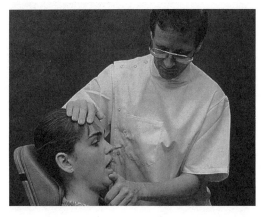

A

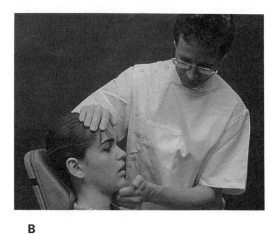

B

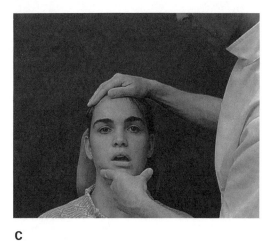

C

Figure 7–38 Coordination. The patient stabilizes the mandible against resistance exerted by the examiner. The intensity and the direction of the resistance change. **A**, Resisted elevation; **B**, resisted depression; **C**, resisted lateral excursion.

Supplementary Examination

Auscultation (Figure 7–39)

Palpation

Palpation of the structures of the masticatory system is important in order to judge soft tissue decondition. First, the skin and the subcutaneous tissue are examined in relation to the pliability and shiftability (Figure 7–40). Next, palpation of the muscles takes place. Attention is given mainly to the muscles that are accessible to palpation: masseter muscles, temporal muscles, and the insertion of the medial pterygoid muscles (Figures 7–41 to 7–43).

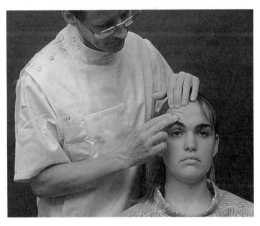

Figure 7–40 Palpation. The skin in the innervation area of the trigeminal nerve is examined for pliability and shiftability.

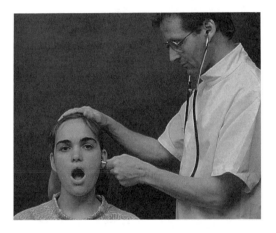

Figure 7–39 Auscultation. By means of a stethoscope, crepitation and/or clicking is detected during movement of the TMJ. The moment of occurrence and the relation with other symptoms are determined.

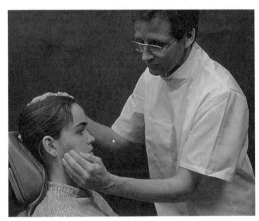

Figure 7–41 Palpation. Determining tenderness and registering structural changes in the masseter muscle, the superficial and deep parts (just in front of the TMJ).

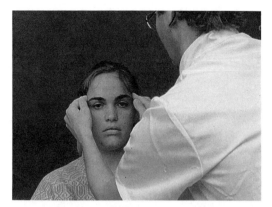

A

Increased tone, structural changes, pain, and trigger points are noted. The examiner is also concerned about localization, degree of provocation, and reproducibility of the signals. In addition, the exiting sites of the trigeminal nerve and the temporal artery are palpated (Figures 7–44 and 7–45). The periarticular structures of the TMJ are palpated from lateral and dorsal aspects (Figure 7–46).

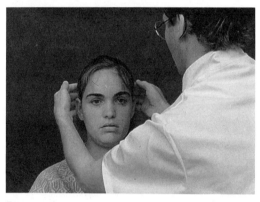

B

Figure 7–42 Palpation. **A**, Temporal muscle, pars ventralis; **B**, temporal muscle, pars medialis and dorsalis.

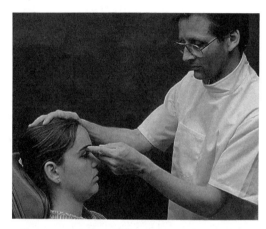

A

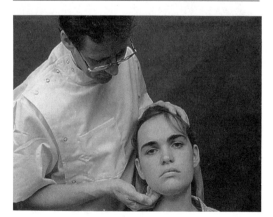

Figure 7–43 Palpation. The insertion of the medial pterygoid muscle is palpated at the medial aspect of the mandibular angle, with the head positioned in slight ipsilateral sidebend.

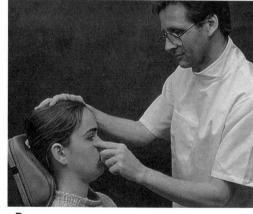

B

Figure 7–44 Palpation of the exiting sites of the trigeminal nerve. **A**, Supraorbital nerve; **B**, infraorbital nerve.

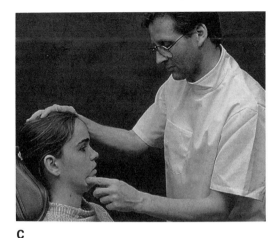

C

Figure 7–44 *C*, mentalis nerve.

Besides the skin corresponding to the trigeminal innervation area, the cutaneous areas innervated by the cutaneous branches of the dorsal rami from the cervical (C2 to C8) and thoracic (T1 to T9) spinal nerves should also be examined. Hagenaars et al[51] describe the tissue-specific changes in the skeletal musculature. Along with the facial and mastication musculature, Oostendorp[40] also studied the intrinsic dorsal back muscles. Sensitivity to pressure of the nerve structures (trigeminal nerve, greater occipital nerve, lesser occipital nerve, and the brachial plexus) can also be the result of this mechanism.

Palpation is performed not only as a pain provocation test, but also to better determine the intra-articular movement behavior (range of motion, sudden shifting). Signs such as clicking and crepitation can also be palpable.

The significance of the sensitivity in palpating cannot be overestimated. Solberg[49] states: "The risk for over-reporting tenderness suggests that palpation might be used most appropriately to augment the findings of the functional test rather than as a 'stand alone' criterion for the temporomandibular disorder."

Frisch[50] writes that tenderness on the trigeminal points is seldom caused by pathology from the nerve itself. These points can be tender as a result of lung disorders, sinus inflammations, or tooth inflammations.

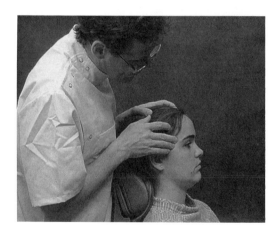

Figure 7–45 Palpation of the temporal artery for tenderness and swelling.

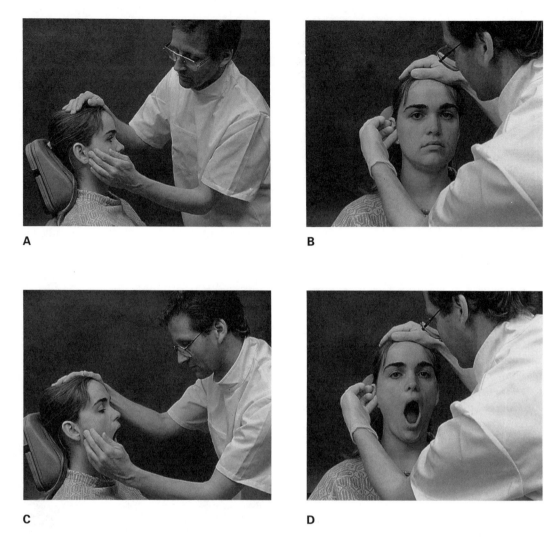

Figure 7–46 Palpation of the periarticular structures of the TMJ. **A**, The level of the lateral pole. **B**, Dorsal via the external acoustic meatus. It is also possible to palpate these structures during movement and in the end-position of the TMJ. **C**, Palpation during movement: lateral and dorsal. **D**, Lateral and dorsal through the external acoustic meatus.

FUNCTIONAL EXAMINATION OF THE SPINAL COLUMN AND SHOULDER GIRDLE

The cervical column plays a significant role in CMD.[8,42,52] Local and projected pain in the head and neck regions can originate from the neck. A number of syndromes are named for this: in the physical therapy and orthopaedic literature,[7,40] it is termed the cervicocephalic syndrome; in the ENT literature,[53] it is called the cervicoesophageal syndrome.

After the functional diagnosis of the masticatory system, a general functional examination of the cervicothoracic spine and the shoulder girdle is performed. In addition, the segmentally directed examination for tissue-specific changes and disturbances is also performed.[40] For the exact description and interpretation of the tests refer to Chapters 5 and 6.

The segmentally directed examination should be performed by an experienced physical therapist. The examination offers additional information that is not discussed in the context of this chapter.[8,41–43,54]

Considering the multifactorial etiology, it is advisable to discuss the findings with the referring dentist. In contemplating the findings, it may also be beneficial to notify the family physician. This physician is often better acquainted with the patient, the social conditions, and the medical background (the viscerogenic and somatogenic aspects).

In complaints of acute pain, it is very possible that the dentist (for example, the onset occurred in a restaurant) or the physical therapist (for instance, the cause lies in the cervical spine) can perform the treatment independently. In chronic pain patients, many factors must be considered. Steenks and de Wijer describe case studies that are based on the above principles.[8] In Table 7–2 a number of abnormalities are described that are important in making a differential diagnosis of CMD.

If the symptoms cannot be provoked in any way, CMD should not be considered. Furthermore, even if aberrations of the TMJ are demonstrated on the radiographic views, these should not be treated if a relation with the patient's complaints cannot be found. In instances of an atypical symptom profile, the patient should be referred back to the primary physician.

The radiological examination by the dentist usually includes an Orthopantomograph and

---

Table 7–2 Several Aberrations That Are Important in the Differential Diagnosis

- Dental abnormalities
  1. Pulpitis
  2. Dentitio difficilis
  3. Parodontal inflammations
- Neurological abnormalities
  1. Neuropathy
  2. Trigeminal neuralgia
  3. Glossopharyngeal neuralgia
- Myopathy
  1. Muscle hypertrophy
  2. Myesthesia
- Blood vessel abnormalities
  1. Temporal arteritis
  2. Migraine
  3. Functional vertebrobasilar insufficiency

- Inflammations
  1. Frontal, maxillary sinusitis
  2. Otitis media
- Tumors
  1. Temporomandibular joint
  2. Sinuses
  3. Maxilla and mandible
  4. Salivary glands
- Traumata
  1. After oral and dental surgery
  2. Contusion
  3. Fracture

Source: Reprinted from Steenk, M.H. and Touw, W.D., *Jaarboek Fysiotherapie*, pp. 314–351, with permission of Bohn, Scheltema and Holkema, © 1987.

several specific views of the TMJ with the mouth closed (maximal occlusion) and if necessary with the mouth open. If a disc displacement is suspected but cannot be clearly diagnosed clinically, use is made of supplementary imaging techniques (computed tomography scan, arthrography, arthroscopy, and MRI).

7.3   TREATMENT

Because of the multifactorial etiology often involved in CMD, the family physician, dentist, and physical therapist should all be included in the treatment team. The family physician is concerned primarily with the viscerogenic and the psychogenic aspects of the disorder. The dentist concentrates on the viscerogenic aspect in regard to dentition and the somatogenic aspect in regard to the musculoskeletal aspect of the masticatory system. The physical therapist is mainly concerned with the somatic side of the dysfunction.

Because of chronic pain, the integrity of the connective tissue in the head-neck region can deteriorate. Intraoral consequences may result, including a dry mouth, warm-cold sensitivity of the teeth, and changes in taste. Even after the primary cause has long been resolved, these signs can occur.

PHYSICAL THERAPY TREATMENT

The literature in relation to physical therapy treatment of CMD is still largely pre-experimental, with only a small number of controlled-effect studies. However, there do appear to be indications for treatment. In addition to dental treatment, relaxation therapy, massage, mobilization, and posture correction, pain-relieving techniques and overall conditioning are important features in the treatment of the patient with CMD. For more detailed information, refer to Chapter 2, General Aspects of Examination and Treatment.

Massage

Of the mastication muscles, the temporal and the masseter muscles are the most accessible for massage therapy. Massage to the head is best applied after introducing techniques and/or treatment to the cervicothoracic region and the shoulder girdle. Massage hand grips in relation to the neck must be performed cautiously. The presence of dentures should be noted and contact lenses should be removed before proceeding with the treatment. Techniques consist of pressure, stroking, kneading, friction, shifting, and vibration.

Connective Tissue Massage

Connective tissue massage begins as low as necessary on the patient's trunk (usually the back) and usually involves only a few dermatomes; palpable relaxation should result. Initially, the massage is indicated daily for 3 or 4 consecutive days. After 2 days' rest, the massage should be administered two to three times per week until the specific changes in the subcutaneous tissue have resolved. The intensity of the treatment and the frequency can be adjusted according to the symptoms and the findings from the functional examination.

Mobilization

The body's posture and the position of the cervical spine also influence the muscles and the forces working on the mandible and the temporomandibular joint.[27,55] Rocabado[28] describes this influence from a mechanical viewpoint. Mobilization of the craniomandibular joint is indicated in order to allow recovery of disturbed joint function. If dysfunction of the cervical spine also plays a role, mobilization of this area is indicated as well.

Manipulation techniques within the masticatory system are seldom needed. In a ventral disc displacement, without reduction, a manipulation may be indicated in the acute phase (Figure 7–47). After the manipulation, the patient should receive a reposition splint from the dentist.

Rocabado[56] describes therapy for the biomechanical dysfunction of the craniocervical and craniomandibular systems in which home exercises play an essential part. The program is based on exercises that are performed in six repetitions, six times per day. The goals of the therapy program are as follows:

- learning good posture, in which the underlying relation among the head, the cervical spine, the shoulder girdle, and the mandible play important roles

- improvement of proprioception
- recovery of muscle length
- recovery of joint mobility
- recovery of muscle balance

Posture

Rocabado[28] discusses the importance of the position of the hyoid bone in relation to the jaw and the cervical spine. He also states that more than 70% of patients with a craniocervical dysfunction also have a CMD. Anterior positioning of the head facilitates dorsal rotation of the cranium. According to Rocabado, this causes a soft tissue (muscle) stretch with a force acting dorsal and downward on the mandible. A reactive increase in tension of the elevator muscles results. Furthermore, Rocabado describes a relation between the class 2 malocclusion and changes in the position of the clavicle and scapula.

Woodside and Linder-Aronson[57] indicate a relationship between an abnormal position of the head, enlarged adenoids, obstruction of the nasal passages, and malocclusion. Solow and Tallgren[58] demonstrate statistically significant ($P > 0.05$) relationships between posture of the head and the craniofacial and dentoalveolar morphology.

Interaction between the upper cervical spine and the TMJ is also described by Trott.[59] The functional interactions between the upper cervical column and the TMJ play an important role in abnormal posture. Adaptive shortening of the suboccipital musculature and lengthening of the longus capitis, rectus capitis anterior, and the suprahyoid muscles results.

The upper cervical region is important for regulating posture. The propriosensors in the upper cervical joints and muscles, the equilibrium organs, and the eye muscles are closely connected to each other via the vestibular core complex. Through these regulating systems, a number of craniocervical functions are made possible.

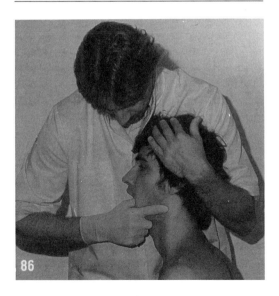

Figure 7–47 Manipulation.

Besides the nocisensoric overlap between the upper cervical region and the trigeminal area, there is also a neuroanatomical relationship between the cervicothoracic junction and the TMJ (Figure 7–48). Autonomic efferent innervation comes from the C8 to T2 seg-

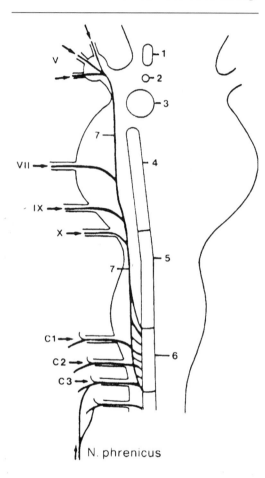

Figure 7–48 Schematic illustration of the running and the projection of the nocisensoric nerve roots via the trigeminal nerve (**V**); the facial nerve (**VII**); the glossopharyngeal nerve (**IX**); the vagus nerve (**X**); the spinal nerves C1, C2, and C3; and the phrenic nerve on the caudal part of the spinal nucleus of the trigeminal nerve, according to Oostendorp.[40] **1**, Mesencephalic nucleus of the trigeminal nerve; **2**, motor nucleus of the trigeminal nerve; **3**, main sensory nucleus of the trigeminal nerve; **4**, pars oralis; **5**, pars interpolaris; **6**, pars caudalis; **7**, spinal nucleus of trigeminal nerve.

ments. A chronic elevation of tonic orthosympathetic activity in the cervicothoracic junction has consequences for all of the soft tissue structures that have a sympathetic innervation from the cervicothoracic junction.

Even in dentistry, attention was called to improving posture. As early as 1958 and 1959, Duyzings, an orthodontist, described the importance of correcting posture in young patients.[26,60]

Pain Relief

Pain relief can be achieved in various ways. In CMD, postisometric relaxation, oscillation and vibration techniques, soft tissue techniques, and various forms of electrotherapy can be applied. When using electrotherapy, important points for elevated orthosympathetic activity are located in the segments C8 to L2. In this region, the spinal component of the orthosympathetic nervous system is situated in the lateral horns of the spinal cord.[61] For problems of the masticatory system, the neuromodulation techniques should be applied within the segmental regions of C8 to T4. Important trigger points are illustrated in Figure 7–49.

In traction and translation techniques, pain relief is particularly achieved with traction grades 1 and 2. In grade 3 traction, a mobilization effect is achieved (Figure 7–50). By alternating the techniques, the direction of translation, and the frequency of the oscillation, the desired effect can be achieved.

The rhythmic stabilization techniques from proprioceptive neuromuscular facilitation can be applied to improve proprioceptive control over the mandible. With these techniques, increased awareness of position and movement is achieved.

Influencing Respiration and Mouth Behavior

In the treatment of CMD, the physical therapist should also pay attention to the in-

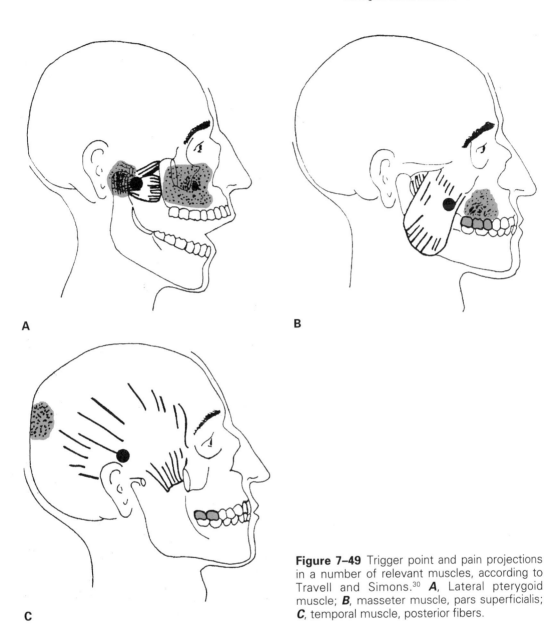

Figure 7–49 Trigger point and pain projections in a number of relevant muscles, according to Travell and Simons.[30] **A**, Lateral pterygoid muscle; **B**, masseter muscle, pars superficialis; **C**, temporal muscle, posterior fibers.

Traction

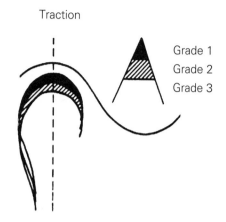

Grade 1
Grade 2
Grade 3

Figure 7–50 Description of the intensities of the traction.

tegrity of the airway passages and the behavior patterns of the mouth.

There is an interaction between form and function in the craniofacial region.[22,62] Two physiological factors appear to be important in the development of the craniomandibular and craniocervical complex: the nasopharyngeal passage and the head and cervical spine posture. Factors that can disturb this development include allergies, enlarged adenoids, disturbances in vision, disturbances in the proprioception of the utricle and semicircular canal system of the ear, anomalies of the cervical column, scar tissue, growth problems of the sutures and the condyle, and a discrepancy between the vertical proportion in the growth of the condyle and the cervical spine.[62]

Other studies[58,63,64] indicate that the mandibular development is dependent on the airway resistance and the craniocervical angle. The causal factor is not mentioned in these studies. There is also a clear relationship between the airway passages and the craniocervical angle. Thus, craniofacial development is also influenced by distant factors such as the patient's posture and breathing.[62] The physical therapist should consider this in the treatment of children with chronic disorders.

The treatment of abnormalities in the behavior patterns of the mouth requires a summation of the knowledge and skills of the dentist, psychologist, speech therapist, and physical therapist. The speech therapist is consulted particularly in disturbed voice production, incorrect tongue position, severely deviated mouth behavior, and speech disorders. If not addressed by the speech therapist, the physical therapist can treat the abnormal mouth behavior, particularly in the form of instruction and exercises. However, voice disorders, speech, and swallowing problems should be dealt with by the speech therapist.

Normally, the tongue should lie against the palate; the anterior one third of the tongue is held with slight pressure against the palate. The tip of the tongue rests behind the upper incisors. In this position, there is a small freeway space, whereby the upper and lower dentition elements do not touch each other. A consistently low position of the tongue during growth can influence the development of the lower and upper jaws. Discrepancies may occur in the width of the lower or upper jaw with possible consequences such as a decreased ability to take load locally. On the basis of occlusion and articular disturbances, CMD can result.

In abnormal mouth behavior, the physical therapist can use the principles of the habit-reversal technique. This technique involves breaking the troublesome habit, such as thumb sucking, nail biting, or grinding or clenching the teeth. If the symptoms can be provoked by clenching the teeth together as hard as possible for a maximum of 60 seconds, then the habit-reversal technique is particularly indicated.[48,65]

According to Duinkerke,[65] five stages can be differentiated in the habit-reversal procedure:

1. describing the habit
2. noticing the habit
3. establishing a warning signal

4. exercising the opposite behavior

5. recognizing the situation in which the habit occurs

Duinkerke[65] also describes five criteria that the habit-reversal exercise program should satisfy:

1. Work preferably with the antagonistic muscles, in other words opposite the movement of the habit.
2. Perform the exercise every few minutes.
3. Work with isometric contraction.
4. Make sure that the exercises are socially acceptable.
5. Use muscle-strengthening exercises for the antagonists.

Electromyographic biofeedback can be used to reinforce the exercises.

Conclusion

In dealing with the various treatable aspects of CMD, it is obvious that the physical therapist has many choices. Due to the absence of controlled-effect studies, it is impossible to be more specific as to the correct therapy. The treatment choice is determined partially by the patient, the professionals involved, the amount of selectivity within the nervous system, the relative contraindications, and the personal preference of the therapist.

DENTAL TREATMENT

To give the physician and physical therapist insight into the dental treatment, a short description regarding the most applied forms of dental therapy follows. After making the diagnosis and determining the etiological factors of the problem, the dentist chooses from several treatment options:

- advice
- occlusion therapy
- exercise therapy

Before beginning the dental treatment, the relation between the patient's complaints and the findings from the examination must be established. If this relationship is not clear after consulting with the patient, it may still be appropriate to initiate a trial treatment for a short duration.

Advice

Advice is usually related to function and parafunction. For instance, the patient should be dissuaded from biting into or eating tough, chewy food. In addition, certain habits must be stopped, such as nail biting, gum chewing, etc. Patients should be made aware of the clenching behavior and/or the existence of other abnormal mouth behavior.

When a multidisciplinary approach is taken, the dentist is usually the coordinator of the treatment program. Based on the examination, advice can include referral to other medical disciplines. It is also important to ensure that the patient is not confronted with differing opinions from the disciplines involved in the treatment program.

Occlusion Therapy

Within the scope of the dental therapy for TMJ dysfunction, occlusion correction plays a significant role. In acute problems, such as a faulty restorative measure, the occlusion correction should be adapted to this restoration. The occlusion will adapt to fill up a gap from a missing tooth in the dental arch. This also happens in situations where the dorsal support zone is deficient. If the vertical dimension has decreased because of a migration of the dentition, not only is the support zone supplemented, but the vertical dimension is elevated a few millimeters as well. This is achieved by allowing the plastic appliance to extend over the chewing surfaces, providing a new occlusion (Figure 7–51). The objective is to unload the TMJ. Such an appliance is called a splint.

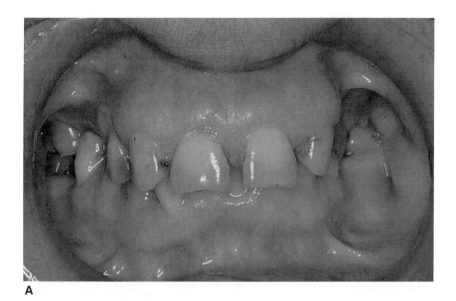

A

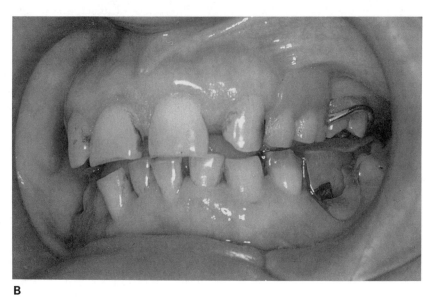

B

Figure 7–51 Plastic splint in the lower jaw to fill in the occlusion at the site of the missing dentition elements, thus resulting in an elevation of the bite. **A**, Mouth view without the splint; **B**, mouth view with the splint.

If the horizontal relation of the lower jaw is involved (for instance, in a discrepancy between the centric occlusion and the maximal occlusion), reversible forms of treatment are applied first rather than directly grinding the occlusal surfaces of the dentition. This reversible form of treatment involves a splint (Figure 7–52). The splint consists of a plastic plate in the lower or upper jaw that covers the chewing surfaces and the incisal edges, as

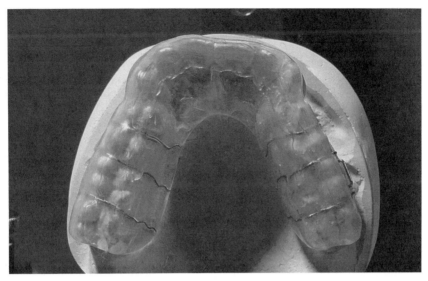

A

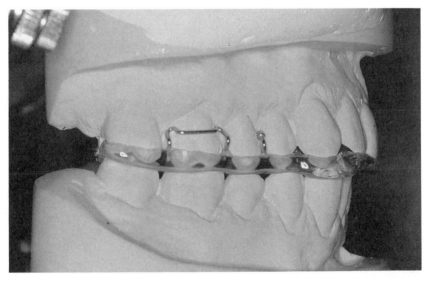

B

Figure 7–52 Stabilization splint. **A,** Occlusal view; **B,** lateral view of the part that lies over the chewing surfaces.

well as a part of the palate or the tongue part of the lower jaw.

By introducing a splint, it is possible to do the following:

- modify the vertical and horizontal relation

- evenly distribute contact in the dental arch, and at the same time
- change the articular pattern.

Such an appliance is called a stabilization splint. The patient should be able to take the splint out of the mouth to maintain proper mouth hygiene. Usually the splint should be worn during the day as well as at night. If nightly bruxism is the significant etiological factor, the patient is advised to wear the splint only at night.

The working mechanism of the splint is not known. The change in the position of the mandibular condyle in the fossa is one of the hypotheses (unloading of the TMJ). Altered input in the central nervous system from the periphery (modified masticatory surfaces, stabilization of the occlusion) is also thought to be responsible for the beneficial results. In addition, the possibility of a placebo effect cannot be ruled out.

If the diagnosis of a ventral disc displacement with reduction is made and there is an indication for treatment (pain, limitation in opening the mouth due to temporary blocking), the reposition splint is applied. This type of splint brings the lower jaw into a slightly more forward position (Figure 7–53). The amount of reposition is determined by judging the contact between the upper and lower dentition elements during closing and during retrusion from a forward position. The patient should wear the splint permanently. Because the goal is to allow the patient to bite down in a more forward position, the reposition splint has a deeper relief than the stabilization splint (Figure 7–53E).

In cases of a ventral disc displacement without reduction, before placing the splint a manipulation should be performed in which the articular disc is brought back into normal relation with regard to the head of the mandible.

Manipulation should not be performed in instances where the disc displacement has already been present for a long period of time. In such a case, the chance for a successful reposition of the articular disc is very small. A stabilization splint can be used to unload the TMJ, relieve pain, and influence the course of the adaptation processes. Surgery is considered in exceptional situations, such as in a severe functional limitation with pain, when

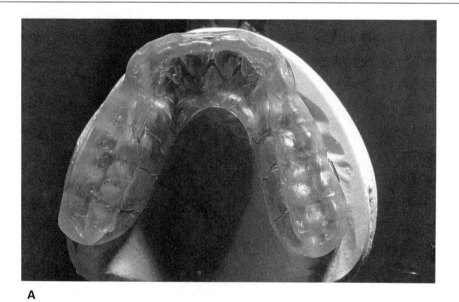

A

Figure 7–53 Reposition splint. **A,** Occlusal view.

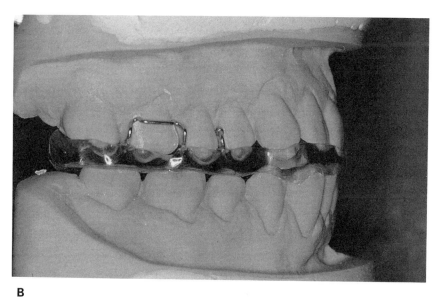

B

Figure 7–53 *B*, Lateral view of the part covering the chewing surfaces.

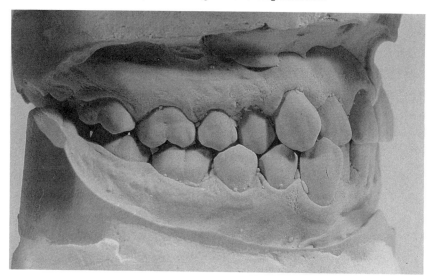

C

Figure 7–53 *C*, Dentition model in maximal occlusion, lateral view.

conservative treatment provides minimal to no improvement. The manipulation maneuver is worthwhile only when a reposition splint is ready. Thus this treatment preferably is performed by an experienced dentist.

After the treatment with the reposition splint is successfully completed, attempts are made to bring the lower jaw gradually back to the original position. In every form of splint therapy, there is a weaning-off phase. At first,

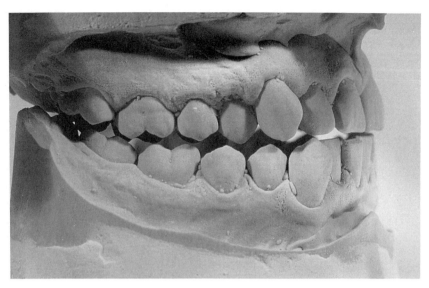

D

Figure 7–53 *D*, Dentition model in a repositioned position. Note the more forward position of the lower model. The space between the elements of the lower and upper jaws are filled by the splint.

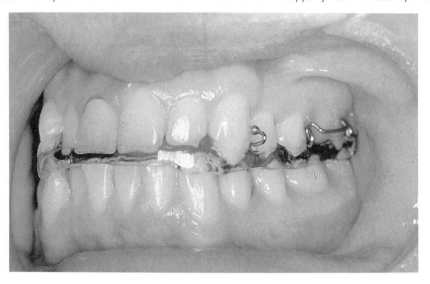

E

Figure 7–53 *E*, Reposition splint in the mouth.

---

the splint is worn gradually less during the day. Afterward, the splint is left out occasionally at night. If necessary, the occlusion is ground down, so that without the splint the centric occlusion corresponds to the maximal occlu- sion, and in maximal occlusion an even and simultaneous contact occurs between the chewing surfaces of the lower and upper jaw.

If the occlusion has not been altered and the symptoms (particularly pain) recur, there may be an indication to adapt the natural dentition similar to what was achieved with the splint. Casted restoration is used to obtain this goal (Figure 7–54).

Exercise Therapy

One goal of exercise therapy is to prevent a proal opening pattern of the mouth (Fig-

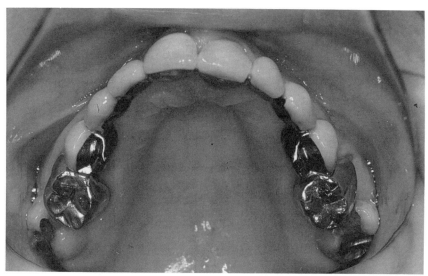

A

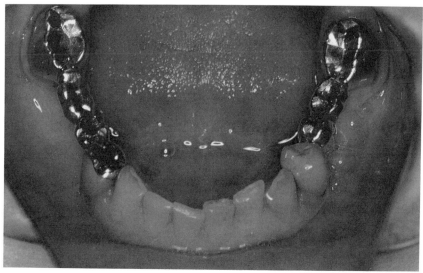

B

Figure 7–54 Casted restoration after treatment with a stabilization splint, indicated by recurrence of complaints as the splint was weaned. ***A***, Overview of the upper jaw; ***B***, overview of the lower jaw.

ure 7–55). The patient is instructed to move the mandible along the trajectory of a hinge motion, which forms almost a pure rotation (Figure 7–2). Coordination is also improved through these exercises. This exercise is also indicated after reposition due to a dislocation of the TMJ, in which the condylar process moved too far in front of the eminences and the patient was unable to close the mandible.

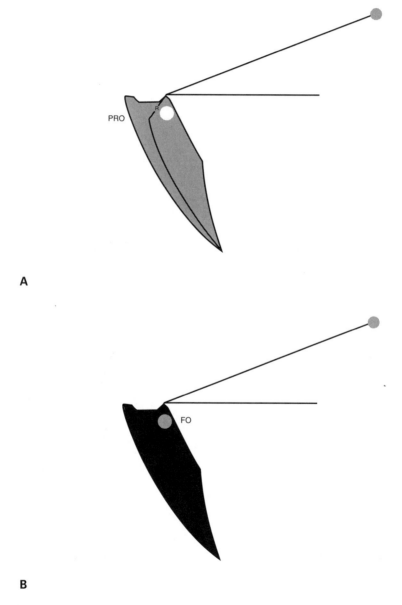

A

B

Figure 7–55 Movement of a point of the mandible at the level of the incisor, projected in the sagittal plane. **A**, grey: proal opening pattern; **B**, black: normal opening and closing movement (see also Figure 7–2).

Conclusion

To date there are relatively few controlled studies about the long-term results in treatment of craniomandibular dysfunction. Carlsson[66] indicates that a large number of patients with CMD can be treated successfully with various simple methods (splint, exercises, grinding, prosthetics). The long-term prognosis is good, not only for neuromuscular dysfunctions but also for osteoarthrosis (articular dysfunction) of the TMJ.

In regard to the prognosis of "internal derangements," the same can be reported. The effect of treatment by means of the reposition splint appears to be mostly due to the quickly achieved comfortable functioning of the musculoskeletal aspect of the TMJ. The symptoms of clicking are difficult to treat. Okeson[67] reports that in 66% of the study's 40 treated patients, the temporomandibular noises remained after 2½ years of treatment with a reposition splint. The treatment contained a "step back" phase, in which the mandible was brought back to the initial relation. However, even in studies regarding the results of treatments in which the patients were rehabilitated in a forward position, similar observations were made. Thus, if the reciprocal click based on a disc displacement with reduction is the only finding, treatment is not indicated.

REFERENCES

1. Costen JB. A syndrome of ear and sinus symptoms dependent upon disturbed function of the temporomandibular joint. *Ann Otol Rhinol Laryngol.* 1934;18:1–15.

2. Schwarz L. Conclusions of the temporomandibular joint: clinic at Columbia. *J Periodontol.* 1958;29:210.

3. Schwarz L. The pain-dysfunction syndrome. In: Schwarz L, Chayes CM, eds. *Facial Pain and Mandibular Dysfunction.* Philadelphia: WB Saunders Co; 1968.

4. Laskin DM. Etiology of the pain dysfunction syndrome. *J Am Dent Assoc.* 1969;79:147.

5. DeBoever JA, Steenks MH. Epidemiologie, symptomatologie en etiologie van craniomandibulaire dysfuncties. In: Steenks MH, Wijer A de, eds. *Craniomandibulaire Dysfunctie vanuit Fysiotherapeutisch en Tandheelkundig Perspectief.* Lochem: De Tijdstroom; 1989.

6. Solberg WK. Epidemiology, incidence and prevalence. Presented at the president's conference on the examination, diagnosis and management of temporomandibular disorders. 1982; Chicago.

7. Krämer J. *Bandscheibenbedingte Erkrankungen.* Stuttgart: Georg Thieme Verlag; 1978.

8. Steenks MH, de Wijer A, eds. *Craniomandibulaire Dysfunctie Vanuit Fysiotherapeutisch en Tandheelkundig Perspectief.* Lochem: DeTijdstroom; 1989.

9. Derksen AAD. *Afwijkingen van het Kauwstelsel.* Utrecht: A. Oosthoek's Uitgeversmaatschappij N.V.; 1970.

10. Derksen AAD. *Inleiding to de Bouw en Functie van het Kauwstelsel.* Utrecht: Bohn, Scheltema & Holkema; 1977.

11. Steenks MH, Bosman F. Reference positions of the mandible. *J Oral Rehabil.* 1985;12:357.

12. Savalle WPM. Some aspects of the morphology of the human temporomandibular joint capsule. *Acta Anat.* 1988;131:292–296.

13. Dawson PE. *Evaluation, Diagnosis and Treatment of Occlusal Problems.* St. Louis: CV Mosby Co; 1974.

14. Lauritzen AG. *Atlas of Occlusal Analysis.* Colorado Springs, Colo: HAH Publications; 1974.

15. Steenks MH. *Referentieposities van de Onderkaak.* Utrecht: Rijks University; 1983. Thesis.

16. Yemm R. The role of time elasticity in the control of mandibular resting posture. In: Anderson DJ, Matthews B, eds. *Mastication.* Bristol, UK; Wright: 1976:81–87.

17. Hanson TL, Oberg T. En kliniskt-bettfysiologisk undersökning av 67-aringar I Dolby. *Tandläkartidn.* 1971;18:650.

18. Agerberg G, Osterberg T. Maximal mandibular movements and symptoms of mandibular dysfunction in 70-year-old men and women. *Swed Dent J.* 1974;57:1.

19. Helkimo M. Studies on function and dysfunction of the masticatory system II: index for anamnestic and clinical dysfunction and occlusal state. *Swed Dent J.* 1974;67:101.

20. Reider CE, Martinoff JT. The prevalence of mandibular dysfunction, Part II: a multiphasic dysfunction profile. *J Prosthet Dent.* 1983;50:237–244.

21. DeBoever JA. Functional disturbances of the temporomandibular joint. In: Zarb GA, Carlsson GE, eds. *Temporomandibular Joint, Function and Dysfunction.* Copenhagen: Munksgaard; 1979.

22. Dibbets JHJ. Groei en craniomandibulaire dysfunctie. In: Steenks MH, Wijer A de, eds. *Craniomandibulaire Dysfunctie vanuit Fysiotherapeutisch en Tandheeldundig Perspectief.* Lochum: De Tijdstroom; 1989.

23. DeBoever JA, Van Steenberghe D. *Occlusie en bewegingsleer van het stomatognatisch stelsel.* Alphen a.d. Rijn: Samson Stafleu; 1988.

24. Rugh JD, Solberg WK. Psychological implications in temporomandibular pain and dysfunction. In: Zarb GA, Carlsson GE, eds. *Temporomandibular Joint Function and Dysfunction.* Copenhagen: Munksgaard; 1979.

25. Meyler WJ. *Preventie van het Chronisch Pijnsyndroom.* Werkgroep preventie chroniciteit; Nederlandse Vereniging ter Bestudering van Pijn. Groningen: Academisch Ziekenhuis, 1984.

26. Duyzings JAC. De betekenis der preventieve orthodontie voor de ontwikkeling van aangezicht en lichaamshouding. *Tijdschr Tandheelkd.* 1958; 65:646–659.

27. Brügger A. *Die Erkrankungen de Bewegungsapparates und seines Nervensystems.* Stuttgart: Gustav Fischer Verlag; 1980.

28. Rocabado M. Biomechanical relationship of the cranial, cervical and hyoid regions. *J Craniomandibular Pract.* 1983;3:62–66.

29. Korr JM. *The Neurobiologic Mechanisms in Manipulative Therapy.* New York: Plenum Press; 1978.

30. Travell J, Simons G. *Myofascial Pain and Dysfunction: The Trigger Point Manual.* Baltimore: Williams & Wilkins; 1983.

31. Hijzen TH, Slangen JL. Myofascial pain dysfunction: subjective signs and symptoms. *J Prosthet Dent.* 1985;54:705–711.

32. Bremer GJ, Janseen JJ, Veenstra A, de Planque BA, Sedee GA. *Hoofdpijn.* Leiden: Stafleu's Wetenschappelijke Uitgeversmaatschappij NV; 1970.

33. Hansson TB, Nordström. Thickness of the soft tissue layers and articular disk in temporomandibular joints with deviations in form. *Acta Odontol Scand.* 1977;35:281.

34. Juniper RP. T.M.J. Dysfunction: a theory based upon electromyographic studies of the lateral pterygoid muscle. *Br J Oral Surg.* 1984:221–228.

35. Steenks MH, Touw WD. In: van Cranenburgh B, den Dekker JB, van Meerwijk GM, Wessel HFM, de Wijer A, eds. *Jaarboek Fysiotherapie.* Utrecht: Bohn, Scheltema & Holkema; 1987:314–351.

36. Steenks MH. De inklemming vaan de discus articularis met betrekking tot het pijndysfunctiesyndroom. *Ned Tijdschr Tandheelkd.* 1974; 81,10:380–387.

37. Farrar WB, McCarthy WL. *A Clinical Outline of Temporomandibular Joint Diagnosis and Treatment.* Normandy Study Group for TMJ Dysfunction. Montgomery, Ala; 1982.

38. van Cranenburgh B. *Inleiding in de toegepaste neurowetenschappen. Deel 3: Pijn.* Lochem: De Tijdstroom; 1987.

39. Schouten JAM. Anamnese en advies. *De Nederlandse bibliotheek der Geneeskunde.* Alphen a.d. Rijn: Stafleu; 1982.

40. Oostendorp RAB. *Functionele Vertebrobasilaire Insufficiëntie.* Nijmegen: Catholic; 1988. Dissertation.

41. Bogduk N. Cervical causes of headache and dizziness. In: Grieve GP, ed. *Modern Manual Therapy of the Vertebral Column.* Edinburgh: Churchill Livingstone; 1986.

42. Janda V. Some aspects of extracranial causes of facial pain. *J Prosthet Dent.* 1986;56:484–487.

43. Lewit K. *Manuelle Medizin im Rahmen der Medizinischen Rehabilitation.* Leipzig: Joh Ambrosius Barth; 1987.

44. van Cranenburgh B. *Segmentale Verschijnselen.* Utrecht: Bohn, Scheltema & Holkema; 1985.

45. Teirich-Leube H. *Grundriss der Bindegewebsmassage.* Stuttgart: Gustav Fischer Verlag; 1968.

46. Dvorak J. *Manuelle Medizin, Therapie.* Stuttgart: Georg Thieme Verlag; 1986.

47. Steenks MH, Bosman F. Various aspects of intercuspal position. *J Oral Rehabil.* 1988;15:209.

48. Krogh-Poulsen WE. Management of the occlusion of the teeth, part 2: examination, diagnosis, treatment. In: Schwarz L, Chayes CM, eds. *Facial Pain and Mandibular Dysfunction.* Philadelphia: WB Saunders Co; 1968.

49. Solberg WK. Temporomandibular disorders: physical tests in diagnosis. *Br Dent J.* 1986;160:273–277.

50. Frisch H. *Programmierte Untersuchung des Bewegungsapparates.* Berlin: Springer Verlag; 1983.

51. Hagenaars LHA, Dekker LJ, van der Plaats J, Bernards ATM, Oostendorp RAB. Effecten van het orthosympatische zenuwstelsel op de dwarsgestreepte spier. *Ned Tijdschr Fysiother.* 1985; 95:77–78.

52. Friedman MH, Weisberg J. *Temporomandibular Joint Disorders, Diagnosis and Treatment.* Chicago: Quintessence Publishing Co; 1985.

53. Seifert K. Peripherer-vestibulare Schwindel und funktionelle Kopfgelenksstörung. *HNO.* 1987;35:363–371.

54. van der El A, Lunacek P, Wagemaker A. *Manuele therapie, wervelkolom onderzoek.* EWI® Uitgenerij Mankwel: Rotterdam; 1983.

55. Kraus SL. T.M.J. Disorders. *Management of the Craniomandibular Complex.* New York: Churchill Livingstone; 1988:367–405.

56. Rocabado M. Diagnosis and treatment of abnormal craniocervical and craniomandibular mechanics. In: Solber WK, Clark GT, eds. *Abnormal Jaw Mechanics. Diagnosis and Treatment.* Chicago; 1984:141–159.

57. Woodside DG, Linder-Aronson S. The channelization of upper and lower anterior face heights compared to population standard in males between ages 6–20 years. *Eur J Orthod.* 1979;1:25–40.

58. Solow B, Tallgren A. Dentoalveolar morphology in relation to craniocervical posture. *Angle Orthod.* 1977;47:157–164.

59. Trott PH. Passive movements and allied techniques in the management of dental patients. In: Grieve G, ed. *Modern Manual Therapy of the Vertebral Column.* Edinburgh: Churchill Livingstone; 1986:691–700.

60. Duyzings JAC. Dento-maxillaire, faciale, craniale en cervicale orthopedie. *Tijdschr Tandheelkd.* 1959:66,10:695–731.

61. Hoogland R. Elektrotherapie als reflextherapie bij pijn en functiestoornessen van de spier. *Geneeskd Sport.* 1987;2:74–78.

62. Solow B, Siersback-Nielsen S, Greve E. Airway adequacy, head posture and craniofacial morphology. *Am J Orthod.* 1984;86:214–244.

63. Linder-Aronson S. Adenoids: their effect on mode of breathing and nasal airflow and their relationship to characteristics of the facial skeleton and the dentition. *Acta Otolaryngol Suppl.* 1979:265.

64. Solow B, Tallgren A. Head posture and craniofacial morphology. *Am J Phys Anthropol.* 1978;44:417–437.

65. Duinkerke ASH. Biofeedback training en "habit reversal" techniek (gewoonte omdraaiing). *Bull N.V.G.* 1985;3.

66. Carlsson GE. Long-term effects of treatment of craniomandibular disorders. *J Craniomandibular Pract.* 1985;3:337–343.

67. Okeson JP. Long-term treatment of disk-interference disorders of the temporomandibular joint with anterior repositioning occlusal splints. *J Prosthet Dent.* 1988;60:611-616.

SUGGESTED READING

Aufdemkampe G, Meijer OG. Effect-onderzoek in verband met TENS. In: Mattie H, ed. *Pijn Informatorium.* Alphen a/d Rijn: Stafleu Samson; 1986.

Aufdemkampe G, Meijer OG, Winkel D, Witmaar GC. Manuele pijnbenaderingen. In: Mattie H, ed. *Pijn Informatorium.* Alphen a/d Rijn: Stafleu Samson; 1985.

Bakker FC. Relaxatietechnieken in de sport: een overzicht. *Geneeskd Sport IV.* 1987:145–151.

Bernards ATM. Relaties tussen belasting en belastbaarheid. *Issue.* 1988;5(4):1–5.

Bernstein DA, Douglas A, Borkovec D, Thomas D. *Progressive Relaxation Training: A Manual for the Helping Professions.* Champaign, Ill: Research Press, X; 1973.

Besse TC. Pijnbehandeling door middel van elektrostimulatie. *Reeks informatiesgidsen voor de gezondheidszorg.* Utrecht: Medifo, Bohn Scheltema & Holkema; 1987:37–45.

Bonica JJ. In: Pauser G, Gerstenbrand F, Gross D. *Gesichtsschmerz.* Stuttgart: Gustav Fischer Verlag; 1979.

Boomsma A. Dictaact Massage. Postbus 14211, Utrecht: SNHC; 1988.

Chung JM et al. Prolonged inhibition of primate spinothalamic tract cells by peripheral nerve stimulation. *Pain.* 1984;19:259–275.

Eriksson MBE, Schuller H, Sjolund BH. Hazard from transcutaneous nerve stimulators in patients with pacemakers. *Lancet.* 1978;1:1319.

Esposito CJ et al. Alleviation of myofascial pain with ultrasonic therapy. *J Prosthet Dent.* 1984:51:106–108.

Evjenth O, Hamber J. *Muscle Stretching in Manual Therapy: A Clinical Manual.* Sweden: Alfta Rehab I/II, 1984.

Fields HL, Basbaum AJ. Brainstem control of spinal pain-transmission neurons. *Annu Rev Physiol.* 1978; 40:217–248.

Friction JR, Hathaway KM, Bromaghim C. Interdisciplinary management of patients with TMJ and craniofacial pain: characteristics and outcome. *J Craniomandibular Disord.* 1987;1:115–123.

Gutmann G, Vele F. *Das Aufrechte Stehen.* Opladen: Westdeutscher Verlag; 1978.

Hargreaves AS, Wardle JJM. The use of physiotherapy in the treatment of temporomandibular disorders. *Br Dent J.* 1983;155:121–124.

Howson DC. Peripheral neural excitability, implications for transcutaneous electrical nerve stimulation. *Phys Ther.* 1978;12.

Ihalainen U, Perkki K. The effect of transcutaneous nerve stimulation on chronic facial pain. *Proc Finn Dent Soc.* 1978;74:86–90.

Kruithof WM. Psychologisch geschrift. Subfaculty Psychology. Utrecht: Rijks University.

Lundeberg T et al. Pain alleviation by vibratory stimulation. *Pain.* 1984;20:25–44.

McCarroll RS, Hesse JR, Naye M, Yoon CK, Hansson TL. Mandibular border positions and their relationship with peripheral joint mobility. *J Oral Rehabil.* 1987;14:125–131.

Melzack R, Stillwell DM, Fox EJ. Triggerpoints and acupuncture points for pain: correlation and implications. *Pain.* 1977:3:3–23.

Mink RJF, ter Veer HJ, Vorselaars JACT. *Extremiteiten, functie-onderzoek en manuele therapie.* Eindhoven: Educational Foundation of Manual Therapy; 1983.

Mitchell L. *Simple Relaxation: The Physiological Method for Easing Tension.* London: Murray; 1985.

Noordenbos W. Prologue. In: Wall PD, Melzack R, eds. *Textbook of Pain.* Edinburgh: Churchill Livingstone; 1984.

Paris SV. Clinical decision making: orthopaedic physical therapy. In: Wolf SL, ed. *Clinical Decision Making in Physical Therapy.* Philadelphia: FA Davis Co; 1985:215–255.

Patist JA. *Massagetherapie.* Lochem: De Tijdstroom; 1982.

Post D. *De Huisarts en Zijn Hoofdpijnpatiënten.* Alphen a/d Rijn: Stafleu's Wetenschappelijke Uitgeversmaatschappij BV; 1980.

Rubin D. Myofascial triggerpoint syndromes: an approach to management. *Arch Phys Med.* 1981;62:107–111.

Sansiesteban A. The role of physical agents in the treatment of spine pain. *Clin Orthop.* 1983;179:24–30.

Schuldes-van de Pol J. Pijn en pijnbehandeling. In: van Cranenburgh B, den Dekker JB, van Meerwijk GM, Wessel HFM, de Wijer A, eds. *Jaarboek Fysiotherapie.* Utrecht: Bohn, Scheltema & Holkema; 1987.

Taube S, Ylipaavalniemi P, Perkki K, Oikarinen VJ. Side-effects of electrical physiotherapy treatment in the orofacial region. *Proc Finn Dent Soc.* 1983;79:168–171.

Tilscher H, Eder M. *Die Rehabilitation von Wirbelsäulen Gestörten.* Berlin: Springer Verlag; 1983.

Wall PD. The gate control therapy of pain mechanisms: a re-examination and re-statement. *Brain.* 1978;101:1–18.

Wijma K, Duinkerek ASH, Reitsma B. Behandeling van patiënten met somatische fixatie in de tandheelkundige praktijk. *Ned Tijdschr Tandheelkd.* 1987;94:101–104.

Winkel D, Fisher S, Vroege C. *Weke Delen Aandoeningen van het Bewegingsapparaat, Deel 2: Diagnostiek.* Utrecht: Bohn, Scheltema & Holkema; 1984.

Part III

Innervation and Kinematics of the Spinal Column

8

Innervation of the Spinal Column and Its Related Structures

EDITOR'S PREFACE

Classic theories regarding structure and function of the nervous system imply that the nervous system consists of nerve fibers that have a distinct course (eg, from point A to point B). Modern studies show that in the central nervous system, when a nerve fiber runs from point A to point B there is almost always a fiber running from point B back to point A.[1] Therefore, the nervous system is increasingly being represented as a model that is not constructed from individual fibers but rather from a network of fibers. Studies about the function of the spinal cord clearly indicate that oscillating plexuses play an important role in controlling movement.[2] Edelman[3] suggests that the functional development of the central nervous system is seen as a competition between networks (plexuses). Recently, psychological models and research on artificial intelligence are also operating on the assumption of the existence of this network.[4,5]

The following chapter written by Dr. Harry Bour concerns the latest developments in studies on the peripheral innervation of the spinal column and its associated structures. As you will see, Bour also describes the nervous system in the sense of multisegmental networks, or plexuses.

INTRODUCTION

Back pain is a common complaint. Four of every five people suffer from back pain at least once in their lifetimes, either for a short time or for a prolonged period. This back pain often leads to a significant negative influence on the quality of life of the person affected.[6,7] Etiology and prognosis are often unknown and uncertain, while chronic back pain is probably too often seen as purely psychological. In many cases, based on clinical and radiological examination, an accurate cause of the pain can be determined.[8] Therefore, a fundamental knowledge about the nociceptive innervation of the spine and its related structures is necessary. In this chapter, innervation of the spinal structures is described with an emphasis on the deeper-lying tissue.

GENERAL CONSIDERATIONS

Segmental Structure of the Spinal Column and Its Related Structures

Except for the head, the body of the vertebrate in the embryonic stage is divided into a number of segments or somatomes. In humans, the vertebrae, ribs, and intercostal musculature are seen as the residual of this segmental system. This segmental arrangement exclusively concerns tissue derived from the mesoderm, such as myotomes and sclerotomes, and not the tissue from endodermal or ectodermal origin, such as the gastrointestinal tract, the nervous system, or the skin.[9]

The embryonic spinal cord is *not* divided into segments, but instead possesses a distinct longitudinal inner organization. Therefore, the gray matter of the spinal cord is composed of uninterrupted columns of neurons (Rexed's laminae), which have consistent functions at different levels of the body (eg, alpha motor neurons in the anterior horn). The white matter of the spinal cord consists mostly of mixed bundles of myelinated and nonmyelinated nerve fibers (axons), which, at various levels of the spinal cord, leave from or lead to synapses in the gray matter. Entering and exiting the spinal cord along its entire length are small nerve fiber (axon) bundles, the dorsal and ventral rootlets (Figure 8–1). The segmentation ascribed to the spinal cord is based on the bundled organization of spinal rootlets confluencing into spinal nerves that exit the vertebral column through the intervertebral foramen.

It is assumed that the synapses that contribute axons to the spinal nerves lie in the gray matter of the spinal cord at the level where the spinal nerve exits. Thus, there are as many functional segments in the spinal cord as there are spinal nerves. However, at the same time, the spinal cord axons, like peripheral sensory axons, seldom restrict their synaptic contacts to one segmental level. In general, the axons fan out over adjacent segments. With the exception of the cervical area, the spinal cord segment with its exiting spinal nerve is localized above its respective vertebra (Figure 8–2). In its exit from the spinal canal through the intervertebral foramen, the nerve root is still surrounded by the spinal dura mater and the arachnoid. Distal from the spinal ganglion, the dura mater becomes the epineurium and the arachnoid becomes the perineurium.

Sunderland[11] points out the following:

- The intervertebral foramen normally offers ample space for all the neural structures passing through.
- Narrowing of the foramen that occurs during extension of the spine does not compromise the passing neural structures.
- In all movements of the vertebrae, the spinal nerve has adequate space to avoid impingement.
- In the foramen, the spinal nerve complex is surrounded by loose connective tissue and fatty tissue in which the spinal arteries, spinal veins, and the sinuvertebral nerve are embedded.
- Venous obstruction of the blood vessels in the neural complexes can hinder the gliding capabilities of the nerve fibers.

Branches of the Spinal Nerves

Shortly after its exit from the intervertebral foramen, the spinal nerve divides into the following:

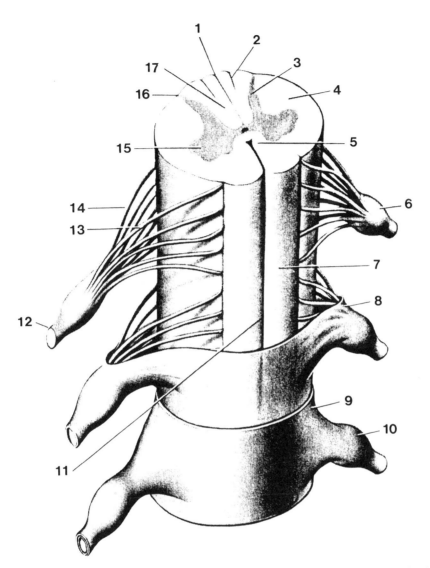

Figure 8–1 The dorsal and ventral rootlets enter and exit the spinal cord along its entire length. Outside the spinal cord they join together to form the spinal nerves, according to Carpenter.[10] *1*, Posterior median septum; *2*, posterior intermediate sulcus; *3*, posterior column; *4*, lateral funiculus; *5*, anterior funiculus; *6*, spinal ganglion; *7*, pia mater; *8*, arachnoid; *9*, dura mater; *10*, dural sleeve; *11*, anterior median fissure; *12*, spinal nerve; *13*, ventral rootlets; *14*, dorsal rootlets; *15*, anterior column; *16*, posterolateral sulcus (entry point for a dorsal root); *17*, posterior funiculus.

- sinuvertebral nerve (recurrent nerve or meningeal nerve)
- dorsal (posterior primary) ramus
- ventral ramus
- white and gray rami communicantes; each has a connection to the para-

vertebral ganglion of the sympathetic trunk (Figure 8–3)

The ventral ramus innervates the ventral trunk musculature, the skin, and the extremities. The dorsal ramus innervates the deep back muscles and the skin from the top of the

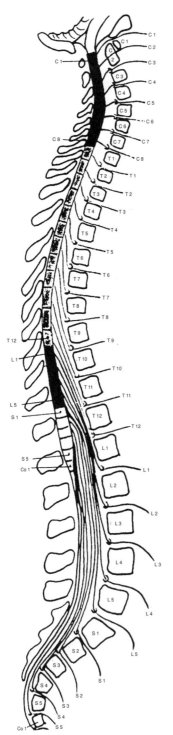

Figure 8–2 Spinal cord segments, spinal nerves, and their corresponding vertebrae.

head, over the dorsal aspect of the trunk to the coccyx. Throughout the back region, a nociceptive system of plexuslike organized nerve fibers and free nerve endings is found. These are located in the skin, the subcutaneous tissue, fasciae, aponeuroses, ligaments, vertebral periosteum, vertebral bodies, blood vessels, fibrous capsules, zygapophyseal joints (except the joint cartilage and synovium), sacroiliac joint, and the intervertebral discs.

Causes of Spinal Pain

Nociceptors are facilitated by mechanical forces that overload, deform, or damage the affected tissue. Furthermore, the various components of this tissue can act as pain-inducing substances, such as lactic acid, potassium ions, plasma kinin, serotonin, prostaglandin, and histamine. These substances are released as a result of trauma, inflammation, necroses, and metabolic disturbances.[12]

The most significant causes of pain in the back region are root irritation, disc degeneration, zygapophseal joint degeneration, and overload of the myofascial elements.[6] Wyke[12] adds to this list referred pain from other regions of the body (eg, urinary tract, prostate, appendix, and the internal female organs).

SPINAL INNERVATION IN DETAIL

The innervation of the spinal column and its surrounding structures comes from the dorsal rami, ventral rami, sinuvertebral nerve (coming from the spinal nerve), communicating rami from the sympathetic trunk, and the perivascular plexus from the vertebral arteries.

Dorsal (Posterior Primary) Ramus

Through a medial branch, the dorsal ramus of each spinal nerve innervates the interspinous muscle and the corresponding ligament. This medial branch has further articu-

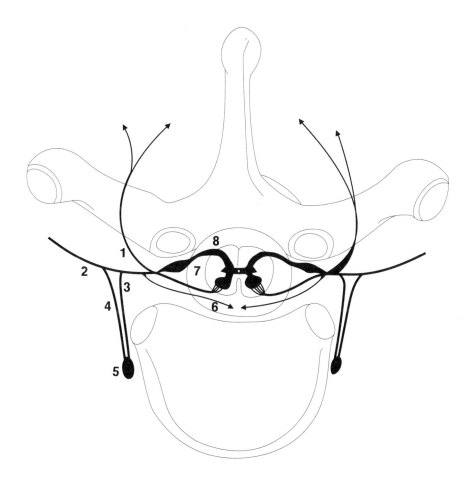

Figure 8–3 Sketch of a segmental spinal nerve and its branches, according to Van der Ende.[6] *1*, Dorsal ramus; *2*, ventral ramus; *3*, white ramus communicans; *4*, gray ramus communicans; *5*, sympathetic ganglion; *6*, sinuvertebral nerve; *7*, ventral root; *8*, dorsal root.

lar branches that supply the vertebral zygapophyseal joint at the level where the spinal nerve exits as well as the zygapophyseal joint one level above and one level below. In the lumbar area and probably also in the other sections, the zygapophyseal joint is innervated by a third branch originating directly from the dorsal ramus.

Moreover, medial branches of the dorsal rami in the lumbar spine supply the sacroiliac joints and the neural arches of the vertebrae (periosteum and fascia). Medial branches of the cervical and upper 10 thoracic dorsal rami project over the back musculature to the skin. Caudal to this level, the skin of the back is innervated through lateral branches of the dorsal rami. From cranial to caudal, the distances between the dermatomes and the originating segments of the corresponding dorsal rami continually increase. The overlapping of the dorsal dermatomes is considerable; four segments innervate the same area of skin.[11,12]

The deep muscles of the back are innervated by the medial, lateral, and—when present—the intermediate branches of the dorsal rami.[11,13]

Ventral Ramus

The ventral rami of the spinal nerves supply the muscles and skin of the ventral and lateral walls of the trunk and the extremities. In the cervical and lumbar regions, the posterolateral aspects of the intervertebral discs are also innervated by the ventral rami through short side branches. There are indications that this is also the case in the thoracic region.[13,14]

Sinuvertebral Nerve

Seen as mixed nerves, the sinuvertebral rami are composed of somatic fibers that originate from the ventral ramus[14] and of sympathetic fibers that originate from the rami communicantes, directly from the sympathetic trunk or from the perivascular plexus of the vertebral artery.[15] The sinuvertebral nerves traverse back through the intervertebral foramen to the spinal canal (Figure 8–3). Several sinuvertebral nerves enter each intervertebral foramen.[15] After entering, the sinuvertebral nerve divides into a long ascending branch, which runs parallel to the posterior longitudinal ligament to the above-lying disc, and into a shorter descending branch, which, at the level of its entry into the spinal canal, innervates the disc and neighboring posterior longitudinal ligament[13,14] (Figure 8–4).

The nerve plexus of the spinal dura mater is also supplied by branches of the sinuvertebral nerve. This innervation occurs exclusively in the lateral and ventral dura mater and in the dural sleeve surrounding the spinal roots. Dorsally, the dura mater has no nerve fibers and therefore is painless during lumbar punctures.

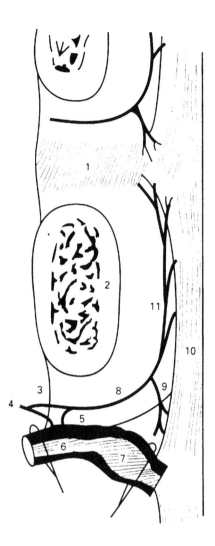

Figure 8–4 Schematic representation of the inside of the vertebral canal. At the level of the uppermost disc, the ventral and dorsal roots and the spinal ganglion are removed so that the disc innervation from both neighboring sinuvertebral nerves can be seen, according to Bogduk.[13] **1**, Disc; **2**, neural arch (cross-section); **3**, autonomic branch; **4**, gray ramus communicans; **5**, somatic branch; **6**, ventral ramus; **7**, spinal ganglion; **8**, sinuvertebral nerve; **9**, descending branch of the sinuvertebral nerve; **10**, posterior longitudinal ligament; **11**, ascending branch of the sinuvertebral nerve.

Sympathetic Trunk

Side branches from the sympathetic trunk and the rami communicantes and branches from the perivascular plexus of the spinal arteries contribute sympathetic fibers to the anterior and posterior longitudinal ligaments, the ventral dura mater, the vertebral bodies, the costovertebral joints, and the discs.

INNERVATION PATTERNS

Anterior Longitudinal Ligament

The nerve plexus of the anterior longitudinal ligament (ALL) is a dense longitudinal network, consisting of a looser structure in the lumbar region. In the thoracic area, this plexus is connected with the plexus from the costovertebral joints. From the plexus of the ALL, radial nerve fibers enter the vertebral body along the blood vessels. At the level of the disc, small branches run in the outermost zone of the annulus fibrosus. The inner zone of the annulus and the nucleus pulposus are not innervated. As described previously, the origin of the ALL nerve plexus comes from three adjacent spinal cord segments.

For a large part, the plexus is composed of nonmyelinated nerve fibers; to a lesser degree, it is composed of thin myelinated nerve fibers. No nociceptive functions are attributed to the ALL nerve plexus. Because the ligament can have a painful irritation at the level of the disc, but not at the level of the vertebral body, it is assumed that nociception possibly may come from the nerves from the disc[15] (Figure 8–5).

Posterior Longitudinal Ligament

The nerve plexus of the posterior longitudinal ligament (PLL) is more loosely organized than the ALL. It contains bilateral side branches from the sinuvertebral nerve (Figure 8–6). Branches from the PLL nerve plexus run to the vertebral structures and the

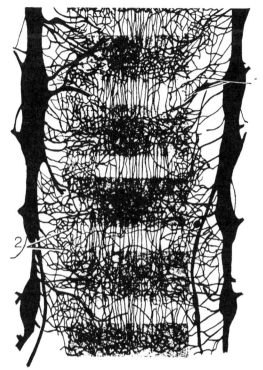

Figure 8–5 Schematic representation of the nerve plexus of the ALL, with the sympathetic trunk on each side, according to Groen.[15] Particularly at the level of the vertebral body (gray rectangle), the plexus receives nerve branches from the sympathetic trunk (**1**) as well as from the plexus innervating the costovertebral joints (**2**).

annulus fibrosus as well as to the epidural blood vessels and the spinal dura mater. Every part of this plexus is innervated from three adjacent spinal segments. The PLL nerve plexus contains not only myelinated and nonmyelinated nerve fibers, but also free nerve endings. Both nociceptive and proprioceptive functions are ascribed to these nerves. Because the PLL is the first structure outside of the annulus fibrosus to be affected by a disc protrusion, it plays an important role in pain elicitation.

Ventrolateral Dura Mater

The ventrolateral dura mater has a dense longitudinal nerve plexus, consisting of side

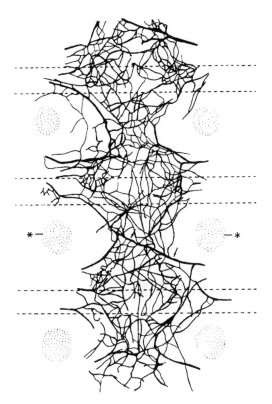

Figure 8–6 Schematic representation of the nerve plexus of the PLL, which is supplied by sinuvertebral nerves entering the spinal canal at the level of the discs (dotted lines), according to Groen.[15] Asterisks indicate position of the neural arch.

branches from the sinuvertebral nerves, the PLL plexus, and the plexus of the radicular branches from the segmental arteries. The branches of this dural plexus can spread out over four segments in either a caudal or a cranial direction. Ventrally, the dural plexus is the most dense; it becomes looser at its lateral aspect and dural sleeve. It contains only non-myelinated fibers with free endings to which nociceptive and vasomotor functions have been ascribed.

Vertebral Body

As previously described, the vertebral body has a radial perivascular innervation from the ALL and PLL nerve plexuses.

Intervertebral Disc

The nerve supply of the disc originates from the ALL and PLL nerve plexuses as well as from two sinuvertebral nerves (see above). In addition, the disc receives side branches from the ventral ramus and branches from the communicating rami[13–15] (Figure 8–7). Functions of nociception and proprioception are attributed to the disc innervation.[14]

Wyke[12] denies disc innervation and postulates that this is present only in the fetal and neonatal stages of development. He argues that the nerves degenerate as soon as children are able to stand erect.

Zygapophyseal Joints

Innervation of the zygapophyseal joint is threefold; it receives a side branch from the medial branch of the dorsal ramus from above and below, as well as a side branch directly from the dorsal ramus. It is assumed that there is an overlapping of three segments per zygapophyseal joint.[8,12] The innervation consists of nonmyelinated and myelinated nerve fibers with free and encapsulated nerve endings, and the function is nociceptive and mechanoreceptive[12] (Figure 8–8).

Neural Arch and Affiliated Structures

The nerve plexuses of the neural arch periosteum, fascia, and the attached aponeurosis

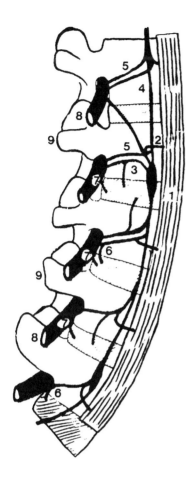

Figure 8–7 Innervation of the outer zone of the lumbar discs, according to Bogduk.[13] *1*, ALL; *2*, branch to the ALL; *3*, branch to the lateral aspect of the disc; *4*, sympathetic trunk; *5*, gray ramus communicans; *6*, side branch of the gray ramus communicans to the disc; *7*, side branch of the ventral ramus to the disc; *8*, ventral ramus; *9*, transverse process.

and tendon are connected with each other. They have a multisegmental innervation from the dorsal rami and are nociceptive and proprioceptive in function.[12]

Sacroiliac Joint

Innervation of the sacroiliac joints is analogous to that of the zygapophyseal joints and includes branches from the medial branch of the dorsal rami. (See Chapter 3, Sacroiliac Joint, section 3.1, Functional Anatomy.)

MULTISEGMENTAL INNERVATION

From the above overview of the innervation of the spinal column and its related structures, it is evident that most of the spinal structures possess a multisegmental innervation. Significant segmental overlapping is found in the spinal dura mater (eight segments), while a threefold innervation is described for the ALL, PLL, and zygapophyseal joints. Thus, identifying a specific segment as the cause of pain is understandably difficult considering the following factors:

- the multisegmental innervation of the spine
- the spatial separation of corresponding structures (eg, lumbar dermatome in relation to its corresponding vertebra)
- the numerous structures, all of which have an innervation through branches of sinuvertebral nerves and dorsal rami[8,15] (Figure 8–9).

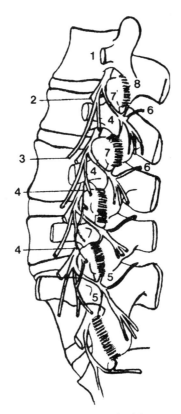

Figure 8–8 Innervation of the zygapophyseal joints. In this representation, the zygapophyseal joint is supplied by two branches from the medial branch of the dorsal ramus from above and below, according to Bogduk.[13] *1*, Transverse process; *2*, ventral ramus; *3*, lateral branch of the dorsal ramus; *4*, intermediate branch; *5*, articular branch; *6*, interspinal side branch; *7*, medial branch of dorsal ramus; *8*, zygapophyseal joint.

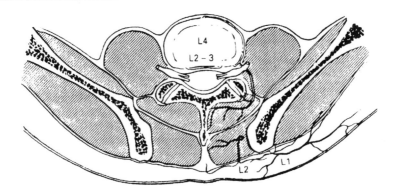

Figure 8–9 Schematic cross section of the spinal column and its associated structures at the level of the fourth lumbar motion segment. Note the complex innervation of the structures. The superficial structures are innervated through L1 and L2. The PLL and the dura mater are innervated through L2 and L3. *Source:* Reprinted from O'Brien, J.P., Mechanics of Spinal Pain, in *Textbook of Pain*, P.D. Wall and R. Melzack, eds., pp. 240–251, with permission of Churchill Livingstone, © 1984.

REFERENCES

1. Crick F, Asanuma C. Certain aspects of the anatomy and physiology of the cerebral cortex. In: McClelland J, Rumelhart DE, PDP Research Group, eds. *Parallel Distributed Processing: Explorations in the Microstructure of Cognition: Psychological and Biological Models.* Cambridge, Mass: MIT Press; 1987; 2.

2. Cohen AH, Rossignol S, Grillner S, eds. *Neural Control of Rhythmic Movements in Vertebrates.* New York: John Wiley & Sons, Inc; 1988.

3. Edelman GM. *Neural Darwinism: The Theory of Neuronal Group Selection.* New York: Basic Books, Inc; 1987.

4. McClelland J, Rumelhart DE, PDP Research Group, eds. *Parallel Distributed Processing: Explorations in the Microstructure of Cognition: Psychological and Biological Models.* Cambridge, Mass: MIT Press; 1987; 2.

5. Rumelhart DE, McClelland J, PDP Research Group, eds. *Parallel Distributed Processing: Explorations in the Microstructure of Cognition: Foundations.* Cambridge, Mass: MIT Press; 1987; 1.

6. Van der Ende N. Degeneratie van facetgewrichten. *Ned Tijdschr Man Ther.* 1986;86:55–57.

7. Wood PMN, Badley EM. Epidemiology of back pain. In: Jayson MIV, ed. *The Lumbar Spine and Back Pain.* 3rd ed. London: Churchill Livingstone; 1987:1–15.

8. O'Brien JP. Mechanisms of spinal pain. In: Wall PD, Melzack R, eds. *Textbook of Pain.* London: Churchill Livingstone; 1984:240–251.

9. Kahle W. *Sesam Atlas van de Anatomie: Zenuwstelsel en Zintuigen.* 4th ed. Baarn: Bosch and Keuning; 1985; 3.

10. Carpenter MB. *Human Neuroanatomy.* 7th ed. Baltimore: Williams & Wilkins; 1976.

11. Sunderland S. The spinal nerves. In: Sunderland S, ed. *Nerves and Nerve Injuries.* 2nd ed. London: Churchill Livingstone; 1978:1021–1031.

12. Wyke B. The neurology of low back pain. In: Jayson MIV, ed. *The Lumbar Spine and Back Pain.* 3rd ed. London: Churchill Livingstone; 1987:56–99.

13. Bogduk N. Innervatie van de wervelkolom. *Ned Tijdschr Man Ther.* 1986;86:50–54. Translated from *Aust J Physiother.* 1985:31–33.

14. Bogduk N. The innervation of the lumbar intervertebral discs. In: Grieve GP, ed. *Modern Manual Therapy of the Vertebral Column.* London: Churchill Livingstone; 1986:146–150.

15. Groen GJ. *Contributions to the Anatomy of the Peripheral Autonomic Nervous System.* Amsterdam: Rodopi; 1986. PhD Dissertation.

SUGGESTED READING

Grieve GP. *Modern Manual Therapy of the Vertebral Column.* London: Churchill Livingstone; 1986.

Noordenbosch W. Prologue. In: Wall PD, Melzack R, eds. *Textbook of Pain.* London: Churchill Livingstone; 1984.

Rothman RH, Simeone FA. *The Spine.* Philadelphia: WB Saunders; 1975.

9

Kinematics of the Spinal Column

EDITOR'S PREFACE

In orthopaedics of the spine, special attention should be given to "kinematic coupling." A kinematic coupling occurs when the motion around one axis (eg, sidebending) forces a motion around another axis (eg, rotation) to occur. Sidebending and rotation are the coupled movements in the spine.

Interpretations of the type and intensity of the coupling vary in the literature. In studying the complex and significant matters of kinematic coupling, several different approaches should be examined. In his dissertation on idiopathic scoliosis and in the following chapter, Dr. Peter Scholten[1] thoroughly addresses this matter.

Between this chapter and the previous "specialized" chapters, terminological as well as factual differences will occur. In this chapter, the direction of an axial rotation is determined by the direction of movement of the spinous process. However, in the previous specialized chapters rotations are named according to the movement direction of the vertebral body.

Obviously this is a difference in terminology. An example of a factual difference can be noted in the description of the coupling during extension in the lower thoracic and lumbar levels. This chapter deals exclusively with the spinal column and purposely does not take the pelvic rotations into consideration. Differences between this chapter and the previous specialized chapters result because pelvic rotations can be superimposed on the coupling in the lower thoracic and lumbar spines. Perhaps there is a connection between this and the important role that the guidance of the pelvic rotation plays in controlling specific movements.[2]

INTRODUCTION

Kinematics are involved with the movements of a system without concern for what causes these movements. Movement of the spinal column can occur either passively by outside forces or actively through the muscles. Seen kinematically, each vertebra has six degrees of freedom: three rotations around and three translations along a transverse, sagittal, or longitudinal axis. Normative data for the amount of movement are unavailable because the amplitude of movement varies with age and is also subject to individual differences.

The movement of the various segments is not the same at every level. Every movement of the spinal column represents a united action of several motion segments in which the various degrees of freedom are more or less coupled together. One speaks of a "kinematic coupling" when the three translatory and the three rotatory motions cannot be performed independently of each another. Particularly obvious in this sense is the sidebending of the spinal column; an axial rotation accompanies the sidebending.

During sidebending of the cervical and upper thoracic segments, a rotation occurs in which the spinous processes turn to the convex side. In other words, during right sidebending the spinous processes turn to the left, and vice versa. This takes place in flexion as well as in extension.

In the lower thoracic region, behavior during flexion is the same as that in the higher segments except that the axial rotation is much less pronounced. Disagreement is noted in descriptions of the kinematic coupling of the lower thoracic spine in an extended position. Feiss,[3] Novogradsky,[4] and Arkin[5] found that the spinous processes rotated to the concave side of the spinal column during sidebending, while Lovett[6] and Gregerson and Lucas[7] state that the vertebrae rotate to the convex side.

The lumbar spine shows the same tendencies as the lower thoracic spine in the flexed position. During sidebending in the extended position, the spinous processes rotate to the concave side. However, Rolander[8] and White and Panjabi[9] have established that the amount of axial rotation is significantly less.

The fact that kinematic coupling during sidebending is not precisely described demonstrates that several factors are working simultaneously, which could bring about the opposite effect. Furthermore, the applied concepts are not always clearly defined in the literature. To a great extent, two main factors determine the kinematic coupling: (1) the form of the spinal column and (2) the position of the zygapophyseal joints. Not taken into account is the influence of the pelvic rotation.

INFLUENCE OF THE FORM OF THE SPINAL COLUMN

The spinal column can be divided in various ways. The classification into cervical, thoracic, and lumbar segments is related to the curvature of the spinal column in the sagittal plane. Its cervical and lumbar curves are lordotic (ventrally convex), and the thoracic curve is kyphotic (dorsally convex). The spinal column can also be classified based on the curvatures in the transverse plane. In the upright position, vertebrae C1 to T6 and L3 to L5 are *proclive*, in other words they have a ventral tilt. On the other hand, vertebrae T7 to L2 are *declive*, meaning they are tilted dorsally (Figure 9–1).

To demonstrate that the form of the spinal column can have an opposite influence on the kinematic coupling, a model dealing exclusively with the form of the spinal column is used. This model begins with a homogeneous cylindrical bar. First, the basic properties of the bar are depicted; then, to bring it closer to an anatomical reality, new characteristics are added. Incorporation of the zygapophyseal joints is dealt with in a later section.

Homogeneous Cylindrical Bar

Consider the spinal column as a homogeneous cylindrical bar that stands vertically on a horizontal surface (Figure 9–2). A shearing force acts upon the bar, creating a bending moment. This moment is equal to the product of force (F) and distance (l) to the projected line of force. The moment works on a horizontal axis, which lies perpendicular to the projected line of force.

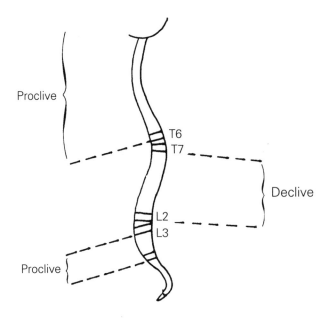

Figure 9–1 Classification according to the inclination of the vertebrae.

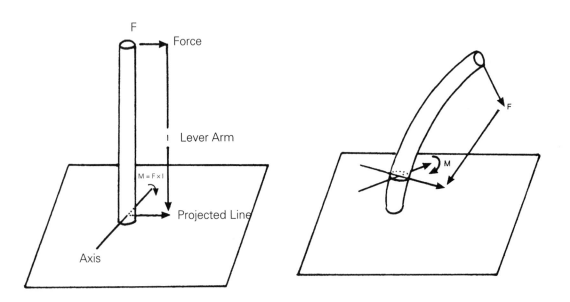

Figure 9–2 Loading of the vertebral column by a force *F* and the corresponding moment *M*: $M = F \times l$.

Figure 9–3 The direction of the axis around which the bending takes place in a bent bar.

Because of the bending moment, the bar bends. The bend in the bar always occurs around the axis that gives the least resistance. In a homogeneous cylindrical bar, this axis and the axis around which the bending moment occurs are the same. The axis lies in the perpendicular cross-sectional plane of the bar.

The same is true for a bent bar, although in this instance the perpendicular cross-section for every point of the bar must be considered. The axis around which the bending takes place lies (for every point, respectively) in the plane with the smallest cross-section. The direction of this plane is determined by the form of the bent bar (Figure 9–3).

Every voluntary translation or rotation can always be divided into two translations or rotations that are perpendicular to each other. Because bending is a rotatory movement, this rotation around one axis that lies in the plane with the smallest cross-section can be divided into two rotatory components that are perpendicular to each other. For the spinal col-

umn as a homogeneous bar, that means that the proclive part of the bar performs a negative axial rotation during sidebending. A negative axial rotation is defined here as a movement in which the spinous process rotates to the convex side. In the declive vertebrae, a positive rotation takes place: the spinous processes turn toward the concave side of the sidebent spinal column (Figure 9–4).

Heterogeneous Cylindrical Bar

If one views the spinal column as a heterogeneous cylindrical bar, the motion axis does not always lie in the plane with the smallest cross-section. (Heterogeneity is determined by the position, form, and physical properties of the structures associated with the motion segment.)

Suppose that a shearing force acts upon the bar (Figure 9–5). In this bar, the shearing force leads to two types of stress and subsequently to two types of deformation. First, a

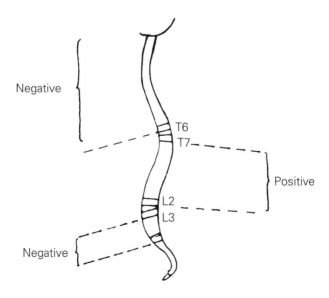

Figure 9–4 Direction of the axial rotation during sidebending (spinal column as a homogeneous bar).

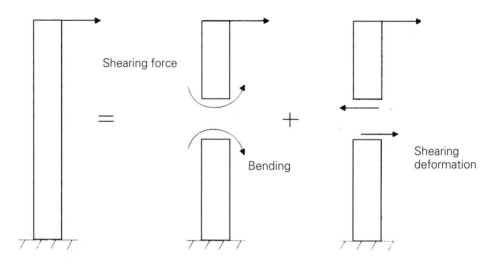

Figure 9–5 Bending and shifting of a heterogeneous bar as a result of a shearing force.

bending moment occurs, causing the bar to bend. The bending axis of this moment lies in the plane with the smallest cross-section. Second, the shearing force acting from the outside causes a shear stress at every level. Depending on the form of the cross-section, it is the shear stress that could cause a deviated movement pattern. This shear stress can be so distributed in the cross-section that a torsion occurs along with the shearing deformation, which means a twisting under the influence of opposite forces.

If the shearing force acts upon the center of gravity of the cross-section but does not act parallel to the cross-section's plane of symmetry, an asymmetrical distribution of the shearing force occurs in the cross-section, leading to a torsion of the bar. In a cylindrical bar, a symmetrical distribution of the shear stress always occurs because there are infinite numbers of symmetrical planes. In reality, however, the spinal column is not a cylindrical bar. Thus, remaining faithful to reality, the ellipsoid-shaped section through a vertebral body with all its related ligaments and muscles as the cross-section is considered. In general, these connected or associated structures lie symmetrically in relation to the median plane, although not in relation to the

frontal plane, which is the plane in which the sidebending takes place (Figure 9–6). For the spinal column, this means that the movement created by a force in the median plane (plane of symmetry) is a pure forward-backward flexion-extension motion. Therefore, flexion or extension of the spinal column can be performed as a rotatory motion.

In general, if the force does not act in the plane of symmetry, then besides a rotation around the bending axis, an axial rotation (torsion) of the spinal column also occurs. In other words, the sidebending cannot be performed as a simple rotational movement. Instead, it is a rotation around a sagittal axis (sidebend) in combination with a rotation around a longitudinal axis (axial rotation or torsion).

However, this does not apply when the force creating the torque moment goes through the point in which the shear stresses are in balance. This point is called the *shearing force middle point*. No torsion occurs when the shearing force acts on this point. Because of the great anatomical variety, both in the location of the associated elements of the motion segment and in the form of the vertebral body, this exception is of minor significance in clinical orthopaedics. For now,

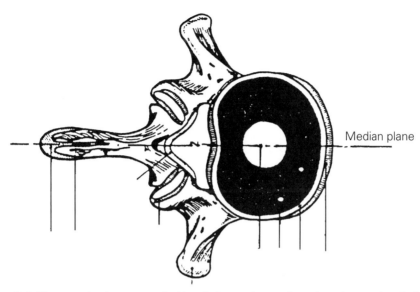

Figure 9–6 The vertebra is symmetrical in relation to the median plane, but not in relation to the frontal plane.

the conclusion that sidebending, unlike flexion and extension, cannot be performed as a pure rotation holds true.

Viewing the spinal column morphology on the basis of the above model, without taking the zygapophyseal joints into account, requires further refinements in the kinematic coupling between sidebending and axial rotation. These refinements can be achieved through the use of a computer model[1] (Figure 9–7).

From Figure 9–7, it follows that the spinous processes of the first eight to nine thoracic vertebrae turn to the convex side during sidebending. In comparison with the behavior of the spine in vivo, the findings in the lower thoracic and lumbar spines need no further confirmation. However, the joint surfaces of the motion segments at the level of the lower thoracic and lumbar spines cause a decrease or even a reversal of the axial rotation during sidebending.

Preliminary Conclusions

For the time being, viewing the spinal column as a cylindrical bar facilitates under-

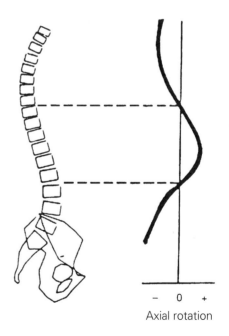

Figure 9–7 Direction of the axial rotation during sidebending of the thoracic spine and the lumbar spine on the basis of a detailed computer model of the spinal column.

standing of the coupling between side-bending and axial rotation. Differences in the behavior of the coupling observed in practice can be caused by existing morphological variations in the spinal column.

Sidebending at the level of the thoracic spine can be induced through a shearing force (this is a passive sidebending). Relatively seen, the bending moment produced diminishes in a caudal direction along the spinal column. Because the shearing force can produce an asymmetrical distribution of shearing stress, the influence of morphological variation on the coupling behavior diminishes in a caudal direction along the spinal column. Since the resulting torsion depends on the asymmetrical distribution of the shearing force, the force introduced—the handgrip to perform the motion—can be of great influence. The fact that the position of the motion segment can influence the axial rotation also accounts for the fact that the initial position of the spine is of great importance in an examination for mobility.

INFLUENCE OF THE POSITION OF THE ZYGAPOPHYSEAL JOINTS

To analyze the influence of the position of the zygapophyseal joints on the kinematic

coupling between sidebending and axial rotation, a computer is again used. In this model, the zygapophyseal joints are described as structures that offer resistance against compression and bending. Because these structures do not give resistance against shearing forces and torsion, they perform a translation and/or axial rotation in relation to each other.

The surfaces of the zygapophyseal joints are not flat at every level of the spinal column. In the computer model, the influence of the forms of the joint surfaces are taken into consideration in the form of a stiffness coefficient.

By using a model of the motion segment (two adjacent vertebrae with their associated structures) and varying the position of the element describing the zygapophyseal joint, the influence on the kinematic coupling can be determined. Thus, it is possible to analyze the influence of the zygapophyseal joints of a motion segment for each level of the spine.

Position of the Zygapophyseal Joints

The position of the zygapophyseal joints is described by means of two parameters. In Figure 9–8, parameter δ_1 (delta 1) reflects the position in relation to the transverse plane

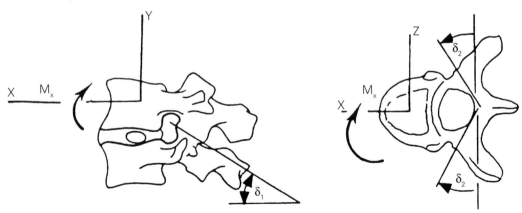

Figure 9–8 Position of the joint facet of the zygapophyseal joints as illustrated by parameter δ_1 in relation to the transverse plane and by parameter δ_2 in relation to the frontal plane.

and parameter δ_2 (delta 2) reflects the position in relation to the frontal plane.

For a normal spinal column, White and Panjabi[9] give a representative value ranging from 45° in the upper thoracic area to 90° at the lumbar level. The value of δ_2 varies from 20° in the upper thoracic region to $-45°$ at the lumbar level. There is a wide range of variation in these values[1] (Figure 9–9).

A load in the form of a pure lateral moment of 10 Newton meters (Nm) is applied on the uppermost vertebra of the motion segment. Due to the function of the zygapophyseal joint position, the response to this moment is defined as a sidebending followed by an accompanying (coupled) axial rotation. First, the δ_1 parameter is varied from 0° to 90° while the δ_2 parameter is kept at 0°. This value is representative of the position of the thoracic vertebral zygapophyseal joints (Figure 9–9). Parameter δ_2 is then varied from 45° to $-45°$, while parameter δ_1 is kept at 90°. This last value is representative of the position of the joint surfaces of the lower thoracic and lumbar vertebrae (Figure 9–9).

Influence of the Angle to the Transverse Plane

Figure 9–10 shows the results of the first computation. The sidebending is indicated by α, the axial rotation by β. These values (α and β) are put along the horizontal axis and parameter δ_1 is placed on the vertical axis. As shown in the figure, with an increase in the angle δ_1, the sidebending (α) increases. This means that an increase in δ_1, which is an increase in the vertical position of the joint surfaces, allows easier performance of sidebending. The resistance against sidebending, due to the position of the zygapophyseal joints, becomes less. When $\delta_1 = 90°$, the zygapophyseal joints no longer offer resistance and sidebending is maximal. This given value is found mostly in the lower thoracic and lumbar regions. At the same time, Figure 9–10 shows that an increase in the angle δ_1, up to a position of

the zygapophyseal joints to an angle of 45°, also leads to an increase in the axial rotation, β. Hereafter, axial rotation again decreases. The direction of the axial rotation is such that the spinous process turns into the direction of the convex side (negative rotation).

In order to represent clearly the coupling between sidebending and axial rotation, the ratio between each motion is displayed in Figure 9–11. The vertical axis δ_1 represents the position of the joint surface. The relation of the axial rotation is represented along the horizontal axis. In relation to sidebending, a relative increase of axial rotation takes place with an increase of the angle δ_1 of the zygapophyseal joint up to approximately 20°. After 20°, a decrease of this coupling occurs. However, under normal circumstances only the area from 45° to 90° is physiologically relevant.

Influence of the Angle in the Frontal Plane

Figure 9–12 describes the influence of the inclination angle δ_2 in relation to the frontal plane. This parameter is represented along the vertical axis, whereby sidebending (α) and axial rotation (β) are represented along the horizontal axis. In an increase of the absolute value of δ_2, a decrease of sidebending takes place. The zygapophyseal joints offer an increasing resistance to sidebending. The value $\delta_2 = 0°$ is in accordance with the position $\delta_1 = 90°$, a position in which the zygapophyseal joints offer no resistance to sidebending. Furthermore, it can be concluded that the coupling with axial rotation, represented by the angle β, is negligibly small with a change in positioning of the zygapophyseal joints around the vertical axis.

RESULTING KINEMATIC COUPLING

When the influence of the form of the spinal column as well as the influence of the posi-

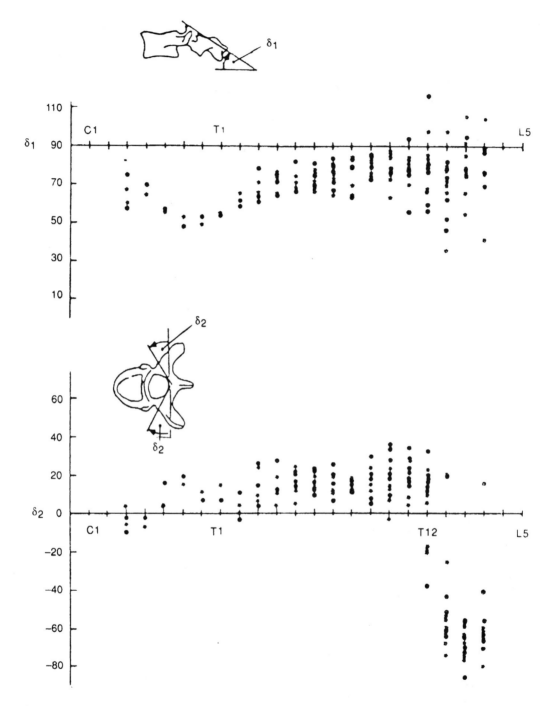

Figure 9–9 The orientation of the joint facets of 100 vertebrae from different spinal columns. Parameter δ_1 indicates the angle with respect to the transverse plane, δ_2 indicates the angle with respect to the frontal plane, according to Scholten.[1] *Source:* Reprinted from *Idiopathic Scoliosis: Some Fundamental Aspects of the Mechanical Behavior of the Human Spine* by P. Scholten with permission of the Free University Press, © 1986.

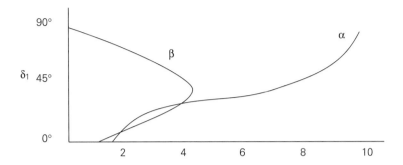

Figure 9–10 The relation between sidebending (α) and axial rotation (β) as a function of the angle δ_1 (with respect to the transverse plane), according to Scholten.[1] *Source:* Reprinted from *Idiopathic Scoliosis: Some Fundamental Aspects of the Mechanical Behavior of the Human Spine* by P. Scholten with permission of the Free University Press, © 1986.

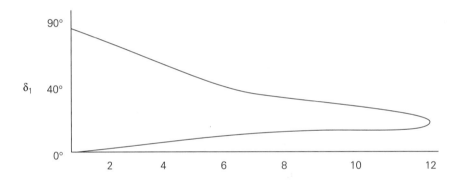

Figure 9–11 The ratio, axial rotation divided by the sidebending, as a function of the inclination angle δ_1 in relation to the transverse plane, according to Scholten.[1]

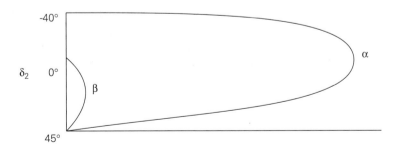

Figure 9–12 The relation between the sidebending (α) and axial rotation (β) as a function of the angle δ_1 (in relation to the frontal plane), according to Scholten.[1]

tions of the zygapophyseal joints between sidebending and axial rotation are taken into consideration, the following conclusion can be drawn. Because of the position of the zygapophyseal joints, an axial rotation of the spinal column takes place during side-bending. The positions of the zygapophyseal joints have an increasing angle of inclination from cranial to caudal, from $\delta_1 = 45°$ to $\delta_1 = 90°$. Figure 9–10 indicates a decrease of the axial rotation from cranial to caudal during sidebending. In the upper thoracic region, the axial rotation is reinforced by the proclive position of the vertebrae. Extending this part of the spinal column prevents the occurrence of too much axial rotation. Vercauteren[10] mentions a "stabilizing" or "neutralizing" function of the proclive vertebrae.

In the lower thoracic and upper lumbar regions, the axial rotation occurring during sidebending is countered by the declive position of the vertebrae. Flexing the spinal column in this area results in less resistance against the axial rotation. Thus the amount of axial rotation increases.

In biomechanical literature, there is no agreement concerning the coupling between sidebending and axial rotation in the lower thoracic spine during extension. The opposite effect of the form of the spinal column, and the positions of the zygapophyseal joints, on the coupling is explained as follows. If the effect of the form of the spinal column is of the same magnitude as the effect of the position of the zygapophyseal joints, the occurring axial rotation will ultimately be positive, negative, or practically zero, depending upon the flexion/extension of the spinal column.

In flexion of the spinal column, the declive vertebrae become proclive vertebrae. Thus,

Table 9–1 Direction of the Axial Rotation of the Spinal Column during Sidebending in Extension and Flexion, Influenced by the Form of the Spinal Column (Left of the Slash) and the Position of the Zygapophyseal Joints (Right of the Slash)

Level	Extension	Flexion
T1	– / – – – –	– / – – – –
|	+ / – – –	– / – – –
|	+ / – –	– / – –
L5	– / –	– / –

the behavior of the vertebrae in axial rotation alters. Instead of opposing each other, the sidebending and the axial rotation will now work together. During sidebending, the spinous processes turn to the convex side, just as in the upper region. Therefore, in flexion of the spinal column, the coupling between sidebending and axial rotation is obvious.

In the lower lumbar region of the spinal column, the axial rotation is reinforced by the proclive position of the vertebrae. This axial rotation is very small as a result of the almost vertical position of the zygapophyseal joints.

In Table 9–1, the direction of the axial rotation during sidebending of the spinal column in extension and flexion is represented. The influence of the pelvis was left out of consideration. A minus sign signifies an axial rotation of the spinous process to the convex side of the lateral curvature of the spinal column. A plus sign denotes a rotation to the concave side. The sign before the slash refers to the influence of the form of the spinal column, while the sign after the slash refers to the influence of the orientation of the zyga-pophyseal joints.

REFERENCES

1. Scholten P. *Idiopathic Scoliosis: Some Fundamental Aspects of the Mechanical Behavior of the Human Spine.* Amsterdam: Free University Press; 1986. Thesis.

2. Wagenaar RC, Beek WJ. Hemiplegic gait: a kinematic analysis of using walking speed as a basis. *J Biomech.* 1992;25(9):1007–1015.

3. Feiss HO. The mechanism of lateral curvature. *Am J Orthop Surg.* 1908;5:152.

4. Novogradsky M. *Die Bewegungsmöglichkeit in der Menschlichen Wirbelsäule.* Bern; 1911. Thesis.

5. Arkin, AM. The mechanism of rotation in combination with lateral deviation in normal man. *J Bone Joint Surg [Am].* 1950;58:180–188.

6. Lovett RW. *Lateral Curvature of the Spine and Round Shoulders.* Philadelphia: Blakiston; 1907.

7. Gregerson GG, Lucas DB. An in vivo study of the axial rotation of the human thoracolumbar spine. *J Bone Joint Surg [Am].* 1967;49:247–262.

8. Rolander SD. *Motion of the Lumbar Spine with Special Reference to the Stabilizing Effect of Posterior Fusion.* Gothenburg: University of Gothenburg Department of Orthopaedic Surgery; 1966. Thesis.

9. White AJ, Panjabi MM. *Clinical Biomechanics of the Spine.* Philadelphia: JB Lippincott Co; 1978.

10. Vercauteren M. *Dorso-lumbale Curven Distributie en Etiopathogenie van de Scoliosis Adolescentium.* Gent: University of Gent; 1980. Thesis.

10

Stability of the Spinal Column

EDITOR'S PREFACE

In the classical sciences, linear models are normally used to explain processes of change. In the linear theory, a doubling of the cause results in a doubling of the effect. The stability theory is an area where linear models obviously do not work. "Instability" occurs when a small cause results in a much larger consequence. Moreover, once this small cause has its onset, the situation changes: the system either collapses or resists further deformation. Thus, these are systems that, at least partially, change (or are changeable) as a function of themselves. Therefore, these systems must be described with the use of nonlinear models.[1]

In the following chapter by Peter Scholten, a linear model describing the stability of the spinal column is presented initially. The limitations of such a model are clarified, and then a nonlinear theory is presented with a simple mathematical analysis.[2]

Without muscles, ligaments, and the thorax, the spinal column is considerably less stable than the intact living spinal column. From the mechanical point of view, the spinal column is less stable in the sagittal plane than in the frontal plane. However, this nor-mally is not accompanied by a clinical instability. From the moment that a force leads to a deformation ("kinking" or bending) of the spinal column, the bending stress increases and counters further deformation. However, local changes of the properties of the material can lead to considerable deformability, which, here also, is not always accompanied by a clinical instability.

INTRODUCTION

Stability can be defined in clinical, anatomical, or biomechanical terms. Biomechanical stability is not the same as clinical or anatomical stability. One speaks of *clinical stability* when a physiological movement or physiological range of motion occurs in reaction to a physiological "nonextreme" load. Symptoms do not accompany this condition. This situation can also be caused by nonmechanical processes. In this instance, there is a diminished or nonoptimal effect of the physiological adapting mechanism. *Anatomical stability* is based on morphometric parameters and does not involve the physiological adaption mechanism. Anatomical stability of a joint can be described as a measure of the motion in that joint. A joint in a close-packed position is in a stable position. Owing to the compression through the surrounding structures, the motion is decreased. Both clinical stability and anatomical stability are more or less qualitative properties, in contrast to mechanical stability.

Mechanical stability, or a mechanically stable position, is a position in which a distinct relation exists between this position and the forces that are necessary for maintaining the position. If there is a large displacement or change in position as the result of a small change in the applied force, one speaks of an unstable position. An example of an unstable position is illustrated in Figure 10–1. A motion segment of the spinal column, without ligaments and muscles, and in which the nucleus pulposus is seen as a ball, has too many degrees of freedom. It is biomechanically unstable. A motion segment with ligaments that hang limply in the neutral position is, within limited terms, unstable. A motion segment in which the ligaments are completely taut is biomechanically stable, but can be clinically unstable.

BENDING THE SPINAL COLUMN AS A ROD

The spinal column can be described as a narrow, straight rod. (One speaks of a narrow

rod because the length is much greater than the cross-section.) If a similar rod is loaded with a compressive force, such as illustrated in Figure 10–2, beyond a certain amount of force the rod suddenly bends or "kinks." An unstable situation occurs. The force required to cause this bending effect is called the bending force or the critical point.

The bending force, P_k, is dependent on the length of the rod, the manner in which the rod is supported, and the bending stiffness, EI. The bending stiffness is dependent on the elasticity module, E, which in turn depends on the material properties and the surface inertia moment of the cross-section (thus, the shape of the cross-section).

The bending force is represented by Euler's bending formula.[2] For a rod that is fixed at one end, the critical point, P_k, is

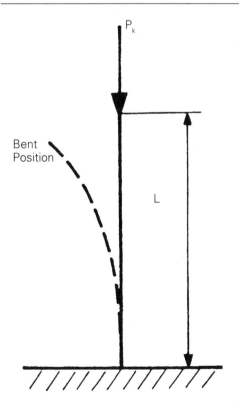

Figure 10–2 The bending of a straight rod, with length, *L*, upon which the bending force, P_k, acts.

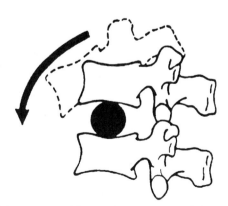

Figure 10–1 The motion segment of the spinal column as an unstable system.

$$P_k = \pi^2 \quad \frac{EI}{4L^2}$$

From this formula, the bending force—or maximally borne load—is determined in large part by the length of the spinal column. The bending force is inversely proportional to the length (L) squared, and is directly proportional to the bending stiffness (EI).

In experiments on cadavers, Lucas and Bresler[3] found a bending force of 20 Newtons (N) on a spinal column without thorax and muscles. This would lead to the conclusion that the spinal column cannot even carry its own weight. However, in vivo the spinal column resists a load much higher that 20 N. This is possible because the bending stiffness of the trunk is determined not only by the mechanical behavior of the spinal column but also by the thorax, the muscles, the abdominal pressure, and the other soft tissue structures. In addition, by contracting the back and abdominal muscles, an extra stiffness is added to the trunk, thus compensating for external load. In their research, Lucas and Bresler[3] initially simulated the body weight by introducing a force that was concentrated at the end of the spinal column. In reality, the weight of the trunk is a load distributed along the entire spinal column. Because of this even distribution of the load, the force under which a bend would occur is twice the initially determined bending force: 2×20 N = 40 N.

With the help of a mathematical model, Andriachi et al[4] demonstrated that the spinal column with thorax has approximately a four times higher bending stiffness than a spinal column without thorax. In another experimental study,[2] the bending stiffness of the trunk in vivo was found to be 10 times that of the isolated spinal column. This means that the spinal column, itself, contributes a minimal amount to the bending stiffness of the trunk. The intact trunk can withstand a load of at least 10×40 N = 400 N before bending.

Euler's bending formula applies only to narrow, straight rods, in which the behavior is assumed to be linear. This means that there must be a linear relationship between the load and the resulting deformation. However, this is not the case when considering the spinal column in the sagittal plane. Because the spinal column is curved in the sagittal plane, if the theoretically calculated bending force is applied to the spinal column, then at part of the spinal column a moment acts in the sagittal plane. In reaction to this moment, a bending in the sagittal plane occurs.

When the bending in the sagittal plane is minimal, the upper vertebrae undergo an almost horizontal forward shift. Because the bending is a rotatory movement, as the bending increases, the shift in a vertical direction increases and the shift in the horizontal direction decreases. This statement implies that there is a nonlinear relation between the load and deviation. In mechanics, the bending force calculated in the bending formula of Euler is defined as the "initial bending force." This is the force that is necessary to bend a rod from an unloaded state. However, Euler's bending formula does not offer any information about the stability of the rod once it has been bent.

INFLUENCE OF THE FORM OF THE SPINAL COLUMN ON STABILITY

Because Euler's bending formula can be applied only to straight rods, it cannot be used to analyze the influence that the form of the spinal column has on stability. This problem is solved by considering the spinal column to be constructed from a large number of small, straight rods, corresponding to the number of motion segments. In this way, a model of the spinal column is composed, with the necessary information about form and position of the motion segments obtained with the help of X-rays. The stability of this system can be determined by looking at the potential energy. Without going further into the mathematical approach, the results of this analysis are discussed.[2]

In Figure 10–3, various forms of the thoracic and lumbar regions of the spinal column are illustrated. The influence of different curves on stability are expressed with regard to stability of the straight rod. The force needed to bend the straight rod is posed as 100%. This force is the initial bending force.

Using calculations from a mathematical model, an increase in lordotic and kyphotic curves results in a decrease in stability (see Figure 10–4). Thus for the spinal column, the stability in the frontal plane, where the spinal column is almost straight, is greater than the stability in the sagittal plane.

In the scoliotic spinal column, curves lie in the frontal plane. Based on the bending theory described above, this means that a scoliotic spinal column cannot be considered to be a bent rod. In instances of a scoliosis,

factors other than mechanical instability play a role.

For a normal, physiologically curved spinal column, the bending force amounts to only 60% of the bending force of the straight rod. This is in contrast to various authorities who have postulated that the stability should increase with the square of the number of curves.[5-7] However, the data from Figure 10–4 apply only for small deviations of the spinal column or for bending in a nonloaded situation.

STABILITY OF THE SPINAL COLUMN IN LARGE DEVIATIONS

Before discussing the stability of the spinal column in large deviations, the stability be-

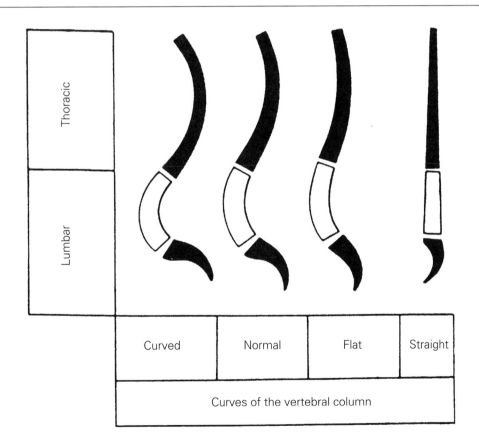

Figure 10–3 Various forms of the spinal column.

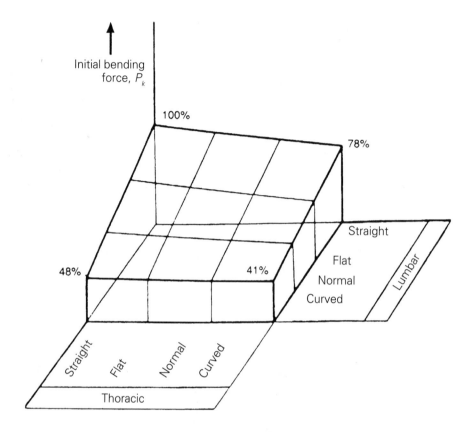

Figure 10–4 The initial bending force as a function of the form of the spinal column.

havior of a straight rod, after bringing it into an unstable situation, is described. This description is based on the nonlinear elasticity theory.[2]

When loading a straight rod just above the bending force, the rod bends. Because of the bend, the rod comes under tension, by which its stiffness increases. In considering the behavior, it can be demonstrated that there is an instability only within a small area. In a larger deviation, due to the applied load, the rod comes into a stable situation again. To bring the rod from this position, again into an unstable situation, the load on the rod has to be increased. This is illustrated in Figure 10–5: in mechanics this is termed the "after-bend effect." As indicated in Figure 10–5, the stabil-ity increases again after the rod is approximately 10% deformed. Apparently the deformation of the rod has a favorable effect with regard to the stability.

Because of its physiological curves in the sagittal plane, it takes only a small load to bend the spinal column. In the spinal column, this deformation increases relatively quickly, without the occurrence of an instability.

From the nonlinear theory (as well as in the linear theory, ie, Euler's bending formula), the chance for a mechanical instability of the spinal column in the frontal plane is smaller than it is in the sagittal plane, where the spinal column has lordotic and kyphotic curves. In a scoliotic spinal column, in which the form of the spinal column is similar to a bent rod, the

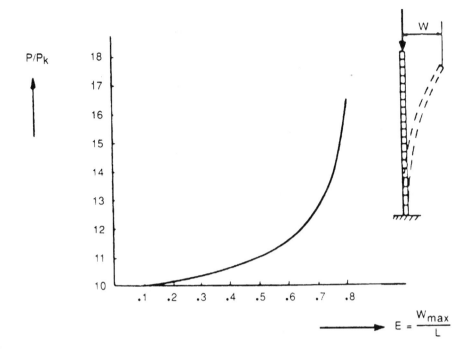

Figure 10–5 The "after-bend effect" of a rod. Horizontal axis: the maximal deformation of the bar, W_{max}, divided by the length, L. Vertical axis: the load, P, divided by the initial bending force, P_k (or critical point, which means the load whereby the rod first comes into an unstable situation).

form is favorable in relation to the mechanical stability.

A summary is illustrated in Figure 10–6: the vertical axis indicates the bending force and the horizontal axis indicates maximal deformation of the rod—one for a straight rod (spinal column in the frontal plane) and one for a curved rod (the spinal column in the sagittal plane). In both situations, the result obtained from the linear theory, as well as from the nonlinear theory, is given.

STABILITY OF THE SPINAL COLUMN IN CHANGING MATERIAL PROPERTIES

The logical step now is to study the stability behavior of a spinal column in which the properties of the material are changed in such a way that the spinal column offers less re-

sistance to bending. This effect is simple to calculate with a mathematical model of the spinal column. In Figure 10–7, the elasticity module, E, lies on the horizontal axis and a measure for the stability, λ, lies on the vertical axis. Instability occurs when $\lambda = 1.$[2]

The results are based on a normally physiologically curved spinal column with its own body weight as a load. It appears that in varying the material properties, a biomechanical instability does not occur. When the value for E is low, the spinal column offers little resistance against bending, and thus deforms significantly. In a large deformation, the compressive load changes into a tensile load.

In this analysis, the elasticity module, E, changes equally along the entire spinal column. In a local reduction of the elasticity, E, a large local deformation occurs (see Figure 10–8). However, the behavior of the spinal

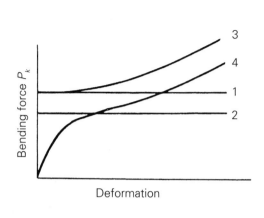

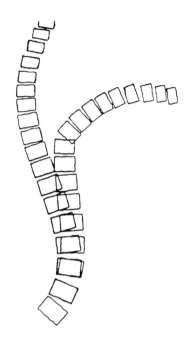

Figure 10–6 The bending force as a function of the deviation of a rod. *1*, Bending force on a straight rod based on the linear theory; *2*, bending force on a curved rod based on the linear theory; *3*, bending force on a straight rod based on the nonlinear theory; *4*, bending force on a curved rod based on the nonlinear theory.

Figure 10–8 The bending pattern of the spinal column with a local weakening.

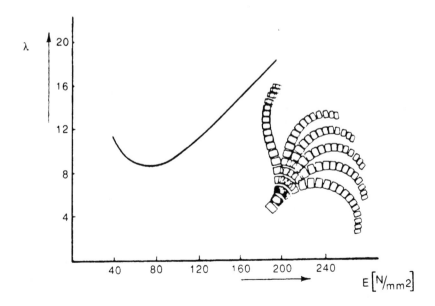

Figure 10–7 The influence of the elasticity module, *E*, on the stability, λ, of the spinal column.

column remains stable, even with a very low value for E. Of course, an exception to this is when $E = 0$. There is no longer a bond between two adjacent vertebrae, and the system has one degree of freedom too much.

However, this is not a realistic situation. With a high value for E, there is little deformation of the spinal column; but, because of the large bending stiffness, biomechanical instability is also prevented here.

REFERENCES

1. Meijer OG. *The Hierarchy Debate: Preliminaries for a Theory and History of Movement Science.* Amsterdam: Free University Press; 1988. Thesis.

2. Scholten P. *Idiopathic Scoliosis: Some Fundamental Aspects of the Mechanical Behavior of the Human Spine.* Amsterdam: Free University Press; 1986. Thesis.

3. Lucas DB, Bresler B. *Stability of the Ligamentous Spine.* San Francisco: Biomechanics Laboratory; 1961; Technical Report 40.

4. Andriachi T, Schultz A, Belytschko T, Galante J. A model for studies of mechanical interactions between the human spine and rib cage. *J Biomech.* 1974; 7:497-507.

5. Fick R. *Handbuch der Anatomie und Mechanik der Gelenke*, Part III. Jena: Gustav Fischer Verlag; 1911.

6. Gelderman PW. *Het Lage Rugsyndroom.* Utrecht: University of Utrecht; 1981. Dissertation.

7. Kapandji IA. *The Physiology of the Joints.* Edinburgh: Churchill Livingstone, 1974.

11

Imaging Techniques for the Spinal Column

EDITOR'S PREFACE

A number of recent developments in imaging techniques have had significant consequences, particularly in diagnosing pathology of the spinal column. Primarily computed tomography and magnetic resonance imaging come to mind. In the fol-

The author especially thanks the following people: Dr. P. Algra (Academic Hospital of the Free University, Amsterdam), for a number of the photographs and for critically reviewing the text, and Dr. J. Peters (Academic Hospital of the Free University, Amsterdam), for a number of the photographs.

lowing chapter, Fred G van den Berg presents an overview of the currently existing imaging techniques for revealing pathology of the spinal column and its associated structures.

Again, it should be emphasized that there is often little or no correlation between the patient's symptoms and the aberrations demonstrated by the imaging. Complaints coinciding with the aberrations should not be taken as absolute proof that the symptoms are "caused" by the aberrations. On the other hand, the absence of aberrations does not mean that the symptoms should not be taken se-

riously. (See Chapter 17, Integrative Approach to Diagnosis and Treatment, for further information.) Koerselman[1] reinforced the fact that medical thinking has too long been restricted to what could be perceived in a material or somatic way.

INTRODUCTION

The most frequent complaints related to the spinal column have to do with pain. However, there is often a poor correlation between the changes seen on the radiographs (X-ray films) and the severity of the symptoms. The radiological examination should be reserved for finding specific aberrations when ruling out significant differential diagnoses. Of course, both preoperatively and postoperatively the clinical functional examination is necessary. Based on the findings, and depending on the pathology to be examined, various imaging techniques can be used.

TECHNIQUES

Conventional Roentgenography

Principles and Methods

Various structures have different translucencies for roentgen rays and thus cast shadows of various intensities on the film. Bone is less roentgen translucent than soft tissue and fat and manifests a higher-intensity shadow. Soft tissue is more roentgen translucent than bone and demonstrates a lower-intensity shadow. Fat is even more translucent than the other soft tissue structures. Along with bony structures, soft tissue structures also can be examined to a greater or lesser extent. This is possible especially when fat and muscle border one another.

To differentiate soft tissue structures, particularly in the anterior neck region, a low-kilovolt view with a minimal penetrating power of the roentgen beams is used; the con-trast in the soft tissue structures is greater. In order to have sufficient exposure, a higher radiation dosage must be administered.

Views of the spinal column are always taken from two directions: anteroposterior and lateral (Figure 11–14B and C). In the cervical and lumbar spine regions, it is also wise to make oblique views. These views are taken at an angle of 45°, from both anteroposterior and lateral. Functional views, performed in maximal extension and flexion, can give information about the stability of the spinal column.

Significance

Generally, conventional radiography is performed as the first imaging examination.

Advantages and Disadvantages

Conventional radiographs can be made in every hospital and clinic. It is an inexpensive and quick diagnostic method. The disadvantage is the harmful ionized effect of the roentgen rays in frequent and lengthy exposures.

Indications and Contraindications

Indications for a roentgenological examination include situations in which nonmyogenic pathology is involved, such as bony fusions, osteoporosis, scoliosis, spondylolisthesis, and traumatic lesions (Figures 11–1 to 11–3). The views should be made in the area in which the suspected cause of the symptoms lies. This often does not correspond to the area where the patient experiences the symptoms. There are no absolute contraindications to radiographic examination. Early pregnancy is a relative contraindication.

Future

In the near future, more use will be made of digital radiology. (See Digital Radiology for more detailed information.)

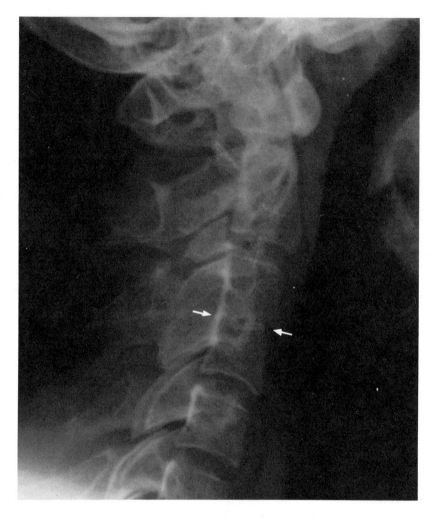

Figure 11–1 Conventional X-ray of the cervical spine. Due to fusion of the C3 and C4 vertebrae *(arrows)*, a block vertebra has developed.

Tomography

Principles and Methods

Tomography signifies the imaging of body sections. In principle, the tomographic effect is obtained by making a sweeping movement with the roentgen tube while the cassette holder with the photographic plate sweeps in the opposite direction. The axis of rotation of both sweeping motions lies in the object being examined. Only one surface, at the level of the axis of rotation and parallel to the photo-graphic plate, is sharply imaged. Structures lying in front of and behind this area are vague. In principle, the greater the sweep angle, the smaller the thickness of the section.

Significance

Tomography diminishes the disturbing overprojection of structures that lie outside the focus surface. A series of adjacent sections gives a clear idea of the three-dimensional relations.

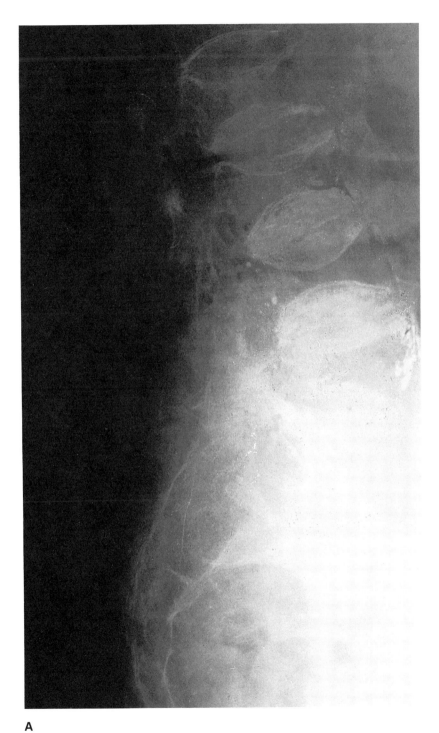

A

Figure 11–2 *A*, Conventional X-ray of the lumbar spine. Due to osteoporosis of the vertebral bodies, the vertebrae appear as "ghost" vertebrae. Because of the simultaneous central impression (the intervertebral discs are almost ball shaped), codfish vertebrae are also visible.

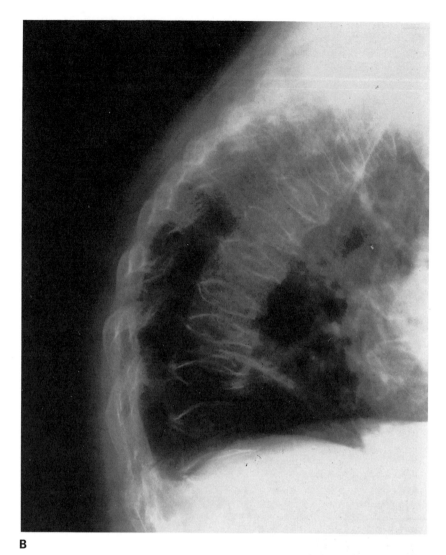

B

Figure 11–2 B, Conventional X-ray of the thoracic spine. The same findings are present here as in view **A**.

Advantages and Disadvantages

The plain linear tomogram is inexpensive and easily accessible. Multidirectional tomograms are very expensive. In both cases, the radiation levels are high.

Indications and Contraindications

Tomographic examinations are indicated when aberrations are visible on plain X-rays, but because of overprojection, the location of the lesion cannot be determined precisely. In principle, there are no absolute contra-indications. However, early pregnancy is a relative contraindication.

Future

As a result of the increased availability of new techniques, such as computed tomography (CT) and magnetic resonance imaging (MRI), the significance of tomograms has

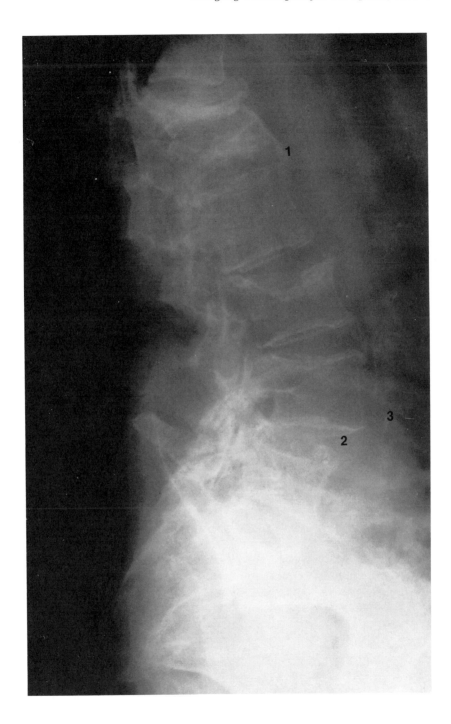

Figure 11–3 Conventional X-ray of the lumbar spine. There is osteoporosis and degeneration. The vertebrae appear as "ghost" vertebrae. There is also an extreme central collapse of T12. *1*, Osteophyte formation; *2*, anterolisthesis (spondylolisthesis ventrally) of L4-5; *3*, ossification of the back wall of the aorta.

decreased. With the help of these methods, cross-sectional views also can be performed, with even more detail and better contrast. Furthermore, in the use of MRI, ionizing radiation beams are not used and the relation with the soft tissue structures can be very well represented.

Radioisotope Examination

Principles and Methods

In radioisotope examination, radioactive material that binds to a carrier molecule is used, such as a phosphorous complex labeled with radioactive technetium, transferrin (or another ferrous bond) labeled with radioactive gallium, or leukocytes labeled with radioactive indium.

Through the exact combination of radioactive material and carrier, a specific image of certain organs can be made. To keep the dosage as low as possible, use is made of radioactive material with a short half-life. In this way, the radiation dose is quickly diminished. Material that can be quickly secreted via the kidneys and the liver is also often used.

Significance

The radioisotope examination is an excellent screening technique for locating bone

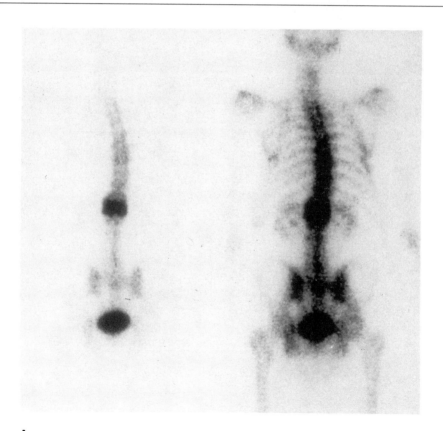

A

Figure 11–4 Solitary metastasis from a prostate carcinoma. **A**, Radioisotope examination. On the fast radioisotope scan (left), a pathological vertebra is visible, as well as elevated activity of the bladder. On the slow radioisotope scan (right), possible metastases in the ribs are demonstrated. (Note the somewhat darker spots laterally to the left and right, at approximately midthoracic level.)

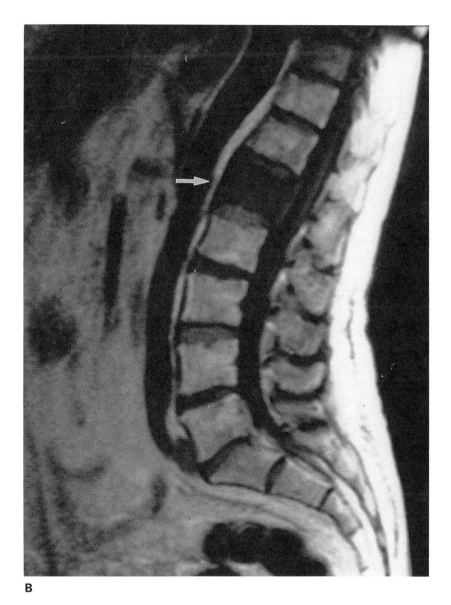

B

Figure 11–4 *B,* MRI view. The pathological vertebra (**arrow**) manifests a reduced signal intensity with a minimal collapse dorsally.

metastases (technetium scan) (Figure 11–4) or certain types of infections in or around the skeleton (gallium or indium scan).

Advantages and Disadvantages

An advantage of the radioisotope examination is that it has a high sensitivity and a large range of vision. An image of the entire body can be made at one time. The radiation dose is low compared with that of most of the roentgen techniques.

By precisely choosing the radioactive material and the complex to which the radioactive material bonds, specific questions can be answered. For instance, information can be obtained regarding metabolic activity and/or vascularization (Figure 11–5). With a gallium scan, particularly an infection or a tumor is best indicated. With an indium scan, acute inflammations can be detected; tumors and chronic inflammations cannot be seen with this examination.

Disadvantages of radioisotope diagnostics are that the examination takes so long and the spatial resolution is low. Only information about global localization, and not about anatomical details, can be obtained. In addition, the examination is nonspecific and is fairly costly.

Indications and Contraindications

Radioisotope examination is indicated chiefly in primary tumors, metastases, chronic infections, metabolic deviations, rheumatoid disorders, stress fractures, and avascular bone necroses. Radioisotope examination is also used in instances of chronic complaints for which plain X-rays are negative. In principle, there are no contraindications to this form of imaging diagnostics.

Future

In the future, the radioisotope examination will probably be further developed in the direction of differentiating physiological processes. Specific carrier molecules can be produced with monoclonal antibodies. These are antibodies that descend from one mother cell and bind to only one specific kind of molecule in the body. For instance, the molecule can be characteristic of a specific tumor. This makes the examination more specific in detecting metastases, resulting in fewer false-positive findings.

Roentgenographic Contrast Examination

Contrast medium can be introduced into a joint cavity (arthrography), the intervertebral disc (discography), the dural sac (myelography and caudography), and the blood vessels (angiography).

Arthrography

Principles and Methods
The joint cavity is pierced via a needle and contrast medium is injected.

Significance
In regard to the spine, this diagnostic technique has no clinical value. In the 1980s, attempts were made to examine the zygapophyseal joints arthrographically. However, this provided a marginal surplus in diagnostic information.

Advantages and Disadvantages
Owing to the invasive character and the minimal diagnostic significance, this examination is no longer performed in the spinal column.

Indications and Contraindications.
To date, there are no indications for performing an arthrography in the spinal column.

Future
The application of arthrography in the region of the spinal column has no future.

Discography

Principles and Methods
In discography, a small amount of contrast medium is injected into the nucleus pulposus of the disc.

Significance
Discography is important in preoperative evaluations to confirm or rule out degeneration of the intervertebral disc. This examination is performed particularly when clear indications cannot be obtained from the standard views.

Advantages and Disadvantages
Few special materials are necessary to perform discography; however, it requires a great deal of technical expertise. Another disadvantage is that the examination is invasive and often very painful.

Indications and Contraindications
Discography is indicated predominantly in cases where surgery is planned for severe disc

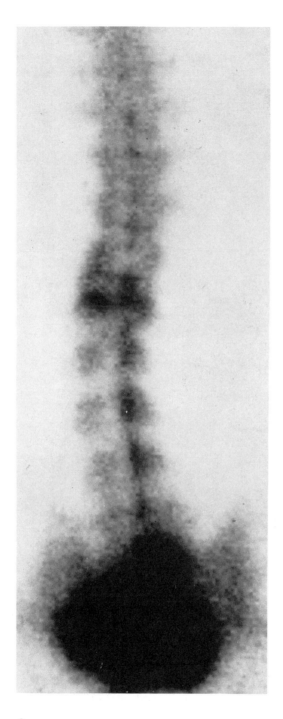

A

Figure 11–5 Osteoporosis with collapse of one vertebra. **A,** Radioisotope examination. Increased activity is visible in one vertebra. As in the conventional X-ray, no differentiation can be made from a metastasis.

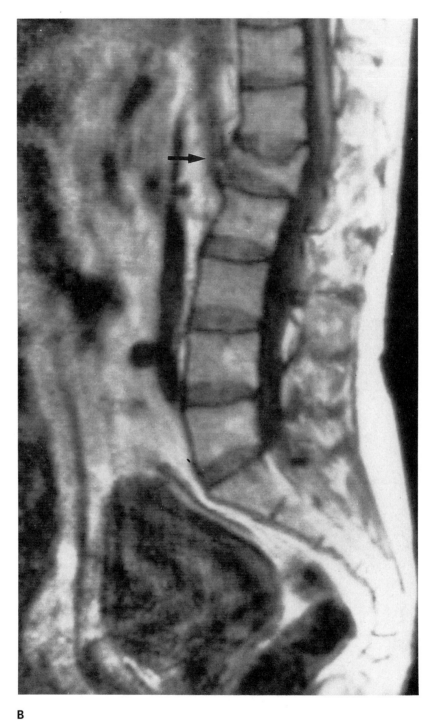

B

Figure 11–5 *B,* MRI view. There is a collapse of L1 with preservation of the normal high-signal intensity. This indicates collapse on the basis of osteoporosis (rather than from a metastasis). At the level of the collapsed vertebra, compression of the spinal cord in the conus is visible.

pathology at one level or at the most two levels. If pathology is suspected at three or more levels, there is little chance that the patient will be completely free of symptoms after the surgery. Furthermore, there is the likelihood of an instability of the spinal column.

Future

With the development of MRI, and particularly if MRI becomes less expensive and more accessible, indications for discography will be minimal.

Myelography

Principles and Methods

Contrast medium can be introduced into the dural sac in three different places: via an occipital puncture, a lateral C1-2 puncture, or, most commonly, a lumbar puncture. When a lumbar puncture is performed, the procedure is termed a caudography. The two former methods are used to examine the cervical myelon or the thoracic myelon. Because of the risk involved in a puncture at the cervical-occipital level, a number of neuroradiologists prefer to obtain images of the cervical and/or thoracic spine through a lumbar puncture.

Presently a water-soluble contrast medium is used in the procedure, versus the previously used oil bond. The latter remains visible for life; occasionally, views of the lumbar spine are still seen in patients who have previously had myelography with an oil-fast contrast medium.

Significance

For many years, the myelogram was the only method for imaging the dural sac and spinal cord. With the increased availability of CT scans and MRI, the significance of myelography has diminished (Figure 11–12).

Advantages and Disadvantages

An advantage of myelography is that the examination can be performed everywhere, in a simple and fast manner. A significant extra advantage of myelography is that, at the same time, lumbar fluid can be drawn for laboratory analysis and the pressure in the dural sac can also be measured. A disadvantage of myelography is that the puncture hole does not close immediately. As a result, the patient may experience a severe headache for 1 to 2 days after the procedure.

Indications and Contraindications

Myelography is indicated in pathology in which the spinal cord is involved, such as in tumors in or around the spinal cord, trauma of the spinal column, congenital abnormalities, degenerative processes in the spinal column (particularly discogenic), vascular aberrations, and inflammatory processes. Myelography is absolutely contraindicated in instances of increased intracranial pressure. If lower distal pressure occurs due to the puncture, parts of the cerebellum and brain stem in the foramen magnum can become "strangled" and an acute life-threatening situation arises. Occipital and C1-2 punctures are contraindicated in tumors at the level of the cervical myelon. In these instances, there is a chance that the compromised spinal cord will be punctured.

Future

Myelography continues to be utilized because of the relative simplicity of the procedure. However, this advantage does not apply to C1-2 and occipital punctures, which must be performed in a specialized neuroradiological center. In many instances where myelography would be indicated, a CT scan is performed instead. Often myelography and CT are performed in combination so that on the CT scans the contrast-filled dural sac becomes visible.

An important breakthrough in imaging techniques is MRI. Without having to administer a contrast medium, the myelon, dural sac, and spinal column can all be imaged from different directions.

Angiography and Digital Subtraction Angiography

Principles and Methods

A venous or arterial puncture in which contrast medium is administered in the arterial or venous system allows for imaging of the arterial and/or venous blood vessels. Presently, computed subtraction techniques, termed digital subtraction angiography, are often used. In this instance, a roentgen view without contrast medium is subtracted from a view with contrast medium, so that only an image of the blood vessels remains.

Significance

Spinal arteriography is significant in diagnosing tumors and arteriovenous malformations in the area of the spinal cord. The epidural phlebography can be used to demonstrate a disc prolapse at the level of L5-S1, where the dural sac does not lie directly adjacent to the spinal column. Using conventional myelography, a disc prolapse at this level is occasionally missed.

Advantages and Disadvantages

Even with the development of MRI, spinal angiography is especially indicated in examining the small blood vessels. Because of the low resolution of MRI, these vessels cannot be depicted. The disadvantage of this procedure is its invasive character.

Indications and Contraindications.

Angiography is indicated in diagnosing tumors and arteriovenous malformation. Of course, if the patient is allergic to the contrast medium, the examination is contraindicated. With the new contrast media, the chance of this occurring is diminished.

Future

At present, epidural phlebography is rarely utilized. However, spinal angiography is performed and likely will continue to be performed in the future.

Ultrasonography

Principles and Methods

In ultrasonography, a transducer emits ultrasound with a frequency of 3.5 to 10 MHz and then registers the reflecting sound waves. The transmission of sound is dependent on the medium. The reflection occurs at the bordering surfaces between tissue layers. The quality of the reflection depends on the angle of the sound beams and the acoustic impedance of the tissue. Air and bone disturb the reflection; these structures cannot be depicted with ultrasonography. This is a significant problem in ultrasonography of the spinal column and the spinal cord. In relation to the spinal column, ultrasonography is useful only in evaluating newborns or fetuses in whom the skeleton is not completely calcified.

Significance

Ultrasonography generally has minimal significance in examination of the spinal column and the dural sac with its contents. However, Doppler ultrasonography, in which the blood-flow velocity can be determined, is important in diagnosing abnormalities in the spinal artery.

Advantages and Disadvantages

The most significant disadvantage of ultrasonography is that the adult spinal column and the myelon cannot be depicted.

Indications and Contraindications

Ultrasonography is used to image the spinal column and the dural sac only in newborns. Furthermore, ultrasonography is very important in ruling out a meningocele in fetuses. There are no contraindications for ultrasonography.

Future

For the time being, the indications for ultrasonography of the spinal column are restricted to newborns and fetuses. In these instances, it is very difficult to perform an examination with MRI.

Computed Tomography

Principles and Methods

Tomography signifies imaging in sections; thus CT means "cutting slices" with the help of a computer. Generally, transverse sections of the body are made through a combination of a ring of detectors and a radiation source that revolves around the patient. The patient is placed lengthwise into the apparatus, so that at different levels, new sections can be made. The images are then reconstructed from the intensity values that have been measured through the detectors.

Significance

In representing the spinal column, the CT scan is of great importance. Particularly in combination with contrast medium in the dural sac, introduced by means of a lumbar puncture, the CT scan gives a clear depiction of the relation of the spinal cord, the exiting roots, and the spinal column.

Advantages and Disadvantages

In performing a CT scan, a routine procedure is followed using standardized examination techniques. Therefore, the resulting images from a CT scan do not depend on the individual examiner's skill. A disadvantage of the CT scan is its expense. CT is much more available than MRI, but still less than conventional roentgenography or myelography.

Indications and Contraindications

Because the relationship among the spinal column, spinal cord, and exiting roots can be so well represented, the CT scan has diagnostic significance in disc prolapses. The CT scan is also very helpful in traumatology as well as in diagnosing tumors of the vertebral spine, the spinal cord, and the exiting roots. A congenital narrowing of the spinal canal (a form of spinal stenosis) can also be diagnosed by use of a CT scan.

Future

Use of a CT scan in examining a scoliosis is problematic because, for the most part, the spinal column is not affected in the transverse plane. With the three-dimensional reconstructions that currently are being developed, this problem will be solved.

Magnetic Resonance Imaging

Principles and Methods

In MRI, instead of roentgen rays, a magnetic field and radio waves are implemented in creating an image. Through use of a magnetic field, all the protons from the examined part of the body initially are directed equally. The net direction of these protons is then changed by sending a radio impulse through a fixed slice. After termination of this radio impulse, all of the protons return to their original direction. Depending on the tissue, some return more quickly, some more slowly. The time it takes for this last stage to occur is measured, and these values are reproduced in a gray hue. Thus, every point in the image has a characteristic gray hue.

Significance

The significance of the MRI lies particularly in the fact that both soft tissue and bony structures can be well represented, with the extra advantage that everything can be visualized in every possible direction.

Advantages and Disadvantages

The different tissue components of the soft tissues (for instance, muscle, fat, tendon, spinal cord, and cerebrospinal fluid) can be well distinguished. In addition, depictions can be made in every possible plane. Of course, another great advantage is that X-rays are not used. A disadvantage of MRI is that the purchase and use of the equipment are very expensive.

Indications and Contraindications

With MRI the spinal canal and lesions lying in it, such as metastases, can be clearly depicted (Figures 11–6 to 11–10). In addition, a disc prolapsing into the dural sac or primary

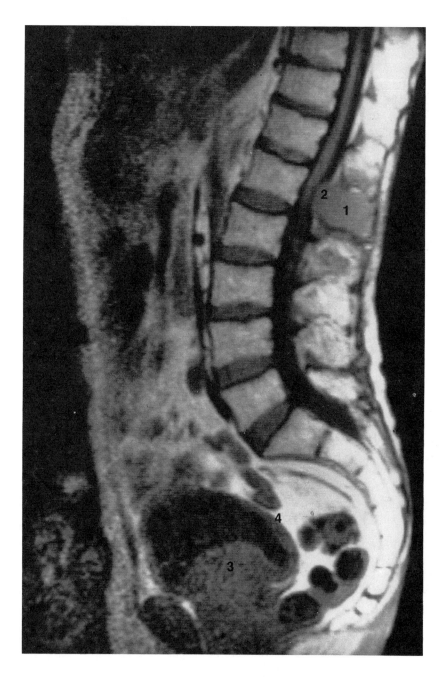

Figure 11–6 MRI. There is a metastasis in the L1 spinous process. **1**, Diminished signal intensity where the metastasis is localized; **2**, impression of the medullary cone; **3**, enlarged prostate; **4**, thickened bladder wall due to urine retention.

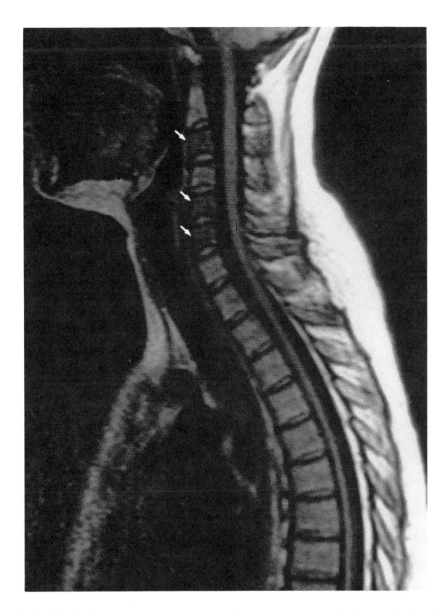

Figure 11–7 MRI. Vertebral metastases due to a breast carcinoma. At the cervical level, there are three vertebrae with a diminished signal intensity due to the metastases *(arrows)*. The spinal cord is clearly identifiable.

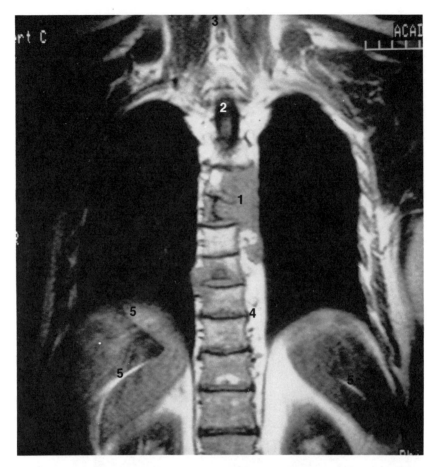

Figure 11–8 MRI. Metastasis from an unknown origin. *1*, Disappearance of the contours of two vertebral bodies with wedge-formed collapses and spreading into the bordering soft tissue structures; *2*, because of the normal curves of the spinal column, a portion of the spinal cord is visible in the upper thoracic region; *3*, in the lower cervical region, a number of spinous processes are visible; *4*, because the vessels are in transverse section and flowing blood has no signal intensity, the paravertebral venous plexus is visible as a gathering of small round areas without signal intensity (imbedded in fat tissue, which has a high signal intensity); *5*, artifacts projected in the liver and spleen.

tumors of the spinal column, the spinal cord, and the surrounding soft tissue structures can be well visualized (Figures 11–11 and 11–12). *The presence of a pacemaker is an absolute contraindication.* The presence of metal prostheses or vessel clips, which can be magnetic, constitute a relative contraindication.

Future

MRI is still in full development and will probably become the most important imaging technique for the spinal column. As it stands today, the use of MRI in evaluating scolioses is not yet optimal. In the future, this may be improved by using a three-dimensional reconstruction or a reconstruction along curved lines.

Digital Radiology

Principles and Methods

In digital radiology, the shadow image obtained by roentgen beams is not recorded on a photographic plate, but instead is received

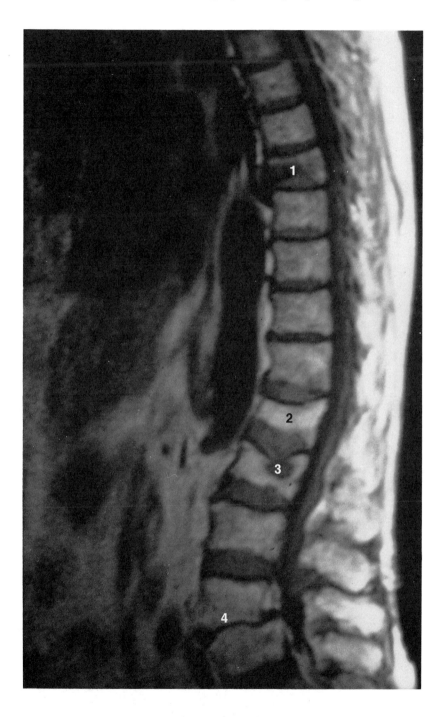

Figure 11–9 MRI. Metastasis and degenerative changes. *1*, Wedge-shaped deformity of the T8 vertebra with minimal signal intensity as the result of a metastasis; *2*, wedge-shaped deformity of the L1
vertebra. The normal signal intensity indicates that the deformity is due to osteoporosis; *3*, Schmorl's
nodule in the L2 vertebral body, characteristic of Scheuermann's disease; *4*, because of degeneration,
there is severe disc narrowing of L4-5, and L4 has an anterior position in relation to L5.

by a series of detectors, which transpose the gray value of every picture point into a number. This number is stored in a computer. From the computer memory, these pictures can then be generated onto a monitor and, if necessary, manipulated.

Significance

In digital radiology, many possibilities exist regarding the exposures, compared with the conventional radiological examination. Large exposure differences in a picture can be corrected. In addition, all kinds of manipulations,

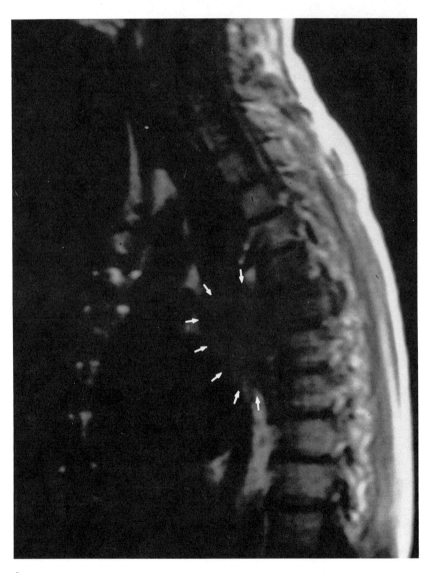

A

Figure 11–10 MRI. **A**, Metastasis from a seminoma. There is lowered signal intensity in the vertebral body where the metastasis is located. The metastasis has spread to the mediastinum **(arrows)**.

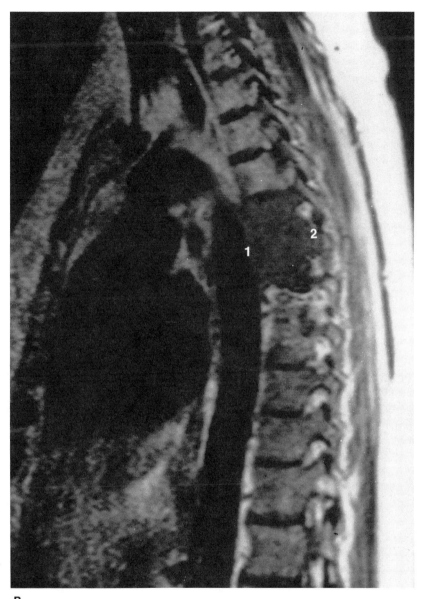

B

Figure 11–10 *B,* The same metastasis in the sagittal plane at the level where the nerve roots exit. The nerve roots are visible as black round structures surrounded by the white fat. ***1***, Spreading to the aorta; ***2***, compression of the exiting nerve roots.

such as measurements, can be performed easily.

Advantages and Disadvantages

The cervicothoracic and the thoracolumbar junctions often are difficult to depict using conventional techniques because of the large exposure differences necessary to illustrate the different parts of the spinal column. The chance for a poor picture is much less with digital techniques. In digital radiology, the pictures seldom have to be redone be-

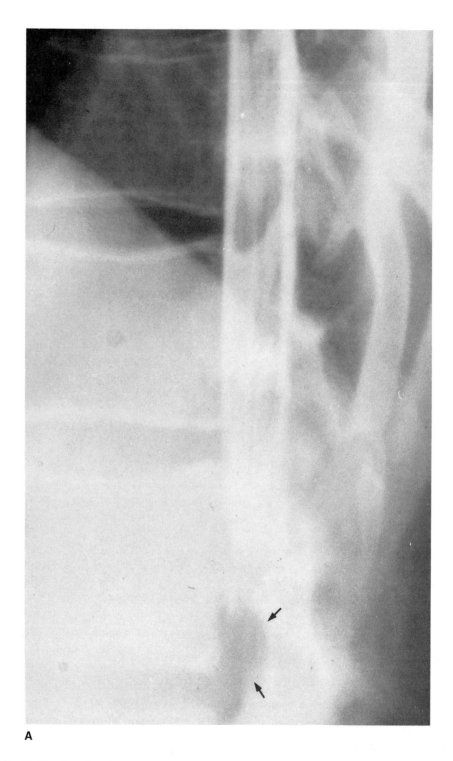

A

Figure 11–11 Herniated nucleus pulposus at the L1-2 level. **A**, Caudography with contrast medium at the level of the disc *(arrows)*.

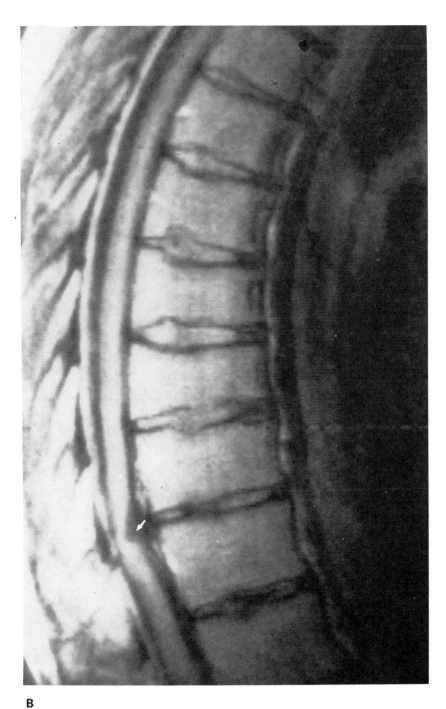

B

Figure 11–11 *B,* MRI.

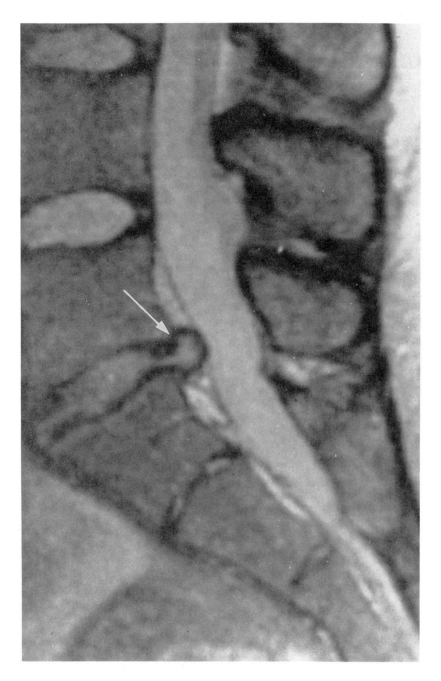

Figure 11–12 MRI. Central herniated nucleus pulposus in the lumbar region. There is obvious compression of the posterior longitudinal ligament and of the dural sac. However, there is no compression of the nerve root. The affected disc has a low signal intensity as a result of the degeneration and decrease in fat content.

cause of bad exposure. In addition, data can be stored on magnetic tapes, computer diskettes, or laser disc ("hard copy"). This is also a solution for the storage problems of the roentgen archive. By using a matrix camera, the most important views can be stored on a photographic plate.

Indications and Contraindications

For the most part, the indications for digital radiology are the same as those for conventional radiology. There are no absolute contraindications. Pregnancy is a relative contraindication.

Future

Although digital radiological techniques are still considered to be experimental, they are being further developed for future commercial use. At this time, use of these techniques is very expensive

PATHOLOGY

The most frequently appearing "pathologies" of the spinal column are degeneration of the vertebrae with the formation of osteophytes (spondylarthrosis) and degeneration of the intervertebral discs (discosis). Tumors and inflammatory processes can cause the collapse of a vertebra. However, most often a collapsed vertebra is due to osteoporosis. There are a number of primary tumors with a preference for metastasizing in the spinal column.

Sacroiliac Pathology

See also Chapter 3, Sacroiliac Joint, section 3.3, Pathology, for more information.

Ankylosing Spondylitis

The diagnosis of ankylosing spondylitis can be confirmed on a conventional radiograph. In the early stages, the sacroiliac joints are vaguely delineated. In later stages, they are completely ankylosed (fused) (Figure 11–13). The entire spinal column is affected in the later stages. The intervertebral joints fuse together, along with an ankylosing of the anterior longitudinal ligament and the ligamentum flavum, giving the characteristic image of the "bamboo spine."

Sacroiliitis of Other Origins

Different systemic disorders, such as psoriasis, Reiter's syndrome, Crohn's disease, and ulcerative colitis, can be accompanied by bilateral sacroiliitis. In other pathology, the sacroiliitis is unilateral, such as in gout and purulent inflammation.

The sacroiliac joint can best be judged by a specific sacroiliac view. The view is made with the patient in prone position, under the assumption that the divergent beams from dorsal are exactly tangent to the bordering surfaces of the sacroiliac joints. Thus the position of the joints is approximately parallel to the divergent course of the beam. The anatomy and pathology of the sacroiliac joint can also be studied with the help of a CT scan.

Asymmetry of the Pelvis

Asymmetry of the pelvis can be judged in a conventional anteroposterior radiograph. A grid is projected over the photograph so that the exact level difference between both pelvic crests can be determined. A leg length difference manifests itself through a difference in the level between both femoral heads.

Lumbar Pathology

For further detailed information refer to Chapter 4, Lumbar Spine, section 4.3, Pathology.

Disc Prolapse and Disc Protrusion

Disc-related disorders in the lumbar region, with or without radicular symptoms, can be evaluated by means of caudography (Figure 11–14). In this way, impression on the

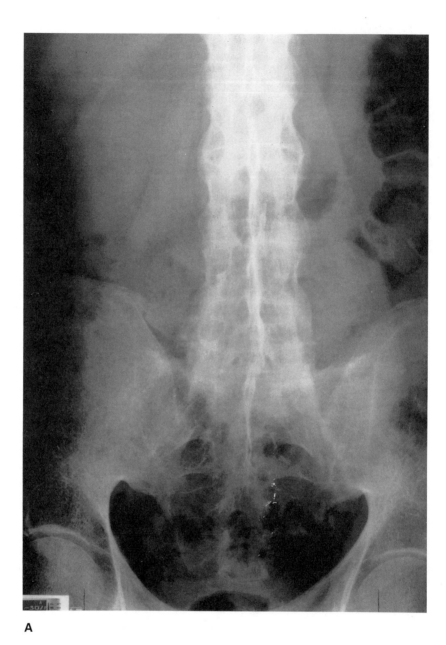

A

Figure 11–13 Conventional radiographs of the spinal column in a patient with ankylosing spondylitis. On each view, the ankylosing (fusing) is obvious. **A**, Lumbar spine.

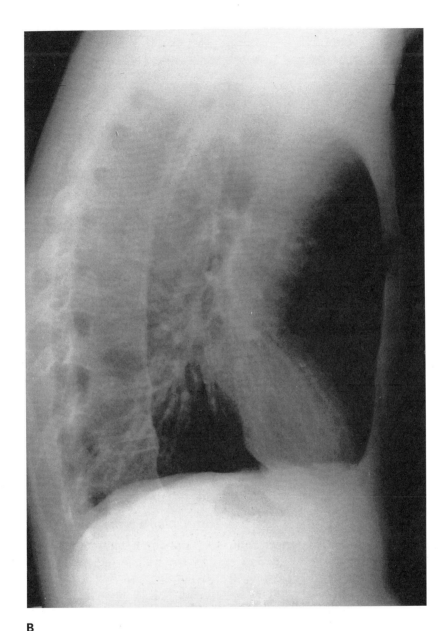

B

Figure 11–13 *B*, Thoracic spine.

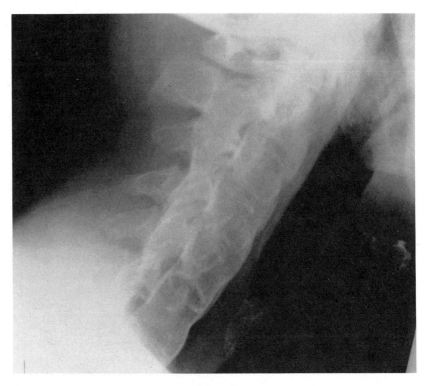

C

Figure 11–13 *C,* Cervical spine.

dural sac and compression on the nerve roots can be examined.

In order to study a disc prolapse or protrusion at L5-S1, some centers utilize epidural phlebography. The CT scan, performed with or without contrast medium in the dural sac, has made this latter technique superfluous. Exact information regarding the disc in relation to the myelon, the cauda equina, and the exiting nerve roots can be obtained from a CT scan. With the help of MRI, disc protrusions and prolapses in relation to the spinal cord also can be clearly depicted (Figures 11–11 and 11–12).

Acute Lumbago

Imaging techniques generally are not required for the examination of acute lumbago. This is a pattern of complaints that are self-limiting and do not require surgery.

Baastrup's Syndrome

Baastrup's syndrome (kissing spine) involves local pain due to the rubbing together of adjacent spinous processes. Usually this syndrome is seen in conjunction with a hyperlordosis. Arthrotic changes can be visible between the spinous process, particularly with densely packed bone tissue (eburnation). These abnormalities are well demonstrated on conventional lateral-view X-rays of the lumbar spine.

Thoracic Pathology

For further detailed information, refer to Chapter 5, Thoracic Spine, section 5.3, Pathology.

Discogenic Lesions

Disc prolapse and degeneration are best examined by use of an MRI. However, because of the expense of the procedure, MRI is indicated only in cases in which surgery is considered.

Scheuermann's Disease

The diagnosis of Scheuermann's disease, also known as *kyphosis dorsalis juvenilis*, can be confirmed with a conventional X-ray of the thoracic spine. The vertebrae collapse into a wedge shape and the characteristic thoracic hyperkyphosis results. The so-called Schmorl's nodules are pathognomonic (Figure 11–9). These nodules are based on a prolapse of the disc into the vertebral body and are found only in Scheuermann's disease. Scheuermann's disease can also be seen in the upper lumbar spine.

Scoliosis

In examining scolioses in which a lateral curve is present along with a torsion of the spinal column, a conventional radiograph of the entire spinal column is made. In this view, the angles can be measured, particularly for a preoperative or postoperative evaluation. The progression of the scoliosis is followed at regular intervals by repeated angle measurements on current X-ray films.

Spondylodiscitis

In spondylodiscitis, an irregular boundary of the intervertebral disc is visible on the conventional X-ray.

Forestier's Disease

Forestier's disease is a form of spondylosis with hyperosseous changes on the ventral and lateral sides of the vertebral bodies (Figure 11–14). Bony bridges between the vertebral bodies, syndesmophytes, can also be seen in the lumbar region.

Cervical Pathology

For further detailed information, refer to Chapter 6, Cervical Spine, section 6.3, Pathology.

Differential Diagnostics of Cervical Syndromes

The local cervical syndrome, the cervicobrachial syndrome, and the cervicomedullary syndrome can all arise as a result of the following:

- a disc protrusion or prolapse
- degenerative changes with narrowing of the intervertebral foramen
- metastases or primary tumors in the vertebral bodies, the spinal cord, or the exiting nerve roots
- inflammatory processes such as rheumatism or tuberculosis
- trauma of the cervical column

In all these forms of pathology, conventional radiographs, in two or more directions, should be performed first. In the future, the conventional radiological examination probably will be replaced by digital radiology.

Tomography (planigraphy) is indicated when traumatic bony aberrations, noted on the X-rays, are obscure. Tomography can also be helpful in determining rheumatic aberrations.

In confirming or ruling out metastases in the spinal column, a radioisotope bone scan is indicated. In this instance, the bone scan is a very sensitive imaging procedure: the chance of a false-negative diagnosis is minimal. However, differentiating between the various forms of pathology (the specificity of the imaging technique) is disappointing: in radioisotope diagnostics, indicated aberrations can be caused by degenerative abnormalities, metastases, or inflammatory processes.

For neurological lesions originating in the cervical spine, myelography can be performed, possibly supplemented by a CT scan. In post-traumatic lesions, a CT scan should be

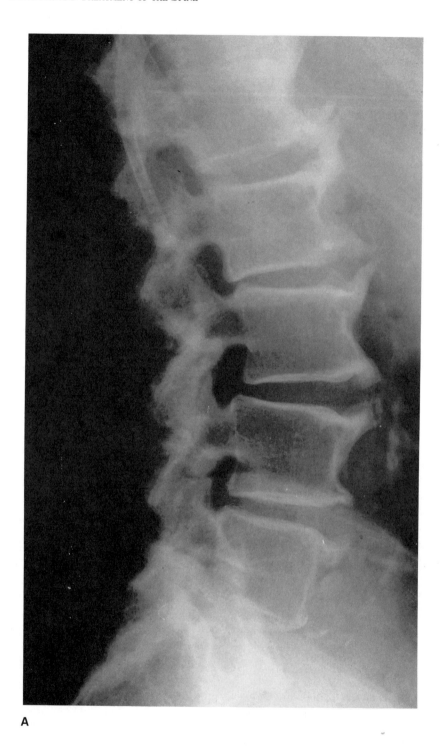

A

Figure 11–14 Forestier's disease. **A**, Conventional X-ray of the lumbar spine. Extensive osteophyte formation is visible on the ventral aspects of the vertebral bodies.

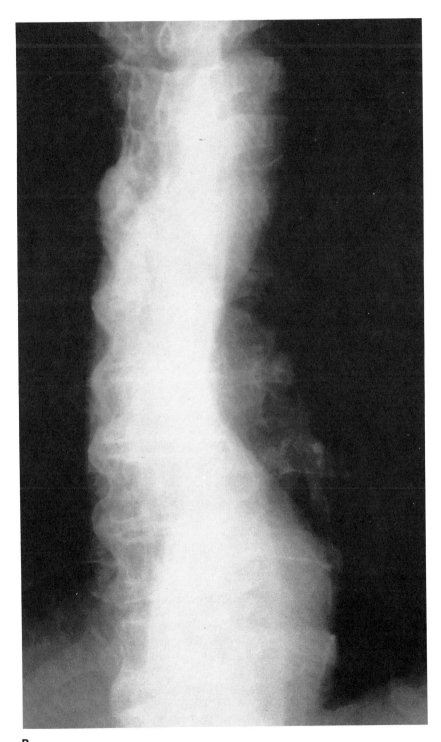

B

Figure 11–14 *B,* Conventional anteroposterior X-ray of the thoracic spine.

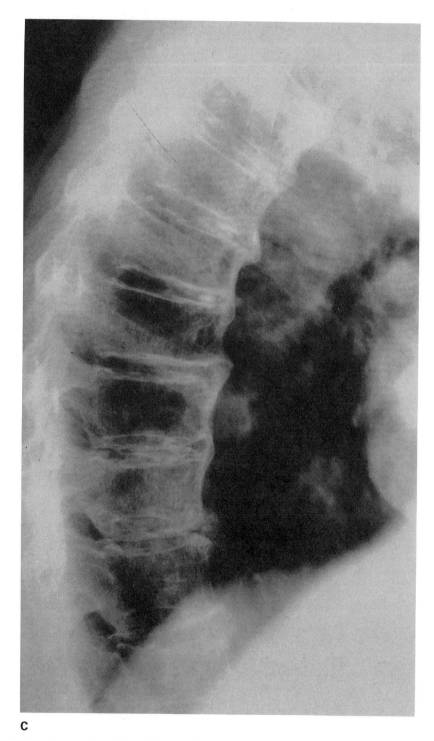

C

Figure 11–14 C, Conventional lateral X-ray of the thoracic spine. Extensive osteophyte formation is visible on the ventral aspects of the vertebral bodies.

performed when the conventional X-ray and/ or tomogram is unclear.

Doppler ultrasonography is useful in examining the vertebral artery in post-traumatic situations or in severe degenerative changes in which stenosis in the vertebral artery is suspected. Of course, the condition of the vertebral artery also can be evaluated by means of angiography, which is performed in preference to digital subtraction angiography.

MRI can be a very important tool in the differential diagnostics of the cervical syndrome. Disc protrusions and prolapses in relation to the spinal cord, as well as metastases or primary tumors in the vertebral bodies, spinal cord, and exiting roots can be depicted clearly (Figure 11–15). MRI can also be well utilized in evaluating inflammatory processes such as rheumatoid arthritis, in which not only the soft tissue structures but also the bony structures are involved (Figure 11–16).

Differential Diagnostics of Thoracic Outlet Syndrome

The typical symptoms of thoracic outlet syndrome can be caused by compression of nerves or blood vessels, or a combination of both. Compression of vessels can be demonstrated with digital subtraction angiography and sometimes also with Doppler ultrasonography. Views are taken with the patient in the provocation position, that is, the position in which the symptoms either arise or worsen. In a suspected thoracic outlet syndrome, it is very important to be able to differentiate among pathologies of the cervical spine, the thorax, and the upper extremities. Cervical pathology usually best can be demonstrated by a conventional X-ray. When pathology of the thorax is suspected, conventional X-rays of the thorax are necessary. These can be supplemented with a view in which there is a specific craniocaudal direction of the beams, particularly in order to rule out a Pancoast tumor in the apex of the lung. Bony aberrations in the upper extremities often can be diagnosed by means of conventional X-rays. To evaluate the soft tissue structures, ultrasonography or even MRI can be performed.

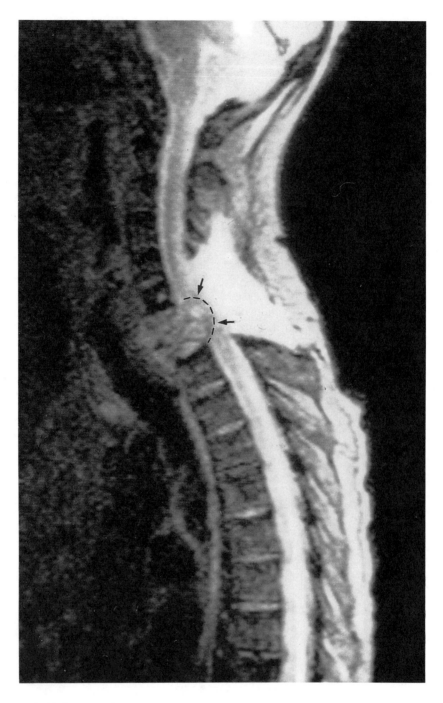

Figure 11–15 MRI. Residual Grawitz tumor. The patient was status post-laminectomy (removal of the posterior vertebral arch). Impression of the dural sac and collapse of the vertebra with a pathological high intensity is visible (probably due to blood or edema).

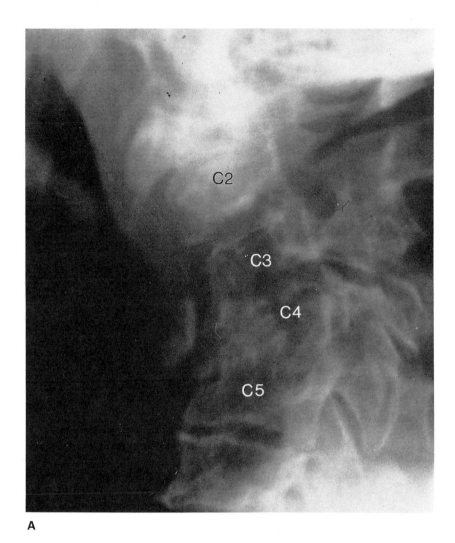

A

Figure 11–16 Rheumatoid arthritis of the cervical column. **A**, Conventional X-ray; there is a lack of calcium in the skeleton, with a wedge-shaped collapse of C4 and C5.

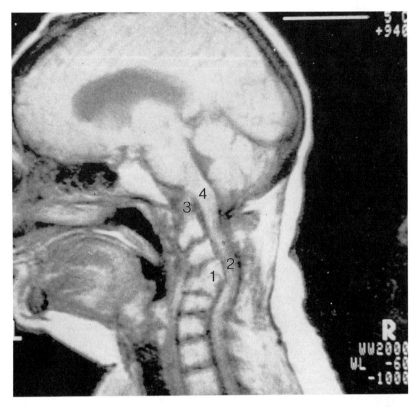

B

Figure 11–16 B, MRI. **1**, Wedge-shaped collapse of C4 and C5; **2**, retroposition of C4 in relation to C5 with resultant compression of the spinal cord; **3**, the dens of the axis protrudes into the foramen magnum; **4**, impression of the dens into the base of the skull with compression of the medulla oblongata.

REFERENCE

1. Koerselman F. *Integratief Medisch Denken: over de psychopathogenetische reconstructie.* Amsterdam: VU Uitgeverij; 1990. Dissertation.

SUGGESTED READING

Dihlmann W. *Gelenke und Wirbelverbindungen.* Stuttgart: Georg Thieme Verlag; 1980.

Gehweiler JA Jr. *The Radiology of Vertebral Trauma.* Philadelphia: WB Saunders; 1980.

Haughton VM, Williams AL. *Computed Tomography of the Spine.* St. Louis: CV Mosby Co; 1982.

Stark DD. *Magnetic Resonance Imaging.* St. Louis: CV Mosby Co; 1988.

12

Prevention of Back and Neck Pain by Improving Posture

EDITOR'S PREFACE

Not only do a large number of people experience one or more incidences of back and/or neck pain in their lifetimes, but a great portion of these symptoms can be prevented. The necessary insights and data to achieve this prevention have been available for a considerable time. Nevertheless, the distance between biomechanical/ergonomic analysis and activities of daily living remains remarkably great. Indeed, in a number of instances ergonomical/biomechanical services are employed; however, outside of the large factory little attention is given to the "loading" and the "loadability" of humans.

Many items are available for purchase to improve comfort; however, few are worth the expense. Little thought is ever given in regard to the height of the working table or the school desk. Chairs are also purchased without consideration. In the same sense, in hospitals one rarely sees patients sitting with optimal posture in wheelchairs. In this chapter, Chris Snijders offers a number of rules for posture and positioning in daily activities, not only in regard to the prevention of complaints but also for achieving comfort.

"Active sitting" is not discussed in this chapter. Active sitting entails sitting on a chair with a declined seat, thus forcing its user into a permanent active sitting. Because of the exertion required in active sitting, it can better be considered a form of exercise therapy than a comfortable form of prevention.

The advice in this chapter is simple but extremely effective. Radical epidemiological consequences could be achieved if these simple recommendations were followed successfully. Thus, it would be wise to give full attention to this chapter.

INTRODUCTION

The concept of prevention can be classified into primary, secondary, and tertiary prevention. Primary prevention in technology entails the prevention of harmful influences on humans during the developing stages of products, technical systems, and processes. For example, this primary prevention occurs when government requirements are placed on certain products or processes. There are protective regulations in relation to noise, radiation, fire, vehicles, harmful materials, and electrical safety of household products. In these instances, there is an obvious relationship between the cause and the possible detrimental result.

Specific legal measures in the prevention of certain chronic, noncontagious, and multicausal symptoms, such as back pain, are much more difficult to find. In addition, such regulations can be challenged because of the dilemma created between forced protection and personal freedom of choice. Prevention here is largely dependent on a series of behavior patterns and living habits, such as consumerism, nutrition, and physical activity. In this chapter, based on a number of biomechanical concepts, suggestions for prevention in regard to daily situations at work, school, and home are given. The practical application of the acquired insight is not achieved through legal measures, but instead must be attained through enlightenment of the public. In this instance, workers in the medical sciences and social health care perform a central role.

Secondary prevention concerns the early detection of physical problems—the early diagnosis. In this sense, periodic preventive examinations are important.

Tertiary prevention can be described as prevention of worsening. Specific technical resources are used in this instance.

FORMS OF LOAD

In 1986, the ad hoc committee of the European Community studied the significance of occupational circumstances on the occurrence of low back problems.[1] The conclusion was that 70% of either the onset or worsening of all low back problems were the result of the working environment. The most important cause of lumbar pathology was related to the various types of mechanical load.

Although uncertainty persists regarding the causal relation, six occupational risk factors can be listed, as follows:

1. physically heavy labor
2. prolonged working postures
3. frequent bending and turning
4. lifting and sudden intense exertion
5. repetitive tasks
6. mechanical vibration

Earlier, the cause for low back pain was generally attributed to lifting heavy objects in a flexed position. Nowadays, the harmful consequences of unfavorable static loads due to work-related, prolonged poor postures are also recognized. Especially in relation to working postures, it is remarkable how many workplaces are incorrectly designed and how simply the situations often can be drastically improved. In illustrating how this can be done, the following activities are differentiated:

- sitting (chairs, working surface)
- standing (bending, lifting)
- walking (shoes)
- lying (hospital beds)
- mechanical vibration.

Sitting

Sitting on chairs should not be taken for granted: still today, in many countries people squat, kneel, or sit on the ground. The origin of chairs probably lies in the boulder or other platform on which the tribal chief sat. As time went on, ornate chairs were made, not to sit on but rather as status symbols. Even today the status element in thrones and directors' chairs can be recognized. The chair was also a symbol indicating the scholarly. In the university setting, one still speaks of a professorial chair.

Western society without chairs is unimaginable. Chairs can be classified roughly into upright (hard) chairs and easy chairs. Sitting for prolonged periods is required in school and office settings. Office workers spend up to three fourths of their working time sitting. Half the working force consists of office workers. There is much to criticize about office chairs. Furthermore, the chairs found in homes are more often bad than good.

Most of the time, the biomechanical requirements that should be incorporated into a chair's body-supporting surfaces (armrest, backrest, seat) to guarantee a posture with minimal muscle activity (passive sitting) are not observed.

Armrest

An advantage of supporting the arms is the unloading of the shoulder girdle and subsequently also of the cervical spine. The height of the armrests should correspond to the level of the elbows with the arms in a slightly abducted position. This also applies to the levels of table tops. Without armrests, the individual crosses the arms in front of the body, leans on the table, or flexes the spine to rest the arms in the lap. In automobiles, an individual often props one arm on the edge at the base of the windowpane in the car door, or with the other arm reaches across the backrest of the passenger seat. Seldom does an individual drive for long periods with the hands in a "ten and two" position. If the work requires that the center of gravity of the arms lie in front of the shoulders rather than underneath, easing the workload can be attained by "hanging up" the arms (Figure 12–1).

Backrest

Sitting straight without a backrest is fatiguing. After a time, the trunk sags and the lumbar spine kyphoses. With the exception of a saddle, this occurs independent of the position of the seat. Prolonged sitting with a kyphotic (C-form) spine is not recommended; the intradiscal pressure increases, collagenous connective tissue lengthens, and there is a passive stretch of the muscles that leads to stimulus of pain at the tendon insertions.

Providing that the support is applied in the lordosis between the iliac crest and the scapulae, the advantage of a backrest is that the spinal column is supported in its normal physiological form (S-form). In addition, because of the support at approximately midback level, the trunk can be held upright without appreciable muscle exertion.

Important provisions of auto seats include an adjustable low back support combined with an adjustable backrest. Seen from above (also in autos), a slightly curved profile of the backrest guarantees sufficient support from the side because backs of various widths still fit into this profile. Auto seats with a straight profile, which have sharply protruding support from the sides, are incorrectly constructed. A seat that is flat when nonloaded with good cushioning is preferred. Considering the maximal velocity with which automobiles make turns (radial velocity is 0.2 to 0.3 times the gravitational velocity), it is impossible to slide off such seats.

Seat

A seat that yields approximately 3 cm offers sufficient cushioning for the ischial tuberosities, which carry the weight of the head, trunk, and arms. Because the weight of the legs is borne by the feet, the seat should not be deeper than about 20 cm. However, seats are usually deeper: approximately 42 cm in straight chairs for adults. This allows for increased pressure on the thighs, which increases stability but also allows the individual to sit in a slouched position. The ability to shift one's position comfortably is an absolute requirement for a good seat. With these factors in mind, the shell-shaped seats and backrests that snugly enclose the body according to its anatomical form—to achieve the maximal contact surface—are indicated only for the severely handicapped.

However, the sitting surface should ensure more than just vertical support for the ischial tuberosities. If the trunk pushes against the backrest in a horizontal direction, there is a balance of forces for the upper body only when an equal but opposite force is exerted in relation to the force of the backrest against the trunk. The friction between the seat and the skin, with the soft tissue structures lying underneath the ischial tuberosities, provides

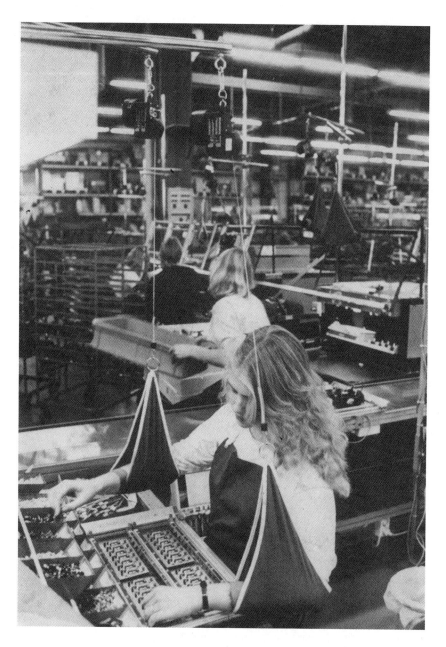

Figure 12–1 "Hanging up" the arms. The force working on the arm (approximately 5% of body weight) is independent of the position and comes from an isotonic spring fixed to the ceiling.

the necessary reaction force. If the seat is smooth, the individual slides down into a slouched position. Because the covering of wheelchairs must be smooth for sanitation purposes, the slouched position is seen frequently. The pelvis tilts posteriorly, and a form of "sacral sitting" occurs. This means that pressure and friction act upon an area of the body that is not made for these forces, thus decubitus ulcers arise. In some countries, a strap resembling a hip safety belt is used to provide counterpressure. Because the device is successful only with a taut strap and a hard seat, in practice this does not appear to be a good solution.

The only correct solution is to give the seat a slope that ensures a pressure force perpendicular to the surface of the seat, working through the ischial tuberosities. This force has to have a horizontal component that is equal to the pressure against the backrest. As the backrest's backward tilt is increased, the horizontal pressure on the back increases and the angle of inclination of the seat also should increase. Thus, straight chairs and automobile seats have a substantial difference in inclination.

The height of the seat should be equal to the length of the lower leg. If the seat is too high, excessive pressure occurs on the thighs, particularly in the blood vessels and nerves. This, along with the difficulty in changing position (due to the height of the seat), causes the legs to fall asleep.

Working Surface

For proper posture, the form of the chair is very important. However, in daily activities such as reading, writing, and drawing it is not the chair but rather the sight direction that is of critical significance in the position of the head and subsequently the position of the entire spine. Upright sitting and reading require an inconvenient "kink" in the cervical spine; at the same time the reading distance is too great. Therefore the individual tends to bend over the reading surface. Disadvantages

of this prolonged slouched position include flexion headaches (school headaches), decreased concentration, dizziness, fatigue, back and neck pain, and hindered breathing. All of these disadvantages can be countered by inclining the working surface. Thus, the working surface is brought closer to the eyes. For example, the Erasmus desk has been developed to be used at home or at work. It is transparent, so that objects and papers do not get lost underneath the working surface. The desk also has an ample groove for pens and similar objects or for an open book (Figure 12–2).

Standing

Prolonged stooped working positions usually indicate a poor working environment. Working surfaces such as desks, treatment and examination tables, and workbenches that are not adjusted to the proper height are all examples of a poor working environment. Because of the increase in height of the general population, the difference in height from individual to individual is now greater than ever before.

Determining the magnitude of the physical load on the back is represented simply in Figure 12–3. On average, forces work to keep upper-lying masses balanced. The total gravitational pull of the earth, F_G, acts upon the body's center of gravity. For the upper body, F_C, this lies approximately at the level of the axillae. Balance of the forces in a vertical direction is realized by means of the reaction force, F_{RC}, which acts in the middle of the intervertebral disc. In this model, the intervertebral disc is considered to be the joint axis. Thus, a coupling occurs. The coupling is formed by two parallel, equal but opposite, directed forces, F_C and F_{RC}. The effect is not a translatory but rather a rotatory motion.

The magnitude of the rotatory effect is given by the moment, M, of the coupling

$$M = F_C \times a \text{ (Newton meter) or (Nm)}$$

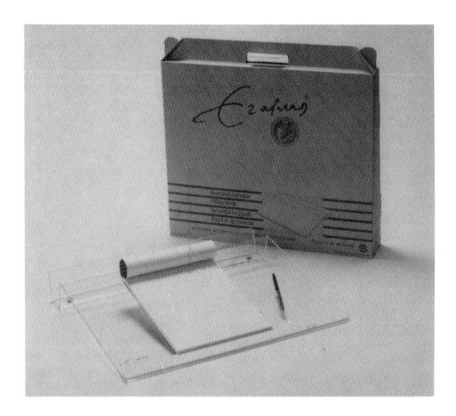

Figure 12–2 Erasmus desk. The angle of inclination is not greater than 10 cm. This amount of inclination has a favorable effect on posture. In addition, with this angle stacked papers do not slide off the working surface.

---

in which a is the moment arm, being the perpendicular distance between the vector of the gravitational force and the vector of the reaction force through the joint axis. Balance is achieved by bringing an equally great, but opposite, moment in the form of force, F_S, in the back muscles. The resultant reaction force on the spine is F_{RS}, such that a coupling with the moment arm, b, occurs. The moment balance is now described as follows:

$$F_S = \frac{a}{b} F_C = \frac{30}{5} \times 500 = 3000 \text{ N}$$

The weight of the upper body and the magnitude of the moment arm of the back muscles are given. The moment arm, a, with regard to the low back (also called lever arm), determines the enlargement factor given through

the relation of a and b (Figure 12–3). Therefore, prolonged stooped positions should be avoided. This is also true for the cervical muscles when considering large moments, proportional to the lever arm of the gravitational force through the center of gravity of the head to the cervical spine.

Constant muscle force can be maintained only for a short period, unless the activity or position requires a force at a level of only approximately 15% of the maximal muscle strength (Figure 12–4).

In the musculoskeletal system, the functions concerning the maintenance of posture and providing movement have a large significance in determining the physical loads occurring at work, at school, and at home. Posture can exist without appreciable move-

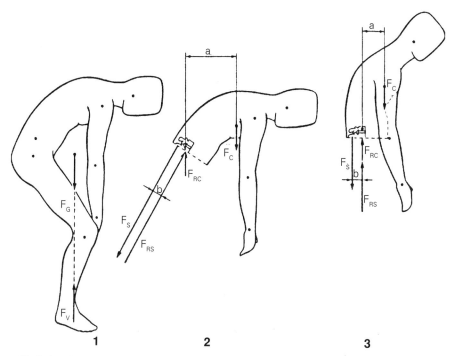

Figure 12–3 Load on the back during stooping. *1*, The center of gravity of the entire body is located above the feet; *2* and *3*, the part of the body above the L5-S1 level is considered separately.

ment, but movement cannot exist without posture. A significant part of physical activity is constantly required to prevent the body from collapsing under the influence of gravity. Thus, the influence of gravity must always be incorporated into this area of biomechanics and in tables showing weight and centers of gravity of body parts. However, such tables are the result of measurements on frozen-sectioned cadavers, which can lead to imprecise deductions when applied to living human beings. Nevertheless, the current standard of technology has progressed in such a way that the workload on structures of the body can be reasonably estimated. These estimations are determined to such a degree that diverse working situations can be compared with each other, and subsequent improvements can be made where necessary. Therefore, decreasing the lever arm, a, for both static and dynamic situations can be interpreted as a measurement to increase comfort and to prevent back and neck pain (Figure 12–3).

One aspect that still carries a lot of uncertainties is the aspect of loadability when certain known harmful processes with a relatively slow course are considered. Most knowledge has been acquired in regard to lifting loads. Normative values for the maximal amount of loads to be lifted are related to the following:

- the distance from the center of gravity of the load to the spinal column
- the trajectory over which the load has to be lifted
- the level of the mid-point of this trajectory
- the amount of lifting movements per time unit

Walking

Regular walking is a good measure for prevention of back pain. Also, the favorable load

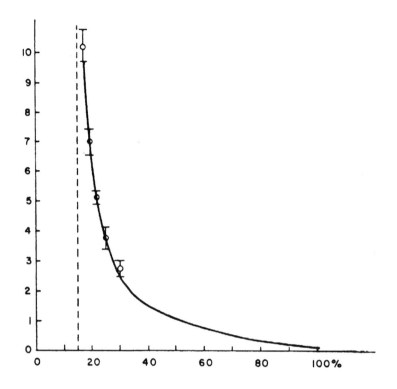

Figure 12–4 Maintaining static muscle activity. The vertical lines indicate the standard deviation.

(lever arm, a) makes walking a therapeutic measure for back patients. Unfavorable factors include wearing heavy clothing and walking on a hard surface such as asphalt and concrete without shock-absorptive soles, particularly at the heel. The abrupt halting of the heel against the ground translates into a repetitive hard impact. These impacts are transferred higher up into the body and have enough force to be able to cause symptoms in the spinal column and even in the head. Viscoelastic or rubber soles act as a spring to provide smoother halting of the moving mass of the foot and the rest of the body. Thus, reaction forces between the foot and the walking surface are reduced by half.

Other relationships between shoes and back pain are not yet proven. However, a relationship could be made between antalgic positions due to pinching shoes or fatigue of back muscles because of standing and walking on high heels (higher than 4 cm).

Lying

A bed is considered to be a body-supporting surface upon which an individual must be able to rest completely for prolonged periods. Generally it consists of a mattress, a mattress support, and a bedstead. Of course, a water bed is a different case.

There are three types of mattresses: polyurethane, foam rubber, and those with inner springs. Foam rubber is proportionately heavy and puts more load on the back when making the bed. On the other hand, polyurethane is less durable and, because of a loss of elasticity, tends to sag.

There are six types of mattress supports: coiled-wire mat, woven steel-wire mat, box spring, lattice support (with straight laths, laths that are slightly convex, and laths that are slightly convex and can be canted), wooden platform, and simple and inexpensive planks (preferably with a distance between the planks of 7 cm).

Many combinations of mattresses and supports are possible; however, not all are equally suitable. A bed with a good combination does the following:

- supports the body's curves
- remains flat
- cushions well
- provides good ventilation
- is not too warm or too cold

The first three qualities are related to supporting the body in such a way that pressure on the prominent bony parts of the body is evenly divided, the spinal column remains straight when sidelying, and in supine the spinal column retains its physiological curves. When individuals with limited hip extension lie on a normal bed with their legs straight out, the low back is pulled into a lordosis. These people prefer a sagging bed or would rather lie on their sides. People with a hyperkyphotic spine, particularly the elderly, like to use a thick pillow so that the head does not lie in too much extension. Pillows should be easily deformable, and at the same time provide good support for the head as well as the neck.

Hospital beds have a special feature in that they are also used for prolonged sitting, as soon as the patient is able to do so. For this reason, the standard hospital bed has one end that can be raised, creating a backrest. The "seat" is completely horizontal; thus the patient gradually slides down into a slouched position. Because of this position, the lumbar spine loses support. Eventually patients complain of back pain. In addition, increased pressure is placed on the sacrum instead of the ischial tuberosities, increasing the risk of developing a decubitus ulcer. A preventive measure would be to raise the bed again at the level of the patient's knees, creating an inclined sitting surface.

Vibration

Musculoskeletal system injury can result from vibration. A combination of the following factors plays a role:

- duration of exposure
- frequency of the vibration
- amplitude of the vibration

The "ascending" part of the vibration is similar to the impact that occurs when the heel strikes the ground. For a given mass, the maximal acceleration is a measure of the force on the body part that has to follow the induced motion. If the body is exposed to a vibratory object, the maximal forces between the body and the object will decrease by placing a spring (for instance, rubber) between both parts. For example, Figure 12–5 shows a blade spring, which is used between the heavily vibrating pneumatic hammer and the hand of the user. At the same time it serves as protection for the spinal column. Such a solution loses its effectiveness, however, when a large amount of force is required to use the tool.

In evaluating the effects of vibration, besides the maximal acceleration (usually this is measured and not the maximal amplitude), the frequency of the periodic movement is also significant. This is stated in hertz (1 Hz = one vibration per second). Mechanical vibrations, particularly within certain frequencies, can be harmful to structures in the body.

Inherent frequency is the frequency of the vibration that occurs in the mass-spring system, when it is left by itself, after impact. The inherent frequencies (resonance frequencies) of structures in the body are known. Some examples are:

- shoulder   4 to 5 Hz
- abdomen   4 to 8 Hz

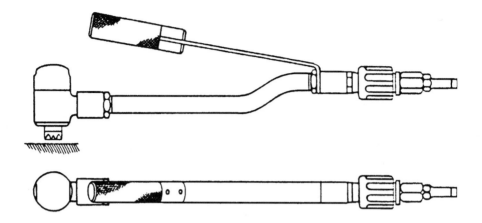

Figure 12–5 The head of the hammer (left) vibrates heavily on the work surface; therefore a blade spring is placed between the grip and hammer. *Source:* Atlas Copco, Stockholm.

- spinal column   10 to 12 Hz
- upper arm   10 to 16 Hz
- forearm   16 to 30 Hz
- head-neck-shoulder   20 to 30 Hz
- head   25 Hz
- eyeball and socket   30 to 80 Hz
- chest   60 Hz
- grip   50 to 200 Hz
- mandible-skull   100 to 200 Hz
- hand-arm   100 Hz and higher

The mass of the skeletal parts and their elastic connections with other parts, which can be seen simply as a spring, determine the inherent frequencies in hertz.

$$F_e = \frac{1}{2\pi}\sqrt{\frac{c}{m}}$$

in which m equals mass in kilograms and c the spring value in newton meters. A high value for c indicates a firm spring.

If an external force with the same frequency is exerted on the mass, amplitude increases significantly due to resonance. Taking into account the frequency, intensity, and duration of exposure, graphs are available indicating limits of comfort and harmfulness of vibrations.

When the entire body is brought into a vibratory state, the following typical symptoms can occur[2]:

- general feeling of
  discomfort   4 to 9 Hz
- head symptoms   13 to 20 Hz
- mandible symptoms   6 to 8 Hz
- problems speaking   13 to 20 Hz
- chest pain   5 to 7 Hz
- calf pain   4 to 10 Hz
- urge to urinate   10 to 18 Hz
- increase in muscle
  tension   13 to 20 Hz

CONCLUSION

Back problems already are seen in young adults. One fourth of all young adults are currently experiencing low back pain, and 60% have experienced it at least once before. In young adulthood, the body experiences so many influences that the precise cause of the back pain often is unknown.

Some general conclusions can be drawn from epidemiological research performed among patients in the United States who underwent surgery for a herniated disc.[3] The greatest chance for prolapsed disc operations was found in people who were between the ages of 30 and 40, smokers, people who lifted objects in a bent and twisted position, and people who drove long distances in old cars. Various models of cars have different influences on the human spine. One of the most often-purchased models was found to have the worst effect.

In another epidemiological study, Kelsey et al[4] described factors that are related to the occurrence of an acute prolapse of a cervical disc. The most common age was also found to be between 30 and 40 years. The disorder was seen in 40% more males than females, and was especially related to lifting heavy objects, smoking cigarettes (not cigars or a pipe), and frequent diving from a diving board. No relation was found with other sports activities. Fewer, hardly significant, correlations were found in working with vibrating tools and with time spent in automobiles.

Regarding measures for the prevention of back pain, much useful information is already available. Unfortunately, introduction of these measures by influencing consumer behavior is not very successful. The potential health endangerments seem to be at too great a distance from the individual consumer. Indicating an immediate realization of comfort and better performance could be a more effective way of getting people to purchase the most biomechanically and ergonomically correct tools for use in daily living, including chairs, working surfaces, and automobiles.

REFERENCES

1. EG. *Report from the Committee to Study Lumbar Risks at the Workplace to the Director-General of DGV in the Commission from the European Community.* Commission from the European Community; document no. 2080/86 NE.

2. Rasmussen G. *Human Body Vibration Exposure and Its Measurement: Technical Review No. 1.* Huddinge: Bruel & Kjar; 1982.

3. Kelsey JL, Githens PB, O'Connor T, et al. Acute prolapsed lumbar intervertebral disk: an epidemiological study with special reference to driving automobiles and cigarette smoking. *Spine.* 1984;9:608–613.

4. Kelsey JL, Githens PB, Walter SD, et al. An epidemiological study of acute prolapsed cervical intervertebral disc. *J Bone Joint Surg [Am].* 1984;66:907–914.

SUGGESTED READING

Williams M, Lissner HR. *Biomechanics of Human Motion.* Philadelphia: WB Saunders; 1976.

13

Mobilization of the Spinal Column

EDITOR'S PREFACE

Conservative treatment of spinal column disorders, for a large part, is manual. In "mobilization," motion is applied slowly after first taking up pre-tension in the joint and soft tissue structures. In "manipulation," a very fast, but small, movement is performed after first taking up the pre-tension. Mobilization is aimed at increasing or restoring a limitation of motion. Manipulation is indicated for a minor limitation of motion or in instances of an altered (excessively hard) end-feel.

An important question remains regarding whether these manual techniques should be performed with a long or a short lever. In techniques with a long lever, a large number of segments are involved. On the other hand, many individuals question whether it is really possible to induce a monosegmental motion when working with a short lever. Strictly seen, it is not possible: movement of one vertebra is generally movement in relation to two other vertebrae. However, on theoretical grounds the term monosegmental mobilization *clearly makes sense: there are tech-niques in which movement takes place particularly in one movement segment. In this chapter, Peter Scholten discusses this theoretical reasoning.*

In performing manual mobilization on the spine, attempts are made to fix (manually) and lock (by means of kinematic coupling) the spinal column to keep the mobilization effect as local as possible. Initially, mobilization with a long lever is applied. However, distinctly local problems are treated with a short lever. In the following theoretical analysis, considerations are presented that lead to a reinforcement of this choice.

As yet there are no effect studies known that differentiate the indications for mobilizing with the long versus the short lever. Research regarding manual therapy in general must be encouraged. Such detailed studies are greatly needed.

INTRODUCTION

In mobilization of the spinal column, mobility of the segments in the spinal column is promoted. Mobilization is performed not only to improve a limitation of motion but also to maintain the present range of motion. There are a number of techniques, both active and passive, for mobilizing the spinal column. These techniques all have one thing in common: a force is applied to achieve the mobilization. In this chapter, the mechanism of *force transmission* in the mobilization of a motion segment is first clarified. The *mobility* of a motion segment then is discussed, and finally the force transmission in the mobilization of several motion segments is examined.

FORCE TRANSMISSION IN MONOSEGMENTAL MOBILIZATION

To clarify force transmission in mobilizations, the concept of force transmission must be explained. For this, the axioms of Newton are applied, specifically, the axiom "action equals reaction" and the axiom "forces acting on a body at rest create balance."

Action Equals Reaction

The axiom "action equals reaction" means that when a body is loaded by a force, another equal force is present, but in the opposite direction. This force is called the reaction force. Thus, forces always occur in pairs (Figure 13–1). For example, during contraction of an arm muscle, the forearm performs a flexion movement in relation to the upper arm (Figure 13–2). Suppose the friction in the muscle and the friction in the elbow joint, as well as the atmospheric resistance, equal zero. If we nullify the mass of the moving parts, this movement does not require force. Therefore, the magnitude of the muscle force is zero. Muscle force is present only if resistance is offered by elements such as friction, atmospheric resistance, the influence of gravity, or an externally applied force. The muscle force can be interpreted as the action force, and the resistance as the necessary reaction force. Furthermore, within the muscle the axiom "action equals reaction" is also taking place. As the muscle exerts a force upon the fore-

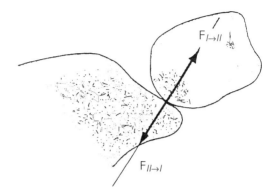

Figure 13–1 If body *I* exerts a force onto body *II*, then body *II* exerts an equal but opposite force onto body *I*. $F_{II\to I}$, the reaction force of $F_{I\to II}$.

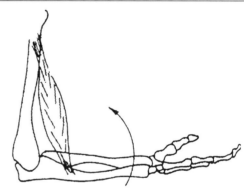

Figure 13–2 Flexion movement of the arm by muscle contraction.

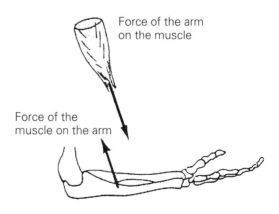

Force of the arm on the muscle

Force of the muscle on the arm

Figure 13–3 The axiom "action equals reaction" applied to the force in a muscle.

arm, the lower arm exerts an equal but opposite force upon the muscle (Figure 13–3).

Forces Acting on a Body at Rest Create Balance

If there is no force working on a body, the body will be at rest. If a system of forces acts upon a body in such a way that the joint reactions of all these forces do not change the resting situation, this system of forces forms a balanced system. Deduced from this are the two requirements for balance: *force balance* and *moment balance*. A body is at rest if the requirements of both force balance and moment balance are met.

In force balance, the sum of the components of the forces in any direction has to be zero. For two-dimensional situations, force balance in two mutually perpendicular directions is sufficient. This is noted with the following formula:

$$F_{x1} + F_{x2} + \cdots + F_{Xn} = 0 \text{ or } \Sigma F_x = 0$$

$$F_{y1} + F_{y2} + \cdots + F_{Xn} = 0 \text{ or } \Sigma F_y = 0$$

For three-dimensional situations, three balance formulas are necessary for the force balance in three mutually perpendicular directions:

$$\Sigma F_x = 0, \quad \Sigma F_y = 0, \quad \Sigma F_z = 0$$

The moment balance implies that the sum of the moments of the forces, in relation to any arbitrary point, has to be zero. For two-dimensional situations, the balance around an axis perpendicular to the plane in which the forces are acting is sufficient. Suppose this plane is the x-y plane, then $\Sigma M_z = 0$. For three-dimensional situations, three balance formulas are necessary and sufficient for the moment balance around three mutually perpendicular axes. The following applies:

$$\Sigma M_x = 0, \quad \Sigma M_y = 0, \quad \Sigma M_z = 0$$

In order to obtain balance in two-dimensional situations, the requirements set by three balance formulas have to be met:

$$\Sigma F_x = 0, \quad \Sigma F_y = 0, \quad \Sigma F_z = 0$$

For three-dimensional situations the requirements set by six balance formulas have to be met:

$$\Sigma F_x = 0, \quad \Sigma F_y = 0, \quad \Sigma F_z = 0$$

$$\Sigma M_x = 0, \quad \Sigma M_y = 0, \quad \Sigma M_z = 0$$

Let us observe the application of these axioms when successively loading first a vertebra and then a motion segment, consisting of two vertebrae and an intervertebral disc.

Loading of a Vertebra

There are two magnitudes of loading: forces and moments. Seen in two dimensions, the load on a vertebra can be described by two mutually perpendicular forces and a moment. Considered in three dimensions, three mutually perpendicular forces and three moments around three mutually perpendicular axes are necessary. In Figure 13–4, several different loading situations of a vertebra are depicted.

In a resting situation, thus a balanced situation, the loading magnitude of the surrounding structures on the vertebra can be determined with the balance formulas. For each situation, the requirements of force balance and moment balance have to be met. Suppose the load is a transverse force parallel to the upper end-plate of the vertebra (Figure 13–5). For the balance of forces, an equal but opposite-directed transverse force has to load the lower end-plate. For the balance of moments, the center of the lower end-plate is significant. In addition, the following requirement has to be met: the moment occurring due to the transverse-force loading of the upper end-plate has to be equal and directed opposite to the moment exerted on the lower end-plate by the caudally located structures. The results of the other loading situations from Figure 13–4 are illustrated in Figure 13–6. It is obvious from these balance situations that an eccentric compressive force will have a moment as a result.

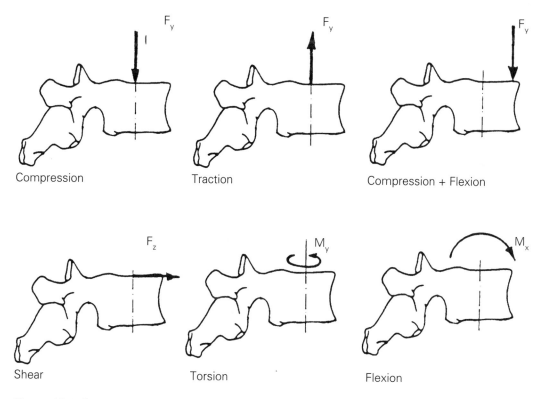

Figure 13–4 Several different loading situations of a vertebra.

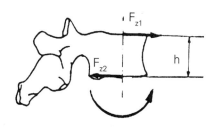

$$F_{z2} = F_{z1}$$

$$M_x = F_{z1} \times h$$

Figure 13–5 The transverse force balance of a vertebra.

Loading of a Motion Segment

Suppose the load on a segment's upper vertebra is an eccentric compressive force (Figure 13–7). To determine the forces and moments exerted by the upper vertebra on the intervertebral disc, as well as the forces and moments exerted by the intervertebral disc on the lower vertebra, we detach the two vertebrae and the intervertebral disc. In biomechanics, this process is known as drafting a free-body diagram (Figure 13–8).

The magnitudes of loading on the lower end-plate of the upper vertebra can be derived from the force and moment balance. These forces and moments are exerted by the intervertebral disc on the upper vertebra. If the axiom "action equals reaction" is now applied, the magnitude of forces and moments influencing the intervertebral disc is also known.

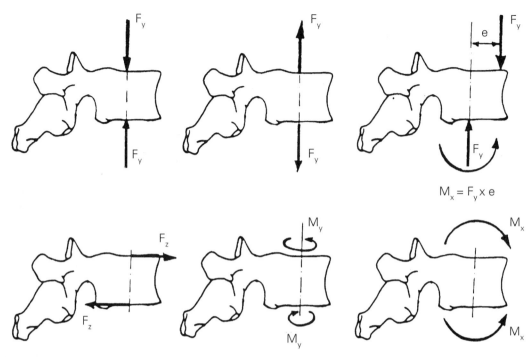

Figure 13–6 Some possible balance situations of a vertebra.

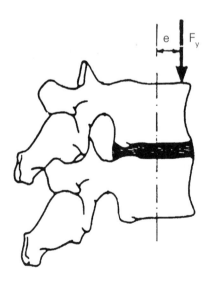

Figure 13–7 The loading of a motion segment.

Thus, these forces and moments are exerted by the upper vertebra on the intervertebral disc. Next the forces and moments exerted by the lower vertebra on the intervertebral disc can be calculated by using the balance formula belonging to the intervertebral disc.

Summary

In summary, the following conclusion can be drawn: with the loading of a vertebra, all caudally located vertebrae are loaded with the same magnitude. If a force influences a vertebral body, this force is transmitted to all lower located vertebrae in such a way that the magnitude and the direction of this force are equal on every vertebra. This also counts for a moment or the combination of both force and moment. However, two exceptions can be proved based on the above-mentioned balance considerations.

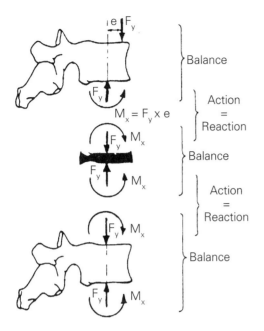

Figure 13–8 The free body diagram of a motion segment.

---

1. If an eccentric compressive force is applied, then besides the force, a moment is transmitted. The magnitude of this moment is determined by the product of the magnitude of the eccentric compressive force and the amount of eccentricity of this force. The direction of the moment depends on the direction of the eccentricity of the force.

2. If a force on a vertebra can be resolved into a compressive force and a shear force (the shear force being a force parallel to the vertebra's end-plate), then the shear force will be the transmitter of the moment. The magnitude of this moment equals the product of the magnitude of the shear force and the distance to the place where the shear force exerts its influence. Thus, this moment does not have a constant magnitude but increases as the distance to the place of exertion of the shear force decreases.

MOBILITY OF A MOTION SEGMENT

The terminology "mobility" or "flexibility" indicates the amount of movement in the spinal column. The mobility or flexibility of a motion segment can be defined as the ratio between the range of motion and the force necessary to achieve this motion. The reciprocal value of flexibility is stiffness. This is defined as the ratio between the load required to attain the movement and the magnitude of the corresponding range of motion.

The stiffness of a motion segment is determined by the resistance of the connecting elements between two adjacent vertebrae. Such structures include ligaments, intervertebral discs, zygapophyseal joints, and muscles.

Because the deformation of a vertebra is much smaller than the deformation of the connecting elements, the vertebra is generally considered to be a rigid and therefore nondeformable body. Thus, in describing the mobility of a motion segment, the mobility caused by the connecting structures is actually meant instead. The influence of the different components of this mobility will not be further clarified in the framework of this text.

When a torsional moment acts on a motion segment, one vertebra rotates axially in relation to the other vertebra (Figure 13–9). The magnitude of the axial rotation depends on the resistance offered by the interposed tissue of the two adjacent vertebrae. The corresponding resistance to the torsion is called torsion stiffness. For example, vertebra 1 is loaded by a torsional moment. If vertebra 2 is fixed, the moment results in an axial rotation of vertebra 1. The relation between the torsional moment and the axial rotation of vertebra 1 can be described by the following formula:

$$M_Y = CR_Y$$

where C is the torsional stiffness of the interposed tissue, M_Y is the torsional moment, and R_Y is the axial rotation. The physical behavior

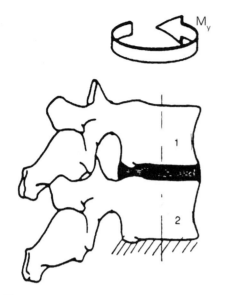

Figure 13–9 A motion segment loaded by a torsional moment (M_y).

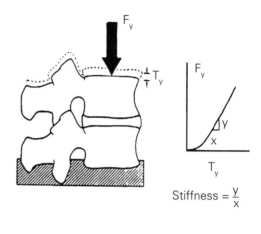

Figure 13–10 The relation between load (F_y) and deformation (T_y) of an intervertebral disc.

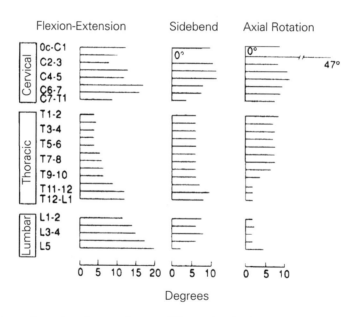

Figure 13–11 Normative values for rotations at different levels of the spinal column.

of biological material can be described by a constant when very small movements are concerned, in this instance, the torsion stiffness, C. In general, the relation between load and deformation in biological material is nonlinear. This means that the physical behavior usually cannot be described by a constant, but instead by a nonlinear function, as illustrated in Figure 13–10.

The terms *flexibility/mobility* and *maximal range of motion* do not have the same meaning. Maximal range of motion is the amount of motion caused by a load, whereby tissue damage or pain arises if this range of motion is increased. Thus, maximal range of motion does not relate to the flexibility; the force necessary for the performance of the maximal motion is not reported. An overview of normative values for the maximal range of motion in various spinal column motion segments is given in Figure 13–11.

As already mentioned in the section dealing with loading of a vertebra, the load on a vertebra in a three-dimensional situation can be entirely described by three mutually per-

pendicular forces and three moments around mutually perpendicular axes (Figure 13–12). The six magnitudes of load are coupled to six magnitudes of motion through six stiffness coefficients: three translations and three rotations. An overview of the most important stiffness coefficients is given in Table 13–1.

The values in Table 13–1 must be interpreted as average values. The values are obtained through experiments on cadavers with isolated motion segments. The in vivo values are probably higher because the stiffness of the spinal column also depends on such factors as the stiffness of the rib cage and the stiffness of the muscles connected to the spinal column and rib cage.

Furthermore, coupled movements occur when the spinal column is loaded. When a motion segment is compressed, an impression takes place. The magnitude of this impression can be estimated by using the column of compression stiffnesses from Table 13–1. With a compression stiffness of 2.0 MN/m, or 2000 N/mm, and a compression force of 500 N, the impression will have a

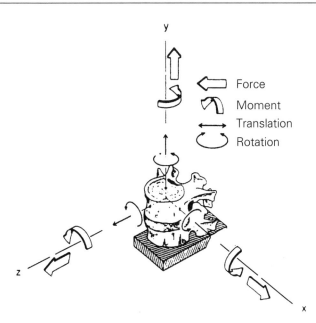

y

Force
Moment
Translation
Rotation

z

x

Figure 13–12 The three-dimensional coordinate system for the loading of a motion segment.

Table 13–1 Stiffness Coefficients of a Movement Segment

Authors	Stiffness Coefficient*	Maximal Load*	Spine Region
Compression (−F_Y)			
Hirsch and Nachemson,[1] 1954	3.0 MN/m	4.5 kN	Lumbar
Rolander,[2] 1966	2.0 MN/m	1.0 kN	Lumbar
Panjabi et al,[3] 1976	1.3 MN/m	160 N	Thoracic
Tension (+F_Y)			
Panjabi et al,[3] 1976	0.80 MN/m	160 N	Thoracic
Shear (F_X, F_Z)			
Liu et al,[4] 1975	0.55 MN/m	450 N	Lumbar
Panjabi et al,[3] 1976	0.10 MN/m	160 N	Thoracic
Flexion (+M_X)			
Markolf,[5] 1972	2.0 NM/degree	7 Nm	T7–8 to L3-4
Panjabi et al,[3] 1976	2.6 NM/degree	8 Nm	Thoracic
Extension (−M_X)			
Markolf,[5] 1972	2.6 NM /degree	7 Nm	T7–8 to L3-4
Panjabi et al,[3] 1976	3.2 NM/degree	8 Nm	Thoracic
Sidebend (M_Z)			
Markolf,[5] 1972	1.8 NM/degree	7 Nm	Thoracic
Panjabi et al,[3] 1976	2.9 NM/degree	8 Nm	Thoracic
Axial Rotation (M_Y)			
Markolf,[5] 1972	6.0 NM/degree	7 Nm	Thoracic
Farfan et al,[6] 1970	4.0 NM/degree	8 Nm	Lumbar
Panjabi et al,[3] 1976	2.5 NM/degree	8 Nm	Thoracic

*N = newton, kN = 1000 N, MN = 1,000,000 N, Nm = newton meter.

magnitude of 500/2000 = 0.25 mm. As a result of the compressive force, a coupled movement takes place, resulting in a shift of the vertebra in a ventral direction along with a flexion motion.

To a large extent, this ventral shift of the vertebra under compression is due to the oblique position of the zygapophyseal joints. The flexion motion results because the center of rotation of a motion segment is not located in the center of the segment but instead more dorsally. Furthermore, in flexion of a motion segment, deformation of the intervertebral disc takes place. This is accompanied by a ventral displacement of the vertebra (Figure 13–13).

Although coupled motions generally are smaller than the main motion, corresponding with the direction of the load, they cannot be ignored. An excellent example of a coupled motion is the axial rotation of a vertebra that accompanies the sidebending motion. An overview of the coupled motions is reported in Table 13–2.

The matrix presented in Table 13–2 is symmetrical. In other words, a torsional moment, M_Y, results in a translation, T_X; an axial rotation, R_Y; and a sidebending, R_Z. But the performance of an axial rotation, R_Y, results in a mediolateral force, F_X; a torsional moment, M_Y, and a sidebending moment, M_Z. Furthermore, every component in Table 13–2 has to be interpreted as a magnitude that is nonlinear for large motions. In Figure 13–14, the different loading situations from Figure 13–4 are shown again, but now with an average value for the corresponding motion of the vertebra. This can be calculated by using the data from Table 13–1.

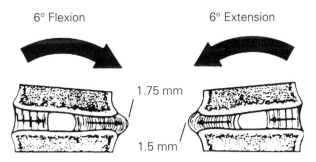

Figure 13–13 Flexion and extension of a motion segment caused by a motion of the intervertebral disc in the horizontal plane.

FORCE TRANSMISSION IN MULTISEGMENTAL MOBILIZATION

The force transmission in different motion segments is discussed above. The result of loading a motion segment is the motion of one vertebra in relation to the other. The magnitude of the motion depends on the magnitude of the load and the stiffness of the motion segment. If the coupled motion is left out of consideration, the direction of the motion is determined by the direction of the load. With the mobilization of several motion segments, a force transmission takes place through all of the motion segments that are part of the chain being mobilized. If the loads upon and the stiffnesses of the relevant motion segments are known, the movement of every motion segment can be determined. The total

Table 13–2 Relation of Load and Motion of a Motion Segment*

Motion	F_X	F_Y	F_Z	M_X	M_Y	M_Z
T_X	X				O	O
T_Y		X	O	O		
T_Z		O	X	O		
R_X		O	O	X		
R_Y	O				X	O
R_Z	O				O	X

*The letter X indicates the main motions. The letter O represents the coupled motions.

change in position between the vertebrae at each end of the chain being mobilized has to equal the sum of the motions in every motion segment.

Imagine a chain of three motion segments. The proximal vertebra is loaded by a torsional moment, M. The distal vertebra is thought to be in a fixed situation (Figure 13–15). Every motion segment is now loaded by a torsional moment, M, of the same magnitude. The axial rotation, a, of vertebra 3, in relation to vertebra 4, is now $a_3 = M/c_3$, with c_3 being the torsional stiffness of the third motion segment. The axial rotation of vertebra 2 in relation to vertebra 3 is $a_{23} = M/c_2$, and the total axial rotation of vertebra 2 is $a_2 = a_{23} + a_3$. For the axial rotation of the proximal vertebra 1, in relation to the distal vertebra 4, the following derivation can be made: $a_1 = M (1/c_1 + 1/c_2 + 1/c_3)$ (Figure 13–16).

If the stiffnesses of every motion segment are of the same magnitude, the axial rotation of the proximal vertebra 1, in relation to the distal vertebra 4, will simply equal three times the axial rotation of one motion segment. Because the stiffnesses of the different motion segments are not mutually equal, the method described above can be used only to make a rough estimation of the occurring motion.

In Figure 13–17, the relative translations and rotations between two adjacent vertebrae are illustrated as a result of a shear force of 10 N and a moment of 0.225 Nm, respectively. These values were determined on a

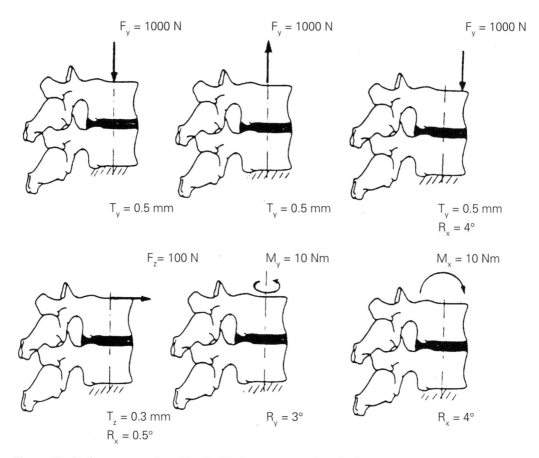

Figure 13–14 Some examples of load with the corresponding displacement.

sectioned spinal column of an 11-year-old child and therefore show less stiffness than the data offered in Table 13–1. However, the differences in stiffnesses between two adjacent motion segments are depicted clearly.

CONCLUSION

The question can now be asked whether there is a difference between monosegmental and multisegmental mobilization. Suppose the motion segment between vertebra 2 and vertebra 3 from Figure 13–15 has a limitation of motion. The question here is in regard to the influence of the torsional moment on the mobilization of the structures between vertebra 2 and vertebra 3. The answer is very simple: the torsional moment is of the same magnitude in

every motion segment. The magnitude of the axial rotation of every motion segment is determined by the torsional moment, M, and the torsional stiffness, c, of the relevant segment: axial rotation equals M/c.

In a limitation of motion, the stiffness increases, resulting in a decreased rotation. Mobilization with the goal of achieving a large amount of motion has the greatest effect on the surrounding motion segments. A greater torsional moment can be applied in order to create a larger rotation. According to the earlier derived formula $a_1 = M(1/c_1 + 1/c_2 + 1/c_3)$, there is an increase of the axial rotation in every motion segment. However, this increase is directly proportional to the flexibility, or inversely proportional to the stiffness, of the motion segment. In this example, be-

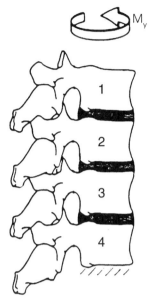

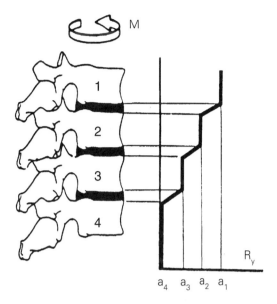

Figure 13–15 A chain of three motion segments loaded by a torsional moment.

Figure 13–16 The axial rotation of three motion segments.

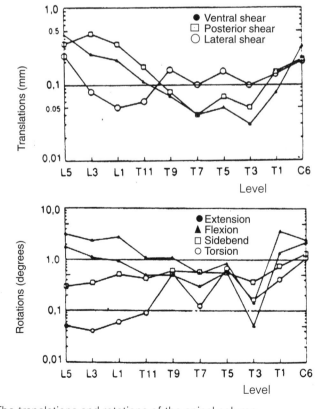

Figure 13–17 The translations and rotations of the spinal column.

cause motion segment 2 possesses a greater stiffness, an increase in the moment will have the most effect on the adjacent motion segments. If the mutual differences in stiffnesses are large, the maximal range of motion in the adjacent motion segments may be reached without achieving the desired effect in the segment that has to be mobilized. Thus, a further increase in the torsional moment can be harmful.

From this, it can be concluded that in instances of minor limitations of motions, multisegmental mobilizations can lead to the desired result. With a major local limitation of motion, a monosegmental treatment is preferred. Obviously, when several adjacent motion segments show a limitation of motion, a multisegmental treatment will have the same significance as a monosegmental treatment.

In testing the mobility of the spinal column, it is wise to include as many motion segments as possible in the chain that has to be examined. Because the total range of motion equals the sum of the separate motions and because a larger range of motion is easier to observe, it will contribute to the preciseness of the examination. When a limited range of motion is found, it will have to be localized by a monosegmental examination.

REFERENCES

1. Hirsch C, Nachemson A. A new observation on the mechanical behavior of lumbar discs. *Acta Orthop Scand.* 1954;23:254.

2. Rolander SD. Motion of the lumbar spine with special reference to the stabilizing effect of posterior fusion. *Acta Orthop Scand Suppl.* 1966;90.

3. Panjabi MM, Brand RA, White AA. Mechanical properties of the human thoracic spine, as shown by three dimensional displacement curves. *J Bone Joint Surg [Am].* 1976;58:642–652.

4. Liu YK, Ray G, Hirsch C. The resistance of the lumbar spine to direct shear. *Orthop Clin North Am.* 1975;6:33.

5. Markolf KL. Deformation of the thoracolumbar intervertebral joints in response to external loads. *J Bone Joint Surg [Am].* 1972;54:511–533.

6. Farfan HF, Cossette JW, Robertson GH, Wells RV, Kraus H. The effects of torsion on the lumbar intervertebral joint: the role of torsion in the production of disc degeneration. *J Bone Joint Surg [Am].* 1970; 52:468.

SUGGESTED READING

Kapandji LA. *The Physiology of the Joints: The Trunk and the Vertebral Column.* Edinburgh: Churchill Livingstone; 1974:3.

Scholten P. Enkele theoretische achtergronden van het mobiliseren van de wervelkolom. *Ned Tijkschr Man Ther.* 1989;8:30–38.

Scholten PJM. *Idiopathic Scoliosis: Some Fundamental Aspects of the Mechanical Behavior of the Human Spine.* Amsterdam: Free University Press; 1986. Thesis.

Skogland LB, Miller JAA. *On the Importance of Growth in Idiopathic Scoliosis: A Biochemical, Radiological, and Biomechanical Study.* Oslo; 1980. Thesis.

White AA, Panjabi MM. *Clinical Biomechanics of the Spine.* Philadelphia: JB Lippincott Co; 1978.

White AA, Panjabi MM. The basic kinematics of the human spine: a review of past and current knowledge. *Spine.* 1978;3:12–20.

14

Research on Effectiveness of Manual Therapy for the Spinal Column

EDITOR'S PREFACE

In reviewing articles related to the various forms of "movement medicine" (orthopaedic medicine, physical therapy, osteopathy, occupational therapy, rehabilitative medicine, etc), conflicting results are often found. A number of true experimental group studies find a significant effect in favor of the researched treatment, while other studies are unable to confirm the same effect.

Because of the significant differences among patients, circumstances, measurement results, and types of treatment, the results of a true experimental group study can be partially coincidental. Repeated experiments rarely, if ever, produce the same results. The situation would be completely different if one or more articles indicated results that were against the experimental treatment. Although a study with such results might be coincidental, it still should not be suppressed.

On the basis of the above considerations, Geert Aufdemkampe reviews the true experimental studies concerning manipulation for low back pain. From these studies, it can be deduced that manipulation has a significant effect in instances of acute symptoms, however, only in the sense that the recovery process is accelerated. Concerning treatment for chronic symptoms, no definite conclusions can be reached.

INTRODUCTION

In this chapter, effect studies and review articles of manual therapy for low back pain are described. Although effect studies are also available for manual therapy for cervical problems,[1-4] these are not described here. At present, there is not enough research literature to detect possible patterns of efficacy.

In view of the relatively large number of published research articles regarding the effectiveness of manual therapy in the treatment of low back pain, only studies with a true experimental design are described in this chapter. The number of "review" articles concerning manual therapy of the spinal column witnesses the fact that a relatively large number of research reports have been published.[5-14] On first impression, the conclusions of the different studies seem to be contradictory.

Aufdemkampe et al[5] find a certain pattern in the research results of seven true and two quasi-experimentally designed studies. In patients with long-standing symptoms, defined as lasting longer than 1 year and/or under treatment of a specialist, manual therapy seems to be ineffective. However, for symptoms of short duration, meaning less than 1 year and not under treatment by a specialist, manual therapy appears to be effective.

Based on six studies, Bouter[15] states that it is not possible to make a solid judgment in relation to the effectiveness of manual therapy in patients with low back pain.

In a review of nine true experimentally designed studies, Deyo[6] writes that manual therapy seems to have some short-term, but no long-term, effects. However, Deyo does not define these "terms" on a time basis.

After examining nine true experimentally designed studies, DiFabio[7] found more questions than answers. One of DiFabio's questions is whether manual therapy is effective in some disorders of the low back and not in others. However, DiFabio did not mention the disorders that might react positively to manual therapy.

Nine true experimentally designed studies are discussed by Evans,[8] with the conclusion that manual therapy is effective in low back pain of recent history in older patients, in whom the cause is almost certainly not a prolapsed intervertebral disc.

Based on 10 true experimentally designed studies, Jull[9] observed two apparent factors from the review. First, in the treatment of low back pain, manual therapy does not lead to results better than those obtained with other conservative methods in the long term (the "term" is not further defined). Second, and partly contradictory to the first conclusion, Jull concludes that manual therapy is significantly more effective than conservative methods (such as shortwave, massage, corset, analgesics, and isometric exercises) in recently occurring low back symptoms. Again, the question arises as to what Jull defines as "recent."

Lankhorst[10] comes to the following three conclusions based on 11 true experimental studies:

1. Manual therapy has a favorable effect in comparison to other forms of treatment on a short-term basis (without indication of time) but not on a long-term basis (again, without indication of time).

2. The pronouncement that manipulation in some patients with low back pain leads to a fast improvement seems justified.

3. One cannot indicate beforehand which patients will react favorably and which ones will not react favorably to manual therapy.

After examining one quasi- and two true experimentally designed studies, Lindahl[25] found that manual therapy seems to be as effective, if not more effective, than other conservative treatment methods.

The above-mentioned concept that manual therapy is effective in symptoms of relatively short duration but not in symptoms of long duration (defined by Aufdemkampe et al[5] as lasting longer than 1 year and/or under treatment of a specialist) is supported by Moritz,[12] based on 13 controlled studies.

O'Donoghue[13] indicates that based on 10 true experimentally designed studies, some proof in favor of the effectiveness of manual therapy in the treatment of low back pain can be found. However, O'Donoghue states that there is less support for the conclusion that fewer treatments are necessary when treating with manual therapy than with other treatment methods.

Finally, Stoddard[14] again states, based on a description of six true experimentally designed studies, that manual therapy is effective in the early stages of low back pain (without defining "early") and that a faster response can be expected with manual therapy in relation to other conservative treatment methods.

In summary, the overall conclusion from the above-mentioned reviews is that manual therapy is an effective treatment in certain low back disorders. The duration of the symptoms seems to make a difference in the outcome of the treatment. It is noteworthy that almost all of the authors plead for true experimental design in research of the effects of manual therapy, in which a blind scoring of the effect variables is of primary concern.

TRUE EXPERIMENTAL RESEARCH ON EFFECTIVENESS OF MANUAL THERAPY IN TREATING LOW BACK PAIN

In the following pages, 17 true experimental studies regarding the effectiveness of manual therapy applied to healthy subjects and to subjects with low back pain are described. The pre- and quasi-experimental research is left out of consideration in this discussion.

In describing the effect variables, special attention is given to the ecological variables. Ecological variables are effect variables related to pain; activities of daily living (ADL), including work and sports; and/or the feeling of well-being.[16] Furthermore, when possible, the "blindness" of the tester is indicated.

Terret and Vernon, 1984

In 1984, Terret and Vernon[17] performed a true experimental study of healthy subjects. By means of 60-Hz interrupted direct current, the pain threshold of each subject was established. After evoking the experimental pain, half of the subjects were treated with manipulation and the other half were not. Afterward, the pain threshold was again determined. The experimental group showed a significantly higher ($P < 0.05$) pain threshold to the experimentally induced pain. Although this research was not performed on patients, manipulation of the spinal column appears to have an influence on the pain threshold.

Coyer and Curwen, 1955

The first true experimental research on patients with low back pain appears to be from Coyer and Curwen.[18] Patients with acute (duration was not specified) low back pain ($N = 136$) were divided at random into two treatment programs: manipulation as described by Cyriax and bed rest with analgesics. The effect variables consisted of increased pain with sneezing, pain during lumbar flexion, and pain with straight leg raising. One week after treatment, 50% of the manipulated group had complete relief of pain, compared with 27% of the control group. Six weeks after the treatment, 12% of the manipulated patients and 28% of the control patients still had symptoms. The authors gave only a descriptive representation of the data and did not perform a statistical analysis. Furthermore, no information was given on whether the straight leg raise was performed by a "blind" tester.

Glover et al, 1974

In 1974, Glover et al[19] published a study involving 84 patients with complaints of pain in the region between T7 and the lowest point of the sacrum. The patients were randomly divided into treatment groups: manipulation and nonactivated shortwave diathermy. The manipulation group received 15 minutes or less of rotation manipulation, followed by 15 minutes of placebo shortwave diathermy. The control group received only the 15-minute placebo shortwave diathermy. The effect variables included the pressure test over the hyperesthetic area of skin, straight leg raise, amount of lumbar flexion, and the subjective experience of pain as rated on a percentage scale (of 0% to 100%). The first three variables were examined by a "blind" tester. In addition, differentiation was made between patients who were experiencing their symptoms for the first time and patients who had had one or more previous episodes of back pain.

The only significant ($P < 0.05$) finding was that directly after the treatment, the manipulated patients reported less pain on the percentage scale than the control group. This was the case for both those with recurrent problems and those experiencing their symptoms for the first time. Also, the authors noted that patients who had had their pain for less than 1 week tended to improve faster than patients who had had symptoms for longer than 1 week. However, this difference was not statistically significant at $\alpha = 0.5$.

This study, in a slightly modified form but with exactly the same data, was also published by Glover et al in 1977.[20]

Doran and Newell, 1975

Doran and Newell[21] performed a study concerning 456 patients with low back pain who were referred to a hospital's rheumatology department for complaints of low back pain. In 36% of the patients, the pain was experienced for the first time, while 25% of the patients had had symptoms for more than 5 years. Of the patients who had previously experienced low back pain, 64%, the average number of previous episodes was seven. This means that a strongly heterogeneous population was involved in this study.

Pain measured by means of a "verbal rating scale," straight leg raise, lumbar flexion, and extension were used as effect variables. The latter three were evaluated by a "blind" tester.

The patients were randomly assigned to four different treatment programs: manipulation as determined appropriate by the physical therapist, other forms of physical therapy as deemed appropriate by the therapist, a brace as chosen by the treater, and medication consisting of two paracetamol tablets (acetaminophen, a weak anti-inflammatory) taken every 4 hours. Sixty-eight patients dropped out during the study, but some of these patients were still included in the follow-up evaluation. Three weeks after treatment, there was no significant difference ($\alpha = 0.05$) among the four treatment groups. Six weeks, 3 months, and 1 year after treatment there also was no significant difference.

This study, too, in a somewhat modified form but with the same data, was again published in 1977 by Newell.

Sims-Williams et al, 1978

In 1978, Sims-Williams et al[23] published a study on the effect of mobilization and manipulation for low back pain. The research group concerned 94 patients who had visited their family doctor because of complaints of back pain, and through the physician were referred for further treatment. The patients were randomly placed either into a group that received mobilization and manipulation as described by Maitland or into a control group that received 15 minutes of microwave set at the lowest possible intensity.

Flexion, extension, and sidebending of the lumbar spine as well as straight leg raise were evaluated by a "blind" tester. In addition, the patients were asked to give an impression about their pain and their ability to perform daily activities.

One month after the treatment ended, 78 patients again were seen in follow-up. The group treated with mobilization and manipulation had the greatest decrease in pain, but the difference was "borderline significant" (without mention of the *P* value). In regard to ADL, the mobilization/manipulation group was significantly better in the ability to perform light work. When questioned whether the patients considered their treatment to be effective, significantly more patients in the mobilization/manipulation group gave a positive response.

In the experimental group, lumbar flexion remained unchanged; however, in the control group the lumbar flexion significantly decreased. Both groups showed a significant improvement in extension, while sidebending stayed the same in both groups. Straight leg raising significantly improved in the experimental group, but not in the control group.

After 3 months, 83 patients were seen in follow-up. When asked whether treatment was successful, there was still a (borderline) statistical difference in favor of the experimental group. The lumbar flexion remained unchanged in the experimental group, and it was still significantly decreased in the control group.

In a 1-year follow-up of 90 patients, there were no effect variables to indicate a significant difference between the two groups.

Sims-Williams et al, 1979

In 1979, Sims-Williams et al[24] repeated their study but this time involving patients with low back pain who had been referred to the hospital's department of orthopaedics or rheumatology. Once again, 94 patients were in the study. Randomly, the patients were di-

vided into the same two treatment programs as in the previous study. The same effect variables were evaluated in this research.

After 1 month, the only significant (*P* < 0.05) difference between both groups was an improvement in the straight leg raise for the experimental group.

In the 3-month follow-up, 82 patients were evaluated. The only significant (*P* < 0.05) difference between both groups was an improvement in sidebending for the control group.

One year later, 80 patients were asked whether they thought their back pain had improved. Significantly (*P* < 0.01) more patients in the control group thought that their symptoms were less.

Both of the above studies are presented together by Jayson et al.[25]

Evans et al, 1978

In a randomized crossover design, Evans et al[26] studied 32 patients with chronic low back pain. Chronic low back pain was defined as pain between T7 and the end of the sacrum, present for at least 3 weeks. The duration of the current low back symptoms varied between 6 and 676 weeks, with a median of 39 weeks. The total period during their lifetimes in which the patients experienced back pain varied from 0.2 to 31 years, with a median of 4 years. All of the patients had received codeine phosphates (analgesics).

In one group of patients, treatment consisted of manipulation (axial separation with rotation) on days 1, 7, and 14, followed by 2 weeks of medication only. The other group was treated first with medication and then with manipulation.

The effect variables evaluated consisted of lumbar flexion, pain score on a numerical rating scale, number of capsules of codeine phosphate taken, the patient's rating of the treatment's effectiveness, the patient's preference for one or the other types of treatment, and the patient's impression as to whether the symptoms had changed.

In both groups, the lumbar flexion increased significantly ($P < 0.017$) during the manipulation period and decreased during the control period.

Since there was a high correlation ($r = 0.92$; $P < 0.001$) between the pain scores and the use of the codeine phosphates, only the pain score was evaluated. After 4 weeks, the group that was first manipulated had a significant ($P = 0.05$) decrease in pain. In the group that was first treated with medication, this was not the case. The effectiveness of the treatment was rated significantly ($P < 0.05$) higher in the group first manipulated than in the other group.

The preference for one or the other treatment was not significantly different ($P > 0.05$). The impression of whether there had been a change in the symptoms led to several conclusions. The patients who did not respond well to the manipulations were significantly ($P < 0.05$) younger than the patients who responded well to the manipulations. The duration of the symptoms was varied but not significant ($P = 0.10$); the patients who did not respond well to the manipulations, on the average, had their symptoms for a longer period of time.

The time frame between the first symptoms and the present symptoms (age of onset) was significantly ($P < 0.01$) longer in patients who did not respond well to the manipulation treatment.

In conjunction with this study, radiological examinations were also performed on the same patients. These data were presented by Roberts et al in 1978.[27] Radiographs were taken three times in all patients over the age of 45 years. These anteroposterior views were scored by two independent reviewers.

There was no significant difference between the two patient groups at the beginning of the study. There appeared to be a significant positive correlation ($r = 0.45$; $P < 0.01$) between the measurement of lumbar flexion on the radiographs and the clinically determined lumbar flexion (validity study). There seemed to be no significant ($\alpha = 0.05$) difference between the radiographs in both groups either before or after the study.

Rasmussen, 1979

Rasmussen[28] performed a true experimental study with 24 patients between 20 and 50 years of age who had low back complaints lasting less than 3 weeks. Randomly, they were divided into two groups: one group received six sessions of manipulation and one group received six sessions of shortwave diathermy. The following "nonblind" variables were determined: the ability to work, degree of pain, and a modified Schober test. The patients were considered to be recovered if they had no more pain, could function normally, and could return to work. After 2 weeks, 92% of the manipulated group had recovered, in contrast to 25% of the shortwave diathermy group. This was statistically significant ($P < 0.01$). In the modified Schober test, there was also a significant ($P < 0.01$) difference in favor of the group treated with manipulation.

This research was also published by Rasmussen in 1985.

Buerger, 1980

Buerger[30] performed a study with 83 patients who had low back pain of less than 1-month duration. These patients were randomly assigned to three treatment groups; one group received rotation manipulation, one received massage, and one received placebo manipulation (intermittent laying on of hands). The effect variables were pain on a numerical rating scale and the number of treatments. Whether or not the examiners could establish an improvement in the patients was established between two testers in a correlation study. The examiners scored the patients on the following scale: much better, somewhat better, no change, somewhat worse, much worse. The calculated

Spearman rank correlation coefficient was 0.14 ($P < 0.01$). Although the "blind" judgment in determining the possible improvement of patients was not satisfied, it was still effective with these variables.

For the effect variable regarding the duration of pain, there appeared to be a significant ($P < 0.025$) difference in favor of the manipulation group. In relation to the number of treatments, there was no significant difference. The examiners' judgment of the patients was not accounted for during analysis of the data.

This research was also published by Buerger in 1985.[31]

Coxhead et al, 1981

Coxhead et al[32] performed a true experimental study with 322 patients divided into the following treatment groups: mechanical traction, exercise program, manipulation (as described by Maitland), and corset. At the same time, all patients received shortwave diathermy and a back school lecture. The authors made no statement about the duration of the complaints.

Improvement of the symptoms was determined by asking whether the patient felt better or worse, rating the pain on a Visual Analogue Scale (VAS) of –100 to +100, and judging the ability to work and perform ADL. After 16 months, an inquiry was made as to whether the patient was still experiencing pain.

After 4 weeks, the manipulation group had experienced the most relief of pain ($P < 0.05$). The other variables appeared to be insignificant. At 16 months, there was no significant difference between any of the variables.

This study was also published by O'Donoghue (formerly Coxhead) in 1985.[33]

Zylbergold and Piper, 1981

The true experimental study by Zylbergold and Piper[34] involved patients who experienced low back pain for the first time. Different treatment modalities were compared: lumbar flexion exercises with moist hot packs, moist hot packs followed by axial separation with rotation mobilization, and a home exercise program. All patients ($N = 28$) also received a back school lecture.

As effect variables, pain on a McGill Pain Questionnaire, flexion, sidebending to the right and left, and ADL were used. The patients were evaluated again after 1 month.

On all five effect variables, the three groups showed a significant difference ($P < 0.01$) between each assessment time. When the three groups were compared, the group with the rotation mobilization seemed to produce a better score than the other two, but these differences were not significant ($\alpha = 0.05$).

Hoehler et al, 1981

In this true experimental study, Hoehler et al[35] included 95 patients with low back pain. Some of the patients had had pain for less than 1 month, while others had had symptoms for longer than 6 months. The experimental group received rotation manipulations of the lumbar spine, and the control group received soft tissue massage in the lumbar region.

Pain with straight leg raising, mobility with straight leg raise, ADL, and lumbar flexion were evaluated by a nonblind tester. In addition, the patients rated their experience of the pain. After the first treatment, there was a significant ($P < 0.05$) difference for the amount of pain and the pain elicited through straight leg raising ($P < 0.01$) in favor of the experimental group. Three weeks after the therapy, however, this difference had disappeared.

Farrell and Twomey, 1982

In the study by Farrell and Twomey,[36] 48 patients between 20 and 65 years of age with pain between T12 and the coccyx were involved. The patients did not experience any pain 6 months before the study, and the duration of the current complaints was 3 weeks or less. The treatment consisted of microwave combined with isometric abdominal exercises, and mobilization/manipulation as described by Stoddard and Maitland. The requirements that had to be met to consider the patient's symptoms as being resolved were as follows: the patient could return to normal ADL and had a low score on a Numerical Rating Scale (NRS), a painless passive lumbar flexion, and a painless passive straight leg raise test.

The mobilized/manipulated group needed significantly (P < 0.001) fewer treatments in order to have complete relief of pain than did the control group.

Godfrey et al, 1984

In 1984, Godfrey et al[37] examined 81 patients with low back pain lasting 1 week or less. A checklist was completed by the patients in order to judge the symptoms. Items on this list included estimation of pain, stiffness, ADL on a five-point scale, localization of the pain, exacerbating factors, and additional medication.

The experimental group received massage and rotation manipulations. One control group received faradic current of 40 Hz and the other control group received a massage. Patients in all three groups showed significant (P < 0.001) improvement. No significant differences were found among the groups.

Gibson et al, 1985

Gibson et al[38] divided the patients in their study into three treatment groups: shortwave diathermy, placebo shortwave diathermy (diathermy without output), and manipulation. The 109 patients had experienced low back pain for a duration of between 2 and 12 months. As effect variables, a VAS, a local pressure test on the spinal column, and lum-

bar flexion were used. The two latter variables were tested in a blind manner. Furthermore, the patients were questioned about their use of analgesics and their ADL.

Although all three groups of patients improved, there were no significant differences between the groups ($\alpha = 0.05$).

Hadler et al, 1987

In the study by Hadler et al,[39] 54 patients were divided into four groups: complaints for less than 2 weeks with mobilization, complaints for less than 2 weeks with manipulation, complaints for 2 to 4 weeks with mobilization, and complaints for 2 to 4 weeks with manipulation. The difference between the mobilization and manipulation groups was that the manipulated patients received a high-velocity thrust with rotation through the slack, and in the mobilization patients this thrust was omitted. All patients were between 18 and 40 years of age.

As an effect variable, the pain questionnaire of Roland and Morris was used. This pain questionnaire has not yet been evaluated for validity and reliability.

In the groups with 2- to 4-week complaints, the reduction in pain was significantly ($P = 0.025$) larger for the manipulated group.

CONCLUSION

The true experimental studies for the effects of manipulations and/or mobilizations described in this chapter show subtle differences. Of the eight studies of complaints of short duration, seven show an advantage of manipulation and/or mobilization, but none of the studies indicates a significant difference (Table 14–1). For the variable pain decrease, the pattern seems to be that manipulation and/or mobilization for complaints of short duration (less than 1 month) offers more pain decrease than a number of other conservative treatments. The difference between the groups does not remain significant: manipula-

Table 14–1 Study of Effectiveness of Manual Therapy for Low Back Pain

Research Study	Treatment	Results
Terret and Vernon, 1984[17]; experimental pain in healthy subjects	a. Manipulation b. No manipulation	A > * b
Coyer and Curwen, 1955[18]; N = 136; short duration	a. Manipulation (Cyriax) b. Bed rest with pain-relieving medication	A > b
Glover et al, 1974[19]; N = 84; mixed	a. Manipulation with placebo shortwave diathermy b. Placebo shortwave diathermy	A > * b
Doran and Newell, 1975[21]; N = 84; mixed	a. Manipulation b. Physical therapy c. Corset d. Paracetamol	a ≈ b ≈ c ≈ d
Sims-Williams et al, 1978[23]; N = 94; short duration	a. Mobilization and manipulation (Maitland) b. Placebo microwave	A > * b
Sims-Williams et al, 1979[24]; N = 94; long duration	a. Mobilization and manipulation (Maitland) b. Placebo microwave	After 1 month: a ≈ b After 1 year: B > * a
Evans et al, 1978[26]; N = 32; mixed	a. Rotation manipulation with axial separation b. Codeine phosphate	AB > * ba Short duration: A > * b Long duration: a ≈ b
Rasmussen, 1979[28]; N = 24; short duration	a. Manipulation b. Shortwave diathermy	A > * b
Buerger, 1980[30]; N = 83; short duration	a. Rotation manipulation b. Massage c. Placebo manipulation	A > * (b ≈ c)
Coxhead et al, 1981[32]; N = 322; not indicated	a. Mechanical traction b. Exercise program c. Manipulation (Maitland) d. Corset	C > * (a ≈ b ≈ d)
Zylbergold and Piper, 1981[34]; N = 28; short duration	a. Moist hot packs and lumbar flexion exercises b. Moist hot packs and rotation manipulation c. Home exercises	B > (a ≈ c)

Table 14–1 continued

Research Study	Treatment	Results
Hoehler et al, 1981[35]; N = 95; mixed	a. Rotation manipulation b. Massage	A > * b
Farrell and Twomey, 1982[36]; N = 48; short duration	a. Mobilization/manipulation (Maitland and Stoddard) b. Microwave and isometric abdominal exercises	A > * b
Godfrey et al, 1984[37]; N = 81; short duration	a. Massage and rotation manipulation b. Faradic current c. Massage	a ≈ b < c
Gibson et al, 1985[38]; N = 109; mixed	a. Shortwave diathermy b. Placebo shortwave diathermy c. Manipulation	a ≈ b ≈ c
Hadler et al, 1987[39]; N = 54; short duration	a. Mobilization b. Manipulation	< 2 weeks: a ≈ b 2 weeks: B > * a
Meade et al, 1990[40]; N = 608; mixed	a. Mostly chiropractic b. Mostly Maitland manipulation	Short duration: a ≈ b Long duration: A > * b

Note: All studies are true experimental in design: only the results for pain are indicated; the best treatment results in the study are indicated with a capital letter. * = Significant; > = better than; < = worse than; ≈ = nonsignificant or different only by means of a tendency, thus possibly (but not proven) equal to.

tion and/or mobilization accelerates improvement.

With other effect variables (such as straight leg raising, lumbar flexion, and ADL), manipulations and/or mobilizations seem to be more effective than a number of conservative therapies in the treatment of symptoms with a duration of less than 1 month.

Of the six studies with a mixed duration of symptoms (short-term and long-term, as well as duration not indicated by the authors), four studies show an advantage in favor of mobilizations and/or manipulations, while two studies indicate no difference (Table 14–1).

In itself, this is a favorable result, in which one could deduce that mobilization and/or manipulation sometimes could be indicated in complaints of long duration. However, since the mentioned studies have an insufficient differentiation for the duration of complaints, the assumption cannot yet be solidified. In relation to this, the only mixed study that makes a differentiation (Evans et al[26]) demonstrates no significant difference in complaints of long duration. The study that deals explicitly with complaints of long duration (Sims-Williams et al[24]) offers the possibility that mobilization and Maitland manipulation, at least in the judgment of the patients, have a less favorable effect than placebo.

Generally, manipulation and/or mobilization seems to be indicated in complaints with a duration of less than 1 month. A possible explanation of the effect with these patients can be found in a publication by Mathews.[41] He examined two patients with caudograms before and after a manipulation (as described by Cyriax). The caudogram was performed before the manipulation, the patients were manipulated, and then the caudogram was repeated. In each patient, the manipulation consisted of a rotation manipulation with an axial separation component. In both cases, the manipulation resulted in pain relief.

In the first patient, bulging of the disc between L4 and L5 was visible, which disappeared after the manipulation (Figure 14–1).

In the second patient, the undulations apparent before the manipulation also disappeared after the manipulation (Figure 14–2).

Unfortunately, the study by Mathews was performed in only two patients. However, if caudography is a reliable technique in assessing changes in an intervertebral disc, one could presume that manipulation can influence anatomical structures.

The absence of a convincing effect of mobilization and/or manipulation with complaints of long duration, and the fact that even a nega-

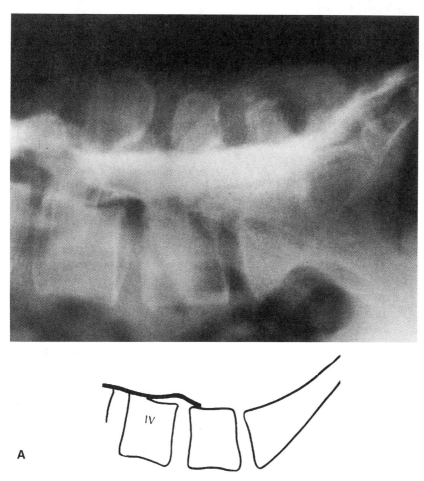

Figure 14–1 The anatomical effects of manipulation in a patient with low back pain.[41] **A,** Before the manipulation, a concavity is visible in the contrast medium at the level of L4-5. *Source:* Reprinted with permission from Mathews, J.A. et al, *Tijdschrift van de Nederlandse en Belgische Vereniging voor Orthopedische Geneeskunde (Cyriax),* Vol. 4, pp. 23–43, © 1984.

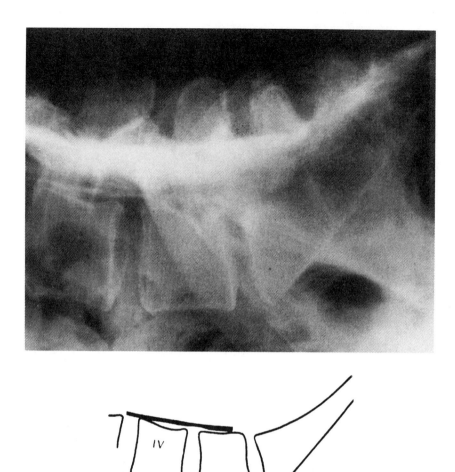

B

Figure 14–1 *B*, After the manipulation, the concavity has almost disappeared.

tive effect was found in one case, could probably be explained by two factors. First, it is usually accepted that in symptoms of long duration, muscle weakness plays an important role. Thus, it is possible that various forms of exercise therapy are mainly indicated here. (See Chapter 16, Exercise Therapy in the Treatment of Low Back Pain, for more detailed information.) Second, a number of different manipulation techniques exist, and in particular regard to this issue, an intensive discussion recently occurred in England.

CONTROVERSY OVER FINDINGS IN THE *BRITISH MEDICAL JOURNAL*

On June 2, 1990, a study by Meade et al[40] regarding the effects of chiropractic was published in the *British Medical Journal*. The 741 patients who participated in the study were first selected for admission criteria. Patients who had radicular irritation and who recently received treatment were excluded from the study. The remaining patients were randomly divided into a group treated by chiropractors and a group treated with physical therapy in a hospital outpatient clinic. The chiropractors mainly administered manipulation with a high-velocity thrust, although in a small number of patients diverse other forms of therapy were used. The outpatient physical therapy consisted mainly of manipulations (as described by Maitland), but more than half the patients also underwent other treatments, such as traction and exercise therapy.

After a period of time, it appeared that the patients treated by the chiropractors were treated more frequently and for a longer period than the outpatient physical therapy group. The effect variables were the Oswestry Scale Score,[42] straight leg raising, lumbar flexion, and absence from work. After 6 weeks, 608 patients were still participating in the study. With time, the dropout rate increased.

After 6 weeks, 6 months, 1 year, 2 years, and 3 years, a significant difference appeared to exist in favor of the chiropractic treatment ($P < 0.05$). These differences concerned pa-

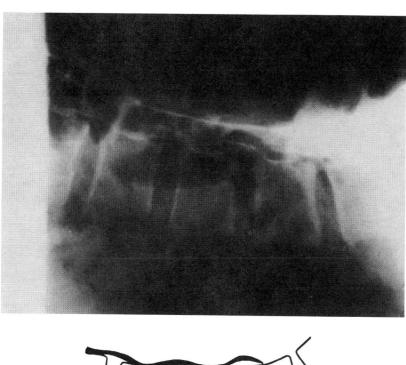

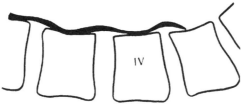

A

Figure 14–2 The anatomical effects of manipulation in a patient with low back pain.[41] **A**, Before the manipulation, concavities are visible in the contrast medium at the levels of L2-5. *Source:* Reprinted with permission from Mathews, J.A. et al, *Tijdschrift van de Nederlandse en Belgische Vereniging voor Orthopedische Geneeskunde (Cyriax)*, Vol. 4, pp. 23–43, © 1984.

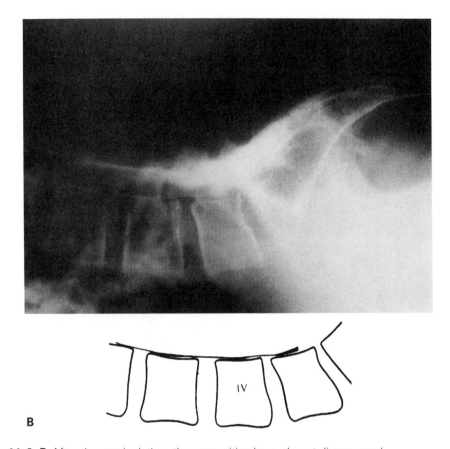

B

Figure 14–2 *B*, After the manipulation, the concavities have almost disappeared.

tients with long-standing complaints, but could not be found for patients with complaints of short duration. This result stirred up controversy in England in the public press, as well as in the *British Medical Journal*.[40]

The most important point of this discussion is that the chosen design does not explain the cause of the difference. A placebo effect is possible, particularly because the chiropractors treated for a longer period and with a higher frequency. It is also possible that indeed the high-velocity chiropractic manipulations (like the Cyriax manipulations) are to be preferred over the more gentle Maitland manipulations, at least for patients with complaints of long duration.

Thus, for the time being, the best treatment for low back pain in patients with long-lasting complaints remains unclear. In order to recognize a more clear pattern, additional true experimental studies are necessary. Research could be directed at the following questions:

- Are there specific manipulative treatment forms for low back complaints of long duration?
- Is it possible to determine a time limit after which manipulation and/or mobilization in general no longer bears a convincing effect on variables such as pain, ADL, and well-being of the patient?
- Besides duration, are there other characteristics of back complaints on which the choice of the exact therapy could be based?

REFERENCES

1. Brodin H. Cervical pain and mobilization. *Man Med.* 1982;20:90–94.

2. Parker GB, Tupling H, Pryor DS. A controlled trial of cervical manipulation for migraine. *Aust N Z J Med.* 1978;8:589–593.

3. Sloop PR, Smith DS, Goldenberg E, Doré C. Manipulation for chronic neck pain. *Spine.* 1982;7:532–535.

4. Vortman BJ. Kinesiologie der Halswirbelsäule vor und nach Manipulation. *Man Med.* 1984;2:49–53.

5. Aufdemkampe G, Meijer OG, Balen JH, et al. De kwaliteit van effectonderzoek in de fysiotherapie. In: Stichting Wetenschap en Scholing Fysiotherapie, ed. *Fysiotherapie, Wetenschap en Beleid.* Utrecht: Bohn, Scheltema & Holkema; 1985:60–99.

6. Deyo RA. Conservative therapy for low back pain. *JAMA.* 1983;250:1057–1062.

7. DiFabio RP. Clinical assessment of manipulation and mobilization of the lumbar spine: a critical review of the literature. *Phys Ther.* 1986;66:51–54.

8. Evans DP. The design and results of clinical trials of lumbar manipulation: a review. In: Buerger AA, Greenman PE, eds. *Empirical Approaches to the Validation of Spinal Manipulation.* Springfield, Ill: Charles C Thomas; 1985:228–238.

9. Jull GA. The management of acute low back pain. In: Grieve GP, ed. *Modern Manual Therapy of the Vertebral Column.* Edinburgh: Churchill Livingstone; 1986:740–749.

10. Lankhorst GJ. Manuele therapie. *Ned Tijdschr Geneeskd.* 1987;131:898–901.

11. Lindahl O. Methods for evaluating the therapeutic effect of non-medical treatment. *Scand J Rehabil Med.* 1979;11:151–155.

12. Moritz U. Evaluation of manipulation and other manual therapy. *Scand J Rehabil Med.* 1979;11:173–179.

13. O'Donoghue CE Manipulation trials. In: Grieve GP, ed. *Modern Manual Therapy of the Vertebral Column.* Edinburgh: Churchill Livingstone; 1986:849–859.

14. Stoddard A. *Manual of Osteopathic Practice.* 2nd ed. London: Hutchinson; 1983.

15. Bouter LM. Het effect van manuele therapie bij lage rugpijn. *Med Contact.* 1985;40:357–360.

16. Aufdemkampe G, Beijer MA, Meijer OG, Obbens HJM, Terlouw TJA. Kwaliteit van effect-meting in de fysiotherapie: ecologische validiteit in het wetenschappelijk onderzoek. *Ned Tijdschr Fysiother.* 1985;95:121–131.

17. Terret ACJ, Vernon H. A controlled study of the effect of spinal manipulation on paraspinal cutaneous pain tolerance levels. *Am J Phys Med.* 1984; 63:217–225.

18. Coyer AB, Curwen IHMM. Low back pain treated by manipulation. *Br Med J.* 1955;2:705–707.

19. Glover JR, Morris JG, Khosla T. Back pain: a randomized clinical trial of rotational manipulation of the trunk. *Br J Ind Med.* 1974;31:59–64.

20. Glover JR, Morris JG, Khosla T. Back pain: a randomized clinical trial of rotational manipulation of the trunk. In: Buerger AA, Tobis JS, eds. *Empirical Approaches to the Validation of Manipulation Therapy.* Springfield, Ill: Charles C Thomas; 1977:271–283.

21. Doran DML, Newell DJ. Manipulation in treatment of low back pain: a multicentre study. *Br Med J.* 1975;2:161–164.

22. Newell DJ. Manipulation in the treatment of low back pain: a multicenter study. In: Buerger AA, Tobis JS, eds. *Empirical Approaches to the Validation of Manipulation Therapy.* Springfield, Ill.: Charles C Thomas; 1977:284–298.

23. Sims-Williams H, Jayson MIV, Young SMS, Baddeley H, Collins E. Controlled trial of mobilization and manipulation for patients with low back pain in general practice. *Br Med J.* 1978;2:1338–1340.

24. Sims-Williams H, Jayson MIV, Young SMS, Baddeley H, Collins E. Controlled trial of mobilization and manipulation for low back pain: hospital patients. *Br Med J.* 1979;2:1318–1320.

25. Jayson MIV, Sims-Williams H, Young SMS, Baddeley H, Collins E. Mobilization and manipulation for low-back pain. *Spine.* 1981;6:409–416.

26. Evans DP, Burke MS, Lloyd KN, Roberts EE, Roberts GM. Lumbar spinal manipulation on trial. part I: clinical assessment. *Rheumatol Rehabil.* 1978;17:46–53.

27. Roberts GM, Roberts EE, Lloyd KN, Burke MS, Evans DP. Lumbar spinal manipulation on trial. part II: radiological assessment. *Rheumatol Rehabil.* 1978;17:54–59.

28. Rasmussen GG. Manipulation in treatment of low back pain: a randomized clinical trial. *Man Med.* 1979;13:8–10.

29. Rasmussen G. A randomized clinical trial of manipulation: diagnostic criteria and treatment techniques. In: Buerger AA, Greenman PE, eds. *Empirical Approaches to the Validation of Spinal Manipulation.* Springfield, Ill: Charles C Thomas; 1985:174–178.

30. Buerger AA. A controlled trial of rotational manipulation in low back pain. *Man Med.* 1980;18:17–26.

31. Buerger AA. A "double-blind" randomized clinical trial of rotational manipulation for low back pain. In: Buerger AA, Greenman PE, eds. *Empirical Approaches to the Validation of Spinal Manipulation.* Springfield, Ill: Charles C Thomas; 1985:193–207.

32. Coxhead CE, Inskip H, Meade TW, North WRS, Troup JDG. Multicentre trial of physiotherapy in the management of sciatic symptoms. *Lancet.* 1981;1:1065–1068. Also presented as: O'Donoghue (formerly Coxhead) CE. A multicentre trial of the physiotherapeutic management of sciatic symptoms. In: Buerger AA, Greenman PE, eds. *Empirical Approaches to the Validation of Spinal Manipulation.* Springfield, Ill: Charles C Thomas; 1985:208–227.

33. O'Donoghue (formerly Coxhead) CE. Multicentre trial of physiotherapy in the management of sciatic symptoms. In: Buerger AA, Greenman PE, eds. *Empirical Approaches to the Validation of Spinal Manipulation.* Springfield, Ill: Charles C Thomas; 1985:208–227.

34. Zylbergold RS, Piper MC. Lumbar disc disease: comparative analysis of physical therapy treatments. *Arch Phys Med Rehabil.* 1981;62:176–179.

35. Hoehler FK, Tobis JS, Buerger AA. Spinal manipulation for low back pain. *JAMA.* 1981;245:1835–1838.

36. Farrell JP, Twomey LT. Acute low back pain: comparison of two conservative treatment approaches. *Med J Aust.* 1982;1:160–164.

37. Godfrey CM, Morgan PP, Schatzker J. A randomized trial of manipulation for low-back pain in a medical setting. *Spine.* 1984;9:301–304.

38. Gibson T, Grahame R, Harkness J, Woo P, Blagrave P, Hills R. Controlled comparison of short-wave diathermy treatment with osteopathic treatment in non-specific low back pain. *Lancet.* 1985;1:1258–1261.

39. Hadler MH, Curtis P, Gillings B, Stinnet S. A benefit of spinal manipulation as adjunctive therapy for acute low-back pain: a stratified controlled trial. *Spine.* 1987;12:703–706.

40. Meade TW, Dyer S, Browne W, Townsend J, Frank AO. Low back pain of mechanical origin: randomized comparison of chiropractic and hospital outpatient treatment. *Br Med J.* 1990;300:1431–1437.

41. Mathews JA. De waarde van epidurography bij de beoordeling van de werking van manipulatie en traktie bij lumbale discusproblemen. *Tijdschrift van de Nederlandse en Belgische Vereniging voor Orthopedische Geneeskunde (Cyriax).* 1984;4:23–43.

42. Fairbank JCT, Davies JB, Couper J, O'Brien JP. The Oswestry low back pain disability questionnaire. *Phys Ther.* 1980;66:271–273.

15

Research on Effectiveness of Traction of the Spinal Column

EDITOR'S PREFACE

In acute complaints of back pain, with at least local symptoms, it appears that mechanical unloading is of great importance in the treatment of the patient. Many forms of treatment involve unloading: manual therapy, traction, rest, and relaxation through medication or relaxation psychotherapy. In view of the favorable results of research on effectiveness of manual therapy, positive effects could also be expected from traction.

In this chapter, Geert Aufdemkampe concludes that there is a disappointingly small number of controlled studies regarding the clinical effectiveness of traction. Furthermore, the few controlled studies do not give rise to optimism. This explains why some people assume that traction is not effective clinically. Of course, it is also possible that the studies mentioned did not apply the most appropriate traction technique, or that significant changes have to be made in establishing the proper indications for traction.

It is still too early to conclude that traction is clinically irrelevant, particularly because in a recently published study it was proved that traction has positive anatomical effects. Onel et al[1] published a study regarding the effects of traction in lumbar disc prolapse. The pre-experimental study was performed in 30 patients. In 28 of the patients, the amount of prolapsed material diminished, as demonstrated through a computed tomography (CT) scan that was performed during the traction. The fact that the examiners also reported positive clinical results cannot yet lead to firm conclusions because the study was only pre-experimental. However, the anatomical findings clearly indicate the positive anatomical effect of traction.

INTRODUCTION

Sometimes traction of the lumbar or cervical spine is the only treatment applied for symptoms in these areas, and sometimes it is used as an adjunct to other forms of therapy. Traction can be performed manually as well as mechanically. The first part of this chapter discusses axial separation studies of the spinal column; the second part is a review of studies on the clinical effectiveness of traction.

The most significant source for axial separation studies is the review by Colachis.[2]

There is no study on effectiveness of traction of the thoracic spine. The same is true for manual therapy of the thoracic spine.

SEPARATION STUDIES

Cervical Spine

According to Colachis,[2] the first study regarding cervical traction was performed by McFarland and Krusen in 1943.[3] In that study, a Sayre traction apparatus was used on healthy subjects between the ages of 55 and 65 years. The amount of traction applied ranged between 20.5 and 45.5 kg. The average increases in distance (separation), measured between adjacent spinous processes, between the posterior edges of the vertebrae, and between the anterior edges of the vertebrae, were 10.9, 6.5, and 2.8 mm, respectively.

In their article, DeSèze and Levernieux[4] discuss the work of Ranier, which is probably the first publication involving cadaver research. In the cervical column, Ranier established a lengthening of 10 mm under 40 kg of traction. DeSèze and Levernieux[4] performed a study on healthy subjects and found that a force of 118 kg of pull was necessary to attain an increase of 2 mm in the distance between C5-6 and C6-7. This increase in distance was determined by means of lateral radiographs.

Because Colachis[2] does not give statistical data for each study, it is difficult to obtain a general overview as to the effect of traction on the cervical column. However, it is possible to establish three conclusions based on the studies reviewed by Colachis:

1. A slight lengthening of the entire cervical spine can be achieved. The maximal separation between two cervical vertebrae is 2.5 mm with 136 kg,[5] and the minimal separation is 0.4 to 0.7 mm with 13.6 kg.[6]
2. From the 12 described studies, only the one from Cyriax[5] was performed with manual traction.

3. In more recent studies, the traction is generally applied with the cervical spine in approximately 20° of flexion and with a relatively small amount of force—2.3 to 13.6 kg. These recent studies indicate a separation between 0.4 and 2 mm.

Lumbar Spine

According to Colachis,[2] Cyriax[5] was the first author (in 1950) to propose using traction for the treatment of disc protrusions. DeSèze and Levernieux[4] conclude that in cadavers a separation of 1.5 mm could be achieved with 9 kg of traction. From the other data listed by Colachis, it is apparent that between two lumbar vertebrae a separation of 0.5 mm (with a pull of 27 to 36 kg) to 2.6 mm (with a pull of 136 kg) can be achieved.

From the reviews by Colachis[2] and Rogoff,[7] it can be concluded that with the use of mechanical traction, axial separation is attainable at both levels of the spinal column. In comparison to the cervical spine, it appears that greater force is necessary to achieve separation between segments in the lumbar spine. More research examining separation in manual traction is necessary to establish the anatomical effect of manual traction.[8]

CLINICAL RESEARCH STUDIES OF TRACTION OF THE SPINAL COLUMN

In spite of the fact that it is anatomically possible to attain separation in the lumbar and cervical spines, it remains questionable whether this separation has noticeable consequences for the patient. There are a number of particularly theoretically inspired articles on traction that are not discussed in this chapter.[9-14] This research review study deals with the effect of traction on the patient's symptoms, and even Hickling,[11] Mathews,[12] and Saunders[14] actually state that the deciding factor in traction is its effect on the patient.

With regard to the previously performed studies, Saunders[14] is rather pessimistic: "The limited number of controlled studies that are available have shown either poor results of treatment or positive effects that were only of limited significance." This opinion is also shared by Larsson et al[15] and Deyo.[16]

Because of the lack of true experimental research, as compared with that for other types of treatments such as manual therapy, the pre- and quasi-experimental studies about traction are also discussed here.

Pre-Experimental Studies

The previously mentioned study by DeSèze and Levernieux[4] contains clinical results concerning a study involving 140 patients with cervical radiculopathy. Using the resolution of pain as the effect variable, 77% of patients indicated a favorable response. In patients in whom the symptoms were present for longer than 2 months, the success rate was 65%. Nevertheless, the authors noted that it is difficult to distinguish beforehand which patients will respond favorably to traction.

Hood and Chrisman[17] studied the effect of intermittent mechanical traction on the symptoms of patients with prolapsed lumbar discs. Fifty-five patients between the ages of 22 and 63 years were treated with traction ranging from 25 to 32 kg. All but two patients had a positive straight leg raise test before treatment. Treatment consisted of the application of warmth followed by traction. After treatment, 21 of the 55 patients had complete relief of their symptoms (38%), in 15 patients the symptoms had improved significantly, and in 19 patients no improvement was noted. The authors hypothesized that intermittent mechanical traction is worthwhile in patients who fall into this category.

Valtonen and Kiuru[18] examined 212 patients, aged 21 to 80 years, with a cervical syndrome. Treatment consisted of the application of warmth, then massage and exercises, followed by traction. Some patients received intermittent traction and other patients received continuous traction, ranging from 3 to 13 kg. Although the authors noted some improvement in the patients, it is not possible, with certainty, to attribute this improvement exclusively to the traction.

Without further description, Rohde[19] determined that manual traction provides pain relief in instances of painful muscular hypertonia.

Quasi-Experimental Studies

In 1955, Christie[20] described a quasi-experimental study in which mechanical traction (23 to 51 kg) was compared with a placebo medication. In order to obtain comparable patients in both groups, matched pairs were used. From each pair, the patients were randomly divided into one of the two groups. In addition, the patients were differentiated into a subgroup with radicular symptoms and a subgroup without radicular symptoms. A numerical rating scale for pain was used as the effect variable. Of the patients with radicular symptoms, 17% improved with the placebo medication and 30% improved with the traction treatment. Of the patients without radicular symptoms, 30% improved with the placebo medication compared with 24% with the traction. Christie did not report any significance analysis of these differences.

Caldwell and Krusen[21] published research regarding 577 patients with a cervical syndrome. All patients received a heat modality, massage, and exercises. In addition, some patients did not receive traction, while various forms of traction were applied to other patients. The forms of traction were continuous traction by means of a simple sling, traction with a Sayre sling (intermittent or continuous), and traction with a combination of these methods. The amount of force applied was not mentioned. The results were represented in terms of improvement of symptoms in relation to the number of treatments with a certain form of traction. Caldwell and Krusen concluded that there was no significant difference in the effectiveness of the various forms of traction. In the authors' opinion, the early initiation of physical therapy was the most important factor in a favorable clinical outcome.

True Experimental Studies

Cervical Spine

The only true experimental study of the cervical column in regard to traction appears to be that by Goldie and Landquist.[22] In this research, 73 patients with cervical pain radiating into the arm were randomly divided into three groups: one group performed isometric exercises, one group received intermittent mechanical traction in 20° flexion (with a force of 14 to 18 kg for men and 11 to 18 kg for women), and the control group was not treated. There was no significant difference in pain relief among the three groups.

Lumbar Spine

Mathews and Hickling[23] studied 27 patients with sciatica or pain radiating into the leg. The experimental group received continuous mechanical traction with a pulling force between 36 and 61 kg, while the control group received "only" 9 kg. The effect variables were pain and the straight leg raise test. There was no significant difference between the two groups. However, this may be explained in that the control group may have received an effective amount of traction.

Larsson et al[15] studied 82 patients with lumbago and/or sciatica. The experimental group received autotraction, whereas rest and a corset were prescribed for the control group. The effect variables were the number of patients recovering within 3 weeks, the straight leg raise test, and the disappearance of neurological symptoms or pain. After 1 week, the traction group was significantly ($P < 0.05$) better than the control group. After 1 month, this was still the case. However,

after 3 months there was no longer a significant difference. Thus, it is possible that traction accelerates the self-healing process.

Coxhead et al[24] compared intermittent mechanical traction (the amount of pull was not mentioned) with manipulation, exercises, and use of a corset. Improvement was determined by means of a questionnaire, which included sense of well-being, pain rated on a Visual Analogue Scale (VAS), and activities of daily living (ADL), 16 months after the study. With regard to the sense of well-being, after 4 weeks 78% of the patients reported improvement; however, there was no significant ($P > 0.05$) difference among the various groups. Only the variable, pain, showed a significant ($P < 0.05$) difference in favor of the manipulation group after 4 weeks. At 16 months, this significant difference had disappeared.

Ljunggren et al[25] performed a study with 49 patients experiencing lumbago and/or sciatica or who were diagnosed with a prolapsed intervertebral disc. Treatment consisted of either autotraction or manual traction by the therapist. None of the effect variables of straight leg raise test, ADL, and self-rating by the patient demonstrated a significant ($P > 0.05$) difference directly after the treatment, 2 weeks later, or 3 months later. Keep in mind that only two traction techniques were compared in this study.

In the research from Gianokopoulos et al,[26] 20 patients with chronic low back pain were treated alternately with different types of inversion traction and traction during upright standing. The treatment sequence was randomized. There were no significant ($P > 0.05$) differences between the forms of treatment in relation to the low back pain.

Dimaggio and Mooney[27] randomly assigned 136 patients to three different treatment groups: McKenzie exercise program, mechanical traction (the amount of pull was not specified), and back school. Results on a VAS and an ADL questionnaire were represented in percentages, without further statistical analysis. The success ratio of the McKenzie group was 97%, the traction group 50%, and the back school group 38%.

CONCLUSION

The above-described clinical studies of the effectiveness of traction of the cervical and lumbar spines appear to demonstrate unclear results (Table 15-1). With regard to traction of the cervical spine only one true experimental study,[22] one quasi-experimental study,[21] and one pre-experimental study (with results that could be interpreted) were found. Although the outcome of the pre-experimental study seemed to be positive, controlled research was unable to confirm this. Obviously, more controlled studies of traction are necessary.

With regard to traction of the lumbar spine, it appears that this treatment may have some effect on patients with low back problems. However, in two true experimental studies, another therapy appeared to be even more effective in the treatment of back pain: manipulation[24] and McKenzie exercises.[27] Until now, comparisons of various forms of traction have indicated no significant differences.

The clinically relevant question of whether mechanical or manual traction is better or whether traction should be applied intermittently or continuously has not yet been answered on the basis of known effect studies. ' Currently, there are no indications from the effect studies that procurement of the very expensive apparatuses would be justified.

Table 15–1 Research on Effectiveness of Traction

Research Study	*Treatment*	*Results*
Goldie and Landquist,[22] 1970: Pain in the cervical region	a Isometric exercises b Intermittent traction c No treatment	a ≈ b ≈ c
Mathews and Hickling,[23] 1975: Sciatica or radiating pain into the leg	Mechanical traction: a 36 to 61 kg b 9 kg	a ≈ b
Larsson et al,[15] 1980: Lumbago/sciatica	a Autotraction b Rest and corset	A > * b
Coxhead et al,[24] 1981: Low back pain	a Mechanical traction b Manipulation (Maitland) c Exercise program d Corset	B > * (a ≈ c ≈ d)
Ljunggren et al,[25] 1984: Lumbago/sciatica or disc prolapse	a Autotraction b Manual traction by therapist	a ≈ b
Gianokopoulos et al,[26] 1985: Chronic low back pain	a Inversion traction b Traction in upright standing	a ≈ b
Dimaggio and Mooney,[27] 1987: Low back pain	a McKenzie exercises b Mechanical traction c Back school	A > b > c

Note: All studies mentioned are true experimental in design; only the results for pain are indicated. The best treatment in the study is indicated with a capital letter. * = Significant; > = better than; < = worse than; ≈ = nonsignificant or different only by means of a tendency, thus possibly (but not proved) equal to.

REFERENCES

1. Onel D, Tuzlaci M, Sari H, Demir K. Computed tomographic investigation of the effect of traction on lumbar disc herniations. *Spine.* 1989;14:82–90. Also published in *J Orthop Med.* 12:6–14.

2. Colachis SC Jr. Traction. In: Leak JC, Gershwin ME, Fowler WM, eds. *Principles of Physical Medicine and Rehabilitation in the Musculoskeletal Diseases.* Orlando, Fla: Grune & Stratton; 1986:121–172.

3. McFarland JW, Krusen FH. Use of the Sayre head sling in osteoarthritis of cervical portion of spinal column. *Arch Phys Med Rehabil.* 1943;24:263–269.

4. DeSèze S, Levernieux J. Les tractions vertébrales: premières études expérimentales et résultats thérapeutiques d'après une expérience de quatre années. *Sem Hop Paris.* 1951;27:2085–2104. (Reference from Colachis)

5. Cyriax JH. *Textbook of Orthopaedic Medicine: Diagnosis of Soft Tissue Lesions.* 7th ed. London: Baillière Tindall; 1977;1.

6. Goldie IF, Reichmann S. The biomechanical influence of traction on the cervical spine. *Scand J Rehabil Med.* 1977;9:31–34. (Reference from Colachis)

7. Rogoff JB. *Manipulation, Traction and Massage.* 2nd ed. Baltimore: Williams & Wilkins; 1981.

8. Hinterbuchner C. Traction. In: Rogoff JB, ed. *Manipulation, Traction and Massage.* 2nd ed. Baltimore: Williams & Wilkins; 1981:184–210.

9. Frazer EH. The use of traction in backache. *Med J Aust.* 1954;2:690–697.

10. Yates DAH. Indications and contra-indications for spinal traction. *Physiotherapy (London).* 1972;58:55–57.

11. Hickling J. Spinal traction technique. *Physiotherapy (London).* 1972;58:58–63.

12. Mathews JA. The effects of spinal traction. *Physiotherapy (London).* 1972;58:64–66.

13. Weinberger LM. Trauma or treatment? The role of intermittent traction in the treatment of cervical soft tissue injuries. *J Trauma.* 1976;16:377–382.

14. Saunders HD. Use of spinal traction in the treatment of neck and back conditions. *Clin Orthop.* 1983;179:31–38.

15. Larsson U, Chöler U, Lidström A, et al. Auto-traction for treatment of lumbago-sciatica: a multicentre controlled investigation. *Acta Orthop Scand.* 1980;51:791–798.

16. Deyo RA. Conservative therapy for low back pain: distinguishing useful from useless therapy. *JAMA.* 1983;250:1057–1062.

17. Hood LB, Chrisman D. Intermittent pelvic traction in the treatment of the ruptured intervertebral disk. *Phys Ther.* 1968;48:21–31.

18. Valtonen EJ, Kiuru E. Cervical traction as a therapeutic tool: a clinical analysis based on 212 patients. *Scand J Rehabil Med.* 1970;2:29–36.

19. Rohde J. Klinishe Untersuchungen zur Wirkung von Traktionen. *Z Physiother.* 1985;37:311–343.

20. Christie BJB. No title. *Proc R S Med Sect Phys Med.* 1955;48:811–814.

21. Caldwell JW, Krusen EM. Effectiveness of cervical traction in treatment of neck problems: evaluation of various methods. *Arch Phys Med Rehabil.* 1962;43:214–221.

22. Goldie I, Landquist A. Evaluation of the effects of different forms of physiotherapy in cervical pain. *Scand J Rehabil Med.* 1970;2:117–121.

23. Mathews JA, Hickling J. Lumbar traction: a double-blind controlled study for sciatica. *Rheumatol Rehabil.* 1975;14:222–225.

24. Coxhead CE, Inskip H, Meade TW, North WRS, Troup JDG. Multicentre trial of physiotherapy in the management of sciatic symptoms. *Lancet.* 1981;1:1056–1068. Also published as O'Donohgue CE. A multicentre trial of the physiotherapeutic management of sciatic symptoms. In: Buerger AA, Greenman PE, eds. *Empirical Approaches to the Validation of Spinal Manipulation.* Springfield, Ill: Charles C Thomas, Publisher; 1985:208–227.

25. Ljunggren AE, Weber H, Larsen S. Autotraction versus manual traction in patients with prolapsed lumbar intervertebral discs. *Scand J Rehabil Med.* 1984;16:117–124.

26. Gianokopoulos G, Waylonis GW, Grant PA, Tottle DO, Blazek JV. Inversion devices: their role in producing lumbar distraction. *Arch Phys Med Rehabil.* 1985;80:187.

27. Dimaggio A, Mooney V. The McKenzie program: exercises effective against back pain. *J Musculoskel Med.* 1987;5:63–72.

SUGGESTED READING

Van der Heiden GJMG, Bouter LM, Terpstra-Lindeman E, Essers AHM. Effectiviteit van tractie bij lage rugklachten. *Ned Tijdschr Fysiother.* 1990;100:168–174.

Exercise Therapy in the Treatment of Low Back Pain

EDITOR'S PREFACE

Research regarding treatment of chronic back pain demonstrates considerably less convincing results than that for acute back pain. Sporadically, very positive results are reported. Ongley et al[1] published strikingly positive findings with sclerosing injections (prolotherapy), and Meade et al[2] had encouraging research results in relation to chiropractic.

A considerable amount of research in chronic low back pain is directed to the possible significance of isometric abdominal exercises, which are based on the assumption that the abdominal muscles are considerably weakened. Unfortunately, it is difficult to perform isolated isometric abdominal exercises without incurring simultaneous activity of the hip flexors, particularly the iliopsoas muscle. During incorrect performance, there is movement of the lumbar spine. Sometimes the exercises even become back exercises, because the back is pulled into a hyperlordosis.

In this chapter, Balm et al[3] establish a critical literature analysis of the currently available research on exercise therapy and back schools in the treatment of low back pain. The number of studies on effectiveness of isometric abdominal exercises in chronic low back pain is meager. The conclusion that isometric abdominal exercises are indicated in chronic low back pain is provisional. Research regarding the effects of low back schools offers a paradoxical picture. Balm et al[3] formulate a hypothesis to explain the phenomenon central to this paradox: they presume that patient compliance is low. Although only a hypothesis is concerned, the importance of intensive contact between therapist and patient in the treatment of chronic low back pain cannot be overemphasized.

RESEARCH ON EFFECTIVENESS OF CLASSIC EXERCISE THERAPY

Back pain research contains a fair number of publications concerning the treatment of low back pain by means of classic exercise therapy: active mobility plus muscle-strengthening exercises. This review is limited to publications in which at least "pain" is measured, because for the patient, pain is the principal complaint. Eight true experimental studies could be found that met this criterion. Because the only studies regarding the Cesar/Mensendieck exercises are pre-experimental, these two are also described. Other quasi- and pre-experimental studies concerning exercises in the treatment of low back pain are not included here.

In the following discussion, low back pain qualifies as being "chronic" when it has been present for longer than 1 year and/or the patient has already received treatment by a specialist. All other cases are considered to be of "short duration." Differences are valued as significant when $P < 0.05$. If a study indicates a difference with P greater than 0.05 but less than 0.02, the difference is understood to be a "trend."

Kendall and Jenkins, 1968

Kendall and Jenkins[4] performed a study with 47 subjects who had chronic low back pain. The patients were divided into three groups undergoing different exercise programs:

1. mobility, abdominal, and back-strengthening exercises
2. isometric abdominal exercises
3. back-strengthening exercises

Although this research attracted a lot of attention in the literature, it is striking that no information is given about the exact exercise program (duration, frequency), the method of measurement, or the statistical analysis. Duration and intensity of the low back pain were evaluated before, 1 month after, and 3 months after the treatment. The authors report that in group 2 significantly more patients had complete relief of their symptoms after the treatment than did patients in groups 1 and 3. Group 3 had the greatest incidence of worsening of symptoms.

This study gives the impression that isometric abdominal exercises are the preferred treatment in chronic low back pain. However, the numbers here are small: after 1 month, 11 patients in group 1, 13 patients in group 2, and 7 patients in group 3 had improved. Thus, based on this study, a generalization does not yet appear to be permissible.

Lidström and Zachrisson, 1970

Lidström and Zachrisson[5] published research regarding a group of 62 patients with chronic nonspecific low back pain (the entire study took place in one orthopaedic clinic). There were three treatment groups:

1. hot packs; massage; and mobility, abdominal, and back-strengthening exercises
2. intermittent pelvic traction, isometric abdominal exercises, isometric hip extension, and the psoas position
3. hot packs and rest

The treatment was administered two or three times per week for a duration of 4 weeks. The use of analgesics and the patient's opinions were recorded. The orthopaedist responsible for the clinical evaluation focused on the question of whether the patient could function normally again.

The groups demonstrated significant differences: during the clinical evaluation, group 2 had more improvement than group 1 ($P < 0.01$) and group 3 ($P < 0.1$; analysis by Balm et al,[3] based on the published raw data). The patients' self-evaluations manifested the same pattern (as analyzed by Balm et al). Group 1 had the most worsening of their symptoms. Group 2 had the strongest decrease in the use of analgesics.

Considering this study, in conjunction with the study by Kendall and Jenkins,[4] the impression arises that isometric abdominal exercises can be beneficial in the treatment of chronic, nonspecific low back pain. At the same time, back-strengthening exercises may even be contraindicated. However, in this study it is possible that the pelvic traction also played a role; in the group concerned, it was applied for 20 minutes during each treatment.

Davies et al, 1979

Davies et al[6] evaluated 43 patients with low back pain of a short duration. There were three treatment groups:

1. placebo shortwave diathermy
2. shortwave diathermy and back-strengthening exercises
3. shortwave diathermy and isometric abdominal exercises

The treatment was applied for 4 weeks. Pain was measured on a Visual Analogue Scale (VAS). In addition, mobility of the spinal column, depth of the lumbar lordosis, and the length of time that the pain interfered with activities of daily living (ADL) were measured. Measurements were registered before treatment and at 2 and 4 weeks after treatment.

The greatest improvement with regard to pain was experienced in group 2; however, the difference between the groups was not significant. In group 3, the most initial worsening appeared. Davies et al emphasized the contrast in data from this research with the results from the study by Kendall and Jenkins.[4] However, the research from Davies et al dealt with symptoms of a short duration, unlike the two previously mentioned studies.

Wiesel et al, 1980

Wiesel et al[7] performed a study by following 80 military people with acute (short duration) lumbago under two conditions:

1. bed rest in the hospital
2. ambulatory with only light activity

The treatment was discontinued when the pain disappeared, or after 14 days at the latest. Pain was rated on a 20-point scale, and the speed of recovery was noted. With regard to the pain, as well as the time it took to return to normal activities, group 1 appeared to have significantly better results.

The authors conclude that bed rest is the preferred treatment in acute lumbago; however, the possible connection of the unpleasantness of this treatment (boredom) to the quick improvement was not controlled.

Zylbergold and Piper, 1981

Zylbergold and Piper[8] performed a study by following 28 people with low back pain of short duration. They were divided into three treatment groups:

1. moist heat and lumbar flexion exercises
2. moist heat and manual therapy
3. instruction in taking load off the lumbar spine and "pelvic tilt" exercises

Groups 1 and 2 were treated twice a week for 4 weeks. Pain was rated by means of the McGill pain questionnaire. In addition, the mobility and the level of ADL were determined. Measurements were taken before and directly after the treatment period.

In terms of the measured variables, there were no significant differences between the groups. However, there was a trend in favor of group 2 with regard to pain as well as forward flexion. Group 2 also demonstrated the best ADL score; according to the authors, this was not significant. Unfortunately, the *P* value could not be calculated because documented data were insufficient. After treatment, all groups were found to be significantly better with regard to all variables.

Martin et al, 1986

Martin et al[9] performed a study by following a group of 36 people with low back pain of various durations, but in every case longer than 6 weeks. There were three chief treatment conditions, and each had a separate subcondition:

1. mobility, abdominal, and back-strengthening exercises
2. isometric abdominal exercises
3. a nonfunctioning ultrasound and short-wave diathermy (placebo), and rest

The groups also received advice as to what to do on nontreatment days:

1. reinforce the treatment at home (ie, group 1-1 and group 2-1 performed a home exercise program, group 3-1 rested and applied a hot water bottle to the back)
2. no reinforcement of the treatment at home

The treatment was performed three times per week for 3 weeks, lasting 20 minutes per session. Measurements were reported regarding muscle strength, mobility, pain, and ADL. Pain was rated throughout the entire study, and the other variables were evaluated 1 week before and 1 week after the treatment period.

Except for an increase in mobility of subgroup 2 (no reinforcement of treatment at home), no significant differences were found between the groups. Group 2 (abdominal exercises) demonstrated an increase in pain, whereas group 1 improved the most in ADL. As in the study by Davies et al,[6] the patients in this study (with symptoms of back pain of various duration) did not benefit from isometric abdominal exercises. Furthermore, at least in this study, it appears that the advice to exercise at home had minimal to no effect.

Evans et al, 1987

Evans et al[10] performed a study with 270 patients with low back pain of short duration. There were four conditions:

1. bed rest, ergonomic advice, and isometric abdominal exercises
2. ergonomic advice and abdominal exercises
3. bed rest
4. no advice (control)

Groups 1 and 2 were treated one time for 50 minutes, with possible follow-up consultations (three times, at the most) during the 8-week duration of the research. Pain (by means of the McGill pain questionnaire), the use of pain-relieving medication, mobility, straight leg raise test, patient's sense of well-being, and ADL were measured before treatment; during the first 15 days of treatment (in a daily diary, and assessed by the physician); and 6, 12, and 52 weeks after treatment. Patient compliance with the therapy was judged by referring to diary annotations.

Patients in groups 1 and 3 spent an average of approximately 8 days in bed, patients in groups 2 and 4 approximately 5 days (group 4 without specific advice to do so). Group 3 required significantly more time to reach a normal ADL level. Moreover, groups 1 and 2 stopped using pain-relieving medication significantly earlier, even though at the first post-treatment evaluation, these groups indicated more pain and showed a decrease in the ADL score. However, this finding was not statistically significant. With regard to returning to normal daily activities, the explicitly prescribed bed rest was the least effective. (Compare this finding with that of the study by Wiesel et al[7] on acute lumbago.)

In our opinion, the use of less medication in the groups with isometric abdominal exercises may be a psychological result of the ergonomic advice: The patients "learn to live with their pain" despite of the fact that they initially had more pain. Research from

Davies et al and Martin et al support the fact that patients with low back pain of short duration seem to have more pain after isometric abdominal exercises. Although in all three instances this finding is not significant, when considered together they suggest a pattern.

In view of the fact that patients obviously do things independent of explicit advice to do so (for instance, the bed rest in groups 2 and 4), and possibly also based on unpublished data from the diaries, Evans et al[10] fear that because of the low patient compliance, interpretation of the findings from this research is questionable.

Manniche et al, 1988

Manniche et al[11] performed a study by following 105 patients with chronic low back complaints. There were three treatment conditions:

1. warmth, massage, mild isometric abdominal and back muscle exercises
2. nonstrenuous back exercises
3. five times more strenuous back exercises than in group 2

Group 1 was treated in eight sessions over a period of 1 month; groups 2 and 3 had 30 treatment sessions over a period of 3 months. Pain was measured by means of Numeral Rating Scale II (NRS II), ADL as reported on a questionnaire, and mobility as tested with the Schober test. These measurements were recorded before the initial treatment and 3 months and 6 months after treatment. At the end of the treatment period, satisfaction was rated on a verbal scale with five categories.

After 3 months and 6 months, patients in group 3 scored significantly better ($P < 0.005$ or less) on all variables than the patients in groups 1 and 2. No significant differences were found between groups 1 and 2. Considering the results reported in the literature until now, the authors were surprisingly pleased about the fact that strenuous back exercises in the treatment of chronic complaints appeared to be so much more effective than the less intensive exercises. The authors have also resolved to research the effects of strenuous abdominal exercises in a later study.

Notice that the study by Kendall and Jenkins[4] demonstrated no effect of back muscle-strengthening exercises in the treatment of chronic low back pain, in contrast to this study in which the exercises were very strenuous and were performed over a long period of time.

Note

The next two studies deal with the exercise therapies of Cesar and Mensendieck (used particularly in the Netherlands). Only pre-experimental results are available on these programs. Both exercise therapies are directed at the improvement of individual postural and movement habits. These treatment programs are applied for pathology generally related to the spine, such as symptoms of back pain (cervical, thoracic, or lumbar), thoracic outlet syndrome, and migraine headaches. Isometric abdominal and back-strengthening exercises, as well as exercises for relaxation, are also part of the therapy. Compliance of the patient is a prerequisite for the exercise program. Theoretically, these programs have their foundation in cognitive learning theories.[12,13] Cesar exercises are more dynamic and directed at total movements. In Mensendieck therapy, the exercises are orally instructed; with Cesar they are also demonstrated. Cesar claims to have established a norm for correct posture and movement.

Hasper, 1986

Hasper[14] performed a retrospective inventorial study about the results of the Cesar therapy program. From 12 physical therapy clinics, data were collected on 1166 patients,

25% of whom had had their complaints less than 6 months. Slightly less than half the patients had been referred to physical therapy because of back pain. According to the judgment of the therapists, in 0.4% the symptoms increased after treatment, in 14.2% there was no change, and in 85.4% the symptoms decreased (Figure 16–1).

In 1988, Hasper and Smit[15] published a further analysis of the data published in 1986. Of 987 patients with back pain, 14% appeared to have a "scoliosis", 16% had "specific" complaints of back pain, 55% had "nonspecific" back complaints, and 15% had "back pain as a result of postural aberrations." The highest percentage of "improvement" was reported in the scoliosis group (93%), and the lowest (77%) was in the group with specific back complaints (Figure 16–1).

Balm and DeLange, 1988

Balm and DeLange[16] performed a retrospective inventorial study in regard to the Mensendieck therapy program. Through 35 Mensendieck exercise therapists, data were gathered from 1129 patients, in whom 60% had complaints of back pain. A questionnaire was sent to 1078 of the patients with a known address; 680 responses were received (63%).

The duration of symptoms before the treatment was less than 6 months in 20% of the patients. From the respondents, 85% were satisfied with the results of the therapy; the same percentage thought that they had received useful information in relation to their complaints. There were 592 respondents who reported having complaints of pain (87%). Of these, 1.7% had an increase in pain after the

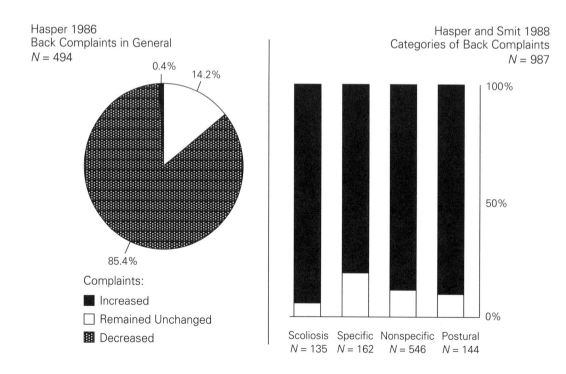

Hasper 1986
Back Complaints in General
N = 494

0.4%   14.2%

85.4%

Complaints:
- ■ Increased
- □ Remained Unchanged
- ▓ Decreased

Hasper and Smit 1988
Categories of Back Complaints
N = 987

100%

50%

0%

Scoliosis   Specific   Nonspecific   Postural
N = 135   N = 162   N = 546   N = 144

Figure 16–1 Judgment of the therapists regarding the effect of the Cesar exercise program in the treatment of back pain.[14,15]

treatment, 16.9% remained unchanged, and 81.4% reported a decrease in their pain (Figure 16–2).

Summary

At first look, it appears that in many studies there were no significant differences found among the groups. It is true that patients usually improve, but often it seems that it does not matter which treatment was administered. Still, specific patterns have emerged from these studies.

Only three of the mentioned studies dealt with chronic low back pain. In two of them, therapy with isometric abdominal exercises was evaluated; these exercises seemed to be more effective than other treatments. In the third study, strenuous back exercises were performed over a long period; these appeared to be much more efficient than less strenuous exercises.

Although only three true experimental studies were concerned, the assumption that isometric abdominal exercises are effective seems justified. Moreover, back exercises could be effective if they are performed strenuously and for a long period (Table 16–1).

The remaining studies were directed mainly at low back complaints of short duration. If isometric abdominal exercises were included in the studies, they resulted in no advantage, compared with other conditions, and in three of the mentioned studies they even produced an increase in pain.

It is possible that back exercises are effective in complaints of short duration.[6] However, in our opinion effect studies dealing with complaints of short duration assume that compression-relieving measures, especially manual therapy and (to a lesser extent) traction, are of a much greater importance than exercise therapy. (See Chapters 14 and 15.) In our view, the effect studies suggest that isometric abdominal exercises would be effective only after successful reduction of compression.

With regard to the Cesar and Mensendieck therapy programs, the only available research is pre-experimental. With the interpretation here, one has to keep in mind the following:

- The research deals not only with low back pain but also with other problems.
- The amount of spontaneous recovery in low back pain can be great.[17]
- All forms of mechanical unloading seem to have a positive effect on low back pain.[18]
- Relaxation may also be an effective treatment technique.[19]

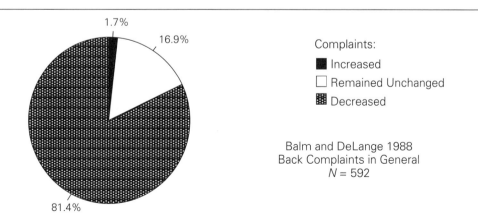

Complaints:

■ Increased
☐ Remained Unchanged
▦ Decreased

Balm and DeLange 1988
Back Complaints in General
N = 592

1.7%
16.9%
81.4%

Figure 16–2 Judgment of the patients regarding the effect of the Mensendieck exercise program in the treatment of back pain, according to Balm and DeLange.[16]

Table 16–1 Research on Effectiveness of Classic Exercise Therapy

Research Study		Treatment	Results
Kendall and Jenkins,[4] 1968; N = 47: Chronic	a	Mobility, abdominal and back-strenghtening exercises	B > * a > c
	b	Isometric abdominal exercises	
	c	Back muscle-strengthening exercises	
Lidström and Zachrisson,[5] 1970; N = 62: Chronic	a	Hot packs, massage, mobility, back- and abdominal-strengthening exercises	a < * B > c
	b	Pelvic traction, isometric abdominal exercises, isometric hip extension, the psoas position	
	c	Hot packs and rest	
Davies et al,[6] 1979; N = 43: Short duration	a	Shortwave diathermy	B > a > c
	b	Shortwave diathermy with back-strengthening exercises	
	c	Shortwave diathermy with isometric abdominal exercises	
Wiesel et al,[7] 1980; N = 80: Short duration: acute lumbago	a	Bed rest in hospital	A > * b
	b	Ambulatory with only light activities	
Zylbergold and Pipeir,[8] 1981; N = 28: Short duration	a	Moist warmth and lumbar flexion exercises	B > (a ≈ c)
	b	Moist warmth and manual therapy	
	c	Information	
Martin et al,[9] 1986; N = 36: Mixed	a	Mobility, abdominal- and back-strengthening exercises	(A ≈ C) > b
	b	Isometric abdominal exercises	
	c	Placebo ultrasound and shortwave diathermy	
	—	With home exercises and rest	
	—	Without home exercises and rest	
Evans et al,[10] 1987; N = 270: Short duration	a	Bed rest, information, isometric abdominal exercises	Analgesics: (A ≈ B) > * (c ≈ d)
	b	Information, isometric abdominal exercises	Pain: (a ≈ b) < (C ≈ D)
	c	Bed rest	
	d	No advice	
Manniche et al,[11] 1988; N = 105: Chronic	a	Warmth, massage, and mild abdominal- and back-strengthening exercises	C > * (a ≈ b)
	b	Nonstrenuous back exercises	
	c	Five times more intensive back exercises	

Note: All studies mentioned are true experimental in design; only the results for pain are indicated. The best treatment in the study is indicated with a capital letter. * = Significant; > = better than; < = worse than; ≈ = nonsignificant or different only by means of a tendency, thus possibly (but not proven) equal to.

However, taking into account that the research is pre-experimental, the percentages of patients showing "improvement" are high.

Although for untreated pain of short duration similar or even higher percentages of improvement have been found,[17] the majority of the patients in the two mentioned studies had chronic complaints. Both therapy programs are intensive (compare with Manniche et al[11]). In addition, the patient compliance is likely very high.

RESEARCH ON EFFECTIVENESS OF BACK SCHOOLS

In the last several years, the popularity of back schools has risen.[20–24] In back schools, exercises are only a part of the total program, where significant attention is given to information, education, ergonomic principles, and/or psychological techniques. Many back schools are presented to groups rather than the individual, and the number of treatment sessions is relatively small. In general, it is claimed that in comparison with other therapies, back schools are less expensive.

For a large part, the Swedish back school was inspired through the work of Nachemson, who emphasized rest and pain-relieving medication in the acute phase, and ergonomic advice to prevent the occurrence of chronic pain.[18] This ergonomic advice is based on the measurements of intradiscal pressure under various mechanical loads.

The Canadian back school[25] is directed more toward the psychological aspect of back pain and gained inspiration from Fordyce.[19] Besides the psychological management, the Canadian back school includes exercises based on biomechanics and techniques for relaxation.

All of the back schools known to us incorporate isometric abdominal exercises and "pelvic tilts."

This effectiveness study review is limited to true experimental research in which at least pain is measured. Although psychological techniques fall outside the scope of this overview, one controlled study of the effectiveness of psychological therapy in chronic pain indicates good results.[26] The following research concerns the effectiveness of the Swedish back school. Only one study, from Keijsers,[27] also includes psychological techniques.

Bergquist-Ullman and Larsson, 1977

Bergquist-Ullman and Larsson[28] researched 217 employees of the Volvo factory who had back pain complaints of short duration. There were three treatment conditions:

1. Swedish back school (A)
2. physical therapy, which included manual techniques (B)
3. placebo shortwave diathermy (C)

The patients in group 1 (A) received four, and in groups 2 (B) and 3 (C) maximally ten, treatments. Effect variables were the time it took to "recover," the number of days absent from work during the initial period of back pain, the severity of the pain, and the number and severity of recurrences in 1 year. This study received wide attention. However, a number of methodological oversights make it difficult to interpret the data.

The "recovery" in groups 1 (A) and 2 (B) was significantly shorter than in group 3 (C): $(A \approx B) > {}^*c$. However, there was no significant difference in the pain index between the "recovered" and the "not yet recovered."

Patients in group 1 (A) averaged significantly fewer absences from work, during the initial period of back pain, than in group 2 (B) or group 3 (C): $A (> b) > {}^* c$. However, group 2 (B) had the least recurrence, followed by group 1 (A) and then group 3 (C)—only the difference between B and C showed an obvious trend (our analysis): $B (> a) > c$. With regard to the other variables, no significant differences were found.

The quicker "recovery" in the experimental groups is difficult to understand considering that the "nonrecovered" group demonstrated no significant difference on the pain index.

Perhaps the "recovered" patients initially still had considerable pain.[10] Nevertheless, the "acceleration of the recovery" in itself is significant.

The advantage of the back school in regard to absence from work is encouraging. The larger number of recurrences in the back school group over the group receiving physical therapy plus manual techniques is disappointing, considering the fact that the Swedish back school directed considerable measures at prevention.

Lindequist et al, 1984

Lindequist et al[29] performed research on 56 patients with complaints of short duration, under two treatment conditions:

1. individualized Swedish back school (A)
2. advice regarding taking load off the back, and pain-relieving medication as necessary (B)

The patients received two treatments and could consult the therapist as necessary in the following 6 weeks (average 2.4 times per patient). Measurements of the duration and severity of the symptoms, absence from work, recurrence, and satisfaction regarding the treatment were registered at the beginning, after 3 and 6 weeks, and in a follow-up 1 year later.

There was a marginal trend for quicker recovery and less recurrence in group 1 (A) (our analysis): A > b. Absence from work due to the back pain did not differ obviously, while the absence from work due to other symptoms was significantly less in group 1 (A) (our analysis). Considered together, there is a trend: A > b. Also, patients were significantly more satisfied in group 1 (A): A > * b.

The researchers concluded that the back school had a psychological effect, but no clear effect on the course of the symptoms. However, considering the trends in this study (on one relatively small heterogeneous group),

there still appears to be a confirmation of the findings of Bergquist-Ullman, which was also performed on patients with complaints of short duration.

Lankhorst et al, 1984

Lankhorst et al[30] performed research on 48 patients with chronic complaints. The two treatment conditions were as follows:

1. Swedish back school (A)
2. placebo shortwave diathermy (B)

The patients were treated four times in 2 weeks. Effect variables included pain intensity and functional ability and were measured before; directly after; and at 3, 6, and 12 months after treatment.

Directly after the treatment, group 2 (B) demonstrated an unexpected worsening in pain and functional ability; however, group 1 (A) did not. After 6 months, group 1 (A) showed a worsening of the pain; however, group 2 (B) did not.

A statistical comparison of the groups was absent in this publication. The authors concluded that the back school in the chronic phase of back pain had little influence and propose that this is in contradiction with the findings of Bergquist-Ullman and Larsson[28] for the subacute phase. However, we attempted to perform a comparison of the groups based on the data given in the study. There appeared to be a trend in favor of A: A > b. Thus, in our opinion there *is* a trend in favor of the back school.

Aberg, 1984

Aberg[31] performed research on 431 patients, of whom 65% were laborers, with chronic symptoms. The two treatment conditions were:

1. institutionalized Swedish back school (A)
2. waiting list (B)

Intensive treatment took place for 6 weeks in a special institution. By means of a questionnaire, measurements were made with respect to pain, ADL, attitude, compliance, sense of well-being, and social activities. These measurements were registered at 2 weeks before, and 4 and 12 months after, treatment.

With regard to attitude, ADL (only after 4 months), and sense of well-being (only after 12 months), the patients in group 1 (A) scored significantly better than group 2 (B): A > * b. With regard to pain and social activities, no significant differences were found: a ≈ b. The author concluded that the back school had mainly a psychological effect.

It is striking that in spite of the intensity of the treatment, after 4 months only 50% of the treated patients were able to perform exercises, in comparison with 29% of the waiting-list group. After 1 year, the percentages were 45% and 26%, respectively.

Klaber-Moffett et al, 1986

Klaber-Moffett et al[32] performed research on 92 patients with chronic back pain. The two treatment conditions of the study were as follows:

1. Swedish back school (A)
2. only exercises from the back school (B)

There were three treatment sessions. Pain, functional activities, degree of disability, and knowledge concerning the back complaints were measured before treatment and at 6 and 16 weeks after treatment.

With regard to pain, no significant difference was found; however, there was a trend: A > b. The effect variable, functional activities, was initially better in group 1 (A). Knowledge about the symptoms initially increased more in group 1 (A). Afterward, the amount of disability was the lowest in group 1 (A): A > b.

The authors concluded that in chronic complaints, back school seems to have not

only a psychological effect but also an effect in relation to pain and functional ability. This conclusion is contrary to the *conclusions* of Lankhorst et al[30] and Aberg,[31] but in our opinion it is not refuted by the *data* of these studies.

Keijsers, 1987

Keijsers[27] published a study of 40 patients with predominantly chronic low back pain. The patients were all under treatment by a specialist. There were two conditions:

1. back school including relaxation exercises (A)
2. waiting list (B)

Eight lessons were given in the back school treatment. The effect variables used were behavior, pain cognition, and pain experience. Preceding, directly after, and 8 weeks after the treatment measurements were made.

In relation to the pain, both groups demonstrated significant, but not different, improvement: a ≈ b. Later, when group 2 (B) was also treated with the back school methods, no significant changes in the pain were perceived. On behavior indices, there were no significant differences; however, a trend was noted (our calculation): A > b. Both pain cognition and the search for social support were significantly better in group 1 (A): A > * b.

The significant improvement in the waiting-list group is surprising. Perhaps because the patients knew that they would be receiving treatment, a placebo effect occurred. The positive effects of the back school were chiefly related to psychological variables, just as in the study by Aberg.[31]

Summary

Two studies were reviewed concerning the Swedish back school in complaints of short duration (Table 16–2).

The research in complaints of short duration leads to the assumption that the Swedish back school is better than placebo in regard to work absence and acceleration of recovery.

Table 16–2 Research on Effectiveness of Back Schools

Research Study		Treatment	Results
Bergquist-Ullman and Larsson,[28] 1977; $N = 217$: Short duration	a	Swedish back school	Recovery: (A ≈ B) > * c
	b	Physical therapy and manual therapy	Absence from work: A (> b) > * c
	c	Placebo shortwave diathermy	Recurrence: B (> a) > c
Lindequist et al,[29] 1984; $N = 56$: Short duration	a	Individualized Swedish back school	Recovery, absence from work, recurrence: A > b
	b	Advice and analgesics	Satisfaction: A > * b
Lankhorst et al,[30] 1984; $N = 48$: Chronic	a	Swedish back school	Pain, functional capacity: A > b
	b	Placebo shortwave diathermy	
Aberg,[31] 1984; $N = 431$: Chronic	a	Institutionalized Swedish back school	Attitude, ADL, sense of well-being: A > * b
	b	Waiting list	Pain, social activities: a ≈ b
Klaber-Moffett et al,[32] 1986; $N = 92$: Chronic	a	Swedish back school	Functional activities, knowledge, disability, pain: A > b
	b	Exercises from the Swedish back school	
Keijsers,[27] 1987; $N = 40$: Chronic	a	Back school plus relaxation exercises	Pain cognition, searching for social support: A > * b
	b	Waiting list	Behavior: A > b
			Pain: a ≈ b

Note: All studies mentioned are true experimental in design; only the results for pain are indicated. The best treatment in the study is indicated with a capital letter. * = Significant; > = better than; < = worse than; ≈ = not significant or different only by means of a tendency, thus possibly (but not proven) equal to.

However, in regard to recovery, there is no advantage in comparison of physical therapy with manual therapy, and the latter treatment scored better on recurrence.

In the research on classic exercise therapy, there seems to be no or even a negative effect of isometric abdominal exercises in complaints of short duration (Table 16–1). Yet the Swedish back school, which recommends these exercises, appeared to have a positive effect on complaints of short duration. It is obvious that in chronic complaints, the back

schools have a psychologically favorable effect, even though they do not specifically aim for that. Some suggest that back schools have a beneficial effect on chronic back pain; however, either that effect is subtle or it does not appear at all. Thus, we conclude that for chronic complaints, back schools may have a possible effect on pain, but this effect is so minimal that it is not of any interest.

In the research on classic exercise therapy for chronic complaints, a possible beneficial effect of isometric abdominal exercises is suggested (Table 16–1). However, back schools, which make use of these exercises, hardly support this suggestion.

Surprisingly, in research on classic exercise therapy for short-duration complaints, isometric abdominal exercises seem to have either no effect or even a negative effect, while in back schools these programs have a positive effect. In the treatment of chronic back pain, this is just the opposite.

The findings of Martin et al[9] about the possible uselessness of home exercises, the doubt by Evans et al[10] about patient compliance, and Aberg's data[31] lead us to the following hypotheses in relation to the back school research:

1. Back schools are less effective in chronic back complaintss because of poor patient compliance in following the *correct* advice of performing isometric abdominal exercises.

2. Back schools are effective in complaints of short duration because of poor patient compliance in following the wrong advice of performing isometric abdominal exercises.

CONCLUSION

In low back pain of short duration, compression-relieving techniques are preferred. (See Chapters 14 and 15.)

In chronic low back pain, back schools mainly have a psychological effect. Isometric abdominal exercises also seem to be effective. From one recently published true experimental study, a positive effect is achieved from intensive back muscle exercises performed over a long period. Pre-experimental research regarding the Cesar and Mensendieck exercise programs (mainly dealing with chronic low back pain) also suggests a beneficial effect; however, true experimentally designed studies are needed in this area.

REFERENCES

1. Ongley MJ, Klein RG, Dorman TA, Eek BC, Hubert LJ. A new approach to the treatment of chronic low back pain. *Lancet.* 1987;2:143–146.

2. Meade TW, Dyer S, Browne W, Townsend J, Frank AO. Low back pain of mechanical origin: randomized comparison of chiropractic and hospital outpatient treatment. *Br Med J.* 1990; 300:1431–1437.

3. Balm MFK, Sybrandi CR, Volman MJM, et al. Oefenen bij lage rugpijn: Een kritische literatuur-analyse. In: Mattie H, Menges LJ, Spierdijk J, eds. *Pijn-Informatorium.* Alphen a.d. Rijn: Stafleu; 1988:44101–44128.

4. Kendall PH, Jenkins JM. Exercises for back ache: a double blind controlled trial. *Physiotherapy (London).* 1968;54:154–157.

5. Lidström A, Zachrisson M. Physical therapy on low back pain and sciatica: an attempt at evaluation. *Scand J Rehabil Med.* 1970;2:37–42.

6. Davies JE, Gibson T, Tester L. The value of exercises in the treatment of low back pain. *Rheumatol Rehabil.* 1979;18:243–247.

7. Wiesel SW, Cuckler JM, DeLuca F, et al. Acute low back pain: an objective analysis of conservative therapy. *Spine.* 1980;5:324–330.

8. Zylbergold RS, Piper MC. Lumbar disc disease: comparative analysis of physical therapy treatments. *Arch Phys Med Rehabil.* 1981;62:176–179.

9. Martin PR, Rose MJ, Nichols PJR, Russell PL, Hughes IG. Physiotherapy exercises for low back pain: process and clinical outcome. *Int Rehabil Med.* 1986;8:34–38.

10. Evans C, Gilbert JR, Taylor W, Hildebrand A. A randomized controlled trial of flexion exercises, education and bed rest for patients with acute low back pain. *Physiother Can.* 1987;39:96–101.

11. Manniche C, Hesselsøe G, Bentzen L, Christensen I, Lundberg E. Clinical trial of intensive muscle training for chronic low back pain. *Lancet.* 1988;2:1473–1476.

12. Fitts PM, Posner MI. *Human Performance.* Belmont, Calif: Brooks/Cole; 1967.

13. Schmidt RA. A schema theory of discrete motor skill learning. *Psychol Rev.* 1975;82:225–260.

14. Hasper HC. *Rapport 1e-Fase Onderzoek naar de Resultaten van de Oefentherapie Cesar.* Den Dolder: Vormingsfonds Cesar; 1986.

15. Hasper HC, Smit J. *Rapport 2e-Fase Onderzoek naar de Resultaten van de Oefentherapie Cesar.* Den Dolder: Opleiding Oefentherapie Cesar; 1988.

16. Balm MFK, DeLange CJ. *Een inventariserend onderzoek naar de patiëntenpopulatie van de oefentherapie—Mensendieck binnen de eerstelijns gezondheidszorg.* Amsterdam: Publication by the authors; 1988.

17. Simms-Williams H, Jayson MIV, Young SMS, Baddeley H, Collins E. Controlled trial of mobilization and manipulation for patients with low back pain in general practice. *Br Med J.* 1978;2:1338–1340.

18. Nachemson A. Work for all. *Clin Orthop.* 1983;179:77–83.

19. Fordyce F. Relationship of patient semantic pain descriptions to physician diagnostic judgements, activity level measures, and MMPI. *Pain.* 1978;5:293–303.

20. Kennedy B. Management of back problems. *Physiotherapy (London).* 1980;66:108–111.

21. Fisk JR, Dimonte P, McKay Cowington S. Back schools. *Clin Orthop.* 1983;179:18–23.

22. Hayne CR. Back schools and total back care programmes: a review. *Physiotherapy (London).* 1984:70:14–17.

23. Linton SJ, Kamwendo KY. Low back schools: a critical review. *Phys Ther.* 1987;67:1375–1383.

24. Terpstra SJ, Bouter LM. Het effect van de rugschool: Overzicht van de literatuur. *Ned Tijdschr Fysiother.* 1988;98:112–114.

25. Hall H. The Canadian back education units. *Physiotherapy (London).* 1980;66:115–117.

26. Linton SJ. Behavioral remediation of chronic pain: a status report. *Pain.* 1986;24:125–141.

27. Keijsers J. *Leren omgaan met rug & pijn.* Rijksuniversiteit Limburg, Maastricht: Rijksuniversiteit Limburg; 1987. Doctoral thesis.

28. Bergquist-Ullman M, Larsson U. Acute low back pain in industry. *Acta Orthop Scand Suppl.* 1977.

29. Lindequist S, Lundberg B, Wikmark R, et al. Information and regime at low back pain. *Scand J Rehabil Med.* 1984;16:113–116.

30. Lankhorst GJ, Van der Stadt RJ, Vogellar TW, Van der Korst JK, Prevo AJH. Het effect van de Zweedse rugschool bij chronische idiopathische lage rugpijn. *Ned Tijdschr Fysiother.* 1984;94:62–65.

31. Aberg J. Evaluation of an advanced back pain rehabilitation program. *Spine.* 1984;9:317–318.

32. Klaber-Moffett JA, Chase SM, Portek I, Ennis JR. A controlled, prospective study to evaluate the effectiveness of a back school in the relief of chronic low back pain. *Spine.* 1986;11:120–122.

17

Integrative Approach to Diagnosis and Treatment

EDITOR'S PREFACE

Traditionally, complaints associated with the spine have led to the following dichotomy: the complaints either are morphologically explainable or are psychologically derived. This dichotomy usually leads to a sequence of treatment procedures. First, the patient is referred to a therapist who thinks in morphological terms. If morphological treatment is unsuccessful, referral to a psychotherapist is considered. For many reasons, we believe that this is a no-win situation. A definitive line separating "body" and "spirit" is philosophically unsound; how, in that case, would there be contact between body and spirit?[1] The different aspects of individual experiences are closely connected. Research has made it clear that it is possible to approach the body on different levels, but an absolute division is unthinkable.[2]

Psychophysiology developed as a reaction to a health care system that is predominantly based on morphology. Moreover, aspects of personal life have been successfully incorporated into the treatment of complaints. However, psychophysiology still carries traces of previous thought: some complaints can be understood morphologically while others can be understood in psychological terms.

In this chapter, Albert de Jong tries to disprove the traditional division theory. Essentially, disorders are not "caused" solely by morphological or psychological factors. However, every approach has its own merits. De Jong advocates simultaneous treatment of symptoms from several different disciplines. If carefully presented, the patient will benefit and we will better understand the complaints expressed by the patient.

INTRODUCTION

Lewit[3] states that many pain complaints related to disorders of the spine are difficult to treat without considering the psychology of the patient. Therefore, it is important for the clinician to recognize patients' normal reactions to significant experiences in their lives. A patient should not just happen to ventilate his or her distress for the first time when he or she is undergoing a computed tomography (CT) scan.

Traditionally, in Western society, there has been a distinction between complaints with a physical (somatic) cause and complaints with a mental (psychological) cause. The normal sequence of treatment is as follows: First, the clinician looks for possible anatomical aberrations. If an anatomical aberration is found, it is considered the cause of the complaints. If an anatomical aberration is not found, the complaint "must be psychological."

For quite some time, there have been objections to this traditional dichotomy. First, there are *logical* objections: the human is a biopsychosocial unit that can be studied through the use of different disciplines, but cannot be separated into different compartments.

Second, there are *empirical* objections. For example, some people have the typical symptoms of a herniated nucleus pulposus but there are no "supporting" radiological findings. Other people have radiological findings without symptoms. Thus, how can we conclude that the symptoms are a result of anatomical "aberrations" in people who have both the symptoms and the radiological findings?

Third, there are *ethical* objections against the dichotomy. After all, in patients with complaints but without demonstrable anatomical aberrations, we quite often assume that the complaints are "psychological." In other words, a patient is assumed to have a psychological dysfunction in addition to his or her somatic complaint.

In response to these objections, a new concept has been developed in which the relationships among the biological, psychological, and social functions are centralized. In clinical psychology and psychiatry, this is called *psychophysiology*. In modern scientific research, it is called *psychoneuroimmunology*. This development is a definite improvement in Western medicine and has immediate clinical consequences. For example, in many cases it is preferable to achieve a cooperation between the orthopaedic specialist and the clinical psychologist in the treatment of symptoms. From a psychosomatic (psychophysiological) standpoint, cooperation between a physiological specialist and a psychological specialist is a requirement in the following three situations:

1. in complaints about physical functioning with specific tissue damage (ie, internal ulcers, local atrophy)

2. in complaints about physical functioning without tissue damage, for example, conversion complaints (a patient spontaneously cannot move his or her arm, but can do so while under hypnosis)

3. in complaints after a severe trauma, for example, post-traumatic stress after a severe traffic accident, after a mutilating surgery, or after the loss of a loved one

Still, the present clinical situation is far from ideal. For example, even in psychophysiology there is an assumption that psychological "causes" can be responsible for somatic complaints, and vice versa. These assumptions are still made as if this separation is actually possible, only now it is termed *multicausal*.

The ideal concept for diagnosis and treatment goes much further than what is addressed in psychophysiology. The human body is a biopsychosocial unit. Not only do physicians have something to contribute, but so do psychologists and so do sociologists. On first impression, the opinions of these specialists do not seem to relate to each other; the same patient can be diagnosed with a herniated nucleus pulposus, a personality disorder, or a social uprooting. Each of these hypotheses leads to its own treatment plan. Most of the time it is preferable to start several of these treatment plans at the same time. In so doing, the purpose is to resolve the patient's complaints and not to find the "cause(s)" of the complaints.

The meeting point of the different specialists involved with the treatment of the patient is not their theories; these can even be incompatible. The focal point of the various clinicians (for example, the orthopaedic specialist and the psychologist) is the patient and his or her complaints. Therefore, in the following discussion, cooperation is stressed.

In this book, much attention is given to the different orthopaedic techniques for the treatment of complaints. In this chapter, an attempt is made to describe the present position of the clinical psychologist. Recently, this position has leaned more toward the psychosomatic and partially toward the ideal "integrative approach." Still, it makes sense to know each other's language, even when realizing the possible limitations of that language. Thus the opinions of the different schools of thought will be described as clearly as possible.

PSYCHOSOMATIC APPROACHES

Psychoanalysis

According to Freud's psychoanalytical theory, psychosomatic illness is seen especially in persons with neurotic signs. The emotional stress of these patients can be reflected in the physical complaints. Famous are Freud and Brauer's first experiments in which they proved that patients could move parts of the body under hypnosis, whereas before the hypnosis they were unable to.

Freud described the existence of the "subconscious." As a result of a traumatic experience, the subconscious can be suppressed; therefore it can be threatening to make the subconscious conscious. As a defense against this threat, the patient shuts out the traumatic experience, in effect ignoring the bad news. According to psychoanalysis, these defense mechanisms explain the origin of somatic illness.

Freud assumed that when a patient is unable to process a traumatic experience effectively, this can lead to a neurosis that can be the cause of, for example, nervousness and increased somatic tension.

Well-known defense mechanisms include projection, denial, and rationalization. These mechanisms give the patient a short-term solution; he or she can live with his or her problem without truly solving it. The patient projects his or her real feelings onto somebody else (projection), denies the (for him or her) insurmountable reality (denial), or comes up with explanations for his or her failures (rationalization). According to the patient, the reason for his or her sorrow lies outside his or her reach. But analyzing these situations is only a partial explanation.

The use of these and other defense mechanisms is completely subconscious. The patients are unable to express their feelings; they do not even have access to their feelings. This can result in the development of physical complaints, such as nervousness, stress, sleep, eating disorders, and even sexual problems.

Freud's vision about psychological regulation in humans may have been historically important, but for modern orthopaedic medicine, the relevance of Freud's theories is minimal, except for his theory of neurosis.

Neurotic Signs

Neurotic signs indicate a disturbed psychological balance. Such signs can be induced temporarily by certain social situations but can also be part of the patient's fixed behavior patterns. In the latter instance, the patient is said to have a "neurosis." Neuroses can be identified by one of the following signs:

- the presence of defense mechanisms, for example, projection, denial, or rationalization
- the repetitive character of failures, for example, chronic lateness or repeatedly not living up to expectations at school
- the refusal to accept responsibility for personal behavior, which results in such situations as frequently changing partners or confrontations and conflicts at work
- the exaggeration of normal reaction, for instance panic in a situation that would not bother somebody else
- the inability to concentrate and the associated malfunction of memory

Often the patient's history reveals that the patient has had childhood problems, which may entail excessive sleepwalking, fearfulness, bed-wetting, nail biting, etc.

During diagnosis and treatment of neurosis, *conversion* can be an important factor. Conversion is a term used when the symptoms are considered to be a transformation of psychological problems into somatic symptoms, for example, the loss of speech (mutism) or the loss of certain active motions (paresis). There is a noticeable attitude of indifference as the patient describes the complaints (belle indifférence); the relaxation during the patient's description does not fit with the intensity of the complaints and the limitations these complaints impose in daily life. (This is also seen in persons without any signs of psychopathology, but who have a desire to organize difficult problems for themselves and others.)

Behavioral Medicine

Behavioral medicine attempts to help patients by taking into account the unique psychological and situational factors involved in each case and directly addressing them. The relationships among three aspects—mind, body, and situation—are responsible for the onset and continuation of complaints. Therefore a three-way treatment is possible: the classic somatic treatment, psychotherapy, and advice regarding the patient's situation. In such a treatment, a patient with nonspecific low back pain would be treated not only according to the Cyriax method, but also with massage and relaxation psychotherapy. In addition, the patient would receive information about lifting and daily exercises. Controlled research has proved that relaxation techniques have a positive effect on patients suffering chronic pain.[4] Good results can be achieved when patients follow recommendations to reduce stress during significant situations, such as with the family or in the love life. On one hand, these treatment options may seem too trivial to mention. But on the other hand, because little serious research has been conducted regarding these options, potentially valuable techniques may be overlooked. Experience has shown that patients have good results with the more integrated approach of behavioral medicine. Helping a patient to lead a healthier lifestyle, be it through improving eating habits, developing a creative hobby, or convincing him or her to take a relaxing vacation, can be more effective than all the classic somatic treatment methods. Generally, patients with a more independent and resilient attitude have a better chance of recovery than patients who feel helpless and dependent.[5]

Learning Theory

Practitioners of behavioral medicine pay close attention to a patient's personal situation. They also encourage a patient's independence. To do so, the therapist utilizes a learning theory based on the premise that people will increase behaviors that are rewarded. Behavior that is not rewarded or reinforced will be gradually "unlearned."

Take the case of a child who is punished for expressing his or her emotions. Even as an adult, this patient may associate the expression of feelings with anxiety. Because every emotion is coupled with anxiety, the patient is likely to avoid the expression of emotion, both verbally and nonverbally. One possibility is that the patient will express his or her emotions by developing somatic symptoms. The direct expression of feelings is taboo, but expressing the feelings in an indirect way (in this example, physical symptoms) does not provoke anxiety and is therefore pleasant. The "pleasure" that comes from this indirect expression of emotions is reinforcement. Thus, the patient is likely to continue this behavior, that is, continue to have somatic complaints.

Treatment based on the learning theory is called behavior therapy. This is a misleading term because all forms of psychotherapy have as a goal a change in the behavior of a patient. The term *behavior therapy* is used for the forms of therapy adhering to the principle that all behavior is learned. Behavior therapy attempts to decrease habitual negative behaviors and teach more appropriate behaviors. For example, cigarette smoking in nervous patients can have a relaxing short-term effect. However, in the long run, the physiological and psychological effect of smoking cigarettes is an increase in tension. This increased tension can lead to hyperventilation and/or chronic increased muscle tone. Chronic increased muscle tone of the postural muscles increases pressure on the intervertebral discs, which can influence a disc prolapse, resulting in low back pain.

Communication Theory

The communication theory states that all behavior, including the manifestation of symptoms, has a communicative function. Therapists using this method seek to understand what a patient's symptoms may be communicating. The symptoms may be purely physiological, but they may also be the result of a patient's interpersonal relationships. For example, a headache can be an excuse not to perform certain duties.

The therapist is interested in the way the patient communicates about his or her complaints and to what extent the complaints play a role in the communication. In this way, attention is shifted toward the social consequences of the symptom and the possible social benefits the patient receives by maintaining the symptom. For example, to understand and to be able to treat certain pareses, it can be useful to realize that the patient benefits from constant family care (at least in the short term). Other examples from the communication theory can easily be seen in certain families in which there is such a strong mutual connection between the family members that it overshadows the growth of an individual's identity. Having a somatic complaint gives the patient an option to have a unique identity.

RECOGNIZING PSYCHOSOMATIC COMPLAINTS

In general, the above-mentioned theories are the basis for different psychological explanations of psychosomatic complaints. A dichotic separation between somatic and psychological complaints does not serve the patient.

Because of the close connections among physiological, psychological, and situational factors, it is difficult to diagnose these problems correctly. Obstinate symptoms are infamous. However, when a thorough medical evaluation does not result in any definitive findings, it is not correct to assume that the cause of the complaints is psychological. Like a somatic diagnosis, a psychological diagnosis needs to be based upon clear, documented evidence. It is important to determine precisely which psychological and situational factors are involved. Several methods are available in order to achieve this determination.

In daily practice, a psychological diagnosis is often a matter of intuition. Currently there are different psychotechnical tests that are reliable and valid. It is a mistake not to use these tests in making a psychological diagnosis. If a therapist believes, based on intuition, that a patient is neurotic, then he or she needs to verify that judgment with reliable and valid testing.

Monitoring

In this text, monitoring refers to keeping a diary of complaints that are charted on a numerical or visual scale. With the help of the therapist, the patient monitors the presence of symptoms in conjunction with relevant experiences (the intake of medication, sleeping pattern, important encounters with other people, physical activities, etc). The patient notes how he or she feels at that time and whether the symptom increases or decreases.

Based on the information from monitoring, the variables can be illustrated on a time-series graph. The relevant experiences are plotted vertically and the time is plotted horizontally. Other special events can be added to the representation (Figure 17–1).

The purpose of this self-monitoring serves to increase the patient's awareness of the problems. In addition, the patient is forced to look at the cause in a context broader than only physiological dysfunction. Using the patient's self-registration of pain in relation to activity gives the therapist the advantage of a multifaceted diagnostic instrument; during the course of the treatment, the effects of the treatment can be measured. Following are tips for the construction of an optimal time-series questionnaire:

- Make the self-registration of the symptom concrete, for example, "intensity of the pain at this moment."

- If there are other significant symptoms besides the intensity of the pain, use a separate scale (for example, listlessness, hypersensitivity to light, cross-eyed, asymmetrical headache, dizziness, nausea, neck stiffness, radiating pain from the back into the legs, problems during daily activities, caffeine addiction, etc).

- In disorders with "attacks" (such as migraine), the frequency and time of the attacks need to be documented; with these disorders, it is wise to let the patient document more than once a day (mornings, afternoons, and nights).

- In patients with cognitive disorders (such as mental retardation), self-registration is not used; in patients with poor motivation, start with only one visual analog scale, once per day. A shortage of accurate data can give an inaccurate picture and hinder treatment.

- Leave space for patients to make special comments: the therapist can suggest that these comments concern the use of medication, sleeping pattern, significant experiences with other people, and the performance of fatiguing activities. By leaving space open, the patient also has the option to name variables other than the ones suggested.

- If several variables are followed, it is wise to let the patient start with the more general ones (for example, "listlessness") and add the more specific ones later (for instance, "the number of cups of coffee").

- The list should be practical; clear instructions are necessary, and the number of variables should be limited (for example, at least one and no more than five).

History

Patients with psychosomatic complaints have a markedly high level of constitutional weaknesses, such as a high frequency of

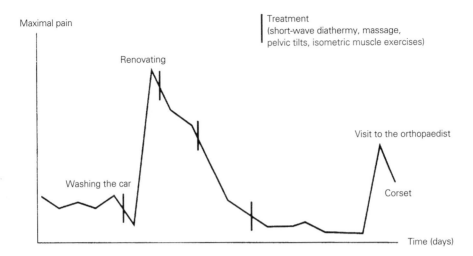

Figure 17–1 Time series graph of a young adult with symptoms of low back pain. Notice that the variations in complaints seem to be related to significant experiences.

colds, in their history. Also, there is a high frequency of doctor visits, medicinal intake, medical examinations, and sometimes previous surgeries.

Neurotic Reactions

Important signs of neurotic reactions include a pattern of a problem-specific situation (for example, always the same complaints at work or at school), depression, and exaggeration of reactions. Due to stress, there is increased muscle tone of the postural muscles and the muscles in the neck, low back, and chest.

Conversion

Conversion means "a transforming." In this situation, the psychological becomes somatic. A patient who loses the ability to stand because of the loss of a loved one but is able to dance at a school dance would be diagnosed as having a conversion disorder. Because the symbolic significance of the inability is so fulfilling for the patient, psychotherapy can be very difficult. However, the opinion that this problem should be dealt with only through psychotherapy is incorrect. In a conversion

paresis, the physical therapist should be consulted to prevent atrophy and contractures.

Depression

Depression is a syndrome that causes both physical problems (such as the inability to sleep well) and psychological problems (such as a decrease in self-esteem). During a period of depression, the patient blames himself or herself for setbacks. Typical symptoms of depression include a decrease in self-esteem, concentration difficulties, libido problems, and a general feeling of gloominess.

If attention is given to both the patient's somatic complaints and psychological complaints, there is a good prognosis for treating depression. With obvious somatic complaints, treatment can be more effective with the assistance of psychotherapy and/or the use of antidepressant medication. Thus, it is possible that symptoms of pain will disappear with the intake of antidepressant medication.[3]

Diminishing Network

It is typical for patients with psychosomatic complaints to have a diminishing of their social network. Almost all patients show a noticeable loss of social contact, because their attention is completely occupied with their symptoms and pain. However, at the same time, their social dependency actually increases; this results in a vicious circle that cannot be broken without help. Re-establishing contact with the social network can be a very satisfying aspect of the therapy. It is a great accomplishment when the patient returns to sports activities or participation in social events.

Life Events

Sometimes a patient is able to indicate exactly which life event precipitated his or her symptoms. For the therapist, the event itself is not as important as the way the patient reacts to the event (coping). For the patient, the event, and not the coping mechanism, is what is important. A patient who loses his or her job and as a reaction develops low back pain realizes the significance of the layoff, but has no idea that it would have been possible to react differently to the situation. Because these life events are so important, the therapist can use them to make the coping mechanism obvious and easier to work with. This gives the patient the opportunity to pick up life again constructively.

Post-Traumatic Stress Reactions

If a patient has experienced an intense trauma such as an accident, a hospital admission, the loss of a loved one, or the loss of a job, symptoms can arise that are not caused by a neurotic personality but instead are based on the experienced trauma. A trauma, such as whiplash, can be an extraordinarily substantial event. In comparison with a severe physical trauma, the day-to-day problems of daily life may seem like a luxury. Directly after a trauma, this is a completely normal reaction and certainly does not qualify as pathological. It becomes pathological only when the reaction to the trauma occurs out of

context, for example, when a patient continues to have nightmares long after the initial suffering from the trauma has disappeared.

Post-traumatic stress reactions that have become pathological are characterized by disturbances in the vital functions and include difficulty in falling or remaining asleep, irritability, bursts of rage, difficulty in concentrating, or excessive reactions of fear to situations that have vague similarities to the initial trauma (such as when a loud noise provokes the same alarm as was expressed during the auto accident).

Reliving the trauma—such as during a guided daydream—can be very beneficial therapeutically. Because successful treatment techniques are available, it is especially important to recognize and correctly diagnose pathological post-traumatic stress reactions.

Personal Experiences of the Therapist

Some patients irritate the therapist. There are a number of reasons for this, and understanding these reasons can be very important for the therapy. Instead of denying his or her own irritation, the therapist can use it in the analysis of the problem.

Irritation can arise because the therapist is not yet able to establish the right diagnosis, or the therapist is not satisfied with the treatment plan. These irritations indicate the need to correct the patient's treatment approach.

Irritation can also result when the therapist has the same problem as the patient. For example, if both the therapist and the patient have alcohol problems, when the patient confides in the therapist the details of the problem the therapist may become upset, seeing a reflection of self. The therapist must be aware that personal problems may interfere in the interaction with the patient.

The onset of irritation or other feelings of displeasure also can indicate the manner in which the patient interacts with other people.

Cautiously presuming that the way in which the patient deals with symptoms in the presence of the therapist is the same way in which the patient deals with symptoms outside the treatment room can be a useful indication of how significant the symptoms are to the patient. For instance, the patient can present the complaint in such a way that another person is always at fault—in the clinic, this person is always the therapist. By rejecting others, the patient becomes isolated; this isolation can be the essence of the patient's problem.

Symbolic Meaning of Pain

In examining the symbolic meaning behind neck and low back pain, one can observe how a cat prepares itself for possible danger. In preparing itself for danger, a cat exhibits increased blood flow to the head, faster breathing, and a change in posture. As the cat initially manifests aggression, tension arises in the neck muscles and the creature bares its teeth (Figure 17–2). In the same way, in humans who are upset, tension in the neck musculature also increases. On the other hand, even if the cat is not planning to attack, a threatening posture is manifested. The cat makes itself bigger to impress the attacker in hopes that the attacker will disappear (Figure 17–3). In human symbolism, this is demonstrated by an individual who does not really grasp a problem, but at the same time shows intentions of dealing with the problem (as if the patient will scare the problem away). In the latter instance, one speaks of a "flight response." However, this "fleeing" is a disregard of the problem rather than a successful escape of the problem.

Persons with low self-esteem may be unusually wary because of the fear that they may not be accepted. Constant aggression, as a result of anger that cannot be ventilated, can lead to chronic increased tension of the neck muscles. On the other hand, being in a constant state of defense without ever actually dealing with the problem can lead to chronic muscle tension of the low back.

These patterns of hypertension can become permanent and after a while can lead to symptoms similar to those experienced by someone who has had a mechanical overloading in this area. Thus during treatment, it is necessary to keep in mind the possible symbolic meaning behind the pain's origin. Of

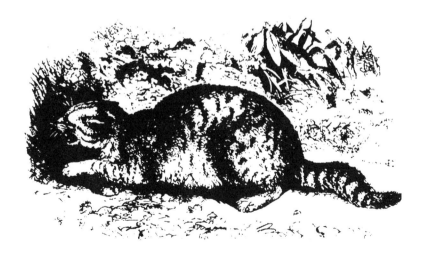

Figure 17–2 Attack posture of a cat.

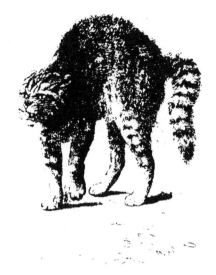

Figure 17–3 Threatening posture of a cat.

course, this does not mean that the somatic pathology should not be treated.

In a clinical situation, it is difficult to explain to patients the connection between psychological and somatic factors without alarming them. When patients are made aware of relevant psychological factors, there is a tendency for them to think that the therapist believes that they are faking their symptoms. In the same way, patients are easily insulted during evaluations for the significant psychological aspects of their problems. Quite often, there is a massive rejection of the psychological examination; some patients do not appreciate the integrative approach to their problems because they do not see the problems as multifactorial. This issue can be remedied easily with the help of the family physician, who can play an essential role in providing health care information and education. The psychotherapist who is confronted with substantial rejection should not insist on continuing. Utmost caution is mandatory here.

Questionnaires

As previously mentioned, questionnaires are useful tools in making psychological diag-

noses. Because standardized questionnaires have been tested for their reliability and validity, they can be used by the clinician recommending psychotherapy to confirm the diagnosis.

Amsterdam Biographical Questionnaire

In the Netherlands, the Amsterdam biographical questionnaire (ABV) is often used to indicate the following:

- neurotic lability (the presence of neurotic signs)
- the neurotic-somatic dimension (the degree to which neurotic lability is manifested in the somatic complaints)
- extroversion (open, focused on other people)
- test attitude (self-criticism versus self-defense)

Approximately 20 minutes are needed to complete the ABV, and another 20 minutes are required for scoring and interpretation.

Luteyn Personality Questionnaire

Because several dimensions are measured, the Luteyn personality questionnaire has many applications. According to Luteyn et al,[6] the "inadequateness" score is the most important in the psychosomatic assessment. In addition, vague somatic complaints, pessimism, and feelings of insufficiency are rated. Approximately 20 minutes are required to complete the entire questionnaire, and another 15 minutes are required for scoring and interpretation.

On the Luteyn personality questionnaire, people with low back pain score significantly higher on the "inadequateness" scale and lower on the "self-esteem" scale than do individuals without low back pain.[6] Zand et al[7] report that men with low back pain score significantly higher on the "aggrieved" and "social inadequacy" scales.

Questionnaires in Headaches

In patients with headaches, questionnaires serve to differentiate among migraine, tension, and mixed headaches. Characteristics of migraines include the following:

- pain that comes in attacks and does not last for more than 1 week
- pain that is throbbing and pulsating
- pain that is usually unilateral
- prodromal signs or indications, such as flickering of light, poor vision, or vomiting

If the headache has two of the first three characteristics and/or only the last, along with, at the most, one of the characteristics of the tension headache, the diagnosis of migraine headache is made.

Typical characteristics of a tension headache include the following:

- pain that is more often present than absent
- pain that feels like pressure or like a band
- pain that is located over the whole head, in the forehead, or just in the neck

If the headache has two or more of the above characteristics and does not qualify as a migraine headache, the diagnosis of tension headache is made.

A mixed headache has characteristics of both migraine and tension headaches.

From a psychosomatic viewpoint, the diagnosis of tension headache is made when signs of psychological tension are found. Thus, a correctly diagnosed tension headache is an indication for psychotherapy.

Diagnosis Based on the *Diagnostic and Statistical Manual of Mental Disorders, Third Revised Edition*

The diagnosis of the psychosomatic aspects of symptoms of the low back, neck, extremities, and head can be made with the help of the *Diagnostic and Statistical Manual of Mental Disorders, Third Revised Edition* (DSM-III-R). The DSM-III-R gives a multidimensional classification of disorders (Table 17–1). It is based on a descriptive system; definitions of the disorders are restricted to the characteristics of the disorders rather than delving into possible causes.[8]

Because of the classifications and the corresponding specific numbering, it is possible to organize the psychopathological symptoms and make them accessible for statistical research. The manual is available in many different languages, which has improved international communication and the exchange of information. The expectation is that the uniform classification of the DSM-III-R will be widely used by therapists and insurance companies.

In using the DSM-III-R classifications, it is possible to describe the somatic, psychological, and situational aspects of the patient. Therefore, a relationship can also be made among these aspects, resulting in an overview of the physical, psychological, and environmental factors that mutually define the illness of the patient.

Because of the unequivocal system of the DSM-III-R, the complex situation of the somatic, physical, and situational factors as a whole can be overlooked.

Examples of the most common diagnostic criteria that are relevant to the diagnosis and probable treatment of psychosomatic complaints, particularly from the low back, neck, and/or head, are given in Tables 17–2 to 17–4.

TREATMENT FROM A PSYCHOSOMATIC VIEWPOINT

Simultaneous Treatment

Human observation tells us that physiological, psychological, and social aspects of human existence form a constant unit. Problems arise when various professionals start to

Table 17–1 Dimensions of the DSM-III-R

Axis	Classification	Assessment
Axis I	Clinical syndromes	Depression in the restricted sense; one-time episode, intense without psychotic signs
		Alcohol dependency
		Marital conflicts
Axis II	Developmental disorders Personality disorders	Dependent personality
Axis III	Somatic diseases or disorders	Alcohol-related liver cirrhosis
Axis IV	Severity of psychosocial stress factors	Expecting retirement and moving with the loss of friends and family
		Intensity: 4 (fair)
		Mainly long-lasting conditions
Axis V	General judgment of patient's functioning	Present "global assessment of functioning" GAF: 44
		Highest GAF from the previous year: 55

Note: Assessment occurs on five axes.[8] In the actual diagnosis, there is a score under each of these axes.

study the different aspects (eg, physical therapists, psychotherapists, social workers) of this existence separately and at different times. When one clinician fails in a treatment of the problem, the individual is sequentially referred to the next professional. Because of this "time-sequential" manner of treatment, an *incorrect* suggestion is given to the patient: "real" complaints can be understood anatomically, and in the absence of anatomical disorders, the psychiatrist has to be consulted. If the latter also fails, the psychologist or social worker has to help the patient learn to live with the symptoms.

In a clinician's personal life, gross separations are not made between the somatic, the psychological, and the social aspects of a problem. Regardless of which discipline, clinicians can often apply their human experience to their interactions with their patients. This should be encouraged. On the other hand, a justifiable argument can be made that professionals should "mind their own business," staying vigilant not to cross the personal boundaries of professional specializations.

Thus, the best situation is one in which specialists with different viewpoints simultaneously offer help to a patient. In this way, the patient can be confident that the many possible aspects

Table 17–2 Hypochondria[8]

A   Preoccupied with the fear of having a serious disease
B   Based on the interpretation of somatic signs that are not purely symptoms of panic attacks
C   Specific physical examination does not give any support
D   Reassurance from the physician has no effect
E   Duration: at least 6 months
F   Persuasion does not have the intensity of the delusion

Source: Excerpted from *Diagnostic and Statistical Manual of Mental Disorders: DSM-III -R*, American Psychiatric Association, © 1987.

Table 17–3 Somatization disorder[8]

A Multiple somatic symptoms or the conviction that one is sick
B Onset before 30 years of age
C Several years' duration
D At least 13 symptoms from a symptom list including
   • Gastrointestinal symptoms (ie, vomiting)
   • Pain (ie, pain in the extremities)
   • Cardiopulmonary symptoms (ie, shortness of breath)
   • Pseudoneurological symptoms (ie, amnesia, swallowing difficulties)
   • Psychosexual symptoms (ie, burning feeling in the genitals or rectum)
   • Symptoms from the female organs (ie, menstrual cramps)
E In relation to the symptoms
   • No organic pathology or pathophysiological mechanisms are found to be responsible for the symptoms; if there is a connection, the complaint or its related dysfunction, is exaggerated
   • Symptoms can also appear outside of panic attacks
   • Medication is taken, physicians are consulted, the lifestyle is affected

Source: Excerpted from *Diagnostic and Statistical Manual of Mental Disorders: DSM-III -R*, American Psychiatric Association, © 1987.

---

of the problems are attended to. However, this ideal situation is sometimes both too expensive and too time consuming for the patient. Fortunately, a great number of patients recover quickly with treatment based only on anatomical considerations.

Many factors in daily life contribute to the occurrence of symptoms, and these symptoms can have consequences on daily life. In low back pain, it is obvious that pain can increase due to stress. Furthermore, pain can also be the cause of stress, such as when the patient is no longer able to work because of real anxiety. Pain can have consequences for sexual behavior, and can also be triggered by certain sexual habits. Role models in a family can experience stress, even if only temporarily, when the normal distribution of tasks no longer takes place. On top of it all, the procedures that have to be followed within the health care system add an extra burden of stress onto the patient. Although theoretically the stress-causing factors are "secondary," in the life of the patient they are by far the most important aspects of the problem. Unfortunately, these secondary aspects of the symptoms are rarely addressed in medical literature.

Table 17–4 Conversion[8]

A Loss or change of physical functions (which can indicate a physical disorder)
B Psychological factors are assumed to have a relationship with the symptom
C The involved person is not aware that he or she manifests the symptom
D No known physical injury can explain the symptom
E The symptom is not a culturally related form of reacting (in the 19th century one "had to faint" or "swoon")
F The symptom is not limited to pain or a sexual problem

Source: Excerpted from *Diagnostic and Statistical Manual of Mental Disorders: DSM-III -R*, American Psychiatric Association, © 1987.

Success can be obtained with a "consultation structure." With this structure, several specialists contribute to a patient's treatment, while one central trust relationship remains. When the patient is involved *early on* in the consultation structure treatment, the disadvantages of the classic time-sequential structure disappear. After the initial examination, a referral into this consultation structure adds an element to the treatment that is missing in the time-sequential treatment: connection is made to the patient's experiences.

Motivation Phase

Examination and treatment from a psychosomatic viewpoint demand patience and tact on the part of the therapist. Referral to a psychiatrist, a psychologist, or a social worker causes problems in itself. It often implies to the patient that the symptoms experienced are really interpreted by the therapist as imaginary. Referrals to psychiatry can be perceived by the patient as a direct insult; the implication is given that besides the low back pain, the patient also has psychological problems. Motivating patients does not consist of searching for and offering arguments in order to try to convince the patient that he or she need this advice. The patient must achieve self-motivation and, in so doing, understand the various aspects of the experienced symptoms.

This situation can be achieved by the following:

- giving clear feedback about behavior and the situation
- offering the possibility of choice
- maintaining good contact with the patient

Experience shows that patients are open to the multidisciplinary approach. Some researchers report good results when they advise the patient to go for a consultation, based on the argument that there may be psycho-logical and situational aspects that could worsen the symptoms. For the patient, it has to be made clear that stress can cause the onset of somatic symptoms. It should be emphasized to the patient that these symptoms really exist. Through this combined consultation structure, the team gives the patient the feeling of being taken seriously.

Specific Treatment Methods

Monitoring

Monitoring of the patient was already described in the discussion of diagnostic tools. An increased matter-of-fact concentration on the problem by the patient is an important way to achieve a change in attitude toward the symptoms. Ask the patient to keep a diary highlighting when and with what severity symptoms occur. This serves to weaken the conviction that the problem entails only anatomical/physiological processes.

Learning how to view the relationship between daily life experiences and physical symptoms can be an important step for the patient. This awareness also creates a remarkably favorable climate for other therapeutic proposals (Figure 17–1). This process of increasing patient awareness is an important role best served by the family physician, as the patient is the most constant factor in a successful treatment.

Relaxation Techniques

Relaxation techniques are an important part of a patient's therapy. Relaxation decreases feelings of fear and worry. Relaxation techniques are used in behavioral therapy and in psychoanalytically oriented therapies.

Relaxation without Mental Imaging. Many patients benefit from yoga exercises, transcendental meditation, progressive relaxation, or the techniques for autogenic training as described by Schultz.[9] Biofeedback, sometimes combined with the option to measure temperature changes during relaxation, provides useful information to the patient about his or her progress. These relaxation techniques provide the best results when they are used in combination with other treatment forms.

Relaxation with Mental Imaging. In relaxation techniques with mental imaging, the patient has to imagine a threatening situation. If the patient is offered relaxation at the moment the uncomfortable situation occurs, a connection develops between this situation and relaxation (instead of fright or anxiety). For the best results, it is essential to provide the patient with clear explanations, especially when using hypnosis (under trance). It is not sufficient to explain a trance as a normal daily state that results from driving on a boring highway for hours or watching a movie. One must explain that there is a change of consciousness, to a more associative level, which gives more access to emotional perception. During hypnosis, the therapist uses the trance to reach a specific result. The patient is constantly aware of what is happening.

Guided Daydreams

In the 1950s, Leuner, a German psychiatrist and psychoanalyst who was familiar with hypnosis and autogenic training, developed a system of daydreams for psychodiagnositic purposes. He noticed that daydreams are often coupled with an emotional release that can have a clear therapeutic effect. Based on this finding, he developed a system that was very successful in short, problem-related treatment.

Patients are challenged to imagine a theme for a daydream during a relaxed situation. These themes come from the psychoanalytic theories of Jung. When the patient reaches a relaxed state, there is a reduction of anxiety or stress that makes it possible for the patient to see a personal repetitive pattern of neurotic anxiety. The combination of emotionally reliving a stressful situation, relaxation, and insight gives the patient who has difficulty expressing feelings a method for improve-

ment. When the symptoms can be understood as a somatic expression of psychological tensions, this kind of treatment can be very beneficial.

Suggestions Given While on the Treatment Table

Making suggestions to the patient while he or she is relaxing on the treatment table can have effects similar to those of suggestions given during hypnosis. Every therapist has a suggestive effect, even when unaware of this effect on the patient. Consciously using this suggestive component can be very helpful in the treatment of the patient. Advice to the patient about the positive effects of a therapeutic home program, or about the importance of consistently performing that program, contains an important suggestive component.

Special Techniques To Change Present Situation

Some problems start during childhood. Patients who develop psychosomatic symptoms later in their lives may do so as a result of inadequate problem-solving techniques throughout their lives. For example, patients who were victims of incest may accept a behavior as a way of coping with their problems. If this solution is not appropriately dealt with, it can lead to choosing a partner with sadistic tendencies in adulthood.

The way people learn to manipulate other family members during their childhood can establish relationship patterns that last for the rest of their lives.[10] To understand a family, one examines not the individuals, but rather the relationships between the individuals.

A common family role is that of the "go-between." This is the person who always tries to stop conflicts between other family members. People who successfully play the role of intermediary have an extra burden to carry. More than the other family members, they feel responsible for the atmosphere in the house, especially in ensuring the peace between other family members. The go-between has the opportunity for control, because the communication within the family goes through this individual. If the problems within a family increase and seem unresolvable, pressure on the go-between becomes intense. Continuing to try to solve the problems can have the opposite effect and may result in an escalation of the problem.

It is possible that the go-between extends this role outside the family circle. Such people feel responsible for the atmosphere in the work environment, as well as at home. When a go-between seeks help and becomes a patient, following the advice not to interfere with other people's arguments can lead to significant changes. The argument intensity remains under control and the patient begins to function better at home and at work. Generally, there is a good prognosis for patients with depression, tension headaches, or low back pain who follow the advice to stop acting as a go-between.[10]

Increase in the Social Network

As previously mentioned, patients whose complaints are psychosomatically based tend to decrease their social contacts. Conversely, increasing social contact, such as participating in sports, can be a positive addition to the treatment.

From a biological point of view, stress can be interpreted as a reaction of the organism to extreme exertion (in most mammals: "fight or flight"). The physiology of the stress reaction is aimed toward processing the bodily functions during this physiological exertion. It is therefore possible that precisely through this physical exertion, toxic by-products of the stress reaction are broken down. After physical exertion, one feels "tired but good" and certainly not stressed.

Therefore, in addition to extending the social network, physical exertion such as sport participation should also be included in the

therapy. Many companies have programs that use some kind of organized sport event to enhance the working atmosphere. Two advantages can be gained from this: (1) the ability to manage stress is improved and (2) the social network is improved. Although some consider these events as lost time, there are in fact indications that such events increase productivity.

Group Therapy

By participating in a group, patients can make contact with fellow sufferers. Besides the positive experience of this mutual contact, another benefit is that information can be given more efficiently by the physical or behavioral therapist. Group therapy is directed at decreasing the somatic complaint and teaching a new, more assertive, behavior. Also, a further decrease in the social network is prevented.

Research on the effectiveness of back schools has been disappointing (see Chapter 16, Exercise Therapy in the Treatment of Low Back Pain); controlled studies hardly demonstrate any positive effects, especially in patients with chronic symptoms. A possible explanation for this is that, in the average back school, intense contacts do not develop because of the impersonal structure of the group. Perhaps if the schools were reorganized into subgroups, the ability to foster intensive contact would be possible.

Treatment after Serious Events

Trauma often occurs in our society in the form of auto accidents, death, or serious illnesses. Medical intervention such as surgery is also interpreted as a serious event. Knowledge and experience related to the consequences of personal calamities and the resulting stress reaction have increased significantly in the last years. In the DSM-III-R, the consequences of the post-traumatic stress disorder are defined (Tables 17–5 and

Table 17–5 Post-Traumatic Stress Disorders[8]

A Traumatic event
B Reliving
C Strong denial of signs associated with the trauma or numbness of the general reactivity
D Constant signs of increased sensitivity with at least two of the following signs:
  • sleeping difficulties
  • irritability or bursts of anger
  • excessive alertness
  • exaggerated fear reactions
  • physiological reactions in situations that symbolize or have similarities to the traumatic experience
E Duration of the disorder is at least 1 month

Note: Vegetative complaints do not come from the neurotic personality, but as a result of the trauma.

Source: Excerpted from *Diagnostic and Statistical Manual of Mental Disorders: DSM-III -R*, American Psychiatric Association, © 1987.

Table 17–6 Intensity Scale for Psychosocial Stress Factors in Adults[8]

Code	Description	Acute Events	Constant Circumstances
1	None	No acute events important to the disorder	No constant circumstances important to the disorder
2	Slight	Broken relationship; started at school or ended at school; child left home	Family fights; unsatisfactory work; living in a high-crime area
3	Moderate	Marriage; broken relationship; loss of job; retirement; miscarriage	Bad marriage; poor finances; conflicts with supervisor; single parent
4	Severe	Divorce; birth of first child	Unemployment; poverty
5	Extreme	Death of partner; diagnosed with serious disease; rape victim	Serious disease in oneself or child; constant sexual abuse
6	Catastrophic	Death of child; suicide of partner; devastating natural disaster	Hostageship; concentration-camp experiences
0	Not enough information or no change in the condition		

Source: Excerpted from *Diagnostic and Statistical Manual of Mental Disorders: DSM-III -R*, American Psychiatric Association, © 1987.

17–6). The most important consequences of serious events usually include a decrease in self-confidence, depression, anxiety, tension, irritability, sleeping disturbances, libido disturbances, eating disturbances, concentration problems, and the like. In addition, the consequences of post-traumatic and other stress factors can severely worsen already existing complaints, even in such cases as rheumatoid arthritis.[11]

The reactions to a physical or psychological trauma are relevant to the treating physician or physical therapist—even if the reactions did not evolve into a problem. Without warning, during a treatment in a safe, calm environment the patient can relive the experience of the sustained trauma; for instance, while the patient is receiving pelvic traction, a previous incident of forced incest might be relived.

Reliving the incident (flashback) is often followed by denial, or avoidance, of memories or feelings about the incident. If a part of the post-traumatic stress reaction occurred in a hospital setting (for instance, during preoperative procedures), later treatment can become severely complicated by the re-experience; flashbacks may be provoked in spaces strongly resembling those of the hospital. Usually, the patient does not realize that the sudden anxiety can be understood as a delayed reaction to the accident or the operation, even if the event took place years previously. Therefore, the therapist has to realize that such reactions can occur especially within the framework of a carefully performed, calming treatment.

Characteristic of a post-stress reaction is that the negation (repression in the form of forgetting) is broken through during relaxation. Thus in the presence of symptoms that may indicate a post-stress reaction, one might want to ask explicitly about serious events (operations, accidents, sudden disability as in whiplash).

Information for the patient is important, such as explaining that the delayed reactions could be a sign of a healthy "dosing out" of the anxieties. Tranquil, personality-supporting behavior; a renewed discussion of the problems; and maintenance of contact (if the patient agrees with it) can be a significant part of the therapy.

REFERENCES

1. Tamboer JWI. Images of the body underlying concepts of action. In: Meijer OG, Roth K, eds. *Complex Movement Behavior: "The" Motor-Action Controversy.* Amsterdam: Elsevier Science Publishers; 1988:439–461.

2. Koerselman F. *Integratief Medisch Denken: over de psychopathogenetische reconstuctie.* Amsterdam: VU-Publishers; 1990.

3. Lewit K. *Manuele Therapie.* Part 1 & 2. Lochem: De Tijdstroom; 1979.

4. Linton SJ. Behavioral remediation of chronic pain: a status report. *Pain.* 1986;24:125–141.

5. Diekstra R. *Hoe Geestelijk is Gezondheid?* Deventer: Van Loghum Slaterus; 1988.

6. Luteyn F, Starren J, Van Dijk H. *Nederlandse Persoonlijkheids Vragenlijst.* Lisse: Swets & Zeitlinger; 1986.

7. Zand JL, Lankhorst GJ, Kolman A. *Psychogene Rugpijn Test.* Lisse: Swets & Zeitlinger; 1987.

8. Koster van Groos GAS. *Beknopte Handleiding bij de Diagnostische Criteria van de DSM III-R.* Lisse: Swets & Zeitlinger; 1988. Dutch translation of the publication from the American Psychiatric Association.

9. Vrolijk A. *Interventie Modellen.* Alphen a.d. Rijn: Samsom; 1985.

10. Minuchin S. *Psychosomatic Families.* Cambridge, Mass: Harvard University Press; 1978.

11. Reedijk J. *Psychiatrie.* Lochem: De Tijdstroom; 1987.

SUGGESTED READING

Brom D, Kleber RJ, Defares DB. *Traumatische Ervaringen en Psychotherapie.* Lisse: Swets & Zeitlinger; 1986.

Darwin C. *The Expressions of the Emotions in Man and Animals.* London: Murray; 1872.

Gay P. *Sigmund Freud: zijn leven en werk.* Baarn: Tirion, translated from English; 1988.

Wilde GJS. *Neurotische Labiliteit Gemeten Volgens de Vragenlijst Methode.* Amsterdam: F van Rossen; 1970.

Zand JL. *Psychogene Rugpijn: dat is andere taal.* Lisse: Swets & Zeitlinger; 1987.

Appendix A

Algorithms for the Diagnosis and Treatment of the Sacroiliac Joint and for General Spine Pathology

DIAGNOSIS AND TREATMENT OF SACROILIAC JOINT PATHOLOGY

Pathology	History	Provocation tests	Vorlauf phenomenon*	Treatment
Arthritis	Spontaneous onset. Usually pain first noted in the gluteal region	Positive only in the active stage	Can be positive on the painful side	Medications (nonsteroidal anti-inflammatory drugs). Injection
Instability	Traumatic onset or during/after pregnancy. Mostly prolonged standing or walking is painful. Carrying heavy loads is also painful	Positive	Positive on the nonpainful side	Stabilization exercises (abdominal and gluteal muscles). Sacroiliac stabilization belt
Locking	Usually traumatic onset. In many instances, found in patients who already have had sacroiliac joint instability problems	Positive	Positive on the painful side	Mobilization. Stabilization exercises and sacroiliac belt in cases where an instability is also present

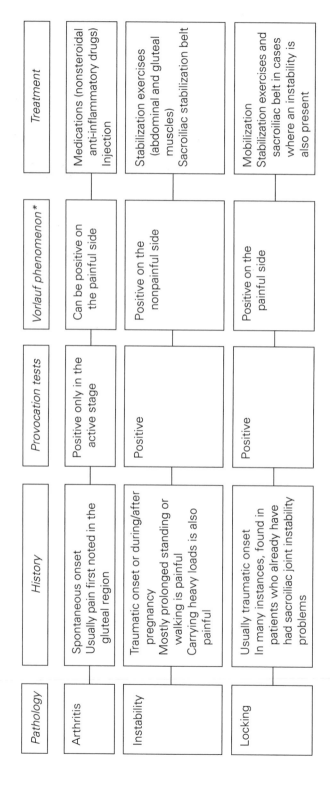

*Vorlauf phenomenon: During forward flexion (either in standing or in sitting) one posterior-superior iliac spine moves earlier and remains in a more cranioventral position at the end of the motion.

INTERPRETATION OF THE VORLAUF PHENOMENON IN SACROILIAC JOINT LOCKING AND INSTABILITY

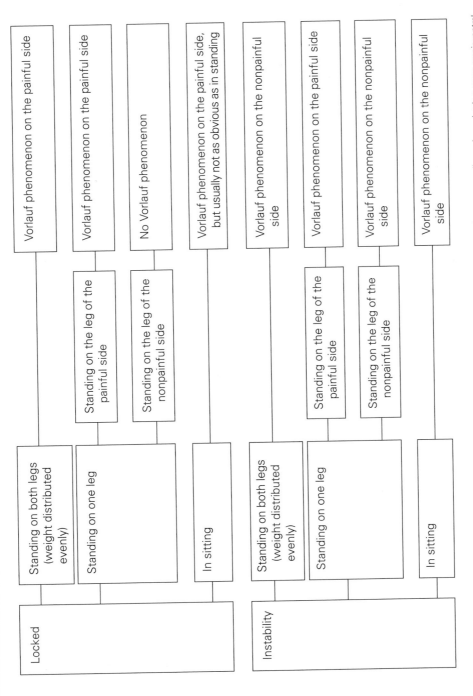

Note: Vorlauf phenomenon: During forward flexion (either in standing or in sitting) one posterior-superior iliac spine moves earlier and remains in a more cranioventral position at the end of the motion.

DISCOSIS (PHYSIOLOGICAL DISC DEGENERATION)

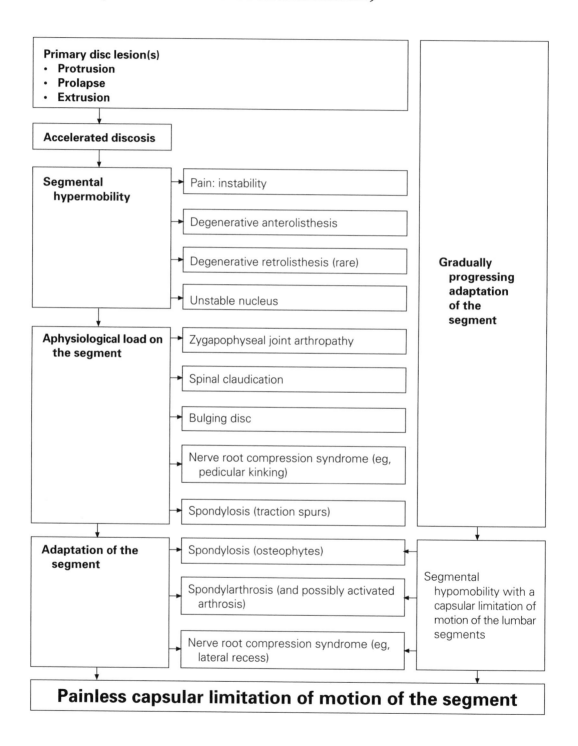

Primary disc lesion(s) • **Protrusion** • **Prolapse** • **Extrusion**	
Accelerated discosis	
Segmental hypermobility	Pain: instability Degenerative anterolisthesis Degenerative retrolisthesis (rare) Unstable nucleus
Aphysiological load on the segment	Zygapophyseal joint arthropathy Spinal claudication Bulging disc Nerve root compression syndrome (eg, pedicular kinking) Spondylosis (traction spurs)
Adaptation of the segment	Spondylosis (osteophytes) Spondylarthrosis (and possibly activated arthrosis) Nerve root compression syndrome (eg, lateral recess)

Gradually progressing adaptation of the segment

Segmental hypomobility with a capsular limitation of motion of the lumbar segments

Painless capsular limitation of motion of the segment

CAPSULAR PATTERN OF THE SPINAL COLUMN

Joint (or joint chain)	Limitation of Motion (passive angular movements)
Cervical spine	Extension > rotation (symmetrical limitation) = lateral flexion (symmetrical limitation) > flexion
Thoracic spine	Rotation (symmetrical limitation) > other motions
Lumbar spine	Extension > Lateral flexion (symmetrical limitation) > flexion
Sacroiliac joint	No capsular pattern; sometimes pain in the end positions

Appendix B

Algorithms for the Diagnosis and Treatment of Lumbar Spine Pathology

DIFFERENTIAL DIAGNOSIS OF LUMBAR SPINE PATHOLOGY

Primary Discogenic Pathology

Factor	Disc protrusion	Disc prolapse
Gender	More often seen in women than in men	More often seen in women than in men
Age	Approximately 30 to 55 years	Approximately 30 to 55 years
Localization of symptoms	Low back and possibly the gluteal area.	Low back, gluteal area, and leg: segmental
Posture	Sometimes flexed posture with/without lateral shift	Sometimes flexed posture, usually with lateral shift
Positions provoking symptoms	Prolonged stooped positions Prolonged sitting	Particularly prolonged stooped positions
Motions provoking symptoms	1. Forward flexion 2. Lateral flexion to one side 3. Rotation in one direction 4. Extension	1. Extension 2. Lateral flexion to one side 3. Rotation in one direction 4. Forward flexion
Neurological findings	None	• Sensation • Motor function • Reflexes
Coughing and/or sneezing	Sometimes positive	Usually positive
Radiological examination	Usually misleading information (degenerative changes)	Usually misleading information (degenerative changes)
Other diagnostic measures	1. MRI 2. CT scan	1. MRI 2. CT scan 3. Myelogram 4. EMG
Treatment	1. Information and ergonomic measures 2. Manual therapy or continuous traction 3. Exercise program 4. Epidural anesthetic	1. Information and ergonomic measures 2. Manual therapy and/or continuous traction (sometimes indicated) 3. Exercise program 4. Epidural anesthetic 5. Surgery or chemonucleolysis

Secondary Discogenic Pathology

Nerve root compression syndrome	*Neurogenic (spinal claudication*	*Segmental instability*
Seen equally in women and men	Seen almost exclusively in men	Seen equally in men and women
50+ years	50+ years	35+ Years
Leg: segmental, usually L5	Heavy and tired feeling in both legs (thighs, calves, and feet); back pain existing for many years	Low back, with or without pain in posterior thigh
Negative	Particularly during walking; after a period, a flexed position of the lumbar spine occurs: the so-called simian (ape) posture	Unremarkable
1. Sitting 2. Sometimes standing 3. Sometimes walking	Walking, extension of the lumbar spine	1. Prolonged standing and walking 2. Particularly leisurely walking with frequent stops and starts (such as in a day of shopping or sightseeing)
Extension, especially in combination with ipsilateral sidebending and rotation	Extension Descending stairs and inclined surfaces	Returning to erect standing from a forward flexed position (the patient "climbs up" the legs with the hands)
None	None	None
Negative	Negative	Negative
Degenerative changes, usually around the intervertebral foramen of the affected nerve root	Degenerative changes: in 50%, a degenerative spondylolisthesis, usually L3-4	Narrowed disc space with osteophytes
CT scan	1. Myelogram 2. CT scan	Much discussion over the value of functional X-ray views
1. Information 2. Epidural anesthetic 3. Surgery	1. Information 2. Medication (calcitonin) 3. Surgery	1. Information 2. Exercise program (aimed at stabilization and decreasing intradiscal pressure) 3. Lumbar corset 4. Surgery: spinal fusion

continues

Secondary Discogenic Pathology continued

Factor	Degenerative spondylolisthesis	Retrolisthesis
Gender	Seen more frequently in women than in men	Seen usually in men
Age	60+ years	Middle age
Localization of symptoms	Low back and thigh	Low back region; in about 45%, referred pain in the leg in one dermatome (L5, L4, or L3)
Posture	Unremarkable	Unremarkable
Positions provoking symptoms	Prolonged standing and walking	Various positions can be painful
Motions provoking symptoms	Extension (very limited) "Climbs up" the legs on returning from forward flexion	Extension is painful and significantly limited
Neurological findings	None	Seldom
Coughing and/or sneezing	Negative	Negative
Radiological examination	Spondylolisthesis without lysis, usually L4-5, seldom more than a 15% forward displacement	Retrolisthesis, L4 > L3
Other diagnostic measures	1. MRI 2. CT scan	1. Rotation provocation (in prone, pressure exerted on the affected vertebra is very painful; "doorbell sign") 2. MRI 3. CT scan
Treatment	1. Information 2. Exercise program (aimed at stabilization and decreasing intradiscal pressure) 3. Surgery (seldom necessary)	1. Information 2. Exercise program (with goals of stabilization and decreasing intradiscal pressure) 3. Epidural anesthetic (only with referred pain to the leg) 4. Surgery (seldom necessary)

Other Pathology

Spondylolytic spondylolisthesis	Facet joint syndrome (usually postlaminectomy and postchemo-nucleolysis)	Traumatic compression fracture
Men to women = 3:1	Seen equally in men and women	Seen equally in women and men
All ages	20 to 50 years	All ages
Low back region, sometimes with referred pain in the thigh and calf	Vague, deeply localized pain in the low back, gluteal area, and thigh, which never radiates more distally than about 10 cm above the knee (nonsegmental/pseudoradicular)	Severe local pain (thoracic or lumbar)
Sometimes very local lordosis ("apparent" hypertrophied paravertebral musculature with a "midline hollow")	Unremarkable	Unremarkable
Prolonged standing and walking Periods of walking interrupted by periods of standing (eg, shopping) Strenuous activities (eg, sports)	Sometimes prolonged sitting in kyphosis	All positions painful in the acute phase
Sometimes, although not painful, a click occurs with various lumbar spine movements	Combined motions of the lumbar spine: both extension with ipsilateral sidebending and rotation, as well as forward flexion with ipsilateral sidebending and contralateral rotation	All motions painful in the acute phase
None	None	Rare
Negative	Negative	Negative
Spondylolysis, L5 > L4 > L3 Usually stable Often more than 30% anterolisthesis	Usually gives misleading information, showing degenerative changes in the lumbar spine	Compression fracture of (mostly) T12 or L1 or L2; sometimes of two or more vertebrae
1. Rotation test in sidelying: the affected spinous process sometimes remains in the same position (in the cases of instability) 2. MRI 3. CT scan	Of little use	CT scan (shows more damage than normal X-ray)
1. Information 2. Exercise program (with goals of stabilization and decreasing intradiscal pressure) 3. Lumbar corset 4. Surgery (spinal fusion)	1. Instruction in proper posture 2. Mobilization/manipulation	1. In the acute stage: bed rest (days to weeks) until pain resolves 2. Information (to include the good prognosis)

continues

Other Pathology continued

Factor	Spontaneous compression fracture	Traumatic ligament sprain
Gender	Seen more frequently in women	Seen equally in men and women
Age	60+ years	Between 20 and 50 years
Localization of symptoms	Usually minimal to no pain at level of the thoracic fracture; compensatory complaints in the cervical and/or lumbar area	Usually just cranial from the posterior-superior iliac spine at the level of the lumbar spinous processes Usually concerns the superior iliolumbar ligament; sometimes it concerns the supra- or interspinal ligaments
Posture	Marked angular thoracic kyphosis	Unremarkable
Positions provoking symptoms	Unremarkable	Stooped standing and sometimes prolonged sitting in kyphosis
Motions provoking symptoms	Sometimes extension of the cervical and/or lumbar spine	Forward flexion and (when the superior iliolumbar ligament is affected) also contralateral lateral flexion
Neurological findings	None	None
Coughing and/or sneezing	Negative	Negative
Radiological examination	Anterior compression fracture of the osteoporotic thoracic vertebrae: codfish vertebrae	Usually gives misleading information (degenerative changes and/or congenital variations)
Other diagnostic measures	Bone biopsy for the differential diagnosis	Palpation
Treatment	1. In the (seldomly seen) acute stage: only a few days of bed rest 2. Early mobilization 3. Encourage movement	Transverse friction and temporarily avoid painful motions

continues

Other Pathology continued

Traumatic muscle strain	Kissing spine (Bastrop's syndrome)	Traumatic kissing spine (compression of the interspinal ligament as a result of a hyperextension trauma)
Seen more frequently in men	Seen more frequently in women	Seen equally in men and women
Between 20 and about 40 years	55+ Years	Mostly young people (15 to 25 years)
Usually between the spinous processes L4-5 and the posterior-superior iliac spine Usually concerns the attachment of the erector spinae muscle	At the level of the lumbar spinous processes	At the level of the lumbar spinous processes
In very acute cases, sometimes a hyperlordosis	Sometimes lumbar kyphosis	Unremarkable
Stooped standing and prolonged sitting in kyphosis	Standing with a hollow back	Taking the position of extreme extension in the lumbar spine
1. Forward flexion 2. Contralateral lateral flexion 3. Resisted extension with ipsilateral lateral flexion	Extension	Maximal extension is more painful than maximal forward flexion
None	None	None
Sometimes positive	Negative	Negative
Almost always gives misleading information (degenerative changes and/or congenital variations)	Degenerative changes of the lumbar spine: sometimes osteoporosis, sometimes the formation of a joint between the spinous processes	Negative
Palpation	Injection with a local anesthetic to differentiate between a local bursitis	Injection of the interspinal ligament with a local anesthetic
1. Transverse friction and cautious stretching 2. Temporarily stop sports activities	1. Information 2. Avoid lumbar extension 3. Injection with a corticosteroid	1. Temporarily avoid maximal lumbar extension 2. Injection with a corticosteroid

INTERPRETATION OF COUPLED AND COMBINED MOTIONS IN THE LOCAL SEGMENTAL LUMBAR EXAMINATION

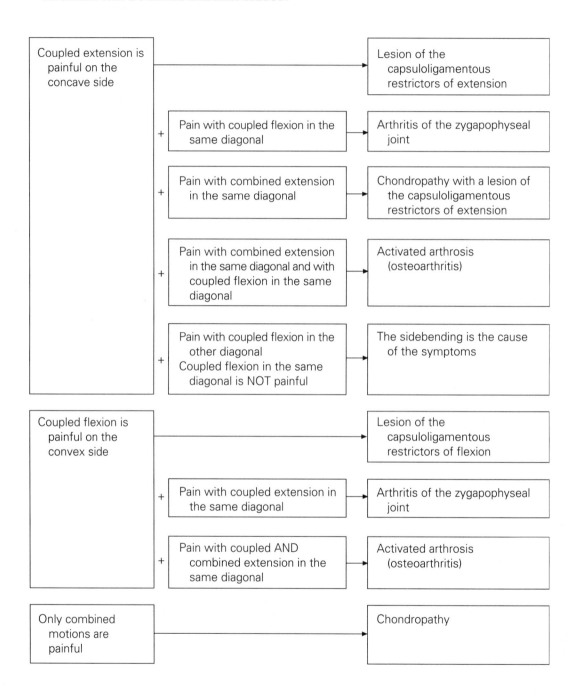

LUMBAR SPINE: TREATMENT DIAGRAM

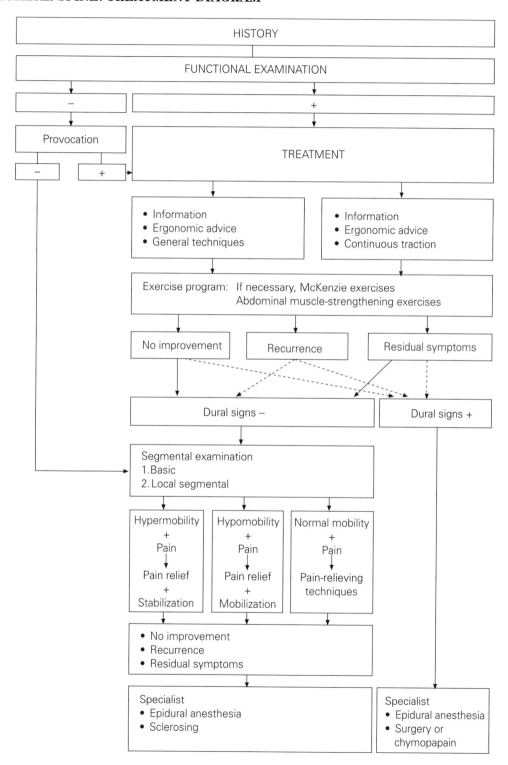

Appendix C

Pathology of the Thoracic Spine

DIFFERENTIAL DIAGNOSIS OF THORACIC SPINE PATHOLOGY

Factor	Thoracic posture syndrome	Posterolateral disc protrusion
Gender	Seen more often in women than in men	Seen more often in women than in men
Age	6 to 40 years	30 to 45 years
Cause	Overload on the dorsal ligaments and muscles due to prolonged sitting in kyphosis	Usually an axial trauma (sometimes years earlier)
Localization of symptoms	Central thoracic pain that disappears during activity and lying (only in the early stages)	Paravertebral pain that disappears during lying and increases during certain motions
Functional examination	Sometimes passive tests are "felt" at end-range	Painful active and passive rotation in one direction Dura test often positive
Neurological signs	None	None
Coughing, sneezing, straining	Negative	Sometimes positive
Imaging examinations	Imaging examinations are negative	Conventional X-rays are usually negative; CT scan and MRI are positive
Differential diagnosis	Early posterocentral disc pathology	Tumors (rare)
Treatment	Primarily Causal: 1. Information 2. Improve work posture and work environment 3. Exercise program to strengthen scapular adductors and thoracic back extensors 4. If necessary, continuous traction; daily for 2 weeks (lasting 15 to 30 minutes)	1. Information 2. Mobilization with axial separation 3. Home program • Mobilizing exercises • Strengthening exercises for the scapular adductors and thoracic back extensors

continues

DIFFERENTIAL DIAGNOSIS OF THORACIC SPINE PATHOLOGY continued

Factor	Posterolateral disc prolapse	Posterocentral disc prolapse
Gender	Seen equally in men and in women	Seen equally in men and in women
Age	30 to 45 years	30 to 45 years
Cause	Trauma	Usually a severe axial trauma
Localization of symptoms	Paravertebral pain with intercostal neuralgia and/or sternal pain	Severe central thoracic pain with extrasegmental radiation and radiation in the corresponding dermatomes The central disc prolapse occurs mostly in the lower thoracic spine (T9 to T12).
Functional examination	Rotation(s), flexion, and extension are painful Dura test often positive	Depends on the severity of the prolapse
Neurological signs	None	Depends on the severity: hypoesthesia to transverse cord lesion
Coughing, sneezing, straining	Positive	Positive (sometimes taking a deep breath is very painful)
Imaging examinations	Conventional X-rays are negative; CT scan and MRI are positive	Myelo-CT scan and MRI are diagnostic
Differential diagnosis	Herpes zoster Malignant tumors	Spondylodiscitis Malignant tumors
Treatment	1. Information 2. Ergonomic advice 3. Mobilization with axial separation 4. Home exercises • Mobilizing exercises • Exercises to strengthen scapular adductors and thoracic back extensors 5. If necessary, continuous traction; daily for 2 weeks (lasting 15 to 30 minutes)	Without spinal cord compression: 1. Bed rest 2. Cautious, continuous traction With spinal cord compression: immediate surgery

continues

DIFFERENTIAL DIAGNOSIS OF THORACIC SPINE PATHOLOGY continued

Factor	Spondylodiscitis	Malignant tumors
Gender	Seen equally in men and in women	Seen equally in men and in women
Age	Over 50 years	All ages
Cause	Hematogenous inflammation of a disc	Usually metastases from bronchial carcinoma or Pancoast tumor
Localization of symptoms	Central thoracic pain with radiation into the side and/or into the legs	Severe central thoracic pain and usually intercostal neuralgia
Functional examination	Limitations of motion in a capsular pattern (rotations symmetrically limited) Often pain on percussion and when falling back onto the heels from a tiptoe position	Severe limitation of motion, often in a capsular pattern Often pain on percussion and when falling back onto the heels from a tiptoe position
Neurological signs	None	Depends on severity: hypoesthesia to transverse cord lesion
Coughing, sneezing, straining	Usually negative	Sometimes positive
Imaging examinations	Conventional X-rays, CT scan, and MRI are positive	Conventional X-rays often negative in early stages; CT scan and MRI are positive
Differential diagnosis	Malignant tumors	Spondylodiscitis
Treatment	1. Bed rest 2. Antibiotics	1. Surgery, if possible 2. Otherwise, dependent on the type of tumor and the stage

continues

DIFFERENTIAL DIAGNOSIS OF THORACIC SPINE PATHOLOGY continued

Factor	Traumatic compression fracture	Spontaneous compression fracture
Gender	Seen equally in men and in women	Seen mostly in women
Age	All ages	Over 60 years
Cause	Axial trauma with a flexed spine	Osteoporosis
Localization of symptoms	Acute local pain (usually lower thoracic)	Severe local pain with an acute fracture; chronic pain with a gradually occurring fracture Often lumbar and/or cervical pain due to an increased compensatory lordosis
Functional examination	Usually impossible to perform because of pain	Varied: extension limitation due to kissing spines Flexion painful and limited due to the flexed position Lateral flexion sometimes painful due to costoiliac compression
Neurological signs	Seldom	None
Coughing, sneezing, straining	Usually negative	Usually negative
Imaging examinations	Conventional X-rays, CT scan, and MRI are positive; CT scan best indicates the severity of the fracture	Conventional X-ray (codfish vertebrae), CT scan, and MRI are positive
Differential diagnosis	None	Spondylodiscitis Tumors
Treatment	1. Bed rest 2. Return to activities as soon as pain allows 3. Usually prognosis is good	1. Acute stage (not often seen): • A few days of bed rest • Return to activity as soon as possible 2. Chronic stage: • Encourage patient to stay active • Medication

continues

DIFFERENTIAL DIAGNOSIS OF THORACIC SPINE PATHOLOGY continued

Factor	Manubriosternal joint arthritis	Tietze syndrome
Gender	Seen most often in women	Seen equally in men and women
Age	Between 20 and 45 years	Adults (seldom older than 50 years)
Cause	Rheumatoid arthritis Ankylosing spondylitis Psoriatic arthritis Reiter's disease Idiopathic	Unknown
Localization of symptoms	Amphiarthrosis between the manubrium and the sternum	Costosternal cartilage of the second rib (less often the first or third rib); left more often affected than right
Functional examination	All movements are painful	Negative; only local tenderness
Neurological signs	None	None
Coughing, sneezing, straining	Positive; taking a deep breath is also painful	Usually positive, as well as taking a deep breath
Imaging examinations	Bone scan	Negative
Differential diagnosis	Angina pectoris	Tumors
Treatment	1. Depending on the cause: often a local injection with a corticosteroid is indicated	1. Usually self-limiting, within a period of weeks to months 2. Injection of the painful swelling is often helpful 3. Mobilization of the thoracic spine and ribs may be indicated

continues

TREATMENT OF DISORDERS OF THE THORACIC SPINE

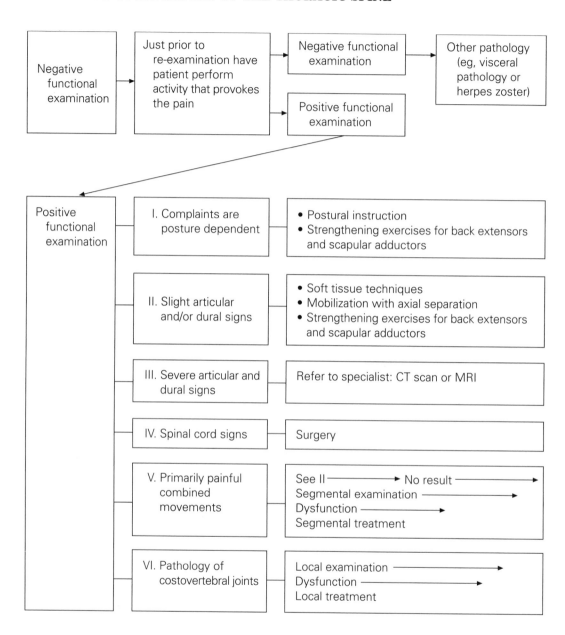

Pathology of the Cervical Spine

DIFFERENTIAL DIAGNOSIS OF CERVICAL SPINE PATHOLOGY

Factor	Cervical posture syndrome	Local cervical syndrome
Gender	Women to men = ±3:1	Women to men = ±2:1
Age	6 to 45 years	30 to 45 years
Cause	Overuse of cervical musculature as a result of frequent prolonged sitting (standing) with forward-bent head posture	Segmental problem? Disc problem? MRI sometimes shows obvious symptomatic disc protrusion
Localization of symptoms	Head (from occiput to forehead), neck, trapezius muscle area (pars descendens), and frequently between the scapulae Bilateral	Unilateral neck and trapezius muscle area (pars descendens) Sometimes between the scapulae
Head posture	Normal	Sometimes an antalgic posture • Flexion • Flexion with slight contralateral sidebending and rotation
Functional examination	Usually minimal to no findings ("it pulls a little")	Pain and a noncapsular limitation of motion
Neurological signs	None	None
Coughing and/or sneezing	Negative	Negative
Radiological examination	Negative, or misleading information (degenerative changes) in patients over 35 years	Misleading information (physiological degenerative changes)
Other diagnostic measures	Not indicated	Seldom indicated
Differential diagnosis	Local cervical syndrome and the differential diagnoses listed there	Sometimes symptoms from tumors can begin as an apparent innocent local cervical syndrome (mainly metastases in the cervical spine from the bronchii, thyroid gland, breasts, and kidneys) Neurinoma (in the beginning stages)
Treatment	1. Information 2. Improve working posture and work environment 3. Treatment of the muscles • Massage • Stretching (also as home exercise program) 4. Modalities (heat, etc)	1. Information (good prognosis) 2. Manual traction 3. When indicated, cervical collar 4. When indicated, medication 5. With recurrent problems: stabilization exercises

continues

937

DIFFERENTIAL DIAGNOSIS OF CERVICAL SPINE PATHOLOGY continued

Factor	Discogenic cervicobrachial syndrome	Nerve root compression syndrome
Gender	Women to men = ±2:1	Women to men = ±1:2
Age	30 to 45 years	45 to 65 years
Cause	Disc protrusion or prolapse	Narrowing of the intervertebral foramen through disc degeneration or uncovertebral osteoarthrosis (osteophytes)
Localization of symptoms	Unilateral pain in the neck with radicular symptoms in the arm, frequently to and including the fingers (usually C6 or C7 dermatome) Usually acute onset	Minimal to no pain in the neck Pain in the C5 dermatome and/or the scapula The symptoms develop gradually over a number of years
Head posture	Forward flexion deviation, sometimes with contralateral sidebending and rotation	Normal
Functional examination	Extension, ipsilateral sidebending, and rotation are the most painful and limited motions	Limitation of motion in the capsular pattern as a result of the spondylarthrosis, although minimal to no pain Sometimes ipsilateral sidebending is painful in the arm
Neurological signs	Protrusion: none Prolapse 1. Sensory deficit 2. Abnormal reflexes 3. Motor deficit Usually C6 or C7 nerve root	Mostly only motor deficit: usually C5 (mainly weakness of the shoulder abductors)
Coughing and/or sneezing	Painful, mainly in the neck	Negative
Radiological examination	In very acute cases, sometimes disc edema (greater distance between two vertebral bodies) Straightened lordosis, often an obvious kyphotic crook at the affected level Further misleading "degenerative" changes	In particular, the oblique view shows the significantly narrowed intervertebral foramen: usually C4–5
Other diagnostic measures	CT scan MRI (best indicator of a protrusion or prolapse)	CT scan
Differential diagnosis	Neurinoma Tumors (particularly metastases from the bronchi, thyroid, breasts, or kidneys) can, in the beginning stages, look like an innocent cervical or cervicobrachial syndrome	Neurinoma

continues

DIFFERENTIAL DIAGNOSIS OF CERVICAL SPINE PATHOLOGY continued

Factor	Discogenic cervicobrachial syndrome	Nerve root compression syndrome
Treatment	1. Information (almost always a good prognosis) 2. In cases without neurological deficit: manual traction 3. Cervical collar 4. Ergonomic advice 5. Home program: cautious extension-rotation exercises 6. When symptoms are (almost) resolved: stabilization exercises (home program) Self-limiting: Recovery seldom takes longer than 6 months	1. Information 2. With significant neurological deficits, consider surgery

Factor	Neurinoma
Gender	Seen equally in men and women
Age	After 20 years
Cause	Neurofibromatosis, or without known cause
Localization of symptoms	Often begins distally (hand) with pain and paresthesia, then radiates proximally and even to the thorax Symptoms are progressive More than one dermatome
Head posture	Normal
Functional examination	Strikingly normal, except cervical spine flexion, which causes an increase in paresthesia
Neurological signs	Motor deficits from more than one root Spinal cord symptoms in a later stage
Coughing and/or sneezing	Pain in the arm
Radiological examination	In an advanced stage, abnormally large intervertebral foramen (from erosion due to the neurinoma)
Other diagnostic measures	Neurologist or neurosurgeon
Differential diagnosis	Other tumors In the early stages, this lesion can look like any other "benign" type of cervical lesion
Treatment	In severe cases, surgery

continues

DIFFERENTIAL DIAGNOSIS OF CERVICAL SPINE PATHOLOGY continued

Factor	Congenital torticollis	Acute torticollis
Gender	Seen equally in boys and girls	Girls to boys = 2:1
Age	From birth	Children and adolescents
Cause	Unknown Fibrosing with shortening of the sternocleidomastoid muscle	Disc protrusion
Localization of symptoms	No pain	Unilateral neck pain and pain in trapezius muscle area (pars descendens)
Head posture	Sidebent to the affected side, rotated to the nonaffected side Slight forward flexion	Sidebent and rotated to the nonaffected side Slight forward flexion
Functional examination	Limited sidebending to the nonaffected side Limited rotation to the affected side Limited extension	Limited sidebending to the painful side Limited rotation to the painful side Limited extension
Neurological signs	None	None
Coughing and/or sneezing	Negative	Negative
Radiological examination	Straightened lordosis	Antalgic posture is obvious
Other diagnostic measures	Not indicated	Not indicated
Differential diagnosis	Klippel-Feil syndrome (congenital malformation such as fused vertebrae or hemivertebrae)	Grisel's disease Spastic torticollis, eg, with encephalitis epidemica, otitis media (inflammation of the middle ear) Juvenile rheumatoid arthritis Hysterical torticollis
Treatment	Surgery	Self-limiting: Recovery in 1 to 2 weeks 1. Information 2. Manual traction in the antalgic posture, and afterward also in the neutral position 3. Cervical collar (also at night) 4. When indicated, medication

continues

DIFFERENTIAL DIAGNOSIS OF CERVICAL SPINE PATHOLOGY continued

Factor	Hysterical torticollis	Spastic torticollis
Gender	Seen more frequently in women than in men	Seen equally in women and men
Age	Adolescents and adults, seldom older than 50 years	Adults
Cause	Psychosomatic	• Psychological • As a result of encephalitis epidemica • Symptom of an extrapyramidal lesion
Localization of symptoms	Diffuse pain in the head, neck, and shoulder, whereby the pain is predominantly on one side	No pain
Head posture	Characteristic: sidebent toward the painful side and the patient holds the shoulder on that same side elevated	Normal, although on involuntary moments, the head turns very briefly to one side (always the same side)
Functional examination	Limitation of motion in all directions. By slowly going through with the passive movement, one can easily win over the muscle contraction	Negative
Neurological signs	None	None
Coughing and/or sneezing	Negative	Negative
Radiological examination	Misleading information ("degenerative changes" in patients over age 35 years)	Misleading information ("degenerative changes" in patients over age 35 years)
Other diagnostic measures	Not indicated	Neurologist
Differential diagnosis	This head-shoulder posture is only seen with hysterical torticollis	See Cause
Treatment	Psychotherapy	Dependent on the cause, although in many cases, without results

continues

DIFFERENTIAL DIAGNOSIS OF CERVICAL SPINE PATHOLOGY continued

Factor	Grisel's disease (spontaneous atlantoaxial subluxation/ dislocation)	Traumatic atlantoaxial subluxation/ dislocation
Gender	Seen equally in men and women	Seen equally in men and women
Age	All ages	All ages
Cause	Congenital or developed weakness, particularly of the transverse ligament of the atlas A normal movement or a minor trauma can cause the dislocation Possibilities: rheumatoid arthritis; ankylosing spondylitis; psoriatic arthritis; regional infections such as lymphangitis, nose or throat infections, etc; primary tumors or metastases; congenital dens anomaly; congenital ligamentous laxity (eg, Down syndrome); previous trauma	Trauma Possibilities: rotatory subluxation, spondylolisthesis of the axis (hangman's fracture), odontoid fracture
Localization of symptoms	Primarily headache (occipital) Neck-shoulder pain and spinal cord symptoms, as well as vertebrobasilar problems, dependent on the severity of the lesion	If the patient survives the trauma, the symptoms and the signs are very severe: all possible results of spinal cord damage and vertebrobasilar problems
Head posture	Flexion deviation	Flexion deviation or flexion, ipsilaterally sidebent, and contralaterally rotated posture with a rotatory subluxation
Functional examination	All motions are very limited and painful, and due to muscle guarding likely unable to be performed	No functional examination performed First, thorough radiological examination
Neurological signs	Due to spinal cord compression, dependent on the severity of the lesion, spastic hemi- and paraparesis Positive Babinski test Ataxia	Significant signs of spinal cord compression • Spastic paraparesis • Ataxia
Coughing and/or sneezing	Very positive	Very positive
Radiological examination	Most important part of the examination, together with the history (infections, etc)	Diagnostic
Other diagnostic measures	CT scan MRI	CT scan MRI
Differential diagnosis	See Cause	See Cause
Treatment	Surgery	Surgery

continues

DIFFERENTIAL DIAGNOSIS OF CERVICAL SPINE PATHOLOGY continued

Factor	*Subacute atlantoaxial arthritis*	*Retropharyngeal tendinitis*
Gender	Seen only in men	Seen equally in men and women
Age	25 to 40 years	25 to 80 years
Cause	Nonspecific inflammation of the atlantoaxial capsuloligamentous complex No fever BSE normal Negative history	Unknown Sometimes slight fever
Localization of symptoms	Increasing pain and stiffness, lasting a few weeks, in the mid- and upper cervical region	Acute onset of severe head and neck pain
Head posture	Neutral position	Head (cervical spine) in slight flexion
Functional examination	Severely limited and painful rotations (symmetrical) Other motions are normal	Extension and both rotations are symmetrically limited and painful Flexion and both rotations are painful against resistance
Neurological signs	None	None
Coughing and/or sneezing	Negative	So painful that the patient has to hold the head steady with both hands Swallowing is painful
Radiological examination	Normal at the level of C1-2	Calcium deposit ventrally from the body of the axis
Other diagnostic measures	No indication for further diagnostic imaging Blood tests are indicated	MRI shows thickening of the longus colli muscle from the normal 3 mm to 10 to 15 mm
Differential diagnosis	Other arthritides Tumors	Retropharyngeal abscess
Treatment	Medications (NSAIDs)	1. Spontaneous healing in 2 to 3 weeks 2. Analgesics for pain relief

continues

DIFFERENTIAL DIAGNOSIS OF CERVICAL SPINE PATHOLOGY continued

Factor	Unilateral facet subluxation/ dislocation	Bilateral facet subluxation/ dislocation
Gender	Rarely seen in both men and women	Rarely seen in both men and women
Age	All ages (seldom over 60 years)	All ages (seldom over 60 years)
Cause	Traumatic, eg: Right sidebending with a forced left rotation (combined coupling pattern) causes a right dislocation and fracture (mostly of the caudal facet) Right sidebending with a forced right rotation (coupled coupling pattern) causes a left dislocation	Traumatic: symmetrical flexion trauma with slight axial compression
Localization of symptoms	Local pain, usually with radicular symptoms mostly of C5-6 or C6-7	All symptoms of severe ligamentous ruptures and disc damage Sometimes also spinal cord symptoms
Head posture	Dependent on the dislocation; eg, with a right dislocation the head is deviated into left sidebending and left rotation; subluxation/dislocation ventrally of the cranial facet	Head (cervical spine) fixed in flexion
Functional examination	Severely limited and painful motions in the directions opposite to the antalgic position	All motions are severely limited and painful
Neurological signs	Without a fracture: usually none With a fracture: frequently neurological signs	Bilateral root irritation but often without deficit
Coughing and/or sneezing	Sometimes positive	Usually positive
Radiological examination	Shows the subluxation/dislocation of the cranial part of the facet joint In some cases, further examination is necessary	Shows the subluxation/dislocation In particular, the lateral view is diagnostic
Other diagnostic measures	CT scan MRI	CT scan MRI
Differential diagnosis	Fractures other than of the facet joint	Fractures
Treatment	1. In the hospital: traction for reduction of the dislocation; afterward, a rigid collar	1. Usually operative

continues

DIFFERENTIAL DIAGNOSIS OF CERVICAL SPINE PATHOLOGY continued

Factor	*First rib fracture (stress fracture)*	*Arthritis of the first costotransversal joint*
Gender	Seen more often in men	Rarely seen in both men and women
Age	20 to 40 years	Adults
Cause	Overuse, mostly due to sports (handball, water polo, or other throwing sports; some power sports)	Overuse (see "first rib fracture") or as a result of a systemic disease
Localization of symptoms	Unilateral, at the base of the neck	Unilateral, at the base of the neck
Head posture	Normal	Sometimes slightly sidebent toward the affected side
Functional examination	Painful flexion and sidebending away from the affected side Painful resisted sidebending toward the affected side Painful active and passive elevation of the scapula Painful active and passive elevation of the arm	Painful sidebending away from the affected side Contracting the scalene muscles against resistance is painful (ipsilateral sidebending with contralateral rotation and flexion) Active arm elevation is sometimes very painful and limited Passive arm elevation is slightly painful but not limited
Neurological signs	None	None
Coughing and/or sneezing	Mostly painful	Sometimes painful
Radiological examination	Shows the stress fracture	Mostly negative
Other diagnostic measures	Not indicated	Injection with a local anesthetic
Differential diagnosis	Stress fracture of spinous process from C7 or T1 Contracture of the costocoracoid fascia Arthritis of the first costotransversal joint	Stress fracture of the spinous process from C7 or T1, or of the first rib Contracture of the costocoracoid fascia
Treatment	1. Reassure: spontaneous recovery within 2 months	1. Usually an injection with a corticosteroid is indicated

continues

DIFFERENTIAL DIAGNOSIS OF CERVICAL SPINE PATHOLOGY continued

Factor	Stress fracture of the spinous process from C7 or T1	Contracture of the costocoracoid fascia
Gender	Seen more often in men	Rarely seen in both men and women
Age	20 to 70 years	25 to 50 years
Cause	Overuse, mostly from digging or raking in the garden	Sometimes as a result of a long-standing tuberculosis in the apex of the lung Mostly unknown cause
Localization of symptoms	Centrally at the level of C7-T1	Unilateral pain in the pectoral and scapular regions as well as at the base of the neck
Head posture	Normal	Normal
Functional examination	Painful flexion and extension of the neck Painful active elevation of the scapula Very painful and very limited active elevation of the arm Passive elevation of the arm is painful but only slightly limited Significant local tenderness	Slightly limited and painful elevation of the scapula on the affected side Painful sidebending away from the affected side Painful resisted sidebending toward the affected side Protraction of the scapula is painful but not limited All resisted tests of the shoulder are painful at the base of the neck
Neurological signs	None	None
Coughing and/or sneezing	Local pain	Negative
Radiological examination	Shows the stress fracture	Negative: misleading information (physiological degenerative changes in patients over 35 years)
Other diagnostic measures	Not indicated	CT scan MRI
Treatment	1. Self-limiting: Recovery within 2 months 2. When indicated, medications for pain relief	1. Physical therapy (to include specific stretching) 2. When physical therapy is not successful: surgical release of the fascia and of the pectoralis minor

Index

Allodynia = Hypersensitive pain from stim. to normal skin

947

DISH = diffuse idiopathic skeletal hyperostosis: bone disease c̄ degeneration.

Thoracic ⊤ ⟋⟑ 441-2